Pocket Atlas of
Human Anatomy

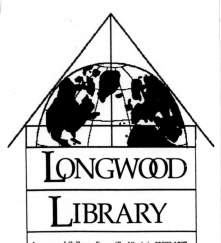

Pocket Atlas of Human Anatomy

Based on the International Nomenclature

Heinz Feneis
in collaboration with Wolfgang Dauber

Translated by David B. Meyer

Third edition, revised and enlarged
810 illustrations by Gerhard Spitzer

1994
Georg Thieme Verlag Stuttgart · New York
Thieme Medical Publishers, Inc. New York

Prof. Dr. Heinz Feneis
Prof. Dr. Wolfgang Dauber
Anatomisches Institut der Universität
Tübingen, Germany

Prof. Gerhard Spitzer
Frankfurt/Main, Germany

David B. Meyer, M. D.
Professor (emeritus), Department of Anatomy
Wayne State University
School of Medicine
Detroit, Michigan, USA

Library of Congress Cataloging-in-Publication Data
Feneis, Heinz.
[Anatomisches Bildwörterbuch der internationalen Nomenklatur. English]
Pocket atlas of human anatomy : based on the international nomenclature / Heinz Feneis in colla-
boration with Wolfgang Dauber : translated by David B. Meyer : 810 illustrations by Gerhard Spit-
zer.—3rd ed., rev. and enl.
Includes bibliographical references and index.
ISBN 3-13-511203-9 (GTV, Stuttgart).—ISBN 0-86577-479-X (TMP, New York)
1. Human anatomy—Nomenclature. 2. Human anatomy—Atlases.
I. Dauber, Wolfgang. II. Title.
[DNLM: 1. Anatomy—nomenclature.   QS 15 F322a 1994a]
QM81.F4513 1994
611'.0014—dc20
DNLM/DLC
for Library of Congress 93-47935

QM
81
.F4513
1994

1st German edition 1967	1st Danish edition 1977	6th German edition 1988
2nd German edition 1970	1st Swedish edition 1979	2nd Italian edition 1989
1st Italian edition 1970	1st Czech edition 1981	2nd Spanish edition 1989
3rd German edition 1972	5th German edition 1982	1st Turkish edition 1990
1st Polish edition 1973	1st Dutch edition 1984	1st Greek edition 1991
4th German edition 1974	2nd Danish edition 1983	1st Chinese edition 1991
1st Spanish edition 1974	2nd Japanese edition 1983	1st Icelandic edition 1992
1st Japanese edition 1974	2nd Swedish edition 1984	2nd Polish edition 1992
1st Portuguese edition 1976	2nd English edition 1985	7th German edition 1993
1st English edition 1976	1st French edition 1986	

This book is an authorized translation of the 7th German edition published and copyrighted 1967,
1993 by Georg Thieme Verlag, Stuttgart, Germany.
Title of the German edition: Anatomisches Bildwörterbuch der internationalen Nomenklatur

© 1976, 1994 Georg Thieme Verlag, Rüdigerstraße 14, D-70469 Stuttgart, Germany
Thieme Medical Publishers, Inc., 381 Park Avenue
South, New York, N.Y. 10016

ISBN 3-13-511203-9 (GTV, Stuttgart)   Typesetting by primustype Hurler GmbH, Notzingen
ISBN 0-86577-479-x (TMP, New York)   Printed in Germany by Clausen & Bosse, Leck.

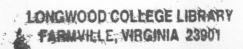

Foreword

The success of Dr. Feneis's "Bildwörterbuch" has been phenomenal. I remember seeing the first edition of it most vividly and wondering why no one else had thought of producing such a useful book. And now it is in its seventh German edition, and has also been translated into many languages. I have several such versions of it on the shelf above my desk, and I refer to it frequently. It is, of course, much more than a dictionary of the official "Nomina Anatomica", for it is also a most valuable working pocket book for anyone in the field of anatomy and medicine. It is its illustration which makes it so useful and, indeed, unique; I know of no other similar dictionary in any language in which the terms are not only defined but also shown in clear, simple pictures. Among the large numbers of books of anatomy which appear year after year, few have the originality and perennial usefulness to become of permanent value. This volume is undoubtedly of this elite quality. It will serve students, academics, and clinicians throughout their working years.

ROGER WARWICK
Professor Emeritus
University of London
(Guy's Hospital Medical School)

Preface to the Third English Edition

This book presents time-saving, concise information on anatomical concepts and indicates which Latin terminology is internationally accepted.

Anatomists in Germany have been striving for a uniform terminology in their specialty since 1895; since 1955, this has also been done on the international level with the Paris nomenclature (INA). The latter has been amended five times, most recently in 1988. More amendments are not expected very soon, therefore, it seems appropriate to update the *Pocket Atlas of Human Anatomy* according to the most recent version, in spite of all of the problems with the INA. It is a difficult job, not only because we had to include 189 new terms without markedly increasing the volume of the book, but also because most of the new terms were provided by the Comittee with no commentary, and our attempts to contact them for more information were in vain. Thus, in a few of these cases we had to leave out an explanation. But since these are not very important items, this minor flaw should be bearable. Incidentally, the new names have been earmarked with a small letter after the old number. A tilde under the number means that the name has been changed. Our intention to indicate the hierarchy of terms by using different typefaces was not always possible, as the number of available typefaces is limited.

As the years progress, it becomes necessary to consider an appropriate successor for further editions of this book. It is a joy and a relief that Professor Dauber has agreed to take on this difficult task and that he prepared most of the work on this edition. Besides being personally suited for the job, Professor Dauber also has the advantage of being from the same university. This was important, for example, when new illustrations and changes to old ones became necessary and could be handled, as always, in excellent cooperation with Professor Spitzer. The fact that this book has attained worldwide distribution—the only major languages into which it has not been translated is Russian and Chinese—is also due to Professor Spitzer's work.

As with the previous editions, we were able to incorporate the suggestions sent to us by readers. One in particular that we must mention is Mr. C. Walter (Marburg, Germany). For years, his tenacious, meticulous reading has led him to make more expert suggestions than anyone else. We thank him and all the others. For the English edition, we would also like to express our thanks to the translator, David Meyer, for his careful translation and suggestions.

And finally, we thank Thieme for its cooperation with this new edition.

Tübingen, January 1994   *Heinz Feneis*

Table of Contents

1 **VERTEBRAL COLUMN.** COLUMNA VERTEBRALIS. A

1 a **Vertebra.**

2 **VERTEBRAL CANAL.** Canalis vertebralis. Canal formed by the individual vertebral foramina lying above one another. It contains the spinal cord. B

3 **Body of vertebra.** Corpus vertebrae (vertebrale).
~ B C D

3 a **Facies intervertebralis.** The surface of a vertebra facing the adjacent vertebra. B

3 b **Ring apophysis (epiphysis).** Apophysis anularis. Ring of bone around the upper and lower surfaces of the vertebral body. It represents a secondary center of ossification. B

4 **Vertebral arch.** Arcus vertebrae (vertebralis). It
~ forms the posterior and lateral boundaries of the vertebral foramen. C D

5 **Pedicle.** Pediculus arcus vertebrae. The portion of the vertebral arch situated anteriorly between the body and transverse process as well as between the superior and inferior vertebral notches. B D

6 **Lamina.** Lamina arcus vertebrae (vertebralis). The portion of the vertebral arch situated posteriorly between the transverse process and the spinous process. C

6 a **Neurocentral junction (synchondrosis).** Junctio neurocentralis. Cartilaginous joint between the left and right fetal neural arches and the centrum. E

7 **Intervertebral foramen.** Foramen intervertebrale. Opening for the passage of the spinal nerve and small vessels. It is bordered by the two adjacent vertebral notches, the vertebral body and the intervertebral disc. A B

8 **Superior vertebral notch.** Incisura vertebralis superior. Notch on the superior aspect of the pedicle. B

9 **Inferior vertebral notch.** Incisura vertebralis inferior. Notch on the inferior aspect of the pedicle. B

10 **Vertebral foramen.** Foramen vertebrale. Space surrounded by the vertebral arch and body. Together, the series of foramina form the vertebral canal. C D

11 **Spinous process.** Processus spinosus. They are bifid in the upper four cervical vertebrae. B C D

12 **Transverse process.** Processus transversus. B C

13 **Costal process.** Processus costalis. The trans-
~ verse process of a lumbar vertebra. It corresponds to a rudimentary rib formed by the embryonic costal element. D

14 **Superior articular process (zygapophysis).** Processus articularis (zygapophysis) superior. Articular process on the superior aspect of the vertebral arch. B C D

15 **Inferior articular process (zygapophysis).** Processus articularis (zygapophysis) inferior. Articular process on the inferior aspect of the vertebral arch. B C

16 **CERVICAL VERTEBRAE.** VERTEBRAE CERVICALES. The seven uppermost vertebrae (Cl-7). A

17 **Uncal process or uncus.** Uncus corporis. Superiorly directed, hook-like process along the lateral margin of the bodies of the cervical vertebrae. It occasionally gives rise to bony proliferations which can exert pressure on the spinal nerve. C

18 **Foramen transversarium.** Hole in the transverse process of cervical vertebrae for the passage of the vertebral artery and vein. C

19 **Anterior tubercle.** Tuberculum anterius. Anterior projection on the transverse processes of cervical vertebrae 2–7 for muscle attachment. C

20 **Posterior tubercle.** Tuberculum posterius. Posterior projection on the transverse processes of cervical vertebrae 2–7 for muscle attachment. C

21 **Carotid tubercle.** Tuberculum caroticum. Well developed anterior tubercle of C6. So named because the common carotid artery can be compressed against it anteriorly. A

22 **Groove for spinal nerve.** Sulcus n. spinalis. Groove on the transverse processes of C3–7 for the spinal nerves exiting from the intervertebral foramina. C

23 **Vertebra prominens (C7).** The seventh cervical vertebra. It is so named because of its especially well-developed spinous process (in 70% of cases). A

24 THORACIC VERTEBRAE. VERTEBRAE THORACICAE. The twelve vertebrae of the thorax (T1–12). A

25 **Superior costal facet.** Fovea costalis superior. Articular facet for the head of the rib. It is located on the vertebral body, above the root of the arch. B

26 **Inferior costal facet.** Fovea costalis inferior. Articular facet for the head of the rib. It is located on the vertebral body below the root of the arch. B

27 **Costal facet of transverse process.** Fovea costa-
~ lis processus transversi. Articular facet on the transverse process for the tubercle of the rib. B

28 LUMBAR VERTEBRAE. VERTEBRAE LUMBALES (LUMBARES). The five vertebrae of the lumbar region (L1–5). A

29 **Accessory process.** Processus accessorius. Rudiment of the original lumbar transverse process. It projects posteriorly from the base of the costal process. D

30 **Mamillary process.** Processus mamillaris. Rudimentary process projecting posteriorly from the superior articular process of the lumbar vertebra. D

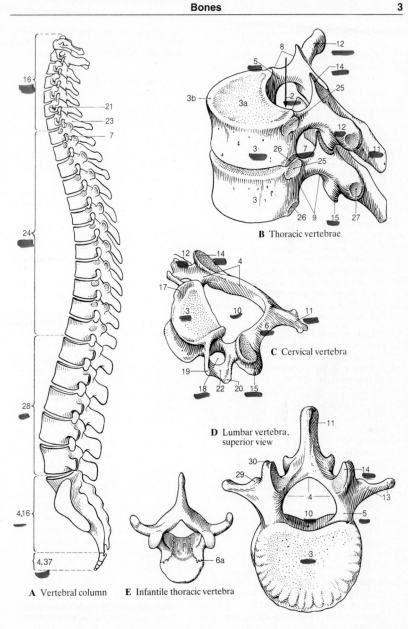

A Vertebral column

B Thoracic vertebrae

C Cervical vertebra

D Lumbar vertebra, superior view

E Infantile thoracic vertebra

1 **Atlas (C1). First cervical vertebra.** It lacks a body. A

2 **Lateral mass of atlas.** Massa lateralis atlantis. The well developed lateral part of the atlas which articulates with the skull. A

3 Superior articular facet. Facies articularis superior. A

4 Inferior articular facet. Facies articularis inferior. A

5 **Anterior arch of atlas.** Arcus anterior atlantis. A

6 Dental fovea of atlas. Fovea dentis. Articular facet for the dens of the axis on the inner surface of the anterior arch. A

7 Anterior tubercle of atlas. Tuberculum anterius. A

8 **Posterior arch of atlas.** Arcus posterior atlantis. A

9 Groove for vertebral artery. Sulcus arteriae vertebralis. It lies on the posterior arch of the atlas behind the articular surfaces. A

10 Posterior tubercle. Tuberculum posterius. It is a rudiment of the spinous process. A

11 **Axis (C2)** *[[Epistropheus]]* The second cervical vertebra. B

12 **Dens** [[odontoid process]] of axis. Dens axis. B

13 **Apex of dens.** Apex dentis. Attachment site of the apical ligament of the dens. B

14 Anterior articular surface of dens. Facies articularis anterior. B

15 Posterior articular surface of dens. Facies articularis posterior. B

16 **Os sacrum (sacrale) [Vertebrae sacrales I–V].** Sacral bone [[sacrum]] consisting of five vertebrae. C D F

17 **Base of sacrum.** Basis ossis sacri. Broad upper end. F

18 Promontory of sacrum. Promontorium. Prominent anterior margin of the body of the first sacral vertebra. It projects quite far into the pelvic inlet. F

19 Ala of sacrum. Ala sacralis. Part of the base of the sacrum situated lateral to the vertebral body. F

20 Superior articular process. Processus articularis superior. C F

21 **Lateral part or mass of sacrum.** Pars lateralis. The portion of the sacrum derived from the transverse processes and rudimentary ribs. C F

22 Auricular surface. Facies auricularis. Ear-shaped articular surface for the ilium. C

23 Sacral tuberosity. Tuberositas sacralis. Rough area behind the auricular surface for the attachment of ligaments coming from the ilium. C

24 **Pelvic surface.** Facies pelvica. Anterior surface of the sacrum facing the pelvis. F

25 Transverse lines. Lineae transversae. Four anteriorly situated fusion lines of the five sacral vertebral bodies. F

26 Intervertebral foramina. Foramina intervertebralia. Openings for the passage of the sacral spinal nerves. They develop from the original superior and inferior notches. D

27 Anterior sacral foramina. Foramina sacralia anteriora (pelvica). Anterior openings for nerves and vessels. D F

28 **Dorsal surface of sacrum.** Facies dorsalis. C

29 Median sacral crest. Crista sacralis mediana. Row of rudimentary spinous processes in the midline. C

30 Posterior sacral foramina. Foramina sacralia posteriora. Openings for nerves and vessels. C D

31 Intermediate sacral crest. Crista sacralis intermedia. Remains of the articular processes located bilateral to the median sacral crest. C

32 Lateral sacral crest. Crista sacralis lateralis. Row of rudimentary transverse processes located on the right and left posteriorly. C

33 Sacral cornu (horn). Cornu sacrale. Downward projecting process to the right and left of the sacral hiatus. C

34 Sacral canal. Canalis sacralis. It corresponds to the lower end of the vertebral canal. C D

35 *Sacral hiatus.* Hiatus sacralis. Inferior opening of the vertebral canal located usually at the level of S3–4. Emergence site of filum terminale and injection site for lower epidural anesthesia (caudal analgesia). C

36 **Apex of sacrum.** Apex ossis sacri. Inferior tip of sacrum which gives attachment to the coccyx. C F

37 **Coccygeal vertebrae I–IV.** Os coccygis.
~ Coccyx consisting of usually 4 rudimentary vertebrae. E

38 **Coccygeal cornu (horn). Cornu coccygeus.**
~ Upward projecting process formed from the articular process. E

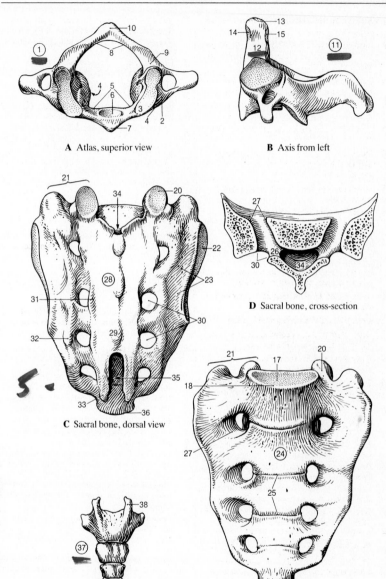

A Atlas, superior view

B Axis from left

C Sacral bone, dorsal view

D Sacral bone, cross-section

E Coccyx, dorsal view

F Sacral bone, anterior view

1 BONES OF THE THORAX. OSSA THORA-
CIS.

2 **Ribs 1–12.** Costae (I–XII). D

3 **True ribs (1–7).** Costae verae (I–VII). The first
seven ribs with individual cartilaginous
connections to the sternum thereby distin-
guishing them from the last five ribs. D

4 **False ribs (8–12).** Costae spuriae (VIII–XII).
The last five ribs which have no direct cartilaginous union with the sternum. D

5 Floating ribs (11–12). Costae fluitantes
(XI–XII). They have no connection with the
costal arch (arch of ribs). D

6 **Costal cartilage.** Cartilago costalis. Cartilage
at the anterior ends of the ribs. D

7 **Bony rib.** Os costale (costa). It is contrasted
with the cartilaginous segment of the rib. D

8 Head of rib. Capit costae. It forms an articular connection with the vertebral column. A

9 *Articular surface on head of rib.* Facies articulares capitis costae. A B

10 *Interarticular crest on head of rib.* Crista capitis costae. Small ridge which separates the two
articular facets. B

11 Neck of rib. Collum costae. It lies lateral to
the head of the rib. A B

12 *Crest of neck of rib.* Crista colli costae. Sharp
ridge on the upper border of the rib's neck. A

13 Shaft (body) of rib. Corpus costae. Main
part of rib adjacent to the neck. A B

14 Costal tubercle. Tuberculum costae. Posterior elevation between the neck and the shaft
of the rib. A B

15 *Articular facet of costa tubercle.* Facies articularis tuberculi costae. Articular surface for the
joint with the transverse process of the thoracic
vertebrae. A B

16 Angle of rib. Angulus costae. Posteriorly
situated bend in the axis of the rib. A B

17 Costal groove. Sulcus costae. Groove for the
intercostal artery, vein and nerve on the lower
margin of the internal surface of the rib. B

17 a **First rib.** Costa prima. It is unique in that only
the marginal curvature exists. A D

18 Tubercle for scalenus anterior muscle.
Tuberculum m. scaleni anterioris. Small prominence on the upper surface of the first rib for
the attachment of the scalenus anterior. A

19 Groove for subclavian artery. Sulcus a.
subclaviae. It is situated on the first rib behind
the tubercle for the scalenus anterior. A

20 Groove for subclavian vein. Sulcus v.
subclaviae. It occupies the first rib in front of
the tubercle for the scalenus anterior. A

20 a **Second rib.** Costa secunda. It attaches to the
sternal angle and can easily be identified in pa-
tients. A D

21 Tuberositas m. serrati anterioris.
Roughness on the outer surface of the shaft of
the second rib for the origin of the serratus
anterior muscle. A D

22 **Cervical rib.** [Costa cervicalis]. Accessory rib
at C7. It can irritate the nerves to the arm.

23 **Sternum.** C D

24 **Manubrium sterni.** The portion of the sternum situated above the sternal angle. C D

25 Clavicular notch. Incisura clavicularis. Indentation for the sternoclavicular joint. C D

26 Jugular notch. Incisura jugularis. Concavity
at the upper border of the manubrium. D

27 **Sternal angle.** Angulus sterni (sternalis) [[Lu-
dovici]]. Angle between the body and manubrium of the sternum palpable through the skin. C
D

28 **Sternal synchondroses.** Synchondroses sternales. The two synchondroses of the sternum
are as follows:

29 *Manubriosternal synchondrosis.* [Synchon-
drosis manubriosternalis]. Cartilaginous joint
between the manubrium and the body of the
sternum. C D

30 Xiphisternal synchondrosis. Synchondrosis xiphisternalis. Cartilaginous joint between the body of the sternum and the xiphoid
process. C D

31 **Body of sternum.** Corpus sterni. It lies between the manubrium and xiphoid process.
C D

32 **Xiphoid process.** Processus xiphoideus. Stout
process below the sternum. C D

33 **Costal notches.** Incisurae costales. Indentations for the costal cartilages. C D

34 **Suprasternal bones.** [Ossa suprasternalia].
Small bony remains of the earlier episternum in
the ligaments of the sternoclavicular joint.

35 **Thoracic skeleton.** Compages thoracis.

35 a **Thoracic cavity. Cavitas thoracis.**

36 **Superior thoracic aperture (thoracic inlet).**
Apertura thoracis superior. Upper thoracic
opening. D

37 **Inferior thoracic aperture (thoracic outlet).**
Apertura thoracis inferior. Lower opening of
thorax. D

38 **Pulmonary sulcus of thorax.** Sulcus pulmonis. Large vertical groove to the right and left
sides of the vertebral column, occupied by the
lungs. D

39 **Costal arch.** Arcus costalis. Arch of ribs
formed by the cartilages of ribs 7–10. D

40 **Intercostal space.** Spatium intercostale.
Space between the ribs. D

41 **Infrasternal angle.** Angulus infrasternalis.
Angle between the right and left costal arch. D

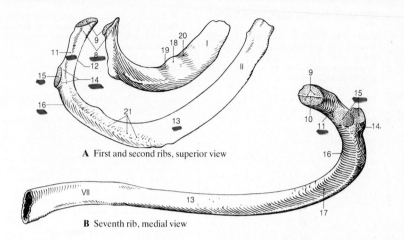

A First and second ribs, superior view

B Seventh rib, medial view

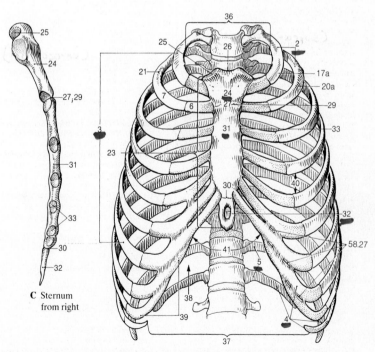

C Sternum
from right

D Thoracic skeleton, anterior view

1 CRANIAL BONES. OSSA CRANII. Bones of the skull.

2 OCCIPITAL BONE. **OS OCCIPITALE.**It lies between the sphenoid, temporal and parietal bones. A B C

3 **Foramen magnum.** Large opening in the occipital bone for the passage of the medulla oblongata, vessels and nerves. A B C

4 Basion. Midpoint of the anterior border of the foramen magnum. B

5 Opisthion. Midpoint at the posterior border of the foramen magnum. A B

6 **Basilar part of occipital bone (basi-occipital).** Pars basilaris. The portion of the occipital bone in front of the foramen magnum, between it and the sphenoid. A C

6a **Clivus.** Sloping superior surface of basiocciput between the foramen magnum and sella turcica. B

7 Groove for inferior petrosal sinus. Sulcus sinus pertrosi inferioris. A

8 **Pharyngeal tubercle.** Tuberculum pharyngeum. Prominence on the inferior surface of the basioccipital for the attachment of the pharyngeal raphe. A C

9 **Lateral (condylar) part of occipital bone.** Pars lateralis. It lies lateral to the foramen magnum. A B *(supra-occipital)*

10 **Squamous part of occipital bone.** Squama occipitalis. It extends behind the foramen magnum. A B C

11 Mastoid margin. Margo mastoideus. The border of the occipital bone united with the temporal bone. A

12 Lambdoid margin. Margo lambdoideus. The border of the occipital bone united with the parietal bone. A

13 Interparietal bone. [Os interparietale]. Separate bone formed as a variant when approximately the upper half of the occipital squama becomes sectioned off by a transverse suture.

14 **Occipital condyle.** Condylus occipitalis. Large protuberance for articulation with the atlas. A B C

15 **Condylar canal.** Canalis condylaris. Located behind the occipital condyle, it transmits an emissary vein from the sigmoid sinus. A B C

16 **Hypoglossal canal.** Canalis hypoglossi. Located anterolateral to the foramen magnum, it transmits cranial nerve XII. A B C

17 **Condylar fossa.** Fossa condylaris. Depression behind the occipital condyle. B

18 **Jugular tubercle.** Tuberculum jugulare. Elevation above the right and left hypoglossal canals on the side of occipital bone facing the brain. A B C

19 **Jugular notch.** Incisura jugularis. Indentation for the jugular foramen. A C

20 **Jugular process.** Processus jugularis. Visible externally and internally, it projects laterally from the jugular foramen. It corresponds to the transverse process of a vertebra. A C

21 **Intrajugular process of occipital bone.** Processus intrajugularis. It occasionally divides the jugular foramen into a lateral portion for the internal jugular vein and a medial segment for nerves. C

22 **External occipital protuberance.** Protuberentia occipitalis externa. Readily palpable bony projection in the middle of the occipital bone. B

23 *Inion.* Anthropological landmark corresponding to the external occipital protuberance. B

24 **External occipital crest.** Crista occipitalis externa. Bony ridge occasionally present between the external occipital protuberance and the foramen magnum. B

25 **Highest (supreme) nuchal line.** Linea nuchalis
~ suprema. Line arching externally from the upper margin of the external occipital protuberance. It gives origin to the occipital belly of the epicranius muscle. B

26 **Superior nuchal line.** Linea nuchalis superior.
~ Transverse ridge at the level of the external occipital protuberance. The field of origin of the trapezius muscle lies between it and the highest nuchal line. B

27 **Inferior nuchal line.** Linea nuchalis inferior.
~ Transverse ridge between the superior nuchal line and the foramen magnum. The semispinalis capitis muscle is attached between it and the superior nuchal line. B

27a **Occipital plane.** Planum occipitale. Outer surface of the occipital bone above the external occipital protuberance. B C *(ex-occipital)*

28 **Cruciform eminence.** Eminentia cruciformis. Cross-shaped bony elevation with the internal occipital protuberance at the center. A

29 **Internal occipital protuberance.** Protuberantia occipitalis interna. Midpoint of the cruciform eminence. A

30 **Internal occipital crest.** [Crista occipitalis interna]. Strongly developed bony ridge occasionally present extending from the internal occipital protuberance to the foramen magnum. A

31 **Groove for the superior sagittal sinus.** Sulcus sinus sagittalis superioris. A

32 **Groove for the transverse sinus.** Sulcus sinus transversi. A

33 **Groove for the sigmoid sinus before its entrance into the jugular foramen.** Sulcus sinus sigmoidei. A C

33a **Groove for the occipital sinus.** Sulcus sinus occipitalis. A

34 **Paramastoid process.** [Processus paramastoideus]. Occasional projection from the jugular process in the direction of the transverse process of the atlas.

34a **Cerebral fossa.** Fossa cerebralis. Depression for the occipital lobes of the cerebrum. A

34b **Cerebellar fossa.** Fossa cerebellaris. Depression for the cerebellum. A

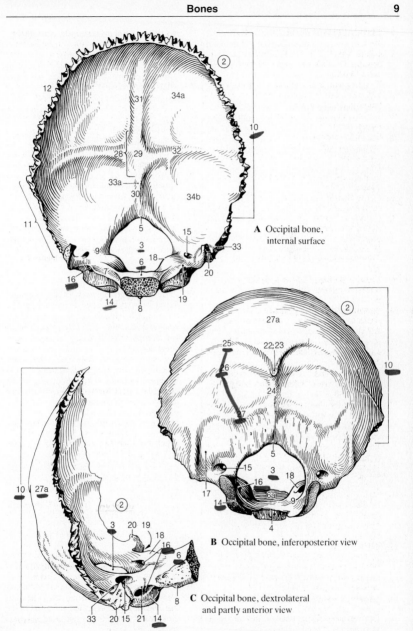

A Occipital bone, internal surface

B Occipital bone, inferoposterior view

C Occipital bone, dextrolateral and partly anterior view

1 SPHENOID BONE. OS SPHENOIDALE. It lies between the frontal, occipital and temporal bones. A B C

2 **Corpus.** Body of sphenoid between the winged processes (pterygoid or alae). A B

3 **Jugum sphenoidale.** Connection between the lesser wings of the sphenoid. A

4 **(Pre)chiasmatic groove.** Sulcus prechiasma-
~ ticus. Groove between the right and left optic canals. A

5 **Turkish saddle.** Sella turcica. It lies above the sphenoidal sinus and contains the hypophysis. A

6 **Tuberculum sellae.** Small process in front of the hypophysial fossa. A

7 Middle clinoid process. [Processus clinoideus medius]. Small protuberance occasionally present bilaterally in the floor of the hypophysial fossa. A

8 Hypophysial fossa. Fossa hypophysialis. Fossa occupied by the hypophysis. A

9 **Dorsum sellae.** Posterior wall of the hypophysial fossa. A C

10 Posterior clinoid process. Processus clinoideus posterior. Bilateral projections of the dorsum sellae. A C

11 **Carotid groove.** Sulcus caroticus. Groove for the internal carotid artery extending anteriorly from the medial aspect of the foramen lacerum. A

12 **Lingula sphenoidalis.** Pointed process lateral to the entrance of the internal carotid artery into the cranial fossa. A

13 **Sphenoidal crest.** Crista sphenoidalis. Median bony ridge on the anterior surface of the body of the sphenoid for articulation with the perpendicular plate of the ethmoid. C

14 **Sphenoidal rostrum.** Rostrum sphenoidale. Continuation of the sphenoidal crest inferiorly. It articulates with the vomer. C

15 **Sphenoidal sinus.** Sinus sphenoidalis. The paired paranasal sphenoidal sinus. C

16 Septum of sphenoidal sinus. Septum intersinuale sphenoidale. It partitions the sinus into right and left parts. C

17 Orifice of sphenoidal sinus. Apertura sinus sphenoidalis. It opens anteriorly into the spheno-ethmoidal recess. C

18 **Sphenoidal concha.** Concha sphenoidalis. Originally paired, concave bony plate which fuses with the body of the sphenoid and forms, among others, a part of the anterior and inferior wall of the sphenoidal sinus. C

19 **Lesser wing of sphenoid.** Ala minor. A B C

20 **Optic canal.** Canalis opticus. Canal for the optic nerve and the ophthalmic artery. A

21 **Anterior clinoid process.** Processus clinoideus anterior. Cone-like process on both sides of the hypophysial fossa anteriorly. A

22 **Superior orbital fissure.** Fissura orbitalis superior. Cleft between the greater and lesser wings of the sphenoid for the passage of nerves and veins. A B C

23 **Greater wing of sphenoid.** Ala major. A B C

24 **Cerebral surface.** Facies cerebralis. Surface of the greater wing facing the brain. A

25 **Temporal surface.** Facies temporalis. Surface of the greater wing directed toward the outside (temporal fossa). B C

26 **Maxillary surface.** Facies maxillaris. Surface of the greater wing facing the maxilla. The foramen rotundum opens here. C

27 **Orbital surface.** Facies orbitalis. Surface of the greater wing facing the orbit. C

28 **Zygomatic border.** Margo zygomaticus. Margin of the greater wing articulating with the zygomatic bone. C

29 **Frontal border.** Margo frontalis. Margin of the greater wing fused with the frontal bone. A

30 **Parietal border.** Margo parietalis. Margin of the greater wing fused with the parietal bone. C

31 **Squamous border.** Margo squamosus. Overlapping articulation with the temporal bone. A

32 **Infratemporal crest.** Crista infratemporalis. Bony ridge between the vertical temporal surface and the horizontally-oriented inferior surface of the greater wing of the sphenoid. B C

33 **Foramen rotundum.** Round opening for the maxillary nerve directed anteriorly into the pterygopalatine fossa. A B C

34 **Foramen ovale.** Oval opening medial to and in front of the foramen spinosum for the passage of the mandibular nerve. A B

35 **[Foramen venosum].** Opening occasionally present medial to the foramen ovale for an emissary vein from the cavernous sinus. A B

36 **Foramen spinosum.** Opening situated lateral to and behind the foramen ovale for the passage of the middle meningeal artery. A B

37 **[Foramen petrosum.** [[Canaliculus innominatus.]] Opening occasionally present between the foramen ovale and the foramen spinosum for the lesser petrosal nerve. A B

38 **Angular spine of sphenoid.** Spina ossis sphenoidalis. Sharp, downward-directed bony spur of the greater wing. A B

39 **Groove for the cartilaginous part of the au-
~ ditory tube.** Sulcus tubae auditoriae (auditivae). Shallow groove on the underside of the greater wing lateral to the root of the pterygoid process. B

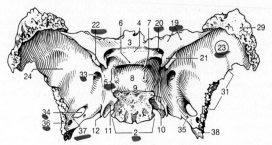

A Sphenoid bone, superior view

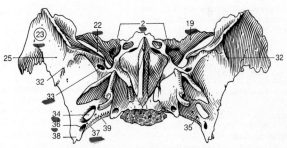

B Sphenoid bone, anteroinferior view

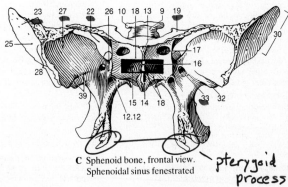

C Sphenoid bone, frontal view.
Sphenoidal sinus fenestrated

pterygoid
process

1 **Pterygoid process of the sphenoid bone.** Processus pterygoideus. A B

2 **Lateral pterygoid plate.** Lamina lateralis [processus pterygoidei]. A B

3 **Medial pterygoid plate.** Lamina medialis [processus pterygoidei]. A B

4 **Pterygoid notch (fissure).** Incisura pterygoidea. Fissure formed inferiorly by the diverging medial and lateral pterygoid plates. It is occupied by the pyramidal process of the palatine bone. A

5 **Pterygoid fossa.** Fossa pterygoidea. Space between the lateral and medial pterygoid plates for the medial pterygoid muscle. A B

6 **Scaphoid fossa.** Fossa scaphoidea. Oblong depression at the root of the medial pterygoid plate for the origin of the tensor veli palatini muscle. A

7 **Vaginal process.** Processus vaginalis. Small bony ridge medial to the root of the medial pterygoid plate. It borders a small furrow laterally. A B

8 Palatovaginal groove. Sulcus palatovaginalis. Groove which, together with the palatine bone, forms the palatovaginal canal. B

9 Vomerovaginal groove. Sulcus vomerovaginalis. Groove at the base of the pterygoid process. Together with the vomer, it forms the vomerovaginal canal. B

10 **Pterygoid hamulus.** Hamulus pterygoideus. Hook-like process at the inferior end of the medial pterygoid plate. A B

11 Sulcus of pterygoid hamulus. Sulcus hamuli pterygoidei. Groove produced by a sharp bend in the hamulus. B

12 **Pterygoid (vidian) canal.** Canalis pterygoideus [[canalis Vidii]]. It passes anteriorly in the base of the pterygoid process carrying the greater and deep petrosal nerves to the pterygopalatine ganglion in the same-named fossa. A see 11 C

13 **Pterygospinous process.** Processus pterygospinosus. Sharp spine on the posterior edge of the lateral pterygoid plate. A

14 TEMPORAL BONE. OS TEMPORALE. It lies between the occipital, sphenoid and parietal bones and consists of three parts: petrous, tympanic and squamous. C D E

15 **Petrous part (pyramid).** Pars petrosa. It houses the inner ear. D

16 **Occipital border.** Margo occipitalis. Margin articulating with the occipital bone. C D

17 **Mastoid process.** Processus mastoideus. It lies behind the external acoustic meatus. C E

18 **Mastoid notch.** Incisura mastoidea. Notch on the inferior side medial to the mastoid process. It gives origin to the posterior belly of the digastric muscle. C

19 **Groove for sigmoid sinus.** Sulcus sinus sigmoidei. It is located internally and posteriorly. D

20 **Groove for occipital artery.** Sulcus a. occipitalis. It lies medial to the mastoid notch and close to the occipital margin. C

21 **Mastoid foramen.** Foramen mastoideum. Opening behind the mastoid process for additional venous drainage from the cranial cavity. C D

22 **Facial canal.** Canalis facialis. Canal for the facial nerve. It begins at the opening of the internal acoustic meatus and ends at the stylomastoid foramen. C D E

23 Genu of facial canal. Geniculum canalis facialis. Sharp bend in the facial canal just below the anterior wall of the petrous temporal near the hiatus of the canal for the greater petrosal nerve. D

24 **Canaliculus of chorda tympani nerve.** Canaliculus chordae tympani. Narrow passageway for the chorda tympani nerve between the facial canal and the tympanic cavity. D E

25 **Apex of petrous temporal.** Apex partis petrosae. It is directed anteromedially. C D

26 Carotid *foramen*. Canalis caroticus. Canal for the internal carotid artery. It begins inferiorly and externally between the jugular foramen and the musculotubal canal. C

27 *Carotidy foramen canaliculi*. Canaliculi caroticotympanici. Small channels in the wall of the carotid canal for arterial and nerve branches to the middle ear from the internal carotid artery and the carotid plexus. C

28 Musculotubal canal. Canalis musculotubarius. Double canal for the auditory tube and tensor tympani muscle. It lies in front of the carotid canal and leads into the tympanic cavity. C E

29 *Semicanal for tensor tympani muscle.* Semicanalis m. tensoris tympani. E

30 *Semicanal for the auditory tube.* Semicanalis tubae auditoriae (auditivae). E

31 *Septum of musculotubal canal.* Septum canalis musculotubarii. Bony partition between the above-mentioned semicanals. E

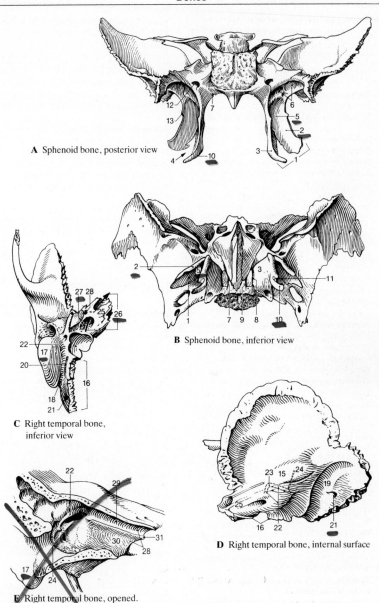

A Sphenoid bone, posterior view

B Sphenoid bone, inferior view

C Right temporal bone, inferior view

D Right temporal bone, internal surface

E Right temporal bone, opened. Anterolateral view

1 **Anterior surface of the petrous part of the temporal bone.** Facies anterior partis petrosae. A C

2 Roof of tympanic cavity. Tegmen tympani. Thin bony plate anterolateral to the arcuate eminence. C

3 Arcuate eminence. Eminentia arcuata. Elevation on the anterior surface of the petrous temporal produced by the underlying anterior semicircular canal. A C

4 Hiatus of canal for greater petrosal nerve. Hiatus canalis n. petrosi majoris. Opening in the anterior wall of the petrous temporal for the same-named branch of the facial nerve. A C

5 Hiatus of canal for lesser petrosal nerve. Hiatus canalis n. petrosi minoris. Opening in the anterior wall of the petrous temporal below the previously mentioned nerve. A C

6 *Groove for greater petrosal nerve.* Sulcus n. petrosi majoris. Its course is from the hiatus anteromedially to the foramen lacerum. C

7 *Groove for lesser petrosal nerve.* Sulcus n. petrosi minoris. Groove for the same-named nerve running from the corresponding hiatus to the foramen lacerum. C

8 Trigeminal impression. Impressio trigeminalis. Shallow depression in the anterior wall of the apex of the petrous temporal for the trigeminal [[semilunar]] ganglion. C

9 **Superior border of petrous temporal.** Margo superior partis petrosae. A C

10 Groove for superior petrosal sinus. Sulcus sinus petrosi superioris. Its course is on the upper margin of the petrous temporal. A C

11 **Posterior surface of petrous temporal.** Facies posterior partis petrosae. A

12 Porus acusticus internus. Opening of internal acoustic meatus on the posterior wall of the petrous temporal. A

13 Internal acoustic (auditory) meatus. Meatus acusticus internus. It transmits cranial nerves VII and VIII and vessels. A

14 Subarcuate fossa. Fossa subarcuata. Depression lateral and superior to the internal acoustic meatus. It was occupied by the fetal flocculus of the cerebellum. A

15 Aqueduct of vestibule. Aqueductus vestibuli. Narrow canal extending from the endolymphatic space of the inner ear to the posterior wall of the petrous temporal.

16 *External opening of vestibular aqueduct.* Apertura externa aqueductus vestibuli. A

17 **Posterior border of petrous temporal.** Margo posterior partis petrosae. A B

18 Groove for inferior petrosal sinus. Sulcus sinus petrosi inferioris. A

19 Jugular notch. Incisura jugularis. Indentation forming the anterior margin of the jugular foramen. A B

20 **Intrajugular process.** Processus intrajugularis. It divides the jugular foramen into a lateral, posterior part for the internal jugular vein and a medial, anterior part for cranial nerves IX, X and XI. A B

21 Cochlear canaliculus. Canaliculus cochleae. Bony canal for the cochlear aqueduct.

22 *External opening of cochlear canaliculus.* Apertura externa canaliculi cochleae. It lies medially in front of the jugular fossa. B

23 **Inferior surface of petrous temporal.** Facies inferior partis petrosae. B

24 Jugular fossa. Fossa jugularis. Enlargement of the jugular foramen for the superior bulb of the internal jugular vein. B

25 *Mastoid canaliculus.* Canaliculus mastoideus. Narrow canal for the auricular branch of the vagus nerve. It begins in the jugular fossa. B

26 Styloid process. Processus styloideus. Long process located laterally in front of the jugular fossa. It is a vestige of the second branchial arch. A B D

27 **Stylomastoid foramen.** Foramen stylomastoideum. External opening of the facial canal behind the styloid process and between the mastoid process and the jugular fossa. B

28 Tympanic canaliculus. Canaliculus tympanicus. Minute canal in the petrosal fossula traversed by the tympanic nerve and inferior tympanic artery. B

29 Petrosal fossula. Fossula petrosa. Slight depression in the bony ridge between the carotid canal and the jugular fossa. It is occupied by the tympanic ganglion of the glossopharyngeal nerve. B

30 **Tympanic (middle ear) cavity.** Cavitas tympanica. Narrow, air-filled space between the osseous labyrinth and the tympanic membrane.

31 **Petrotympanic fissure [Glaserian fissure].** Fissura petrotympanica. Fissure situated dorsomedially from the fossa of the temporomandibular joint between the tympanic part and the evident petrosal strip. The chorda tympani nerve exits from it. B D

32 **Petrosquamous fissure.** Fissura petrosquamosa. It lies on the skull base in front of the petrotympanic fissure between the evident petrous strip and the squamous part of the temporal bone. B C

33 **Squamotympanic fissure.** Fissura tympanosquamosa. Lateral continuation of the two above mentioned fissures after their union. B D

34 **Tympanomastoid fissure.** Fissura tympanomastoidea. Suture between the tympanic part of the temporal bone and the mastoid process. Exit site for the auricular branch of the vagus nerve. B D

(see p. 317)

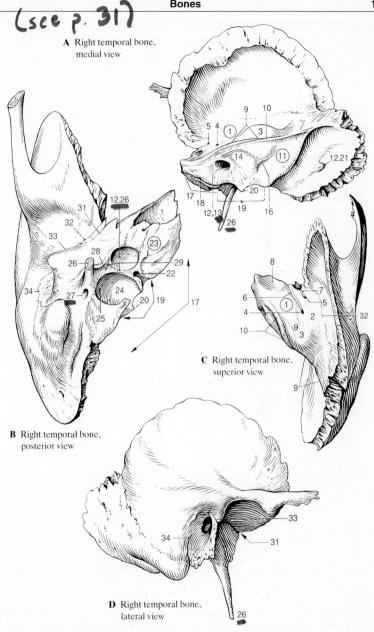

A Right temporal bone,
medial view

B Right temporal bone,
posterior view

C Right temporal bone,
superior view

D Right temporal bone,
lateral view

1 **Tympanic part of temporal bone.** Pars tympanica. Wall of the bony external acoustic meatus with the exception of the posterior, upper wall (tympanic notch). B

2 **Tympanic ring.** Anulus tympanicus. Bony ring which is the developmental precursor of the tympanic part of the temporal bone. At birth it is still open superiorly. A

3 **External acoustic (auditory) meatus.** Meatus acusticus externus. B

4 **Opening of external acoustic meatus.** Porus acusticus externus. B

5 **Greater tympanic spine.** Spina tympanica major. Anteriorly situated end of the incomplete tympanic ring formed by the tympanic part of the temporal bone. A

6 **Lesser tympanic spine.** Spina tympanica minor. Posteriorly situated end of the incomplete ring formed by the tympanic part of the temporal bone. A

7 **Tympanic groove.** Sulcus tympanicus. Groove for the attachment of the tympanic membrane. A

8 **Tympanic notch.** Incisura tympanica. Notch between the greater and lesser tympanic spines. In the newborn it is the space situated superiorly between the free ends of the still open tympanic ring. A

9 **Sheath of styloid process.** Vagina processus styloidei. Ridge formed by the tympanic part of the temporal and partially enclosing the root of the styloid process. A

10 **Squamous part.** Pars squamosa. Part of the temporal bone inserted between the sphenoid, parietal and occipital bones. B

11 **Parietal border.** Margo parietalis. Upper margin articulating with the parietal bone. B

12 **Parietal notch.** Incisura parietalis. Indentation posteroinferior to the temporal line. B

13 **Sphenoidal border.** Margo sphenoidalis. Anterior margin articulating with the sphenoid bone. B

14 **Temporal surface.** Facies temporalis. External surface covered primarily by the temporalis muscle. B

15 **Groove for the middle temporal artery.** Sulcus arteriae temporalis mediae. B

16 **Zygomatic process of temporal bone.** Processus zygomaticus. It contributes to the formation of the zygomatic arch. B

17 **Supramastoid crest.** Crista supramastoidea. Ridge forming the posterior boundary of the field of attachment of the temporalis muscle. B

18 **Suprameatal pit.** Foveola suprameatica (suprameatalis). Small pit above the spine and lateral to the mastoid antrum. B

19 **Suprameatal spine.** [Spina suprameatica].
~ Projection for the attachment of the auricular cartilage. B

20 **Mandibular fossa.** Fossa mandibularis. Depression for the head of the mandible. B

21 **Facies articularis.** Articular surface for the temporomandibular joint. B

22 **Articular tubercle.** Tuberculum articulare. Cylindrical elevation in front of the mandibular fossa. B

23 **Cerebral surface.** Facies cerebralis. Inner surface of squamous temporal facing the brain. B

24 PARIETAL BONE. OS PARIETALE. It is located between the frontal, sphenoid and temporal bones. C D

25 **Internal surface.** Facies interna. Surface turned toward the brain. C

26 Groove for sigmoid sinus. Sulcus sinus sigmoidei. It lies in the vicinity of the mastoid angle. C

26 a **Groove for superior sagittal sinus.** Sulcus sinus sagittalis superioris. C

26 b **Groove for middle meningeal artery.** Sulcus arteriae meningeae mediae. C

27 **External surface.** Facies externa. Surface facing the scalp. D

28 Superior temporal line. Linea temporalis superior. Curved line for the attachment of the temporal fascia. D

29 Inferior temporal line. Linea temporalis inferior. Curved line for the attachment of the temporalis muscle. D

30 *Parietal tuber.* Tuber parietale. Prominence located at about the middle of the external surface of the parietal bone. D

31 **Occipital border.** Margo occipitalis. Margin facing the occiput. C D

32 **Squamous border.** Margo squamosus. Margin directed inferiorly on the temporal bone. C D

33 **Sagittal border.** Margo sagittalis. Upper margin lying in the midsagittal plane. C D

34 **Frontal border.** Margo frontalis. Anterior margin articulating with the frontal bone. C D

35 **Frontal angle.** Angulus frontalis. Upper, anterior angle of the parietal bone. C D

36 **Occipital angle.** Angulus occipitalis. Upper, posterior angle of the parietal bone. C D

37 **Sphenoidal angle.** Angulus sphenoidalis. Lower, anterior angle of the parietal bone. C D

38 **Mastoid angle.** Angulus mastoideus. Lower, posterior angle of the parietal bone. C D

39 **Parietal foramen.** Foramen parietale. Opening for an emissary vein from the cranial cavity located usually posterosuperiorly. C D

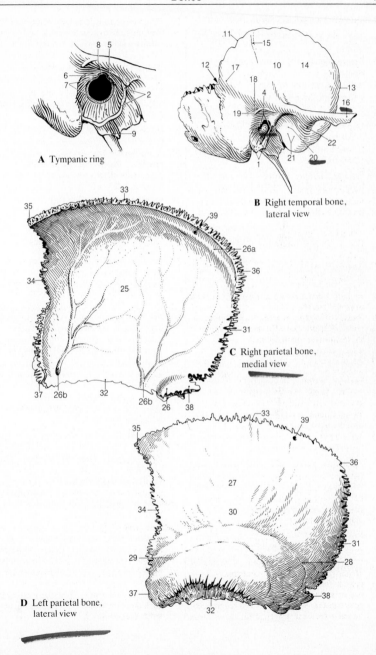

A Tympanic ring

B Right temporal bone, lateral view

C Right parietal bone, medial view

D Left parietal bone, lateral view

1 FRONTAL BONE. OS FRONTALE. A B C

2 **Squama of frontal bone.** Squama frontalis. A C

3 **External surface of frontal bone.** Facies externa. A

4 Frontal tuber (tuberosity). Tuber frontale (eminentia frontalis). A

5 *Superciliary arch.* Arcus superciliaris. Bony elevation above the upper margin of the orbit. A B

6 Glabella. Landmark between the two superciliary arches. A

6 a **Frontal (metopic) suture.** [Sutura frontalis]. It has usually grown together in the adult.

7 Supra-orbital border. Margo supra-orbitalis. Upper orbital margin of frontal bone. A B

8 *Supra-orbital notch or foramen.* Incisura supraorbitalis/foramen supraorbitale. Notch or hole in the supra-orbital margin for the supra-orbital artery and lateral branch of the supra-orbital nerve. Pressure point for the first branch of the trigeminal nerve. A B

9 *Frontal notch or foramen.* Incisura frontalis/foramen frontale. Notch or foramen medial to the supra-orbital foramen for the supratrochlear artery and the medial branch of the supra-orbital nerve. A B

10 **Temporal surface.** Facies temporalis. External, lateral surface of the frontal bone. A B

11 **Parietal border.** Margo parietalis. Posterior margin which articulates with the parietal bone. A C

12 **Temporal line of frontal bone.** Linea temporalis. Continuation of the line formed by the union of the superior and inferior temporal lines of the parietal bone. A

13 **Zygomatic process of frontal bone.** Processus zygomaticus. Process situated lateral to the orbit for articulation with the zygomatic bone. A B C

14 **Internal surface.** Facies interna. Inner surface of the frontal bone facing the brain. C

15 **Frontal crest.** Crista frontalis. Bony ridge located anteriorly in the midline of the inner surface of the frontal bone for the attachment of the falx cerebri. C

16 **Groove for superior sagittal sinus.** Sulcus sinus sagittalis superioris. Its margins come together as it passes downward and become continuous with the frontal crest. C

17 **Foramen cecum.** Foramen caecum. Canal behind the frontal crest. It usually ends blindly but when patent, it contains an emissary vein. C

17 a **Sutura frontalis metopica.** Persistent frontal suture in the adult. A

18 **Nasal part of frontal bone.** Pars nasalis. Middle segment between the two orbital parts. A B

19 **Nasal spine.** Spina nasalis. Median pointed projection. A B C

20 **Nasal border.** Margo nasalis. Serrated lower margin of the nasal part of the frontal bone. Here it articulates with the right and left nasal bones. A B C

21 **Orbital part.** Pars orbitalis. The part of the frontal bone forming the roof of the orbit. A B C

22 **Orbital surface.** Facies orbitalis. The surface facing the orbit. B

23 **Trochlear spine.** [Spina trochlearis]. Small bony spicule occasionally present anterosuperiorly in the medial angle of the orbit for the attachment of the trochlea of the superior oblique muscle. A

24 **Trochlear fovea.** Fovea trochlearis. Small depression for the attachment of a cartilaginous sling (trochlea or pulley) through which passes the tendon of the superior oblique muscle. A B

25 Ethmoidal foramina. Foramina ethmoidalia. Openings for the ethmoidal vessels and nerves. B

26 Fossa for lacrimal gland. Fossa glandulae lacrimalis. Depression for the lacrimal gland in the lateral angle of the orbit. B

27 **Ethmoid notch.** Incisura ethmoidalis. Space between the right and left orbital parts of the frontal bone in which the ethmoid bone is lodged. B

28 **Frontal sinus.** Sinus frontalis. It averages 3 cm high and 2.5 cm wide and often extends 1.8 cm posteriorly thereby forming a part of the orbital roof. A

29 Opening of frontal sinus. Apertura sinus frontalis. Opening located medially in the floor of the frontal sinus for the discharge of secretions into the nasal cavity at the ethmoidal infundibulum below the middle nasal concha. B C

30 Septum of frontal sinus. Septum intersinuale frontale. Partition between the right and left frontal sinuses. A

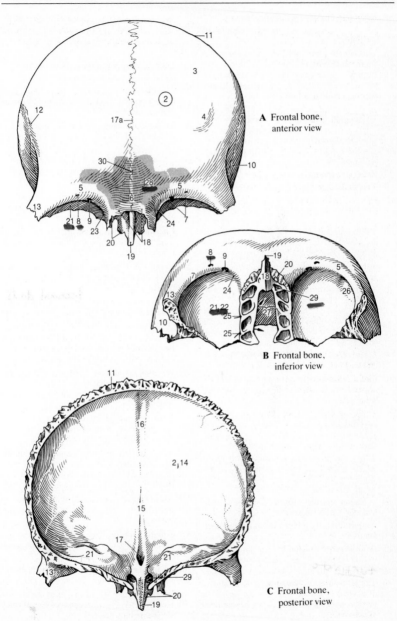

A Frontal bone, anterior view

B Frontal bone, inferior view

C Frontal bone, posterior view

1 ETHMOID BONE. OS ETHMOIDALE. Unpaired bone inserted into the ethmoid notch of the frontal bone. A B C D

2 **Cribriform plate and foramina.** Lamina et foramina cribrosa. Elongated horizontal plate occupying the median plane between the nasal cavity and the anterior cranial fossa. Its numerous foramina transmit the olfactory nerve fibers. B

3 **Crista galli.** Small bony process that projects upward from the anterior cranial fossa and gives attachment to the falx cerebri. A B C D

4 Ala of crista galli. Ala cristae galli. Winglike, paired tip for the connection of the crista galli to the frontal crest. A B C D

5 **Perpendicular plate.** Lamina perpendicularis. It extends downward from the ethmoid bone and forms the upper part of the nasal septum. A B C

6 **Ethmoidal labyrinth.** Labyrinthus ethmoidalis. Collective term for the ethmoidal air cells situated between the orbital and nasal cavities.

7 **Ethmoidal air cells.** Cellulae ethmoidales. A C

8 **Ethmoidal infundibulum.** Infundibulum ethmoidale. Narrow, oblong canal below the middle nasal concha and between the uncinate process and ethmoidal bulla. It receives the openings of the frontal and maxillary sinuses as well as the anterior ethmoidal air cells. A C

9 **Hiatus semilunaris.** Opening of the infundibulum situated toward the nose. C

10 **Bulla ethmoidalis.** An anterior elevation formed by an especially large and wide ethmoidal air cell which compresses the ethmoidal infundibulum. A

11 **Orbital plate.** Lamina orbitalis. An especially thin bony plate which forms a part of the medial wall of the orbit. *[[Lamina papyracea]]*. C

12 **Ethmoidal foramina.** Foramina ethmoidalia. Holes or grooves at the border to the frontal bone for the passage of ethmoidal nerves, arteries and veins to or from the orbit. C

13 **[Concha nasalis suprema].** Highest, rudimentary nasal concha. D

14 **Superior nasal concha.** Concha nasalis superior. A D

15 **Middle nasal concha.** Concha nasalis media. A C D

16 **Uncinate process.** Processus uncinatus. Hook-like process directed postero-inferiorly. It is almost entirely concealed by the middle nasal concha and partially closes the semilunar hiatus. A C

17 INFERIOR NASAL CONCHA. CONCHA NASALIS INFERIOR. Independent lowest nasal concha attached to the lateral nasal wall. E

18 **Lacrimal process.** Processus lacrimalis. It is directed anterosuperiorly. E

19 **Maxillary process.** Processus maxillaris. Lateral process which forms a part of the medial wall of the maxillary sinus. E

20 **Ethmoidal process.** Processus ethmoidalis. It is united with the uncinate process of the ethmoid bone. E

21 LACRIMAL BONE. OS LACRIMALE. It lies in front of the orbital plate of the ethmoid bone. F

22 **Posterior lacrimal crest.** Crista lacrimalis posterior. Ridge forming the posterior border of the entrance into the nasolacrimal canal. F

23 **Lacrimal sulcus of lacrimal bone.** Sulcus lacrimalis. Groove-like beginning of the nasolacrimal canal. F

24 **Lacrimal hamulus.** Hamulus lacrimalis. Hook-like lower margin of the entrance into the nasolacrimal canal. F

25 **Fossa for lacrimal sac.** Fossa sacci lacrimalis. Enlarged area for the nasolacrimal sac located at the beginning of the nasolacrimal canal. F

26 NASAL BONE. OS NASALE. It lies between the right and left halves of the maxilla and articulates with the frontal bone superiorly. G

27 **Ethmoidal sulcus.** Sulcus ethmoidalis. Groove on the undersurface of the nasal bone for the external nasal branch of the anterior ethmoidal nerve. G

27 a **Nasal foramina.** Foramina nasalia. Inconstant openings for branches of the external nasal and anterior ethmoidal nerves and vessels. G

28 VOMER. Unpaired bone forming a part of the nasal septum and lying between the sphenoid, maxillary and palatine bones as well as the perpendicular plate of the ethmoid. H

29 **Ala of vomer.** Ala vomeris. Wing-like process for articulation with the sphenoid and palatine bones. H

30 **Sulcus vomeris.** Obliquely-running groove for the nasopalatine nerve and its accompanying vessels. H

30 a **Choanal crest of vomer.** Crista choanalis vomeris. Posterior edge of vomer separating the two choanae. H

30 b **Cuneiform** Pars cuneiformis vomeris. Wedge-shaped part of vomer. H

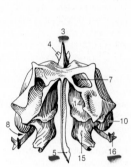

A Ethmoid bone, posterior view

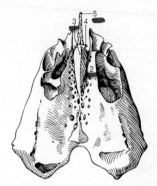

B Ethmoid bone, superior view

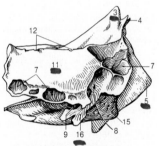

C Ethmoid bone, dextral view

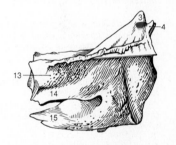

D Ethmoid bone, left half without
perpendicular plate, medial view

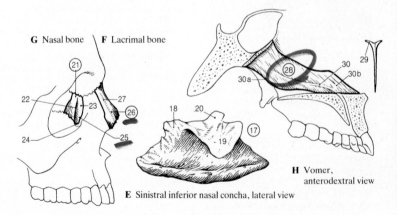

G Nasal bone   **F** Lacrimal bone

E Sinistral inferior nasal concha, lateral view

H Vomer,
anterodextral view

1   FACIAL BONES. OSSA FACIEI.

2   MAXILLA. Upper jaw. A B

3   **Body of maxilla.** Corpus maxillae. Central part of the maxilla enclosing the maxillary sinus. A

4   **Orbital surface.** Facies orbitalis. Surface of the maxilla forming a portion of the floor of the orbit. A

5   Infraorbital canal. Canalis infraorbitalis. Canal for the infraorbital artery and nerve. A

6   Infraorbital groove. Sulcus infraorbitalis. Groove at the beginning of the infraorbital canal. A

7   **Infraorbital margin.** Margo infraorbitalis. Lower margin of the orbit formed in part by the maxilla. A

8   **Anterior surface.** Facies anterior. A

9   Infraorbital foramen. Foramen infraorbitale. Opening of the infraorbital canal traversed by the infraorbital nerve and its accompanying artery. Pressure point for the second division of the trigeminal nerve. A

10 Canine fossa. Fossa canina. Depressed area below the infraorbital canal. Origin site of levator anguli oris muscle. A

11 Nasal notch. Incisura nasalis. Curved margin of the bony anterior nasal (piriform) aperture. A

12 Anterior nasal spine. Spina nasalis anterior. Spinous projection at the lower boundary of the anterior nasal aperture. Attachment site of the cartilaginous nasal septum. A B

13 Zygomaticomaxillary suture. Sutura zygomaticomaxillaris. Suture occasionally present from the infraorbital margin to the infraorbital foramen. A

14 **Infratemporal surface.** Facies infratemporalis. Surface of the maxilla situated behind the zygomatic process. A

15 Alveolar foramina. Foramina alveolaria. Small openings on the infratemporal surface for the passage of nerves and vessels to the teeth. A

16 Alveolar canals. Canales alveolares. Canals leading to the alveolar foramina for the transport of nerves and vessels for the teeth. A

17 Tuber of maxilla. Tuber maxillare (eminentia maxillaris). Thin walled tuberosity at the posterior wall of the maxillary sinus. A

18 **Nasal surface.** Facies nasalis. Medial surface of maxilla forming a portion of the lateral nasal wall. B

19 Lacrimal sulcus. Sulcus lacrimalis. Groove for the nasolacrimal duct. B

20 Conchal crest. Crista conchalis. Oblique ridge for the attachment of the inferior nasal concha. B

21 Lacrimal margin. Margo lacrimalis. Border of the maxilla articulating with the lacrimal bone. A B

22 Maxillary hiatus. Hiatus maxillaris. Large opening in the medial bony wall of the maxillary sinus. B

23 **Greater palatine sulcus [[pterygopalatine sulcus]].** Sulcus palatinus major [[sulcus pterygopalatinus]]. Groove at the posterior border of the maxilla. It combines with a similar groove on the palatine bone to form a canal for the greater palatine nerve and descending palatine artery. B

24 **Maxillary sinus.** Sinus maxillaris. Paranasal cavity within the body of the maxilla. It measures over 3 cm vertically and sagittally and 2.5 cm in the frontal plane. Its floor usually lies at least 1 cm below the floor of the nasal cavity. B

25 **Frontal process of maxilla.** Processus frontalis. A B

26 **Anterior lacrimal crest.** Crista lacrimalis anterior. Bony ridge in front of the entrance into the nasolacrimal canal. A

27 **Lacrimal notch.** Incisura lacrimalis. Crescent-shaped notch at the entrance into the nasolacrimal canal. B

28 **Ethmoidal crest.** Crista ethmoidalis. Oblique ridge on the medial surface of the frontal process for the attachment of the middle nasal concha. B

29 **Zygomatic process.** Processus zygomaticus. Lateral process of the maxilla for articulation with the zygomatic bone. A

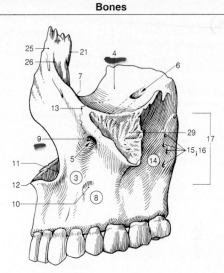

A Left maxilla, lateral view

Inferior
Turbinates (2)

- interior side of nasal
  cavity

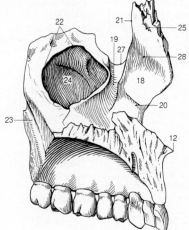

B Left maxilla, medial view

1   **Palatine process** (plate). Processus palatinus. Horizontal plate which forms the largest part of the hard palate. A B

2   **Nasal crest.** Crista nasalis. Midline bony ridge for the attachment of the nasal septum. B

3   **Incisive bone (premaxilla).** [Os incisivum]. Separate fetal bone which becomes incorporated into the adult maxilla and houses the incisor teeth. A

4   **Incisive canal.** Canalis incisivus. Canal for the passage of the greater palatine artery and the nasopalatine nerve. It is doubled on the nasal side, single on the palatine side. A B

5   **Incisive suture.** [Sutura incisiva]. Suture – visible only during development – between the premaxilla and the palatine process of the maxilla. It usually extends from the incisive foramen to the space between the canine and the second incisor tooth. A

6   **Palatine spines.** Spinae palatinae. Bony ridges along the palatine grooves. A

7   **Palatine grooves.** Sulci palatini. Grooves running from posterior to anterior along the inferior surface of the palate for the passage of nerves and vessels from the greater palatine foramen. A

8   **Alveolar process.** Processus alveolaris. Crested process for carrying the teeth. A

9   **Alveolar arch.** Arcus alveolaris. Curved free border of the alveolar process. A

10 **Dental alveoli.** Alveoli dentales. Sockets in the alveolar process for housing the roots of the teeth. A

11 **Interalveolar septa.** Septa interalveolaria. Bony ridges between adjacent alveoli. A

12 **Interradicular septa.** Septa interradicularia. Bony partitions forming compartments for the roots of a tooth. A

13 **Alveolar juga.** Juga alveolaria. Eminences on the external surface of the jaw produced by the protrusion of the tooth sockets. A B

14 **Incisive foramen.** Foramen incisivum. Opening of the incisive canal into the oral cavity. A

15 PALATINE BONE. OS PALATINUM. Bone forming the posterior continuation of the maxilla. A B D E

16 **Perpendicular plate.** Lamina perpendicularis. Vertical plate which forms part of the medial wall of the maxillary sinus. B C D E

17 **Nasal surface.** Facies nasalis. Surface of the perpendicular plate facing the nasal cavity. E

18 **Maxillary surface.** Facies maxillaris. Lateral surface of the perpendicular plate bordering partly the pterygopalatine fossa and partly the maxillary sinus. D

19 **Sphenopalatine notch.** Incisura sphenopalatina. Part of the sphenopalatine foramen at the superior margin of the perpendicular plate. D E

20 **Greater palatine sulcus** (pterygopalatine sulcus). Sulcus palatinus major [[sulcus pterygopalatinus]]. Groove which combines with the greater palatine sulcus of the maxilla to form the greater palatine canal for the greater palatine nerves and the descending palatine artery. D E

21 **Pyramidal process.** Processus pyramidalis. Process inserted into the pterygoid notch (fissure). A C D E

22 **Lesser palatine canals.** Canales palatini minores. Canals in the pyramidal process for the same-named arteries and nerves. A

23 **Conchal crest.** Crista conchalis. Ridge for attachment of the inferior nasal concha. D E

24 **Ethmoidal crest.** Crista ethmoidalis. Ridge for the attachment of the middle nasal concha. D E

25 **Orbital process.** Processus orbitalis. Forward and upward directed process between the maxillary, ethmoid and sphenoid bones. D E

26 **Sphenoidal process.** Processus sphenoidalis. Upper process behind the sphenopalatine notch. D E

27 **Horizontal plate.** Lamina horizontalis. It forms the posterior portion of both the hard palate and the floor of the nasal cavity. A B D E

28 **Nasal surface.** Facies nasalis. Surface facing the nasal cavity. B D

29 **Palatine surface.** Facies palatina. Surface facing the oral cavity. A D

30 **Lesser palatine foramina.** Foramina palatina minora. Openings of the lesser palatine canals. A

31 **Posterior nasal spine.** Spina nasalis posterior. Posteriorly projecting tip of the nasal crest along the median plane at the junction with the palatine bone of the opposite side. A B E

32 **Nasal crest.** Crista nasalis. Median bony ridge at the union with the palatine bone of the opposite side. B D E

33 **Palatine crest.** Crista palatina. Ridge frequently present on the inferior surface of the horizontal plate behind its anterior margin. A

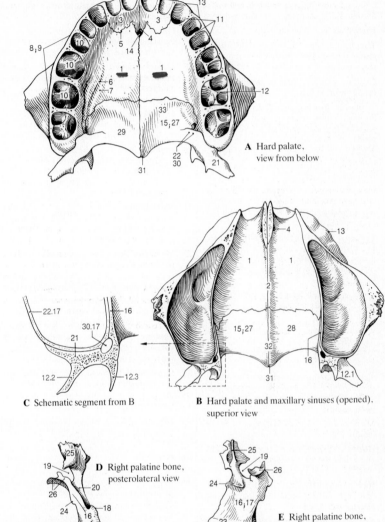

A Hard palate, view from below

C Schematic segment from B

B Hard palate and maxillary sinuses (opened), superior view

D Right palatine bone, posterolateral view

E Right palatine bone, medial view

1 ZYGOMATIC BONE. OS ZYGOMATICUM. It forms a large part of the lateral wall of the orbit and a part of the zygomatic arch. A B

2 **Lateral surface.** Facies lateralis. A

3 **Temporal surface.** Facies temporalis. Surface forming much of the anterior wall of the temporal fossa. B

4 **Orbital surface.** Facies orbitalis. Surface facing the orbit. A B

5 **Temporal process.** Processus temporalis. Posteriorly directed process which combines with the zygomatic process of the temporal bone to form the zygomatic arch. A B

6 **Frontal process.** Processus frontalis. Process which unites with the zygomatic process of the frontal bone. A B

6 a **Orbital eminence.** Eminentia orbitalis. Small tubercle just within the lateral margin of the orbit. Attachment site of lateral palpebral ligament, among others. A B

7 **Marginal tubercle.** [Tuberculum marginale]. Prominence usually present on the posterior margin of the frontal process. Attachment site of the temporalis muscle. A B

8 **Zygomatico-orbital foramen.** Foramen zygomatico-orbitale. Foramen on the orbital surface leading into a bony canal for the zygomatic nerve. A

9 **Zygomaticofacial foramen.** Foramen zygomaticofaciale. Opening on the lateral surface for the passage of the zygomaticofacial nerve. A

10 **Zygomaticotemporal foramen.** Foramen zygomaticotemporale. Foramen on the temporal surface for the passage of the zygomaticotemporal nerve. B

11 MANDIBLE. MANDIBULA. Lower jaw bone. C D E

12 **Body of mandible.** Corpus mandibulae. Horizontal part of the mandible to which the mandibular rami are attached. C

13 **Base of mandible.** Basis mandibulae. Lower portion of the body of the mandible minus the alveolar part. C

14 **Symphysis menti.** Symphysis mandibulae (medialis). Median connective tissue bridge between the right and left halves of the mandible. It becomes ossified in the first postnatal year.

15 **Mental protuberance.** Protuberantia mentalis. Prominence of the chin. C

16 Mental tubercle. Tuberculum mentale. Prominence on each side of the mental protuberance. C

17 **Gnathion.** Most inferior point (landmark) of the mandible in the midline. A cephalometric measuring point. C

18 **Mental foramen.** Foramen mentale. Opening for the mental nerve below the second premolar. Pressure point for the third division of the trigeminal nerve. C

19 **Oblique line.** Linea obliqua. Oblique ridge extending from the mandibular ramus to the external surface of the body of the mandible. C

20 **Digastric fossa.** Fossa digastrica. Pea- to bean-sized depression at the inner and inferior aspect of the body of the mandible near the symphysis. Attachment site of the digastric muscle (anterior belly). D

21 **Mental spine.** Spina mentalis. Bony elevation at the back of the symphysis projecting toward the tongue. Origin site of the genioglossus and geniohyoid muscles. D

22 **Mylohyoid line.** Linea mylohyoidea. Oblique ridge extending from the posterosuperior to the anteroinferior aspect of the body of the mandible. Origin site of the mylohyoid muscle. D

23 **[Torus mandibularis].** Bony outgrowth above the mylohyoid line at the level of the premolars. Possible hindrance to prostheses. D

24 **Sublingual fovea.** Fovea sublingualis. Depression for the sublingual gland located anteriorly above the mylohyoid line. D

25 **Submandibular fovea.** Fovea submandibularis. Depression for the submandibular gland on the posterior half of the body of the mandible below the mylohyoid line. D

26 **Alveolar part.** Pars alveolaris. Pectinate process sitting on the base of the mandible and housing the roots of the teeth. C

27 Alveolar arch. Arcus alveolaris. Curved free margin of the alveolar part. E

28 Dental alveoli. Alveoli dentales. Sockets for the reception and fixation of the roots of the teeth. E

29 Interalveolar septa. Septa interalveolaria. Bony ridges between the dental alveoli. E

30 *Interradicular septa.* Septa interradicularia. Bony partitions between the roots of a tooth. E

31 Alveolar juga. Juga alveolaria. Elevations on the external surface of the mandible caused by the roots of the teeth. C E

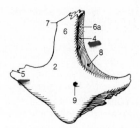

A Zygomatic bone, lateral view

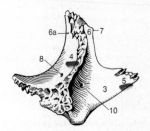

B Zygomatic bone, medial view

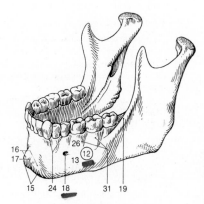

C Mandible

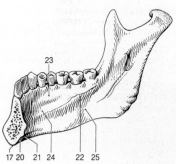

D Mandible, medial view

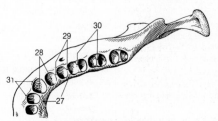

E Mandible, superior view

1 **Ramus of mandible.** Ramus mandibulae. Ascending, posterior process. A

2 **Angle of mandible.** Angulus mandibulae. Angle between the body and ramus of the mandible. It is most upright in the adult, especially shallow (obtuse) in the newborn and edentulous in the elderly (about 140°). A

3 Gonion. Most laterally directed point on the angle of the mandible. A

4 **Masseteric tuberosity.** Tuberositas masseterica. Roughened area occasionally present on the external surface of the angle of the mandible. Attachment site of the masseter muscle. A

5 **Pterygoid tuberosity.** Tuberositas pterygoidea. Roughened area occasionally present on the internal surface of the mandible in the vicinity of the angle. Attachment site of the medial pterygoid muscle. A

6 **Mandibular foramen.** Foramen mandibulae. Opening on the inner aspect of the mandibular ramus leading into the mandibular canal. A

7 Lingula of mandible. Lingula mandibulae. Bony projection medial to the mandibular foramen. Attachment site of the sphenomandibular ligament. A

8 Mandibular canal. Canalis mandibulae. Bony canal within the mandible for the passage of the inferior alveolar nerve. It begins at the mandibular foramen and passes beneath the roots of the teeth up to the vicinity of the median plane. A

9 **Mylohyoid groove.** Sulcus mylohyoideus. Groove extending forward and downward from the mandibular foramen and housing the mylohyoid nerve and the mylohyoid branch of the inferior alveolar artery. A

10 **Coronoid process.** Processus coronoideus. Muscular process that is separated from the posteriorly situated condylar process by the mandibular notch. Attachment site of the temporalis muscle. A

10a **Temporal crest.** Crista temporalis. Sharp bony ridge at the anterior margin of the coronoid process for the attachment of the temporalis muscle. A

11 **Mandibular notch.** Incisura mandibulae. Indentation between the condylar and coronoid processes. A

12 **Condylar process.** Processus condylaris. Articular process. A

13 Head of mandible. Caput mandibulae. Articular head of the mandible. A

14 Neck of mandible. Collum mandibulae. Narrow segment below the mandibular head. A

15 Pterygoid fovea. Fovea pterygoidea. Pit on the front of the neck of the mandible for the attachment of the lateral pterygoid muscle. A

16 HYOID BONE. OS HYOIDEUM. Ossification commences before birth. B

17 **Body of hyoid.** Corpus ossis hyoidea. Anterior segment between the right and left (greater and lesser) horns. B

18 **Lesser horn (cornu).** Cornu minus. B

19 **Greater horn (cornu).** Cornu majus. B

20 **Skull.** CRANIUM. D E F

20a **Cranial cavity.** Cavitas cranii.

21 **Periosteum of the external skull surface.** Pericranium. C

22 **External table (lamina).** Lamina externa. Outer layer of bone comprising the skull cap (calvaria). C

23 **Diploë.** Layer of spongy bone (spongiosa) between the external and internal tables, especially in the cranial bones. C

24 Diploic canals. Canales diploici. Large venous canals in the diploë. C

25 **Internal table (lamina).** Lamina interna. Inner layer of bone comprising the skull cap. C

26 Groove for the superior sagittal sinus. Sulcus sinus sagittalis superioris. C

27 *Granular pits (pacchionian granulations).* Foveolae granulares [[Pacchioni]]. Small pits occupied by the arachnoid granulations. C

28 NORMA VERTICALIS (calvaria). Normal
~ outline of skull cap as viewed from above. F

29 **Bregma.** Point of intersection of the sagittal and coronal sutures. F

30 **Crown of head.** Vertex. Highest point of the vault of the skull. E

31 **Occiput.** Back part of the head. E F

32 NORMA FACIALIS. Normal outline of skull as viewed from in front. D

33 **Forehead.** Frons. Front of calvaria above the eyes. D E

34 **Nasion.** Median point between the intersection of frontal and nasal bones. D E

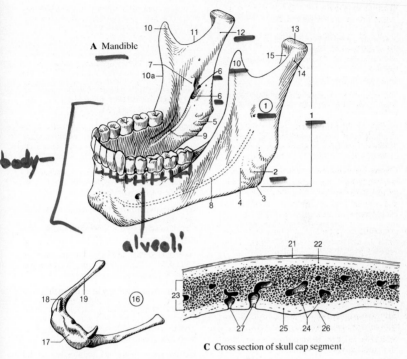

A Mandible

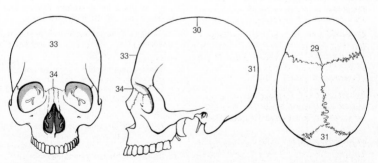

B Hyoid bone, anterosuperior view

C Cross section of skull cap segment

D Norma facialis

E Norma lateralis

F Norma verticalis

1 INTERNAL BASE OF CRANIUM. BASIS CRANII INTERNA. Superior aspect of skull base and its cranial cavities. A

2 **Anterior cranial fossa.** Fossa cranii [cranialis] anterior. Cranial cavity extending from the wall of the frontal bone to the lesser wing of the sphenoid. A

3 **Middle cranial fossa.** Fossa cranii [cranialis] media. Cranial cavity extending from the lesser wing of the sphenoid to the petrous ridge of the temporal bone. A

4 **Posterior cranial fossa.** Fossa cranii [cranialis] posterior. Cranial cavity extending from the petrous ridge to the posterior (occipital) wall of the skull. A

5 **Clivus.** Posteriorly descending segment of bone between the sella turcica and foramen magnum. It is formed by the occipital and sphenoid bones. A B

6 **Digital impressions.** Impressiones digitatae (gyrorum). Flat indentations corresponding to cerebral gyri which produce them. A

7 **Venous grooves.** Sulci venosi. Grooves for meningeal veins occasionally present on the inner wall of the parietal bone.

8 **Arterial grooves.** Sulci arteriales. Grooves on the inner wall of the skull produced primarily by the middle meningeal artery and its branches. A

9 **Sutural (wormian) bones.** Ossa suturalia. Bones occasionally present in cranial sutures. C

10 NORMA LATERALIS. Normal outline of skull as viewed laterally. C

10a **Pterion.** Field where the frontal, parietal, temporal and sphenoid bones meet. It is an important cephalometric measuring point. C

10b **Asterion.** Meeting point of the lambdoid, parietomastoid and occipitomastoid sutures. C

11 **Temporal fossa.** Fossa temporalis. Area lying between the temporal line and the zygomatic arch. C

12 **Zygomatic arch.** Arcus zygomaticus. Bony arch formed by the union of the zygomatic process of the temporal bone with the temporal process of the zygomatic bone. C

13 **Infratemporal fossa.** Fossa infratemporalis. Inferior continuation of the temporal fossa lying between the ramus of the mandible and the greater wing of the sphenoid. It contains the pterygoid muscles and the masseter, among others. C

14 Pterygopalatine fossa. Fossa pterygopalatina. Medial diverticulum of the infratemporal fossa lying between the pterygoid plates of the sphenoid and the perpendicular plate of the palatine bone. Its lateral boundary is the pterygomaxillary fissure through which it communicates with the infratemporal fossa. C

15 Pterygomaxillary fissure. Fissura pterygomaxillaris. Cleft located between the maxilla and the lateral pterygoid plate. C D

16 NORMA BASILARIS (BASIS CRANII EXTERNA). Normal outline of skull base as viewed from below. External base of cranium. B

17 **Greater palatine canal.** Canalis palatinus major. Canal formed by the palatine bone and maxilla for the descending palatine artery and the greater palatine nerve. B E see 25 C

18 **Jugular foramen.** Foramen jugulare. Large opening between the occipital and the petrous portion of the temporal bone for the passage of the internal jugular vein and cranial nerves IX, X and XI. A B

19 **Sphenopetrosal fissure.** Fissura sphenopetrosa. Medial continuation of the petrosquamous fissure. Its expansion forms the foramen lacerum. A B

20 **Petro-occipital fissure.** Fissura petro-occipitalis. Cleft between the petrous temporal and occipital bones extending medially from the jugular foramen. A B

21 **Foramen lacerum.** Irregularly bound opening in the middle cranial fossa between the apex of the petrous temporal and the sphenoid bone. A B

22 **Bony (hard) palate.** Palatum osseum. B E

23 **Greater palatine foramen.** Foramen palatinum majus. Opening into the greater palatine canal located near the posterior margin of the bony palate between the palatine bone and maxilla. B E

24 **Incisive fossa.** Fossa incisiva. Depression, the size of a match head, which receives the incisive canals with their incisive foramina. E

25 Incisive canal. Canalis incisivus. One of several canals for the incisive nerves. E

26 Incisive foramina. Foramina incisiva. Two or four openings for the incisive canals. E

27 **[Torus palatinus].** Longitudinal elevation occasionally present in the midline of the hard palate projecting toward the oral cavity. E

28 **Palatovaginal canal.** Canalis palatovaginalis. Small canal between the vaginal process of the sphenoid and the palatine bone for branches of the maxillary artery and the pterygopalatine ganglion. see 12.8

29 **Vomerovaginal canal.** Canalis vomerovaginalis. Small canal occasionally present between the vomer and the vaginal process of the sphenoid for a branch of the sphenopalatine artery. see 12.9

30 **Vomerorostral canal.** Canalis vomerorostralis. Small canal between the vomer and sphenoidal rostrum.

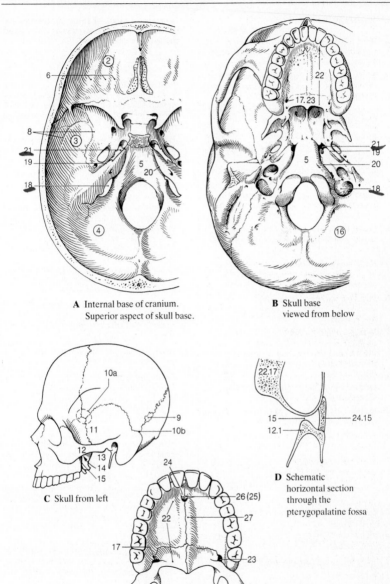

A Internal base of cranium. Superior aspect of skull base.

B Skull base viewed from below

C Skull from left

D Schematic horizontal section through the pterygopalatine fossa

E Hard palate viewed from below

1 **Nasal cavity.** Cavitas nasi. A C

~

2 **Bony nasal septum.** Septum nasi osseum. Bony partition formed by the vomer and the perpendicular plate of the ethmoid. C see 136;4

3 **Piriform aperture.** Apertura piriformis (nasalis anterior). Pear-shaped anterior nasal opening in the bony skull. A C D

4 **Superior nasal meatus.** Meatus nasalis superior. Space above the middle nasal concha. A

5 **Middle nasal meatus.** Meatus nasalis medius. Space between the middle and inferior nasal conchae. A

6 **Inferior nasal meatus.** Meatus nasalis inferior. Space below the inferior nasal concha. A

7 Nasolacrimal canal. Canalis nasolacrimalis. Passageway for the nasolacrimal duct which opens beneath the inferior nasal concha. C

8 **Sphenoethmoidal recess.** Recessus sphenoethmoidalis. Space above the superior nasal concha. A

9 **Nasopharyngeal meatus.** Meatus nasopharyngeus. Posterior portion of the nasal cavity from the posterior margin of the conchae to the choana. A

10 **Posterior apertures of the nose.** Choanae. Bilateral openings between the nasal cavity and the nasopharynx. A

11 **Sphenopalatine foramen.** Foramen sphenopalatinum. Superior opening in the pterygopalatine fossa leading into the nasal cavity. The greatest part is formed by the palatine bone, a lesser part by the sphenoid. A

12 **Orbit.** Orbita. Bony cavity that contains the eyeball. C D

13 **Orbital aditus.** Aditus orbitalis. Anterior opening (base) of the orbit. D

14 Orbital margin. Margo orbitalis. Bony margin of orbit.

15 *Supraorbital margin.* Margo supraorbitalis. Upper margin of orbital aditus. C

16 *Infraorbital margin.* Margo infraorbitalis. Lower margin of orbital aditus. C

16a *Lateral margin.* Margo lateralis. Lateral border of orbital aditus.

16b *Medial margin.* Margo medialis. Medial border of orbital aditus.

17 **Superior wall.** Paries superior. Roof of the orbit. C

18 **Inferior wall.** Paries inferior. Floor of the orbit. C

19 **Lateral wall of orbit.** Paries lateralis. C

20 **Medial wall of orbit.** Paries medialis. C

21 Anterior ethmoidal foramen. Foramen ethmoidale anterius. Anterior opening in the medial wall of the orbit between the frontal and ethmoid bones for the passage of the anterior ethmoidal nerve and vessels from the anterior cranial fossa. C

22 Posterior ethmoidal foramen. Foramen ethmoidale posterius. Posterior opening in the medial wall of the orbit between the frontal and ethmoid bones for the passage of the posterior ethmoidal vessels and nerve. C

22a **Lacrimal sulcus.** Sulcus lacrimalis. Groove-like beginning of the nasolacrimal canal. C

22b **Fossa of lacrimal sac.** Fossa sacci lacrimalis. Expanded depression for the lacrimal sac at the beginning of the nasolacrimal canal. C

23 **Superior orbital fissure.** Fissura orbitalis superior. Fissure in the posterior part of the lateral wall of the orbit between the greater and lesser wings of the sphenoid. It leads from the cranial cavity to the orbit and transmits the ophthalmic, oculomotor, trochlear and abducens nerves, as well as the superior ophthalmic vein. C

24 **Inferior orbital fissure.** Fissura orbitalis inferior. Cleft between the greater wing of the sphenoid and the orbital surface of the maxilla for the passage of the zygomatic nerve and the infraorbital nerve and vessels. C

25 NORMA OCCIPITALIS. Normal outline of skull viewed from behind. B

25a **Inion.** Cephalometric measuring point at the center of the external occipital protuberance.

26 **Lambda.** Junction point of the lambdoid and sagittal sutures. B

27 **Cranial fontanelles.** Fonticuli cranii. Membrane-closed gaps between the developing skull bones (fetal and infant). D E

28 **Anterior fontanelle.** Fonticulus anterior. Rhomboid-like, large space located anteriorly in the sagittal suture between the temporal and frontal anlagen. It is obliterated in the 2nd and 3rd postnatal year. D E

29 **Posterior fontanelle.** Fonticulus posterior. Small triangular gap at the junction of the sagittal and lamboid sutures, thus between the paired temporal bones and the occipital bone. It is closed 3 months after birth. D E

30 **Sphenoidal (anterolateral) fontanelle.** Fonticulus sphenoidalis (anterolateralis). Lateral gap between the frontal, parietal, temporal and sphenoid bones, thus at the site of the pterion. D

~

31 **Mastoid (posterolateral) fontanelle.** Fonticulus mastoideus (posterolateralis). Lateral space between the parietal, occipital and temporal bones, thus at the site of the asterion. D

~

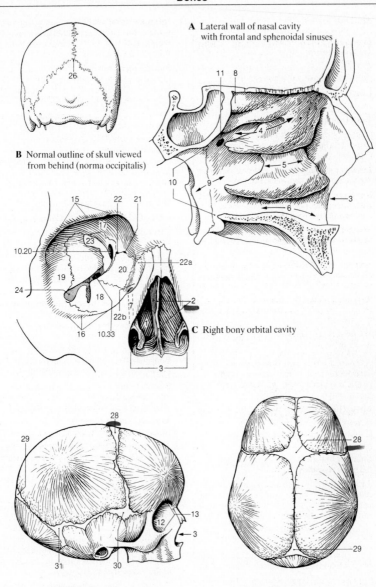

A Lateral wall of nasal cavity
with frontal and sphenoidal sinuses

B Normal outline of skull viewed
from behind (norma occipitalis)

C Right bony orbital cavity

D Skull of newborn,
dextrolateral view

E Skull of newborn,
superior view

APPENDICULAR SKELETON. SKELETON APPENDICULARE. Bones of the limbs.

1   BONES OF THE UPPER LIMB. OSSA MEMBRI SUPERIORIS.

2   SHOULDER (PECTORAL) GIRDLE. CINGULUM MEMBRI SUPERIORIS (Cingulum pectorale).

3   **SCAPULA.** Shoulder blade. A B

4   **Costal (anterior) surface.** Facies costalis (an-
~   terior). Scapular surface facing the ribs. B

5   Subscapular fossa. Fossa subscapularis. Concavity on the costal surface. B

6   **Posterior surface.** Facies posterior. Scapular surface facing the skin of the back. A

7   Spine of scapula. Spina scapulae. Long bony ridge on the posterior scapular surface extending into the acromion. A B

8   Supraspinous fossa. Fossa supraspinata (supraspinosa). Scapular surface above the spine of the scapula. A

9   Infraspinous fossa. Fossa infraspinata (in-
—   fraspinosa). Scapular surface below the spine of the scapula. A

10 **Acromion.** Free end of the scapular spine projecting over the head of the humerus. A B

11 Acromial articular surface. Facies arti-
~   cularis acromii. Articular facet for the clavicle. B

12 Acromial angle. Angulus acromialis. Sharp bend in the spine of the scapula where it becomes continuous with the lateral margin of the acromion. A

13 **Medial margin.** Margo medialis. Border of the scapula facing the vertebral column. A B

14 **Lateral margin.** Margo lateralis. Border of the scapula facing the humerus. A B

15 **Superior margin.** Margo superior. Upper border of the scapula. A B

16 Scapular notch. Incisura scapulae (scapularis). Indentation in the superior margin of the scapula just medial to the coracoid process. It is traversed by the suprascapular nerve. A B

17 **Inferior angle.** Angulus inferior. Lower angle of the scapula. A B

18 **Lateral angle.** Angulus lateralis. Lateral angle of the scapula bearing the glenoid cavity. A B

19 **Superior angle.** Angulus superior. Upper medial angle of the scapula. A B

20 **Glenoid cavity.** Cavitas glenoidalis. Articular cavity of the shoulder. B

21 **Infraglenoid tubercle.** Tuberculum infraglenoidale. Small tubercle at the inferior margin of the glenoid cavity for the origin of the long head of the triceps. A B

22 **Supraglenoid tubercle.** Tuberculum supraglenoidale. Small tubercle at the superior margin of the glenoid cavity for the origin of the long head of the biceps. B

23 **Neck of scapula.** Collum scapulae. The portion of the scapula situated medial to the margin of the glenoid cavity. A B

24 **Coracoid process.** Processus coracoideus. Hook-shaped process projecting anteriorly from the superior margin of the scapula just lateral to the scapular notch. Attachment site of the pectoralis minor, coracobrachialis and short head of the biceps muscles. A B

25 CLAVICLE. CLAVICULA. Collar bone. C

26 **Extremitas sternalis.** Sternal (medial) end of the clavicle facing the sternum. C

27 Sternal articular surface. Facies articularis sternalis. Articular surface on the medial end of clavicle for articulation with the sternum. C

28 Impression for the costoclavicular ligament. Impressio ligamenti costoclavicularis. Roughened area on the inferior surface of the clavicle near the sternal end for the attachment of the costoclavicular ligament. C

29 **Body (shaft) of clavicle.** Corpus claviculae (claviculare). Middle portion of the clavicle. C

30 Subclavian groove. Sulcus musculi subclavii. Elongated groove representing the deep attachment field of the subclavius muscle. C

31 **Acromial (lateral) end.** Extremitas acromialis. End of the clavicle facing the acromion. C

31 a **Tuberosity for the coracoclavicular ligament.** Tuberositas ligamenti coracoclavicularis. Roughness for the attachment of the two portions of the coracoclavicular ligament (conoid and trapezoid ligaments). C

32 Acromial articular surface. Facies articularis acromialis. Joint surface for the acromion. C

33 Conoid tubercle. Tuberculum conoideum. Small eminence on the inferior surface of the acromial end of the clavicle for the attachment of the conoid ligament. C

34 Trapezoid line. Linea trapezoidea. Attachment site for the trapezoid ligament on the inferior surface of the acromial end of the clavicle. C

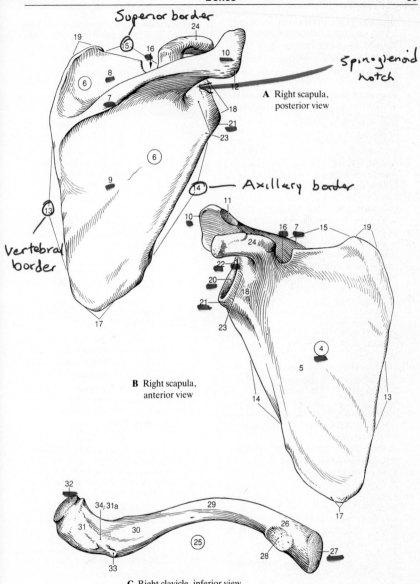

Superior border

Spino-glenoid notch

A Right scapula, posterior view

Axillary border

Vertebral border

B Right scapula, anterior view

C Right clavicle, inferior view

1 FREE PART OF UPPER LIMB. PARS LIBE-RA MEMBRI SUPERIORIS. Skeleton of the free portion of the upper limb.

2 **HUMERUS.** The bone of the upper arm. A B

3 **Head of humerus.** Caput humeri (humerale). A B

4 **Anatomical neck.** Collum anatomicum. Area between the head and the tubercles (greater and lesser) of the humerus. A B

5 **Surgical neck.** Collum chirurgicum. Tapering region distal to the tubercles and continuous with the shaft. A B

6 **Greater tubercle.** Tuberculum majus. Large prominence directed posterolaterally from the upper end of the humerus. Site for muscle insertions. A B

7 **Lesser tubercle.** Tuberculum minus. Smaller prominence directed anteriorly from the upper end of humerus. Site for muscle attachments. A

8 Intertubercular groove. Sulcus intertubercularis. Groove located between the two tubercles for the passage of the tendon of the long head of the biceps. A

9 *Crest of greater tubercle.* Crista tuberculi majoris. Bony ridge extending downward from the greater tubercle. Attachment site for the pectoralis major. A

10 *Crest of lesser tubercle.* Crista tuberculi minoris. Bony ridge extending downward from the lesser tubercle. Attachment site for the teres major and latissimus dorsi. A

11 **Body of humerus.** Corpus humeri. Shaft of the humerus between the two ends. A B

12 Anteromedial surface. Facies anterior medialis (anteromedialis). Surface of the humerus lying medial to the prolongation of the crest of the greater tubercle. A

13 Anterolateral surface. Facies anterior lateralis (anterolateralis). Surface of the humerus located lateral to the prolongation of the crest of the greater tubercle. A

14 Posterior surface of humerus. Facies posterior. B

15 *Groove for radial nerve.* Sulcus nervi radialis. Oblique groove descending laterally on the posterior surface of the humerus. B

16 Medial margin. Margo medialis. Inner margin of the humerus continuous distally with the medial supracondylar ridge. A B

17 *Medial supracondylar ridge.* Crista supracondylaris medialis. Lower, sharp-edged end of the medial margin. It terminates at the medial epicondyle. A B

18 *Supracondylar process.* [Processus supracondylaris]. Bony spur, phylogenetically conditioned, and occasionally present (1%) at the medial margin of the distal humerus. A

19 Lateral margin. Margo lateralis. Outer margin of the humerus continuous distally with the lateral supracondylar ridge. A B

20 *Lateral supracondylar ridge.* Crista supracondylaris lateralis. Lower, sharp-edged terminal portion of the lateral margin ending at the lateral epicondyle. A B

21 Deltoid tuberosity. Tuberositas deltoidea. Rough area on the anterolateral surface of the humerus just above its middle for the attachment of the deltoid muscle. A B

22 **Condyle of humerus.** Condylus humeri. Distal end of the humerus comprising the olecranon fossa, coronoid fossa, radial fossa and the articular surfaces. A B

23 Capitulum of humerus. Capitulum humeri. Rounded projection at the distal end of the humerus for articulation with the radius. A

24 Trochlea of humerus. Trochlea humeri. Articular cylinder at the distal end of the humerus for articulation with the ulna. A B

25 Olecranon fossa. Fossa olecrani. Deep pit above the trochlea on the posterior aspect of the humerus for the reception of the olecranon during extension of the elbow joint. B

26 Coronoid fossa. Fossa coronoidea. Depression on the anterior aspect of the humerus proximal to the trochlea for the reception of the coronoid process of the ulna during flexion of the elbow joint. A

27 Radial fossa. Fossa radialis. Depression above the capitulum on the anterior aspect of the humerus for the reception of the head of the radius in the case of strong flexion of the elbow joint. A

28 **Medial epicondyle.** Epicondylus medialis. Medially directed protuberance which gives origin to the flexor muscles of the forearm. A B

29 Groove for the ulnar nerve. Sulcus nervi ulnaris. It occupies the posterior surface of the medial epicondyle. B

30 **Lateral epicondyle.** Epicondylus lateralis. Protuberance lateral to the capitulum giving origin to the extensor muscles of the forearm. A B

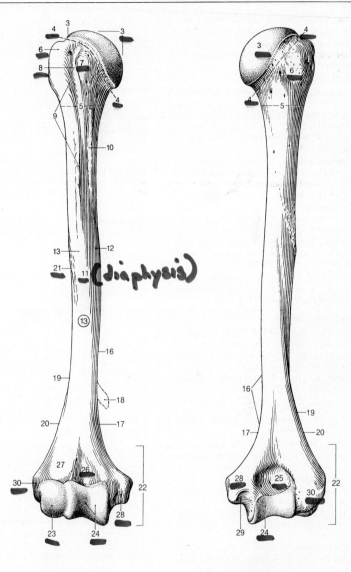

A Right humerus,
anterior view

B Right humerus,
posterior view

1   RADIUS. The lateral of the two forearm bones. A B

2   **Head of radius.** Caput radii (radiale). Proximal end of the radius which articulates with the capitulum of the humerus. A B

3   Articular fovea. Fovea articularis. Concavity for the reception of the capitulum of the humerus. B

4   Articular circumference. Circumferentia articularis. Rim-like surface on the head of the radius for articulation with the radial notch of the ulna. A B

5   **Neck of radius.** Collum radii. More slender region at the proximal end of the radius between the head and tuberosity. A B

6   **Body of radius.** Corpus radii. Radial shaft. A B

7   Radial tuberosity. Tuberositas radii. Roughened prominence on the medial aspect of the radius about 2 cm distal to the proximal end. Attachment site for the biceps tendon. A B

8   Interosseous margin. Margo interosseus. Border facing the ulna and giving attachment to the interosseous membrane. A B

9   Posterior border. Facies posterior. B

10   Anterior border. Facies anterior. A

11   Lateral border. Facies lateralis. A B

11 a   **Pronator tuberosity.** Tuberositas pronatoria. Roughened area at the middle of the lateral surface. Attachment site for the pronator teres muscle. B

12   Posterior margin. Margo posterior. B

13   Anterior margin. Margo anterior. Margin facing anterolaterally. A

14   **Styloid process.** Processus styloideus. Downward projection of the lateral surface of the radius at its distal end. A B

15   **Dorsal tubercle.** Tuberculum dorsale. Bony ridge on the posterior aspect of the lower end of the radius between the grooves for the extensor pollicis longus and extensor carpi radialis brevis muscles. It is often palpable through the skin. B

16   **Ulnar notch.** Incisura ulnaris. Concavity forming the medial surface at the end of the radius for articulation with the ulna. A B

17   **Articular carpal surface.** Facies articularis carpalis. Joint surface on the inferior surface of the lower end of the radius for articulation with the carpus. A

18   **ULNA.** Medially located forearm bone. A B

19   **Olecranon.** Proximal, posterior end of the ulna. Attachment site for the extensor muscles of the elbow joint. B

20   **Coronoid process.** Processus coronoideus. Anteriorly directed projection at the anterior end of the trochlear notch. A

21   Ulnar tuberosity. Tuberositas ulnae. Roughened area on the anterior surface of the upper part of the ulnar shaft for attachment of the brachialis muscle. A

22   **Trochlear notch.** Incisura trochlearis. Articular surface at the proximal end of the anterior surface of the ulna for articulation with the trochlea of the humerus. A

23   **Radial notch.** Incisura radialis. Joint surface on the lateral aspect of the ulna at the level of the coronoid process for articulation with the articular circumference of the radius. A

24   **Body of ulna.** Corpus ulnae. Ulnar shaft. A B

25   Posterior surface. Facies posterior. B

26   Anterior surface. Facies anterior. A

27   Medial surface. Facies medialis. Surface facing the trunk. B

28   Interosseous border. Margo interosseus. Margin providing attachment for the interosseous membrane. A B

29   Posterior margin. Margo posterior. B

30   Anterior margin. Margo anterior. Margin directed anteromedially. A

31   Supinator crest. Crista m. supinatoris. Bony ridge extending distally from the radial notch for attachment of the supinator muscle. A B

32   **Head of ulna.** Caput ulnae. Distal end of the ulna. A B

33   Articular circumference. Circumferentia articularis. Joint surface situated anterolaterally at the head of the ulna for articulation with the ulnar notch of the radius. A

34   Styloid process. Processus styloideus. Peg-like process projecting downward from the posteromedial aspect of the lower end of the ulna. Attachment site for the articular disc and the ulnar collateral ligament. A B

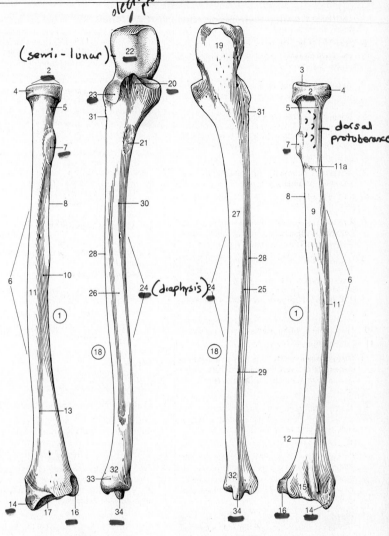

olecranon process

(semi-lunar)

(diaphysis)

dorsal protuberance

A Right radius and ulna,
anterior view

B Right ulna and radius,
posterior view

1 CARPUS. The wrist, comprising eight carpal bones situated between the forearm bones and the metacarpal bones. A B C

2 **Carpal bones.** Ossa carpi (carpalia). Wrist
~ bones. A B C

3 **Accessory carpal bone (ossicle).** [Os centrale]. It is occasionally found between the capitate, scaphoid and trapezoid bones. It is usually fused with the scaphoid. C

4 **Scaphoid.** Os scaphoideum [[Os naviculare]]. Proximal carpal bone situated between the lunate and trapezium. A B

5 Scaphoid tubercle. Tuberculum ossis scaphoidei. Elevation on the anterior surface of the scaphoid. It protrudes visibly with radial abduction of the hand. A

6 **Lunate.** Os lunatum. Proximal carpal bone located between the scaphoid and triquetrum. A B

7 **Triquetrum.** Os triquetrum. Proximal carpal bone situated between the hamate and the lunate, dorsal to the pisiform. A B

8 **Pisiform.** Os pisiforme. Proximal carpal bone residing on the palmar aspect of the triquetrum with which it articulates. It represents a true sesamoid bone within the tendon of the flexor carpi ulnaris. A B

9 **Trapezium.** Os trapezium [[Os multangulum majus]]. Distal carpal bone located between the 1st metacarpal and the scaphoid. A B

10 Tubercle of trapezium. Tuberculum ossis trapezii. Elevation on the palmar side of the trapezium distal to the scaphoid tubercle and radial to the groove for the flexor carpi radialis. A

11 **Trapezoid.** Os trapezoideum [[Os multangulum minus]]. Distal carpal bone positioned between the 2nd metacarpal and the scaphoid, as well as between the trapezium and capitate. A B

12 **Capitate.** Os capitatum. Distal carpal bone situated centrally between the 3rd metacarpal and the lunate. A B

13 **Hamate.** Os hamatum. Distal carpal bone located between the 4th and 5th metacarpals, capitate and triquetrum. A B

14 Hamulus (hook) of hamate. Hamulus ossis hamati. Hook-shaped process on the palmar aspect of the hamate distal to the pisiform. A

15 **Carpal groove.** Sulcus carpi. Palmar concavity between the tubercles of the scaphoid and trapezium on the radial side, and the hamulus and pisiform bone on the ulnar side. A transverse ligament converts it into a closed canal (carpal tunnel) for the flexor tendons of the fingers. A

16 METACARPUS. Region of the hand between the fingers and the wrist. A B

17 **Metacarpal bones I–V.** Ossa metacarpi
~ (metacarpalia) [I–V]. A B

18 Base of metacarpal bone. Basis metacarpalis. Proximal, broad end of a metacarpal bone. A B

19 Body (shaft) of metacarpal bone. Corpus metacarpale. A B

20 Head of metacarpal bone. Caput metacarpale. Distal articular end of a metacarpal bone. A B

21 Third metacarpal bone. Os metacarpale tertium [III]. Metacarpal bone lying proximal to the middle finger. A B

22 Styloid process. Processus styloideus. Pointed process at the base of metacarpal III, radial to the capitate. B

23 **Fingers (digits).** Ossa digitorum (Phalanges). A B

24 **Phalanges.** Bony segments comprising the fingers. A B

25 Proximal phalanx. Phalanx proximalis. Proximal bone of a finger. A B

26 Middle phalanx. Phalanx media. Middle bone of a finger. A B

27 Distal (terminal) phalanx. Phalanx distalis. Distal, nail-bearing segment of a finger. A B

28 *Tuberosity of distal phalanx.* Tuberositas phalangis distalis. Roughened expansions at the distal flexor side of each terminal phalanx for anchoring the tactile pads. A

29 Base of phalanx. Basis phalangis. Proximal, thickened, articular end of the phalanx. A B

30 Body (shaft) of phalanx. Corpus phalangis. A B

31 Distal end (trochlea) of phalanx. Caput (trochlea) phalangis. A B

32 *Sesamoid bones.* Ossa sesamoidea. Bones embedded in tendons or ligaments. A

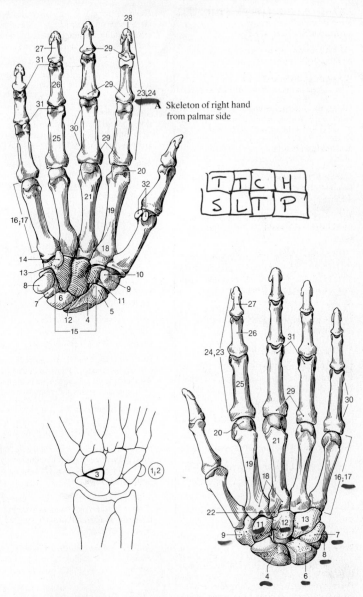

A Skeleton of right hand from palmar side

C Central bone of right hand

B Skeleton of right hand from dorsal side

1 **BONES OF THE LOWER LIMB**. Ossa membri inferioris.

2 PELVIC GIRDLE. CINGULUM MEMBRI INFERIORIS (Cingulum pelvicum). It is composed of the sacrum and the two ilia.

3 HIP BONE. OS COXAE (pelvicum). It is comprised of the ilium, ischium and pubis. A B C

4 **Obturator foramen.** Foramen obturatum (obturatorium). Large opening formed between the pubis and ischium. A C

5 **Acetabulum.** Hip joint socket. It is formed by the ilium, ischium and pubis. A

6 **Margin of the acetabulum.** Limbus acetabuli (margo acetabularis). Margin interrupted by the acetabular notch. A

7 Acetabular fossa. Fossa acetabuli (acetabularis). Deeper part embraced by the lunate surface. A

8 Acetabular notch. Incisura acetabuli (acetabularis). Notch in the lunate surface of the acetabulum facing the obturator foramen and continuous with the acetabular fossa. A

9 Lunate surface. Facies lunata. Cartilage covered, sickle-shaped articular surface of the acetabulum. A

10 **Ilium.** Os ilii (ilium, os iliacum). A B C

11 **Body of the ilium.** Corpus ossis ilii. The central portion of the ilium situated near the acetabulum. A B C

12 Supra-acetabular sulcus. Sulcus supra-acetabularis. Groove formed between the acetabular margin and the body of the ilium. A

13 **Wing (or ala) of the ilium.** Ala ossis ilii. A C

14 Arcuate line. Linea arcuata. Prominent bony ridge at the boundary between the greater and lesser pelvis. C

15 Iliac crest. Crista iliaca. A C

16 *External lip of the iliac crest.* Labium externum. Bony ridge for attachment of the external abdominal oblique muscle. A

17 *Tubercle of iliac crest.* Tuberculum iliacum. Palpable projection on the external lip of the iliac crest about 5 cm behind the anterior iliac spine at the junction of the anterior gluteal line with the iliac crest. A

18 *Linea intermedia.* Rough bony area between the external and internal lips of the iliac crest. Origin site of the internal abdominal oblique muscle. A

19 *Internal lip of the iliac crest.* Labium internum. Bony ridge on the inner margin of the iliac crest for attachment of the transversus abdominis muscle. A C

20 *Anterior superior iliac spine.* Spina iliaca anterior superior. Bony projection marking the anterior limit of the iliac crest. Origin site of the sartorius muscle. A C

21 *Anterior inferior iliac spine.* Spina iliaca anterior inferior. Bony process at the anterior margin of the ilium. Origin site of the rectus femoris muscle. A C

22 *Posterior superior iliac spine.* Spina iliaca posterior superior. Bony process at the posterior end of the iliac crest. A C

23 *Posterior inferior iliac spine.* Spina iliaca posterior inferior. Bony process at the superior end of the greater sciatic notch. A C

24 Iliac fossa. Fossa iliaca. A concavity forming the internal surface of the ala of the ilium. C

25 Gluteal surface. Facies glutealis. External surface of the ala of the ilium. A

26 *Anterior gluteal line.* Linea glutealis anterior. A flat ridge situated somewhat in the middle of the ala of the ilium between the fields of origin of the gluteus medius and minimus muscles. A

27 *Posterior gluteal line.* Linea glutealis posterior. Bony ridge between the fields of origin of the gluteus medius and maximus muscles. A

28 *Inferior gluteal line.* Linea glutealis inferior. Bony ridge above the acetabulum between the fields of origin of the gluteus minimus and rectus femoris muscles. A

29 Sacropelvic surface. Facies sacropelvina. Surface of the dorsal segment of the ilium facing the sacrum and consisting of the following two parts: C

30 *Auricular surface.* Facies auricularis. The ear-shaped surface which articulates with the sacrum. C

31 *Iliac tuberosity.* Tuberositas iliaca. Roughened area behind and above the auricular surface. Attachment site for the sacroiliac ligaments. C

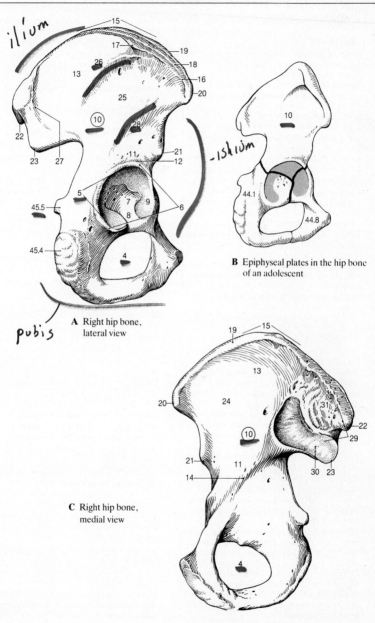

ilium

13

26

15

17

19

18

16

20

25

10

28

22

23 27

11

12

21

5

7 9

8

6

45.5

45.4

4

A Right hip bone,
lateral view

pubis

10

-ishium

44.1

44.8

B Epiphyseal plates in the hip bone
of an adolescent

19 15

13

24

20

3

22

10

29

21

11

14

30 23

4

C Right hip bone,
medial view

1 **Ischium.** Os ischii. Bone which forms the posterior and inferior boundary of the obturator foramen. A B

2 **Body of ischium.** Corpus ossis ischii. That portion of the ischium situated behind the obturator foramen. A B

3 **Ramus of ischium.** Ramus ossis ischii. That portion of the ischium situated below the obturator foramen. It unites with the inferior ramus of the pubis anteriorly. A B

4 Ischial tuberosity. Tuber ischiadicum (ischiale). Ischial process at the lower end of the lesser sciatic notch. B

5 **Ischial spine.** Spina ischiadica (ischialis). Bony prominence between the greater and lesser sciatic notch. B

6 **Greater sciatic notch.** Incisura ischiadica (ischialis) major. Large notch between the posterior inferior iliac spine and the ischial spine. B

7 **Lesser sciatic notch.** Incisura ischiadica (ischialis) minor. Notch between the ischial spine and the ischial tuberosity. B

8 **Pubis.** Os pubis. Bone which forms the anterior and inferior border of the obturator foramen. A B

9 **Body of the pubis.** Corpus ossis pubis. A B

10 Pubic tubercle. Tuberculum pubicum. Protuberance located anterolateral to the symphysis. A B

11 Symphyseal surface. Facies symphysialis. The median surface of the symphysis facing the pubis of the opposite side. B

12 **Pubic crest.** Crista pubica. Ridge extending medially from the pubic tubercle to the symphysis. Attachment site of the rectus abdominis muscle. A B

13 Superior ramus of the pubis. Ramus superior ossis pubis. The part of the pubis situated above the obturator foramen. A B

14 *Iliopubic (iliopectineal) eminence.* Eminentia iliopubica [e. iliopectinea]. Flat prominence at the proximal portion of the pubis. A B

15 Pecten (pectineal line) of the pubis. Pecten ossis pubis. Sharp bony ridge which, as a continuation of the arcuate line, passes to the pubic tubercle. Origin site of the pectineus muscle. A B

16 Obturator crest. Crista obturatoria. It extends from the pubic tubercle to the acetabulum. Origin site of the pubofemoral ligament. A

17 Obturator groove. Sulcus obturatorius. Sulcus above the obturator foramen. A B

18 Anterior obturator tubercle. Tuberculum obturatorium anterius. Small protuberance anterior to the obturator groove. A B

19 *Posterior obturator tubercle.* [Tuberculum obturatorium posterius]. Prominence occasionally present behind the obturator groove. A B

20 Inferior ramus of pubis. Ramus inferior ossis pubis. The portion of the pubis located anteriorly below the obturator foramen between the symphysis and the suture line with the ischium. A B

21 PELVIS. It comprises the sacrum, ilium, pubis and ischium. C D E F

21 a **Pelvic cavity.** Cavitas pelvis (pelvica).

22 **Pubic arch.** Arcus pubis. The arch below the symphysis formed by the right and left pubic bones. D

23 Subpubic angle. Angulus subpubicus. The angle between the right and left inferior ramus of the pubis (in men, 75° on average; in women, 90°–100°). C

24 **Greater pelvis.** Pelvis major. The space between the two alae of the ilium above the linea terminalis.

25 **Lesser pelvis.** Pelvis minor. The space below the linea terminalis.

26 **Linea terminalis.** It extends along the arcuate line from the promontory to the upper margin of the symphysis and marks the boundary between the greater and lesser pelvis as well as the plane of the pelvic inlet. C D E

27 **Upper pelvic aperture (pelvic inlet).** Apertura pelvis (pelvica) superior. Upper opening of the lesser pelvis in the plane of the linea terminalis. D

28 **Lower pelvic aperture (pelvic outlet).** Apertura pelvis (pelvica) inferior. Lower opening of the lesser pelvis between the coccyx, pubic arch and sacrotuberous ligaments. F

29 **Pelvic axis.** Axis pelvis. At the intersection of all the median connecting lines between the symphysis and the anterior surface of the sacrum. F

30 **Conjugate diameter.** Diameter conjugata. Anteroposterior diameter passing from the sacral promontory to the posterior surface of the symphysis, about 11 cm. E F

31 **Transverse diameter of pelvis.** Diameter transversa. Widest part of the inlet, about 13 cm. E

32 **Oblique diameter.** Diameter obliqua. It passes from the iliosacral joint obliquely forward to the iliopubic eminence of the opposite side, about 12.5 cm. E

33 **Pelvic inclination.** Inclinatio pelvis. The angle between the plane of the pelvic inlet and the horizontal plane. F

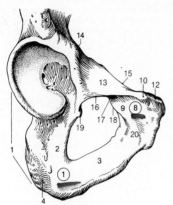

A Lower half of right hip bone, external surface

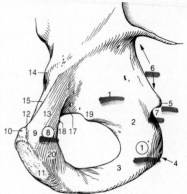

B Lower half of right hip bone, internal surface

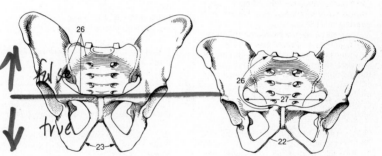

C Male pelvis, anterior view

D Female pelvis, anterior view

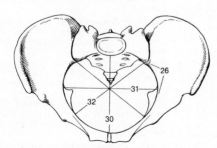

E Pelvis, superior view

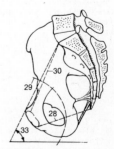

F Pelvis, medial view

1   FREE LOWER LIMB. Pars libera membri inferioris.

2   FEMUR Thigh bone. (Os femoris). A B

~
3   **Head of femur.** Caput femoris. A B

~
4   Pit (fovea) in the head of the femur. Fovea
~   capitis femoris. It is for attachment of the ligament of the head of the femur. A B

5   **Neck of femur.** Collum femoris. Between the head and greater trochanter. A B

6   **Greater trochanter.** Trochanter major. Large prominence on the superolateral aspect of the shaft for attachment of the gluteus medius, gluteus minimus, piriformis, obturator and gemelli muscles. A B

7   Trochanteric fossa. Fossa trochanterica. Depression medial to the root of the greater trochanter. A B

8   **Lesser trochanter.** Trochanter minor. Small prominence on the posteromedial aspect of the proximal shaft for attachment of the iliopsoas muscle. A B

9   **[Trochanter tertius].** Process occasionally present posteriorly at the lateral end of the linea aspera at the level of the lesser trochanter for attachment of a part of the gluteus maximus. B

10 **Intertrochanteric line.** Linea intertrochanterica. Anterior rough line between the shaft and neck extending from the greater to the lesser trochanter. A

10 a **Quadrate tubercle.** Tuberculum quadratum. Rounded elevation on the intertrochanteric crest. B

11 **Intertrochanteric crest.** Crista intertrochanterica. Posterior bony ridge between the shaft and neck running from the greater to the lesser trochanter. B

12 **Shaft of femur.** Corpus femoris. A B

~
13 Linea aspera. Rough double line on the posterior aspect of the femur for attachment of two vasti muscles, the adductors and the short head of the biceps. B

14 *Lateral lip of the linea aspera.* Labium laterale. B

15 *Medial lip of the linea aspera.* Labium mediale. B

16 Pectineal line. Linea pectinea. Bony ridge extending downward from the lesser trochanter almost as far as the linea aspera. Attachment site for the pectineus muscle. B

17 Gluteal tuberosity. Tuberositas gluteaelis. Rough, oblong field continuous with the linea aspera superolaterally. B

18 Intercondylar fossa. Fossa intercondylaris. Posteriorly situated notch between the femoral condyles. B

19 Intercondylar line. Linea intercondylaris. Ridge located posteriorly between the roots of the condyles. B

20 Popliteal surface. Facies poplitea. Triangular field on the posterior aspect of the femur between the intercondylar line and the diverging lips (supracondylar lines) of the linea aspera. B

20 a **Medial supracondylar line.** Linea supracondylaris medialis. Continuation of the medial lip of the linea aspera toward the medial condyle. B

20 b **Lateral supracondylar line.** Linea supracondylaris lateralis. Continuation of the lateral lip of the linea aspera toward the lateral condyle. B

21 **Medial condyle.** Condylus medialis. Articular surface of the femur at the medial aspect of the knee joint. A B

22 Medial epicondyle. Epicondylus medialis. Bony elevation on the medial aspect of the medial condyle. A B

23 Adductor tubercle. Tuberculum adductorium. Small process situated above the medial epicondyle for the attachment of the adductor magnus muscle. A B

24 **Lateral condyle.** Condylus lateralis. Articular surface of the femur at the lateral aspect of the knee joint. A B

25 Lateral epicondyle. Epicondylus lateralis. Bony elevation on the lateral aspect of the lateral condyle. A B

25 a **Groove for popliteus.** Sulcus popliteus. Groove between the lateral condyle and the lateral epicondyle. B

26 **Patellar surface.** Facies patellaris. Articular surface for the patella. A

27 TIBIA. C D

28 **Superior articular surface.** Facies articularis superior. Tibial articular surface of the knee joint. C D

29 **Medial condyle.** Condylus medialis. Medial expansion at the proximal end of the tibia. C D

30 **Lateral condyle.** Condylus lateralis. Lateral expansion at the proximal end of the tibia. C D

31 Articular facet for the fibula. Facies articularis fibularis. Articular surface for the head of the fibula located on the posterolateral aspect of the lateral condyle. C D

32 **Anterior intercondylar area.** Area intercondylaris anterior. The field between the knee joint surfaces of the tibia and in front of the intercondylar eminence. C D

33 **Posterior intercondylar area.** Area intercondylaris posterior. The region between the knee joint surface of the tibia and behind the intercondylar eminence. D

34 **Intercondylar eminence.** Eminentia intercondylaris. Bony elevation between the articular surfaces for attachment of the cruciate ligaments and menisci. C D

35 **Medial intercondylar tubercle.** Tuberculum intercondylare mediale. Elevation of the medial articular surface at the margin facing the intercondylar eminence. C D

36 Tuberculum intercondylare laterale. Elevation of the lateral articular surface at the margin facing the intercondylar eminence. C D

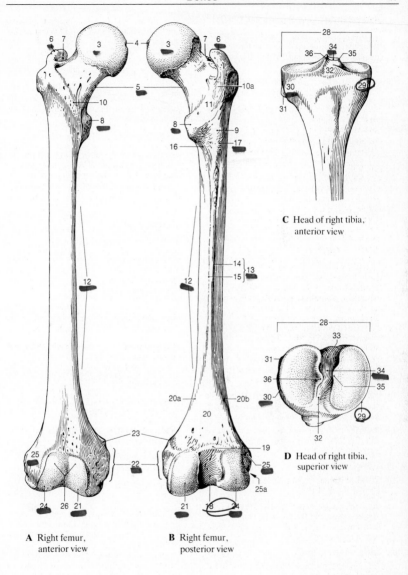

C Head of right tibia,
anterior view

D Head of right tibia,
superior view

A Right femur,
anterior view

B Right femur,
posterior view

1 **Shaft of tibia.** Corpus tibiae (tibiale). A B D

2 Tibial tuberosity. Tuberositas tibiae. Roughness on the upper end of the anterior margin. Attachment site for the patellar ligament. A

3 Medial surface. Facies medialis. Surface of tibia directed anteromedially. A D

4 Posterior surface of tibia. Facies posterior. B D

5 *Soleal line of tibia.* Linea musculi solei. Oblique ridge on the upper third of the posterior surface of the tibia extending downward from the articular facet for the fibula to the medial border. Attachment site for soleus muscle. B

6 Facies lateralis. Lateral surface of tibia facing anterolaterally. A D

7 Medial (inner) margin. Margo medialis. A B D

8 Anterior margin. Margo anterior. A D

9 Interosseous margin. Margo interosseus. Border facing the fibula and providing attachment for the interosseous membrane along most of its margin. A B D

10 **Medial malleolus.** Malleolus medialis. A B

11 Malleolar groove. Sulcus malleolaris. Small groove on the posterior aspect of the medial malleolus for the tendon of the tibialis posterior muscle. B

12 Articular surface of malleolus. Facies articularis malleoli. Lateral surface of the medial malleolus facing the talus. A B

13 **Fibular notch.** Incisura fibularis. Depression on the lateral surface of the0 distal end of the tibia. Articular surface for the fibula. B

14 **Inferior articular surface.** Facies articularis inferior. Inferior joint surface facing the talus. A B

15 FIBULA. A B D

16 **Head of fibula.** Caput fibulae (fibulare). The proximal end. A B

17 Facies articularis capitis fibulae. Articular surface for the proximal end of the fibula facing the tibia. A B

18 Apex (styloid process) of head of fibula. Apex capitis fibulae. Upward prolongation of the head of the fibula. A B

19 **Neck of fibula.** Collum fibulae. A

20 **Shaft of fibula.** Corpus fibulae. A

21 Facies lateralis. Lateral surface directed somewhat anteriorly. A D

22 Facies medialis. Medial surface between the anterior and interosseous margins. It faces the tibia. A B D

23 Facies posterior. Posterior surface between the posterior and interosseous margins. B D

24 *Medial crest.* Crista medialis. Bony ridge on the posterior surface at the border between the origins of the tibialis posterior and flexor hallucis longus muscles. B D

25 Anterior margin. Margo anterior. A D

26 Interosseous margin. Margo interosseus. Osseous ridge located between the anterior margin and the medial crest for the attachment of a portion of the interosseous membrane. A B D

27 Margin posterior. Margo posterior directed posterolaterally. B D

28 Lateral malleolus. Malleolus lateralis. A B

29 *Articular surface of malleolus.* Facies articularis malleoli. Joint surface on the lateral malleolus facing the talus. A B

30 *Lateral malleolar fossa.* Fossa malleoli lateralis. Depression on the posteromedial aspect of the lateral malleolus for attachment of the posterior talofibular ligament. B

30 a **Sulcus malleolaris.** Groove lateral to the malleolar fossa.

31 PATELLA. The knee cap embedded in the quadriceps tendon. C

32 **Base of patella.** Basis patellae. Broad, superior border of the patella. C

33 **Apex of patella.** Apex patellae. Inferior, pointed border of the patella. C

34 **Facies articularis.** Cartilage covered articular surface of the patella facing the femur.

35 **Facies anterior.** Anterior surface of the patella. C

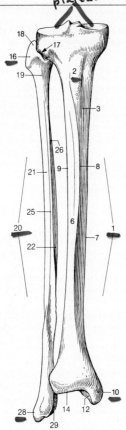
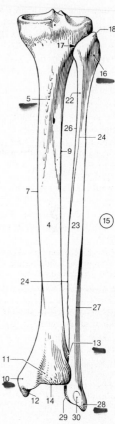

A Right tibia and fibula, anterior view

B Right tibia and fibula, posterior view

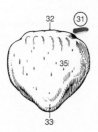

C Patella, anterior view

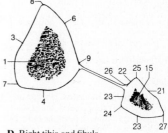

D Right tibia and fibula in cross section

1 TARSUS. It comprises seven bones (calcaneus, talus, navicular, cuboid and three cuneiforms) extending from the heel to the metatarsals. E

2 **Tarsal bones.** Ossa tarsi (tarsalia).

3 **Talus.** Tarsal bone located between the tibia, calcaneus and navicular. A B E

4 Head of talus. Caput tali (talare). It articulates with the navicular. A B

5 *Neck of talus.* Collum tali. Proximal tapering off of the head of the talus. A B

6 Body of talus. Corpus tali. B

7 Trochlea tali (talare). Cylinder-like articular surface for the tibia and fibula. A

8 *Superior surface.* Facies superior. Site of the articular facet for the inferior articular surface of the tibia. A

9 *Medial malleolar surface.* Facies malleolaris medialis. Almost sagittally oriented articular surface for the medial malleolus. A

10 *Lateral malleolar surface.* Facies malleolaris lateralis. Articular surface for the lateral malleolus on the lateral side of the trochlea. A

11 *Lateral process of the talus.* Processus lateralis tali. Bony projection below the lateral malleolar surface. A

12 *Posterior calcanean facet.* Facies articularis calcanea posterior. Postero-inferior articular surface for the calcaneus. B

13 *Sulcus of talus.* Sulcus tali. A groove between the middle and posterior articular facets for the calcaneus. B

14 *Middle calcanean facet.* Facies articularis calcanea media. Middle articular surface for the calcaneus. B

15 *Anterior calcanean facet.* Facies articularis calcanea anterior. Anterior articular surface for the calcaneus below the head of the talus. B

16 *Facies articularis navicularis.* Articular facet for the navicular on the front of the head of the talus. A B

17 Posterior process of talus. Processus posterior tali. Broad process below the posterior margin of the trochlea. It bears the medial and lateral tubercles and the groove for the tendon of the flexor hallucis longus between them. A B

18 *Sulcus tendinis m. flex. hall. longi.* Groove for the tendon of the flexor hallucis longus posteromedial to the posterior process of the talus. A B

19 *Medial tubercle.* Tuberculum mediale. Bony process anteromedial to the groove for the flexor hallucis longus tendon. A B

20 *Lateral tubercle.* Tuberculum laterale. Bony process lateral to the groove for the flexor hallucis longus tendon. A

21 [Os trigonum]. Independent bone occasionally formed from the lateral tubercle of the posterior process of the talus by a separate ossific center. E

22 **Calcaneus.** Heel bone. C D E

23 Tuber calcanei. Tuberosity on the posterior aspect of the calcaneus. C D

24 *Medial process of calcaneus.* Processus medialis tuberis calcanei. Weak process anterior, medial and inferior to the tuberosity of the calcaneus. D

25 *Lateral process of calcaneus.* Processus lateralis tuberis calcanei. Weak process inferolateral to the tuberosity of the calcaneus. C

26 Anterior tubercle of calcaneus. Tuberculum calcanei. Eminence on the anterior aspect of the inferior surface of the calcaneus. Attachment site of the plantar calcaneocuboid ligament. C

27 Sustentaculum tali. Medial prolongation of the calcaneus bearing the middle calcanean articular facet. D E

28 *Sulcus tendinis m. flex. hall. longi.* Groove for the flexor hallucis longus tendon. Bony groove below the sustentaculum tali. D

29 Sulcus calcanei. Groove between the middle and posterior articular facets for the talus. C D

30 Sinus tarsi. A depression between the head of the talus and the calcaneus laterally. Palpation site for the inferior ankle joint. B C

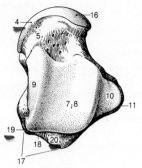

A Right talus, superior view

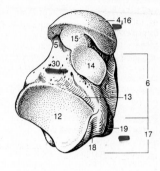

B Right talus, inferior view

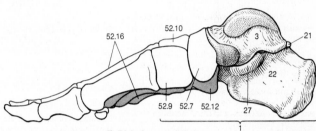

E Right foot, medial view

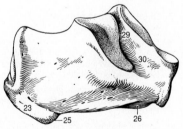

C Right calcaneus, lateral view

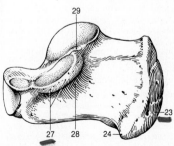

D Right calcaneus, medial view

1 Anterior facet for the talus. Facies articularis talaris anterior. Small anterior articular surface for the head of the talus. A B

2 Middle facet for the talus. Facies articularis talaris media. Middle articular surface for the talus separated from the posterior facet by the sulcus calcanei. A B

3 Posterior facet for the talus. Facies articularis talaris posterior. Large articular surface for the talus located posteriorly. A B

4 Sulcus tendinis m. peronei (fibularis) longi. Groove for the tendon of the peroneus longus muscle on the lateral aspect of the calcaneus below the peroneal trochlea. B

5 Peroneal trochlea. Trochlea peronealis (fibularis). Bony eminence above the groove for the tendon of the peroneus longus. It functions pulley-like for this muscle and serves for the attachment of a part of the peroneal retinaculum. The peroneal brevis runs cranial to the trochlea. B

6 Facies articularis cuboidea. Cuboid articular surface forming the anterior aspect of the calcaneus. A B

7 **Navicular bone.** Os naviculare. It lies medially between the head of the talus and the three cuneiform bones. C D

8 Tuberosity of navicular. Tuberositas ossis navicularis. Rough area located inferomedially for the attachment of the tibialis posterior muscle. It is palpable through the skin. D

9 **Medial cuneiform.** Os cuneiforme mediale. Most medial of the cuneiforms between the navicular and the 1st metatarsal. Its wedged-shaped base is directed downward. C D

10 **Intermediate cuneiform.** Os cuneiforme intermedium. Middle cuneiform between the navicular and the 2nd metatarsal with its wedge-shaped base directed upward. C D

11 **Lateral cuneiform.** Os cuneiforme laterale. Laterally situated cuneiform between the navicular and the 3rd metatarsal with its wedge-shaped base directed upward. C D

12 **Cuboid bone.** Os cuboideum. It is found between the calcaneus and the fourth and fifth metatarsals. C D

13 Groove for tendon of peroneus longus. Sulcus tendinis musculi peronei (fibularis) longi. Lying at the inferolateral aspect of the cuboid, it serves to guide the tendon. D

14 Tuberosity of cuboid. Tuberositas ossis cuboidei. Bony elevation on the inferior aspect of the cuboid proximal to the groove for the peroneus longus. D

15 Calcanean process. Processus calcaneus. Plantar process of the cuboid with an inferior segment of the proximal articular surface directed obliquely upward for the support of the calcaneus. D

16 METATARSUS. The part of the foot situated between the tarsus and the toes. It comprises five metatarsal bones. C D

17 **Metatarsal bones.** Ossa metatarsi (metatarsalia) [I–V]. D

18 **Base of metatarsal bone.** Basis metatarsalis. The thickened proximal end. D

19 **Shaft of metatarsal bone.** Corpus metatarsale. D

20 **Head of metatarsal bone.** Caput metatarsale. C D

21 **Tuberosity of first metatarsal.** Tuberositas ossis metatarsalis primi (I). Proximal, inferolateral bony projection from the first metatarsal bone. D

22 **Tuberosity of fifth metatarsal.** Tuberositas ossis metatarsalis quinti (V). Proximal, lateral bony projection from the fifth metatarsal bone. Attachment site of the peroneus brevis muscle. C D

23 **Phalanges of toes.** Ossa digitorum. C D

24 **Phalanges.** Osseous segments of toes. C D

25 **Proximal phalanx.** Phalanx proximalis. Proximal toe segment. D

26 **Middle phalanx.** Phalanx media. Middle toe segment. D

27 **Distal phalanx.** Phalanx distalis. Distal, nail-bearing toe segment. D

28 Distal tuberosity of toes. Tuberositas phalangis distalis. Roughness located on the plantar aspect of the distal end of the distal phalanx for anchoring of the tactile pads. D

29 **Base of phalanx.** Basis phalangis. Proximal end of phalanx with an acetabular-like articular surface. D

30 **Shaft of phalanx.** Corpus phalangis. D

31 **Head of phalanx.** Caput phalangis. Distal, articular end of the phalanx. D

32 **Sesamoid bones.** Ossa sesamoidea. Wormian bones embedded in tendons or ligaments. They occur regularly below the head of metatarsal I on both sides of the tendon of the flexor hallucis longus muscle. D

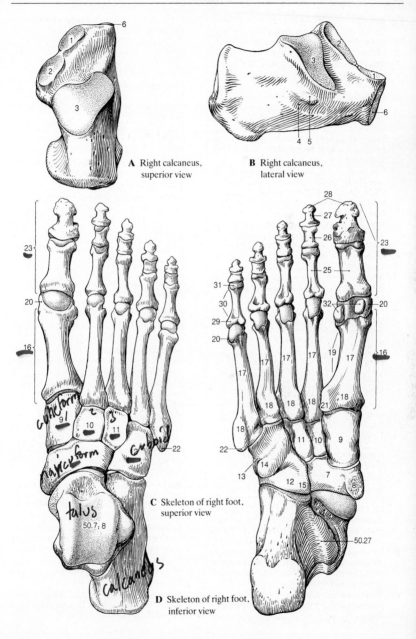

A Right calcaneus,
superior view

B Right calcaneus,
lateral view

C Skeleton of right foot,
superior view

D Skeleton of right foot,
inferior view

1　SUTURES OF THE SKULL. SUTURAE CRA-
　　NII (CRANIALES).

2　**Coronal suture.** Sutura coronalis. It lies between
　　the frontal and both parietal bones. A C D

3　**Sagittal suture.** Sutura sagittalis. The median
　　suture situated between the right and left parietal
　　bones. C

4　**Lambdoidal suture.** Sutura lamboidea. It is lo-
　　cated between the occipital and both parietal
　　bones. A D

5　**Occipitomastoid suture.** Sutura occipitoma-
　　stoidea. Continuation of the lambdoidal suture as
　　far as the base of the skull. A D

6　**Sphenofrontal suture.** Sutura sphenofrontalis.
　　Smooth suture ascending posteriorly between the
　　greater wing of the sphenoid and frontal bone lat-
　　erally in the skull and between the lesser wing of
　　the sphenoid and the frontal bone in the skull
　　base. A B D

7　**Sphenoethmoidal suture.** Sutura sphenoethmoi-
　　dalis. Short suture in front of the jugum sphenoi-
　　dale, internally between the body of sphenoid and
　　the ethmoid. D

8　**Sphenosquamosal suture.** Sutura sphenosqua-
　　mosa. Suture between the squamous portion of the
　　temporal bone and the greater wing of the spheno-
　　id. A C D

9　**Sphenoparietal suture.** Sutura sphenoparietalis.
　　Suture between the greater wing of the sphenoid
　　and the parietal bone. A C D

10　**Squamous suture.** Sutura squamosa. Suture be-
　　tween the squamous temporal and parietal bones.
　　A C D

11　**Frontal (metopic) suture.** [Sutura frontalis (Su-
　　tura metopical)]. Suture between the right and left
　　halves of the frontal bone. It generally fuses in the
　　6th postnatal year. C

12　**Parietomastoid suture.** Sutura parietomastoidea.
　　Suture posteriorly between the parietal bone and
　　the mastoid process of the temporal bone. A

13　**Squamosomastoid suture.** [Sutura squamoso-
　　mastoidea]. Precociously fusing suture between
　　the squamous and mastoid portions of the tempo-
　　ral bone. A

14　**Frontonasal suture.** Sutura frontonasalis. Suture
　　between the frontal and nasal bones anteriorly. C

15　**Frontoethmoidal suture.** Sutura frontoethmoi-
　　dalis. Suture between the ethmoid and frontal
　　bones internally. B D

16　**Frontomaxillary suture.** Sutura frontomaxilla-
　　ris. Suture lateral to the nasal bone between the na-
　　sal portion of the frontal bone and the frontal pro-
　　cess of the maxilla. A B C

17　**Frontolacrimal suture.** Sutura frontolacrimalis.
　　Suture between the frontal and lacrimal bones. A
　　B C

18　**Frontozygomatic suture.** Sutura frontozygoma-
　　tica. Suture at the lateral margin of the orbit be-
　　tween the frontal and zygomatic bones. A B C

19　**Zygomaticomaxillary suture.** Sutura zygomati-
　　comaxillaris. Suture in the floor of the orbit be-
　　tween the zygomatic bone and the maxilla. A B C

20　**Ethmoidomaxillary suture.** Sutura ethmoido-
　　maxillaris. Suture in the medial wall of the orbit
　　between the orbital plate of the ethmoid and the
　　maxilla. B C

21　**Ethmoidolacrimal suture.** Sutura ethmoido-
　　lacrimalis. Suture in the medial wall of the orbit
　　between the ethmoid and lacrimal bones. B

22　**Sphenovomerine suture.** Sutura sphenovomeri-
　　ana. Suture at the nasal septum between the sphe-
　　noid bone and the vomer.

23　**Sphenozygomatic suture.** Sutura sphenozygo-
　　matica. Suture in the lateral wall of the orbit be-
　　tween the greater wing of the sphenoid and zygo-
　　matic bone. B C

24　**Sphenomaxillary suture.** Sutura sphenomaxilla-
　　ris. Inconstant suture between the pterygoid pro-
　　cess and the maxillae lateral to the palatine bone.
　　A

25　**Temporozygomatic suture.** Sutura temporozy-
　　gomatica. Suture between the zygomatic process
　　of the temporal bone and the zygomatic bone on
　　the lateral aspect of the zygomatic arch. A

26　**Internasal suture.** Sutura internasalis. Suture be-
　　tween the right and left nasal bones. C

27　**Nasomaxillary suture.** Sutura nasomaxillaris.
　　Suture between the nasal bone and the frontal pro-
　　cess of the maxilla. A C

28　**Lacrimomaxillary suture.** Sutura lacrimomaxil-
　　laris. Suture between anterior margin of the lacri-
　　mal bone and the maxilla. A B C

29　**Lacrimoconchal suture.** Sutura lacrimoncha-
　　lis. Suture within the nasal cavity between the
　　lacrimal bone and the inferior nasal concha.

30　**Intermaxillary suture.** Sutura intermaxillaris.
　　Median suture between the right and left maxilla
　　anteriorly. C

31　**Palatomaxillary suture.** Sutura palatomaxillaris.
　　Suture between the palatine bone and the maxilla
　　situated posteriorly in the orbit and on the lateral
　　wall of the nasal cavity. B

32　**Palatoethmoidal suture.** Sutura palatoethmoida-
　　lis. Suture in the back of the orbit between the pa-
　　latine and ethmoid bones. B

33　**Median palatine suture.** Sutura palatina media-
　　na. Suture within the oral cavity between both
　　halves of the palatine bone. E

34　**Transverse palatine suture.** Sutura palatina
　　transversa. Suture between the palatine process of
　　the maxilla and the palatine bone. E

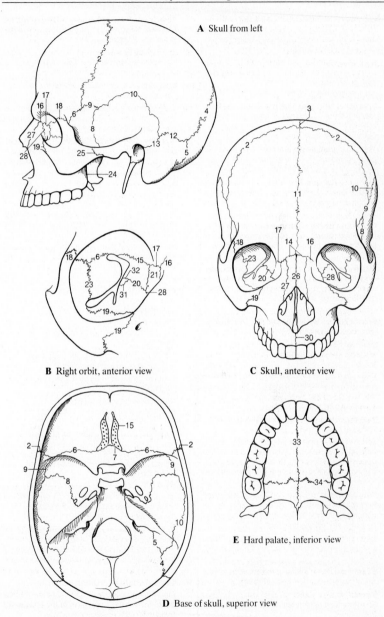

A Skull from left

B Right orbit, anterior view

C Skull, anterior view

D Base of skull, superior view

E Hard palate, inferior view

1 CRANIAL SYNCHONDROSES. SYNCHON-DROSES CRANII (CRANIALES). Cartilaginous joints between skull bones. Most are temporary and become ossified.

2 **Spheno-occipital synchondrosis.** Synchondrosis spheno-occipitalis. Developmental cartilaginous joint postero-inferior to the sella turcica between the sphenoid and occipital bones. A

3 **Sphenopetrosal synchondrosis.** Synchondrosis sphenopetrosa. Cartilaginous union between the sphenoid and petrous bones in the lateral continuation of the foramen lacerum. A

4 **Petro-occipital synchondrosis.** Synchondrosis petro-occipitalis. Anteromedial cartilaginous continuation of the jugular foramen. A

4 a **Intraoccipital synchondroses.** Synchondroses intraoccipitalis. Cartilaginous joints between developmental parts of the occipital bone.

5 **Posterior intraoccipital synchondrosis.** [Synchondrosis intra-occipitalis posterior]. Developmental synchondrosis between the posterior and both lateral ossific centers of the occipital bone. A

6 **Anterior intraoccipital synchondrosis.** [Synchondrosis intra-occipitalis anterior]. Developmental cartilaginous joint between the anterior and both lateral ossific centers of the occipital bone beginning at the anterior circumference of the foramen magnum. A

7 **Sphenoethmoidal synchondrosis.** Synchondrosis spheno-ethmoidalis. Cartilaginous precursor of the spheno-ethmoidal suture. See 54.7.

8 JOINTS OF VERTEBRAL COLUMN, THORAX AND SKULL. ARTICULATIONES COLUMNAE VERTEBRALIS, THORACIS ET CRANII. The connections of the vertebral column, thorax and skull.

9 **Intervertebral symphysis.** Symphysis intervertebralis. Union between adjacent vertebral bodies.

10 **Intervertebral disc.** Discus intervertebralis. Fibrocartilage plate between two adjacent vertebral bodies consisting of circular connective tissue lamellae surrounding a central gelatinous nucleus. B C

11 Anulus fibrosus. Annular fibrous connection between two vertebral bodies consisting of obliquely oriented connective tissue fibers arranged in alternating directions. B

12 Nucleus pulposus. Gelatinous, semifluid mass forming the central core of an intervertebral disc. B

13 **Ligamenta flava.** Yellow, predominantly elastic ligaments between the vertebral arches. B

14 **Zygapophysial joints.** Articulationes zygapo-
~ physiales. Joints between articular processes of vertebrae. C

15 **Intertransverse ligaments.** Ligg. intertrans-
~ versaria. Narrow ligaments between transverse processes of vertebrae. C

16 **Interspinal ligaments.** Ligg. interspinalia. Broad
~ ligaments between adjacent spinous processes. B

17 **Supraspinal ligaments.** Ligg. supraspinalia.
~ Longitudinal ligaments connecting the tips of the spinous processes. C

18 **Ligamentum nuchae.** Backwards projecting expansion of the supraspinal ligaments in the upper neck region. B

19 **Anterior longitudinal ligament.** Lig. longitudinale anterius. Longitudinal ligament uniting mainly the anterior surfaces of the vertebral bodies. B

20 **Posterior longitudinal ligament.** Lig. longitudinale posterius. Longitudinal ligament connecting mainly the intervertebral discs. It lies on the posterior surface of the vertebral bodies and thus on the anterior wall of the vertebral canal. It fuses with the tectorial membrane from the 3rd cervical vertebrae upward. B

21 **Sacrococcygeal joint.** Articulatio sacrococcygea.
~ Union between the sacrum and coccyx; it is frequently a true joint, but often also in the form of a synchondrosis. D

22 Superficial dorsal sacrococcygeal ligament. Lig. sacrococcygeum posterius (dorsale) superficiale. D

23 Deep dorsal sacrococcygeal ligament. Lig. sacrococcygeum posterius (dorsale) profundum. D

24 Ventral sacrococcygeal ligament. Lig. sacrococcygeum anterius (ventrale).

25 Lateral sacrococcygeal ligament. Lig. sacrococcygeum laterale. D

26 **Atlanto-occipital joint.** Articulatio atlanto-occipitalis. Joint between the atlas and the occipital bone. 59 A B

27 **Anterior atlanto-occipital membrane.** Membrana atlanto-occipitalis anterior. Membranous connection between the arch of the atlas and the occipital bone. It lies in front of the apical ligament of the dens. B

28 Anterior atlanto-occipital ligament. [Lig atlanto-occipitale anterius]. Reinforced portion of the atlanto-occipital membrane emanating from the anterior tubercle.

29 **Posterior atlanto-occipital membrane.** Membrana atlanto-occipitalis posterior. Connection between the arch of the atlas and the occipital bone situated in the posterior wall of the vertebral canal. B

30 **Lateral atlanto-occipital membrane.** Lig. atlanto-occipitale laterale. Oblique tract of fibers from the transverse process of the atlas to the jugular process of the occipital bone.

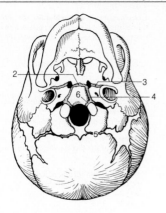

A Skull of newborn,
inferior view

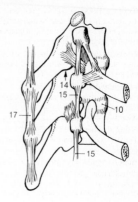

C Ligaments of vertebral column
and ribs, lateral view

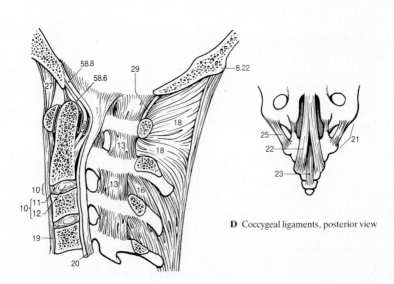

B Ligaments of cervical vertebral column,
medial view

D Coccygeal ligaments, posterior view

1   **Lateral atlanto-axial joint.** Articulatio atlanto-axialis lateralis. Joint between the inferior articular facet of the atlas and the superior articular facet of the axis. A B

2   **Median atlanto-axial joint.** Articulatio atlanto-axialis mediana. Articulation between the atlas and the dens of the axis. C

3   **Alar ligaments.** Ligg. alaria. Paired ligaments from the dens of the axis to the lateral margin of the foramen magnum. A B

4   **Apical ligament of the dens.** Lig. apicis dentis. Unpaired ligament extending from the apex of the dens to the anterior margin of the foramen magnum. A C

5   **Cruciform ligament of atlas.** Lig. cruciforme atlantis. Cruciate ligament consisting of the two following ligamentous bands (6,7) extending between the dens and the tectorial membrane. B

6   **Longitudinal fasciculi of cruciform ligament.** Fasciculi longitudinales. Connective tissue tracts from the body of the axis to the anterior margin of the foramen magnum. They are situated behind the dens and its apical ligament. B C

7   **Transverse ligament of atlas.** Lig. transversum atlantis. Part of the cruciform ligament of the atlas passing behind the dens and extending transversely from one side of the atlas to the other. It maintains the dens in position. B C

8   **Tectorial membrane.** Membrana tectoria. Bilayered continuation of the posterior longitudinal ligament. It passes from the axis to the anterior margin of the foramen magnum and is continuous with the dura-periosteal layer of the skull base. C

9   JOINTS OF THORAX. Articulationes thoracis.
~   Articular connections of the skeleton of the thorax.

10 **Costovertebral joints.** Articulationes costovertebrales. Joints between the ribs and vertebrae. D

11 **Joints of rib heads.** Articulatio capitis costae (costalis). Articular unions of the heads of the ribs with the vertebral bodies and intervertebral discs. D

12 **Radiate ligament of head of rib.** Lig. capitis costae radiatum. Ligament radiating predominantly from the anterior side of the head of the rib to the adjacent vertebral body and intervertebral disc. D E

13 **Intra-articular ligament of head of rib.** Lig. capitis costae intra-articulare. Ligament extending from the crest of the head of the rib to the intervertebral disc. It lies between the two articular facets of the head of the rib. E

14 **Costotransverse joint.** Articulatio costotransversaria. Joint between the articular surface of the tubercle of the rib and the transverse process of the corresponding vertebra. D

15 **Costotransverse ligament.** Lig. costotransversarium. Ligament between the neck of a rib and the transverse process of the corresponding vertebra. D

16 **Superior costotransverse ligament.** Lig. costotransversarium superius. Ligament from the rib to the next higher transverse process. E

17 **Lateral costotransverse ligament.** Lig. costotransversarium laterale. Ligament from the end of the transverse process to corresponding rib. D

18 **Lumbocostal ligament.** Lig. lumbocostale. The upper end of the thoracic fascia attaching to the 12th rib.

19 **Costotransverse foramen.** Foramen costotransversarium. Opening for the intercostal nerves between the superior costotransverse ligament and the neck of the rib. E

20 **Sternocostal joint.** Articulationes sternocostales. Articulation between the costal cartilage and sternum. F

21 **Intra-articular sternocostal ligament.** Lig. sternocostale intra-articulare. Ligament within the articular cavity between the costal cartilage and sternum, especially pronounced at the 2nd rib. F

22 **Radiate sternocostal ligaments.** Ligg. sternocostalia radiata. Fiber tracts located in front of the sternocostal joint and radiating from the end of the costal cartilage to the sternum. F

23 **Sternal membrane.** Membrana sterni. Membranous-like covering of the anterior surface of the sternum derived in part from fibers of the radiate sternocostal ligaments. F

24 **Costoxiphoid ligaments.** Ligg. costoxiphoidea. Fiber tracts extending downward from the 7th costal cartilage to the xiphoid process.

25 **External intercostal membrane.** Membrana intercostalis externa. Continuation of the external intercostal muscles at the sternal end of the intercostal space. F

26 **Internal intercostal membrane.** Membrana intercostalis interna. Continuation of the internal intercostal muscles near the vertebral end of the intercostal space. E

26 a **Sternocostal synchondrosis of the first rib.** Synchondrosis sternocostalis costae primae.

27 **Interchondral joints.** Articulationes interchondrales. Articulations between the costal cartilages, usually between those of ribs 6–9. See 7 D

28 **Costochondral joints.** Articulationes costochondrales. Unions between the bony and cartilaginous parts of a rib without an articular cavity.

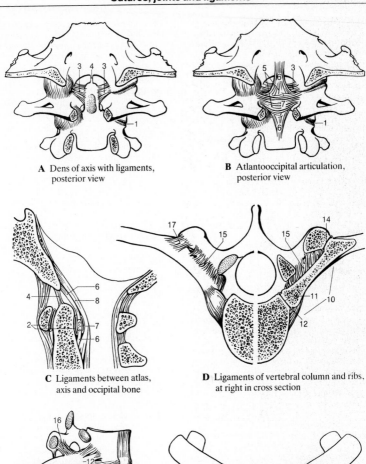

A Dens of axis with ligaments, posterior view

B Atlantooccipital articulation, posterior view

C Ligaments between atlas, axis and occipital bone

D Ligaments of vertebral column and ribs, at right in cross section

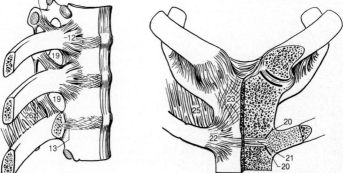

E Ligaments of vertebral column and ribs

F Sternocostal articulations

1 SYNOVIAL JOINTS OF THE SKULL. ARTICULATIONES SYNOVIALES CRANII.

2 **Temporomandibular joint.** Articulatio temporomandibularis. A B C

3 **Articular disc.** Discus articularis. Biconcave connective tissue disc between the head of the mandible and the articular fossa. It divides the joint into two cavities. C

4 **Lateral (temporomandibular) ligament.** Lig. laterale. Often strong connective tissue tracts on the lateral surface of the joint passing obliquely upward and forward from the neck of the mandible. A

5 **Medial ligament.** Lig. mediale. Reinforcement of the medial wall of the capsule. B

6 **Superior synovial membrane.** Membrana synovialis superior. Synovial lining of the superior articular cavity. C

7 **Inferior synovial membrane.** Membrana synovialis inferior. Synovial lining of the inferior articular cavity. C

8 **Sphenomandibular ligament.** Lig. sphenomandibulare. Flat ligament on the inner aspect of the mandibular ramus extending from the mandibular foramen to the spine of the sphenoid bone lateral to the foramen spinosum. B

9 **Stylomandibular ligament.** Lig. stylomandibulare. Ligament passing from the anterior surface of the styloid process to the angle of the mandible. A B

10 **Pterygospinal ligament.** Lig. pterygospinale. Broad connective tissue band extending from the upper part of the lateral plate of the pterygoid process to the spine of the sphenoid. B

11 **Stylohyoid ligament.** Lig. stylohyoideum. Ligament running between the styloid process and the lesser horn of the hyoid bone. Vestige of the second pharyngeal arch. B

12 **JOINTS OF THE SHOULDER GIRDLE.** Articulationes cinguli pectoralis. D E F G

13 **Coracoacromial ligament.** Lig. coracoacromiale. Strong band extending from the coracoid process to the acromion. It roofs the shoulder joint. D

14 **Superior transverse scapular ligament.** Lig. transversum scapulae superius. Ligament lying medial to the coracoid process and bridging the scapular notch. D

15 **Inferior transverse scapular ligament.** [Lig. transversum scapulae inferius]. Weak fibrous band passing from the root of the spine of the scapula to the posterior margin of the glenoid cavity. F

16 **Acromioclavicular joint.** Articulatio acromioclavicularis. Joint between the acromion and the clavicle. D

17 **Acromioclavicular ligament.** Lig. acromioclaviculare. Strong band within and above the articular capsule serving to protect and hold together the clavicle and acromion. D

18 **Articular disc.** Discus articularis. Fibrocartilaginous interarticular disc. D

19 **Coracoclavicular ligament.** Lig. coracoclaviculare. Strong band connecting the coracoid process and the clavicle. It consists of two components. D

20 **Trapezoid ligament.** Lig. trapezoideum. The portion of the coracoclavicular ligament taking an upward and lateral course from the coracoid process to the clavicle. It lies between the conoid and coraco-acromial ligaments. D

21 **Conoid ligament.** Lig. conoideum. The portion of the coraco-clavicular ligament lying medial to the trapezoid ligament and arising from the root of the coracoid process. D

22 **Sternoclavicular joint.** Articulatio sternoclavicularis. Two-chambered joint between the sternum and clavicle. G

23 **Articular disc.** Discus articularis. Interarticular disc anchored below to the first rib and above to the clavicle. G

24 **Anterior sternoclavicular ligament.** Lig. sternoclaviculare anterius. Reinforcing band on the anterior wall of the joint capsule. G

25 **Posterior sternoclavicular ligament.** Lig. sternoclaviculare posterius. Reinforcing band on the posterior wall of the joint capsule.

26 **Costoclavicular ligament.** Lig. costoclaviculare. Ligamentous union between the first rib and the clavicle lateral to the sternoclavicular joint. G

27 **Interclavicular ligament.** Lig. interclaviculare. Ligament passing across the suprasternal notch and uniting both clavicles. G

28 JOINTS OF THE FREE UPPER LIMB. AR-
~ TICULATIONES MEMBRI SUPERIORIS LIBERI.

29 **Shoulder (glenohumeral) joint.** Articulatio humeri (glenohumeralis). D E F

30 **Glenoid lip.** Labrum glenoidale. The fibrocartilaginous margin of the bony glenoid cavity. E

31 **Coracohumeral ligament.** Lig. coracohumerale. Thickened portion of the capsule passing from the root of the coracoid process to the upper margin of the greater and lesser tubercles. D E

32 **Glenohumeral ligaments.** Ligg. glenohumeralia. Three thickenings (superior, middle, inferior) within the anterior wall of the capsule. D E

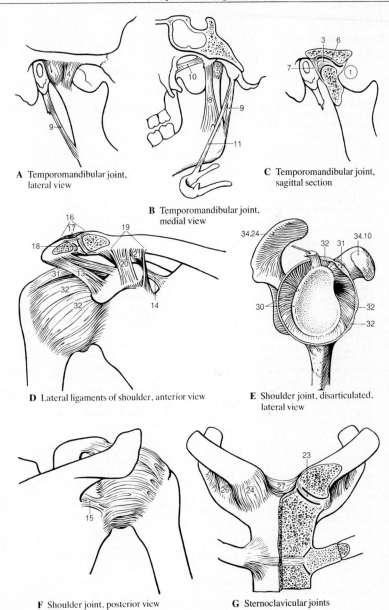

A Temporomandibular joint, lateral view

B Temporomandibular joint, medial view

C Temporomandibular joint, sagittal section

D Lateral ligaments of shoulder, anterior view

E Shoulder joint, disarticulated, lateral view

F Shoulder joint, posterior view

G Sternoclavicular joints

1 **Elbow joint.** Articulatio cubiti (cubitalis). Articular connection between the upper arm and forearm. A

2 **Humeroulnar joint.** Articulatio humeroulnaris. Joint between the humerus and ulna.

3 **Humeroradial joint.** Articulatio humeroradialis. Joint between the humerus and radius.

4 **Proximal radioulnar joint.** Articulatio radioulnaris proximalis. Joint formed by the articular circumference of the radius and the radial notch of the ulna.

5 **Ulnar collateral ligament.** Lig. collaterale ulnare. Collateral ligament at the medial side of the arm between the ulna and humerus. A

6 **Radial collateral ligament.** Lig. collaterale radiale. Ligament which spreads out from the lateral epicondyle into the annular ligament of the radius and also into the ulna. A

7 **Annular ligament of the radius.** Lig. anulare
~ radii. Circular band embracing a part of the articular circumference of the radius. It is attached to the anterior and posterior margins of the radial notch of the ulna. A

8 **Quadrate ligament.** Lig. quadratum. Thin band of fibers passing from the distal margin of the radial notch of the ulna to the neck of the radius.

9 **Radioulnar syndesmosis (joint).** Syndesmosis [articulatio] radioulnaris. Fibrous joint between the radius and ulna.

10 **Interosseous membrane of forearm.** Membrana interossea antebrachii. Membranous sheet which spreads out between the interosseous margins of the radius and ulna. A

11 **Oblique cord.** Chorda obliqua. Ligamentous band extending obliquely downward from the ulnar tuberosity to the radius. It runs in an opposite direction to most fibers of the interosseous membrane. A

12 **Distal radioulnar joint.** Articulatio radioulnaris distalis. B

13 **Articular disc.** Discus articularis. Interarticular disc between the ulna and carpus. It is attached at the radius and styloid process of the ulna and, as an intra-articular ligament, anchors the radius and ulna to one another. B

14 **Recessus sacciformis.** Proximal extension of the flaccid articular capsule. B

15 **Radiocarpal joint.** Articulatio radiocarpalis. Proximal wrist joint between the proximal row of carpal bones and the radius including the articular disc. B

15a **Carpal joints.** Articulationes carpi.

16 **Intercarpal joints.** Articulationes intercarpales. Joints between the carpal bones permitting only slight movements. B

17 **Midcarpal joint.** Articulatio mediocarpalis. The distal wrist joint between the proximal and distal rows of carpal bones. B

18 **Dorsal radiocarpal ligament.** Lig. radiocarpale dorsale. Ligament on the dorsum of the wrist spreading out from the radius to the triquetrum bone. C

19 **Palmar radiocarpal ligament.** Lig. radiocarpale palmare. Ligament on the flexor side radiating from the radius to the lunate and capitate bones. D

20 **Palmar ulnocarpal ligament.** Lig. ulnocarpale palmare. Ligament extending from the flexor side of the head of the ulnar chiefly to the capitate bone. It often unites with fibers of the palmar radiocarpal ligament. D

21 **Radiate carpal ligament.** Lig. carpi radiatum. Groups of fibers radiating to both sides of the wrist mainly from the head of the capitate. D

22 **Ulnar carpal collateral ligament.** Lig. collaterale carpi ulnare. Collateral ligament extending from the styloid process of the ulna to the triquetrum and pisiform bones. C D

23 **Radial carpal collateral ligament.** Lig. collaterale carpi radiale. External collateral ligament passing from the styloid process of the radius to the scaphoid bone. C D

24 **Dorsal intercarpal ligaments.** Ligg. intercarpalia dorsalia. Ligamentous bands extending between the proximal and distal rows of carpal bones on the dorsum of the wrist. C

25 **Palmar intercarpal ligaments.** Ligg. intercarpalia palmaria. Groups of ligaments between the carpal bones on the palmar aspect below the radiate carpal ligament. D

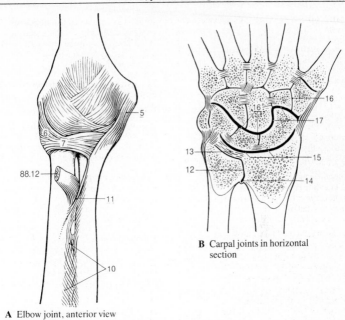

A Elbow joint, anterior view

B Carpal joints in horizontal section

C Carpal ligaments, dorsal view

D Carpal ligaments, palmar view

1 JOINTS OF THE HAND. ARTICULA-
TIONES MANUS. A B C

2 **Interosseous intercarpal ligaments.** Ligg. intercarpalia interossea. Ligaments penetrating
directly through the joint clefts between the
carpal bones within a row. A

3 **Pisotriquetral joint.** Articulatio ossis pi-
siformis. Articulation between the pisiform
and triquetrum bones. A

4 **Pisohamate ligament.** Lig. pisohamatum.
Medial continuation of the tendon of the flexor
carpi ulnaris to the hook of the hamate bone. B

5 **Pisometacarpal ligament.** Lig. pisometacar-
pale. Laterally situated continuation of the tendon of the flexor carpi ulnaris to the base of the
fifth metacarpal. B

6 **Carpal canal or tunnel.** Canalis carpi
(carpalis). Palmar canal located between the
tubercles of the scaphoid and trapezium on the
one side and the pisiform, as well as the hook
of the hamulus on the other side. It is bridged
over by the flexor retinaculum (93.26). B

7 **Metacarpal articulations.** Articulationes carpometacarpales. Slightly movable
joints between the distal carpal bones and the
metacarpals. A

8 **Dorsal carpometacarpal ligaments.** Ligg.
carpometacarpalia dorsalia. Rigid ligaments
on the dorsum of the hand between the distal
carpal bones and the metacarpal bones. C

9 **Palmar carpometacarpal ligaments.** Ligg.
carpometacarpalia palmaria. Ligaments on the
palmar side of the hand between the distal carpal bones and the metacarpal bones. B

10 **Carpometacarpal joint of the thumb.** Articulatio carpometacarpalis pollicis. Saddle
joint between the first metacarpal and the trapezium. A B

11 **Intermetacarpal joints.** Articulationes
intermetacarpales. Joints between the bases of
the metacarpal bones. A

12 **Dorsal metacarpal ligaments.** Ligg. metacarpalia dorsalia. Ligaments between the proximal ends of the metacarpals on the extensor
side. C

13 **Palmar metacarpal ligaments.** Ligg. metacarpalia palmaria. Ligaments between the
bases of the metacarpal bones on the palmar
side. B

14 **Interosseous metacarpal ligaments.** Ligg.
metacarpalia interossea. Short, tense ligaments
at the bases of the metacarpal bones. They lie
intracapsularly between the dorsal and palmar
metacarpal ligaments. A

15 **Interosseous spaces of metacarpus.** Spatia
interossea metacarpi. Spaces between the
metacarpal bones. A C

16 **Metacarpophalangeal joints.** Articulationes metacarpophalangeales. Joints between
the heads of the metacarpal bones and the bases
of the proximal phalanges. B

17 **Collateral ligaments.** Ligg. collateralia.
Collateral ligaments of the metacarpophalangeal joints. They slacken during extension of
the fingers and become tense when making a
closed fist. B

18 **Palmar ligaments.** Ligg. palmaria. Fibers in
the floor of the tendon sheaths extending from
the root of the collateral ligaments to the palmar side. These should not be confused with
the annular parts of the fibrous sheaths. 92.28
B

19 **Deep transverse metacarpal ligament.** Lig.
metacarpale transversum profundum. Transversely oriented fibrous tracts on the palmar
side of the heads of the metacarpal bones at
the level of the joint spaces. They hold the
distal parts of the metacarpus together. B

20 **Interphalangeal joints.** Articulationes
interphalangeales. Middle and distal joints between the phalanges. B

21 **Collateral ligaments of the interphalangeal
joints.** Ligg. collateralia. B

22 **Palmar ligaments.** Ligg. palmaria. Fibers
which pass into the floor of the tendon sheaths
above the interphalangeal joints. B

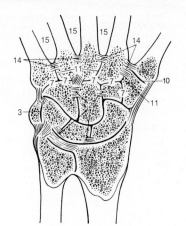

A Carpal joints in horizontal section

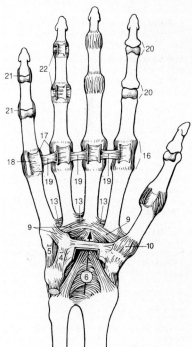

B Carpal joints, palmar view

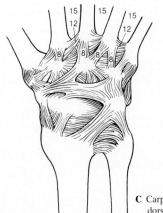

C Carpal joints of right hand, dorsal view

1   **JOINTS OF THE PELVIC GIRDLE.** Articulationes cinguli pelvici.

2   **Obturator membrane.** Membrana obturatoria. Membrane which closes off the obturator foramen except for the obturator canal. It is covered by the obturator externus and internus muscles. A B C D

3   **Obturator canal.** Canalis obturatorius. Opening present in the obturator membrane superolaterally. It corresponds to the obturator groove between the two obturator tubercles and is traversed by the obturator artery, vein and nerve. A C D

4   **Lumbosacral joint.** Articulatio lumbosacralis.
~   Articulation between the sacrum and lumbar vertebra 5 (4). A

5   **Iliolumbar ligament.** Lig. iliolumbale. Strong ligament that passes to the ilium mainly from the transverse processes of L4 and 5. A B

6   **Sacrotuberous ligament.** Lig. sacrotuberale. Strong ligament that extends from the medial margin of the ischial tuberosity to the sacrum and ilium. B D

7   **Falciform process.** Processus falciformis. Slender extension of fibers from the sacrotuberous ligament to the inner aspect of the ischium. B

8   **Sacrospinous ligament.** Lig. sacrospinale. Situated medial to the sacrotuberous ligament, it passes from the ischial spine to the sacrum and coccyx and separates the greater from the lesser sciatic foramen. B D

9   **Greater sciatic foramen.** Foramen sciaticum (ischiadicum) majus. It lies between the greater sciatic notch, sacrum, sacrospinous ligament and the upper part of the sacrotuberous ligament. It is traversed by the piriformis muscle, superior and inferior gluteal arteries, veins and nerves, the internal pudendal vein, pudendal nerve, sciatic nerve and posterior femoral cutaneous nerve. A B D

10   **Lesser sciatic foramen.** Foramen sciaticum (ischiadicum) minus. It lies between the lesser sciatic notch and the sacrospinous and sacrotuberous ligaments. It transmits the obturator internus muscle as well as the internal pudendal artery and vein and the pudendal nerve on their way back into the ischiorectal fossa. B D

11   **Sacroiliac joint.** Articulatio sacroiliaca. The barely movable joint (syndesmosis) between the sacrum and ilium. A

12   **Ventral sacroiliac ligaments.** Ligg. sacroiliaca anteriora (ventralia). Thin, but broad band of fibers extending from the anterior side of S1 and 2 to the ilium. A D

13   **Interosseous sacroiliac ligaments.** Ligg. sacroiliaca interossea. Very strong dorsal ligaments that pass from the tuberosity of the sacrum to the tuberosity of the ilium. B

14   **Dorsal sacroiliac ligaments.** Ligg. sacroiliaca posteriora (dorsalia). Superficial ligamentous mass attached dorsally to the interosseous sacroiliac ligaments between the sacrum and ilium. B

15   **Pubic symphysis.** Symphysis pubica. A

16   **Superior pubic ligament.** Lig. pubicum superius. Fibrous connection between the two halves of the symphysis emanating from the pecten pubis of both sides. A

17   **Arcuate pubic ligament.** Lig. arcuatum pubis. Strong, curved ligament below the symphysis. A

18   **Interpubic disc.** Discus interpubicus. Fibrocartilaginous mass between the right and left pubis with a median fissure in its upper half. A

19   JOINTS OF THE FREE LOWER LIMB.
~   ARTICULATIONES MEMBRI INFERIORIS LIBERI.

20   **Hip joint.** Articulatio coxae (iliofemoralis). It is formed by the acetabulum and the head of the femur. A B C

21   **Joint capsule.** Capsula articularis. It is attached anteriorly to the intertrochanteric line, posteriorly above to the intertrochanteric crest. A fracture of the neck of the femur can therefore lie within the capsule anteriorly and outside of the capsule posteriorly. A

22   Orbicular zone. Zona orbicularis. Ligamentous fibers encircling the neck of the femur. B

23   **Iliofemoral ligament.** Lig. iliofemorale. Strong anterior ligament of the hip joint capsule from the ilium to the intertrochanteric line. A B

24   Ischiofemoral ligament. Lig. ischiofemorale. It radiates into the orbicular zone from the posterior margin of the acetabulum and is also attached to the anterior margin of the greater trochanter and to the intertrochanteric line. B

25   Pubofemoral ligament. Lig. pubofemorale. It extends from the pubis medially in the joint capsule to the orbicular zone and to the femur proximal to the lesser trochanter. A

26   **Acetabular lip.** Labrum acetabulare. Annular lip, partly fibrocartilaginous, partly connective tissue, it completes and deepens the bony acetabulum. C

27   Transverse acetabular ligament. Lig. transversum acetabuli. It bridges the acetabular notch. C

28   **Ligament of head of femur.** Lig. capitis femoris. A smooth ligament from the acetabular notch to the pit on the head of the femur. It transmits blood vessels and has no direct mechanical action. C

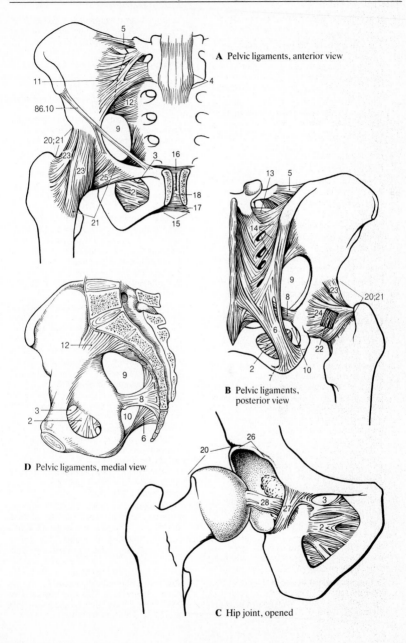

A Pelvic ligaments, anterior view

B Pelvic ligaments, posterior view

D Pelvic ligaments, medial view

C Hip joint, opened

1 **Knee joint.** Articulatio genus [genualis]. A
B C D E

2 **Lateral meniscus.** Meniscus lateralis. Almost
circular ring consisting of connective tissue
similar to fibrocartilage with low points standing close together below the lateral femoral
condyle. When not fused with the lateral collateral ligament, it is relatively movable. B D E

3 **Anterior meniscofemoral ligament.**
Lig. meniscofemorale anterius. Fibrous band
occasionally present connecting the posterior
part of the lateral meniscus with the anterior
cruciate ligament. It passes in front of the
posterior cruciate ligament. D E

4 **Posterior meniscofemoral ligament.**
Lig. meniscofemorale posterius. It passes
posterior to the lateral meniscus to the fibular
surface of the medial femoral condyle behind
the posterior cruciate ligament. D E

5 **Medial meniscus.** Meniscus medialis. C-
shaped ring of fibrocartilage and connective
tissue located below the medial femoral condyle. When fused with the medial collateral ligament, it is not very movable. B D E

6 **Transverse ligament of knee.** Lig. transversum genus [genuale]. Transverse ligament between the lateral and medial menisci anteriorly. B D

7 **Cruciate ligaments of knee.** Ligg. cruciata genus [genualia]. B E

8 **Anterior cruciate ligament.** Lig. crucia-
tum anterius. It passes from the inner surface of
the lateral femoral condyle obliquely forward
and inferomedially to the anterior intercondylar area and among other functions, prevents
the sliding forward of the tibia against the femur. B D E

9 **Posterior cruciate ligament.** Lig. crucia-
tum posterius. It passes from the inner surface
of the medial femoral condyle to the posterior
condylar area and prevents a backward sliding
of the tibia against the femur. B D E

10 **Infrapatellar synovial fold.** Plica synovialis
infrapatellaris. Synovial fold projecting from
the fat pad point-like into the intercondylar fossa. B

11 **Alar folds.** Plicae alares. Paired fat pads from
the infrapatellar synovial folds; deformable
filled body of the anterior knee joint cavity. B

12 **Fibular collateral ligament.** Lig. collaterale
fibulare. Lateral collateral ligament passing
from the head of the fibula to the lateral epicondyle. A B C D E

13 **Tibial collateral ligament.** Lig. collaterale tibiale. Medial collateral ligament extending
from the tibia to the medial epicondyle. A B C
D E

14 **Oblique popliteal ligament.** Lig. popliteum
obliquum. Fibrous expansion in the posterior
wall of the capsule passing upward and outward from the tendon of the semimembranosus. C

15 **Arcuate popliteal ligament.** Lig. popliteum
arcuatum. Bow-shaped fibrous tract above the
entrance of the popliteus muscle into the
posterior capsule of the knee joint from its
origin at the lateral epicondyle. C

16 **Ligamentum patellae.** Very strong band-like
continuation of the tendon of the quadriceps
from the apex of the patella to the tibial tuberosity. A

17 **Medial retinaculum of patella.** Retinaculum
patellae mediale. Aponeurosis of a part of the
vastus medialis medial to the patella. It is attached medial to the tibial tuberosity. A

18 **Lateral retinaculum of patella.** Retinaculum
patellae laterale. Aponeurosis of a part of the
vastus lateralis lateral to the patella with attachment lateral to the tibial tuberosity. A

19 **Infrapatellar fat pad.** Corpus adiposum in-
frapatellare. Large fat body in front of the knee
joint space. The alar and synovial folds form
part of it. A

20 **Tibiofibular joint.** Articulatio tibiofibularis. Articulation between the tibia and the
head of the fibula. E

21 **Anterior ligament of head of fibula.** Lig. capitis fibulae anterius. Group of fibers passing
anteriorly from the head of the fibula to the tibia. It holds both bones together. A

22 **Posterior ligament of head of fibula.** Lig. capitis fibulae posterius. Weaker group of fibers
extending posteriorly from the head of the fibula to the tibia. C D E

23 **Tibiofibular syndesmosis [joint].**
Syndesmosis [articulatio] tibiofibularis. Distal
union of tibia with fibula.

24 **Interosseous membrane.** Membrana interossea cruris. Membrane attached to the interosseous margins of the tibia and fibula. A C F G

25 **Anterior tibiofibular ligament.** Lig. tibiofi-
bulare anterius. Anteriorly situated ligaments
connecting the tibia and fibula providing stability to the malleolar fork. F

26 **Posterior tibiofibular ligament.** Lig. tibiofi-
bulare posterius. Posterior ligamentous
connections between the tibia and fibula, again
providing stability to the malleolar fork. G

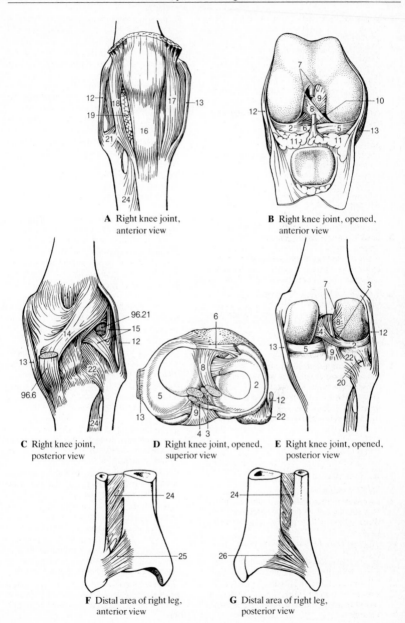

A Right knee joint,
anterior view

B Right knee joint, opened,
anterior view

C Right knee joint,
posterior view

D Right knee joint, opened,
superior view

E Right knee joint, opened,
posterior view

F Distal area of right leg,
anterior view

G Distal area of right leg,
posterior view

1 **Ankle (talocrural) joint.** Articulatio talocruralis. Upper ankle joint between the talus, tibia and fibula. D

2 **Medial or deltoid ligament.** Lig. mediale (deltoideum). Inner ligament of the ankle consisting of the following four segments: D

3 Tibionavicular part. Pars tibionavicularis. Fiber groups from the medial malleolus to the dorsal and medial surface of the navicular bone. D

4 Tibiocalcaneal part. Pars tibiocalcanea. Fiber tracts from the medial malleolus to the sustentaculum tali. B D

5 Anterior tibiotalar part. Pars tibiotalaris anterior. Segment of the deltoid ligament passing from the medial malleolus to the medial surface of the talus as far as the neck of the talus. D

6 Posterior tibiotalar part. Pars tibiotalaris posterior. Fibers passing posteriorly from the medial malleolus almost as far as the posterior process of the talus. B D

7 **Anterior talofibular ligament.** Lig. talofibulare anterius. Ligament from the lateral malleolus to the lateral surface of the neck of the talus. A

8 **Posterior talofibular ligament.** Lig. talofibulare posterius. It originates in the lateral malleolar fossa and inserts at the lateral tubercle of the posterior process of the talus. A B

9 **Calcaneofibular ligament.** Lig. calcaneofibulare. It passes from the apex of the lateral malleolus obliquely backward to the calcaneus. A B

10 **Intertarsal joints.** Articulationes intertarseae. Joints between the tarsal bones.

11 **Joints of the foot.** Articulationes pedis.

12 **Talocalcaneonavicular joint.** Articulatio talocalcaneonavicularis. The anterior portion of the lower ankle joint. In it the talus articulates with the calcaneus and navicular bones. A C

13 **Subtalar joint.** Articulatio subtalaris (talocalcanea). Joint between the talus and calcaneus. It represents the posterior part of the lower ankle joint. A B C D

14 **Lateral talocalcaneal ligament.** Lig. talocalcaneum laterale. It passes from the trochlea of the talus to the lateral surface of the calcaneus covered partially by the calcaneofibular ligament. A

15 **Medial talocalcaneal ligament.** Lig. talocalcaneum mediale. Situated on the medial side of the foot, it extends from the medial tubercle of the posterior process of the talus to the sustentaculum tali. B D

16 **Transverse tarsal (midtarsal) joint** [[Chopart's joint]]. Articulatio tarsi transversa. Joint situated in front of the talus and calcaneus but proximal to the cuboid and navicular bones. C

17 **Calcaneocuboid joint.** Articulatio calcaneocuboidea. Joint situated between the calcaneus and cuboid bones. A C

17a **Cuneocuboid joint.** Articulatio cuneocuboidea. Articulation between the cuboid bone and lateral cuneiform bone. C

18 **Cuneonavicular joint.** Articulatio cuneonavicularis. Joint between the navicular bone and cuneiform bones. C D

18a **Intercuneiform joints.** Articulationes intercuneiformes. Joint between the cuneiform bones.

19 **Interosseous ligaments of the tarsus.** Ligg. tarsi interossea. The following three interosseous ligaments are present between the tarsal bones:

20 Interosseous talocalcaneal ligament. Lig. talocalcaneum interosseum. Strong ligamentous mass in the sinus tarsi. A C

21 Interosseous cuneocuboid ligament. Lig. cuneocuboideum interosseum. Taut connection between the lateral cuneiform bone and the cuboid. A C

22 Interosseous intercuneiform ligaments. Ligg. intercuneiformia interossea. Taut ligaments between the three cuneiform bones. C

23 **Dorsal ligaments of the tarsus.** Ligg. tarsi dorsalia. The following eight dorsal ligaments are present between the tarsal bones.

24 Talonavicular ligament. Lig. talonaviculare. Dorsal ligament between the head of the talus and the navicular bone. A D

25 Dorsal intercuneiform ligaments. Ligg. intercuneiformia dorsalia. Dorsal ligaments between the cuneiform bones. A

26 Dorsal cuneocuboid ligament. Lig. cuneocuboideum dorsale. Dorsal ligaments between the lateral cuneiform bone and the cuboid bone. A

27 Dorsal cuboideonavicular ligament. Lig. cuboideonaviculare dorsale. Ligament between the cuboid and navicular bones. A

28 Bifurcate ligament. Lig. bifurcatum. V-shaped double ligament situated on the dorsum of the foot in front of the sinus tarsi. It passes forward from the calcaneus and consists of the following two parts. A

29 *Calcaneonavicular ligament.* Lig. calcaneonaviculare. It passes laterally from the head of the talus to the navicular bone. A

30 *Calcaneocuboid ligament.* Lig. calcaneocuboideum. It extends from the calcaneus to almost the middle of the cuboid bone. A

31 Dorsal cuneonavicular ligaments. Ligg. cuneonavicularia dorsalia. Broad group of ligaments on the dorsum of the foot connecting the navicular bone with the three cuneiform bones. A

31a **Dorsal calcaneocuboid ligament. Lig. calcaneocuboideum dorsale.** Moderate strengthening of the joint capsule lateral to the bifurcate ligament.

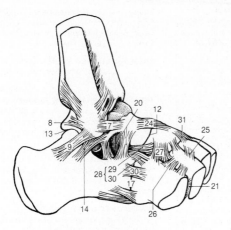

A Ligaments of right foot, lateral view

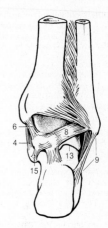

B Ligaments of right ankle (talocrural) joint, posterior view

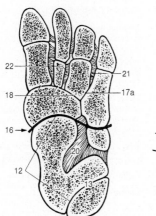

C Tarsometatarsal bones of right foot, horizontal section

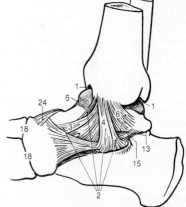

D Ligaments of right foot, medial view

1 **Plantar ligaments of tarsus.** Ligg. tarsi plantaria. Ligaments on the palmar aspect of the foot. They are particularly important for the bracing of both plantar arches of the foot.

2 Long plantar ligament. Lig. plantare longum. Stout ligament which passes from the calcaneus closely in front of its tuber to the cuboid bone and to the bases of metatarsals II–V. It supports the longitudinal arch. A

3 Plantar calcaneocuboid ligament or short plantar ligament. Lig. calcaneocuboideum plantare. Shorter portion of the long plantar ligament. A

4 Plantar calcaneonavicular (spring) ligament. Lig. calcaneonaviculare plantare. It lies medial to the preceding ligament and supports, according to more traditional view, the articular cavity for the head of the talus. Since, however, the talar side of the ligament is quite loose and moreover contains no fibrocartilage, this concept is questionable. A

5 Plantar cuneonavicular ligaments. Ligg. cuneonavicularia plantaria. Groups of ligaments that connect the navicular bone with the cuneiform bones lodged in front of it. A

6 Plantar cuboideonavicular ligament. Lig. cuboideonaviculare plantare. A plantar ligament coursing somewhat obliquely to the axis of the foot connecting the cuboid and navicular bones. It supports the transverse plantar arch of the foot. A

7 Plantar intercuneiform ligaments. Ligg. intercuneiformia plantare. Fibrous bands lying on the plantar aspect of the foot between the cuneiform bones. They support the transverse plantar arch of the foot. A

8 Plantar cuneocuboid ligament. Lig. cuneocuboideum plantare. Fibrous brace on the plantar aspect of the foot between the lateral cuneiform and cuboid bones. A

9 **Tarsometatarsal joints.** Articulationes tarsometatarsales. Joints between the tarsal and metatarsal bones of the foot. A B C

10 **Dorsal tarsometatarsal ligaments.** Ligg. tarsometatarsalia dorsalia. Ligaments located on the dorsum of the foot between the tarsal and metatarsal bones. B

11 **Plantar tarsometatarsal ligaments.** Ligg. tarsometatarsalia plantaria. Ligaments located on the plantar aspect of the foot between the tarsal and metatarsal bones. A

12 **Interosseous cuneometatarsal ligaments.** Ligg. cuneometatarsalia interossea. Ligaments occupying the joint spaces between the cuneiform and metatarsal bones. C

13 **Intermetatarsal joints.** Articulationes intermetatarsales. Joints between the bases of the metatarsal bones. B C

14 **Interosseous metatarsal ligaments.** Ligg. metatarsalia interossea. Ligaments between the bases of the metatarsal bones. They limit the articular spaces between the metatarsal bones distally. C

15 **Dorsal metatarsal ligaments.** Ligg. metatarsalia dorsalia. Ligaments residing between the bases of the metatarsal bones on the dorsum of the foot. B

16 **Plantar metatarsal ligaments.** Ligg. metatarsalia plantaria. Ligaments found between the bases of the metatarsal bones on the plantar aspect of the foot. A

17 **Metatarsal interosseous spaces.** Spatia interossea metatarsi. Spaces between the shafts of the metatarsal bones. They are occupied by muscles of the same name. A

18 **Metatarsophalangeal joints.** Articulationes metatarsophalangeales. A

19 **Collateral ligaments.** Ligg. collateralia. A

20 **Plantar ligaments.** Ligg. plantaria. Connective tissue reinforcement of the capsule of the metatarsophalangeal joint. It is more firmly fused with the proximal phalanx than with the head of the metatarsals and forms a stroma for the flexor tendons. A

21 **Deep transverse metatarsal ligament.** Lig. metatarsale transversum profundum. Transversely oriented ligament connecting the heads of the metatarsal bones. A

22 **Interphalangeal joints of the foot.** Articulationes interphalangeales pedis. A

23 **Collateral ligaments.** Ligg. collateralia. A

24 **Plantar ligaments.** Ligg. plantaria. Connective tissue reinforcements on the plantar aspect of the interphalangeal articular capsules.

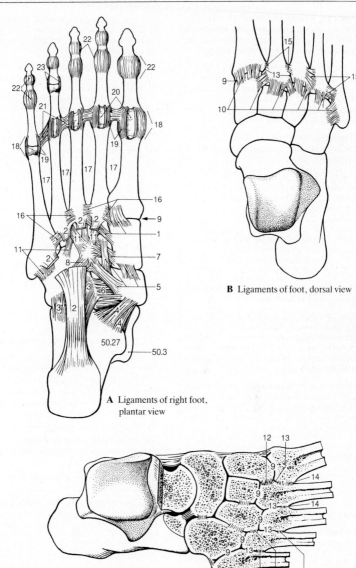

A Ligaments of right foot,
plantar view

B Ligaments of foot, dorsal view

C Ligaments of sectioned foot, dorsal view

1 DORSAL MUSCLES. MUSCULI DORSI. The muscles of the back. True back muscles are innervated by the dorsal rami of spinal nerves; muscles of the shoulder girdle are not. A B C

2 **M. trapezius.** o: Spinous processes of T1–12 and C7, ligamentum nuchae, occipital protuberance and superior nuchal line. i: Spine and acromion of scapula, clavicle. F: Rotates, raises, lowers and adducts scapula, rotates head. I: Accessory nerve, cervical plexus. A

3 **M. transversus nuchae.** (Rare, 25%). Muscle situated between the insertions of the trapezius and sternocleidomastoid. It passes transversely superficial or deep to the trapezius. A

4 **M. latissimus dorsi.** o: Spinous processes of T7–L5, sacrum and ilium. i: Crest of lesser tubercle of humerus. F: Dorsiflexion and medial rotation of arm. I: Thoracodorsal nerve. A

5 **M. rhomboideus major.** o: Spinous processes of T1–4. i: Medial margin of scapula. F: Medial and upward movement of scapula. I: Dorsal scapular nerve. A

6 **M. rhomboideus minor.** o: Spinous processes of C6–7. i: Medial margin of scapula above its spine. F: Medial and upward movement of scapula. I: Dorsal scapular nerve. A

7 **M. levator scapulae.** o: Posterior tubercle of transverse processes C1–4. i: Superior angle of scapula: F: Elevates superior angle of scapula and rotates neck. I: Dorsal scapular nerve. A

8 **M. serratus posterior inferior.** o: Spinous processes of T11–L2. i: Lower 4 ribs. F: Backward rotation of lower 4 ribs. I: Intercostal nerves. A

9 **M. serratus posterior superior.** o: Spinous processes of C6–T2. i: Ribs 2–5. F: Accessory muscle of inspiration. I: Intercostal nerves. A B

10 M. erector spinae. Collective term for the muscles of the lateral and medial tracts of the back. I: Dorsal rami of spinal nerves.

10 a [[Lateral tract]]. [Tractus laterale].

11 M. longissimus. It consists of three parts. B

12 M. longissimus thoracis. o: Iliac crest, spinous processes of L1–S4, mamillary processes of L1–2, transverse processes of T7–12. i: Costal and accessory processes of lumbar vertebrae, angle of lower 11 ribs, all thoracic transverse processes. F: Lateral and backward flexion of vertebral column. B C

13 M. longissimus cervicis. o: Transverse processes T1–6. i: Transverse processes C2–7. It lies between the iliocostalis cervicis and longissimus capitis muscles. C

14 M. longissimus capitis. o: Transverse processes C3–T3. i: Mastoid process. It lies between the longissimus cervicis and semispinalis capitis muscles. F: Lateral and backward flexion of the head. It rotates the face toward the same side. C

15 M. iliocostalis. It consists of three segments.

16 M. iliocostalis lumborum. o: Iliac crest. i: Angle of ribs 5–12. F: Extension and lateral flexion of lower vertebral column. B C

17 M. iliocostalis thoracis. o: Medial sides of 6 lower rib angles. i: Six uppermost rib angles. F: Flattening of thoracic kyphosis, lateral flexion. B C

18 M. iliocostalis cervicis. o: Upper and middle ribs. i: Transverse processes of middle cervical vertebrae. C

19 **M. splenius cervicis.** o: Spinous processes of T3–5. i: Posterior tubercle of transverse processes of C1–2. F: Backward flexion and rotation of head. B

20 **M. splenius capitis.** o: Spinous processes of C4–T3. i: External half of superior nuchal line and mastoid process. F: Backward flexion and rotation of head. A B

21 **Mm. intertransversarii.** Muscular connection of adjacent transverse processes. F: Lateral flexion. see 77 C D E

22 **Mm. intertransversarii laterales lumborum.** Between adjacent costal processes. I: Ventral rami of spinal nerves. see 77 C

23 **Mm. intertransversarii mediales lumborum.** Between the mamillary processes. see 77 C

24 **Mm. intertransversarii thoracis.** Usually absent. see 77 C

25 **Mm. intertransversarii posteriores cervicis.** Between the posterior tubercles of transverse processes of cervical vertebrae. see 77 D

26 *Pars medialis.* Medial part of 25.

27 *Pars lateralis.* Lateral part of 25. I: ventral ramus of spinal nerves.

28 **Mm. intertransversarii anteriores cervicis.** They connect the anterior tubercles of the cervical transverse processes. I: Ventral ramus of spinal nerves. see 77 E

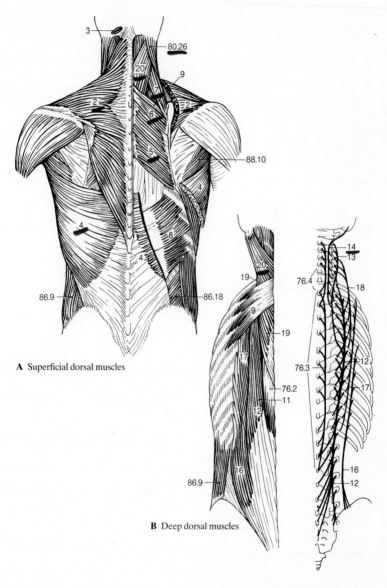

A Superficial dorsal muscles

B Deep dorsal muscles

C Autochthonous
dorsal muscles, schematic view

1 [[**Medial tract**]]. [Tractus mediale].

2 **M. spinalis.** Muscular system attached to the spinous processes and consisting of the following three segments: see 75 B

3 *M. spinalis thoracis.* o: Transverse processes of T11–L2. i: Spinous processes of T2–11. F: Back flexion. see 75 C

4 *M. spinalis cervicis.* o: Transverse processes of C6–T2. i: Spinous processes of C2–4. F: Back flexion. see 75 C

5 *M. spinalis capitis.* Inconstant part of semispinalis capitis with additional origins from the upper thoracic and lower cervical spinous processes.

6 **Mm. interspinales.** In contrast to the spinal muscles, these muscles extend only between the spinous processes of contiguous vertebrae. F: Dorsiflexion. C D

7 **Mm. interspinales cervicis.** These are doubled because of the bifid cervical spinous processes. D

8 **Mm. interspinales thoracis.** Usually absent. C

9 **Mm. interspinales lumborum.** These are especially strong. C

10 **Mm. transversospinales.** Collective term for the following nine muscles. A B C

11 **M. semispinalis.** The longest superficial portion of the transversospinales. It spans four or more vertebrae and comprises the following three segments:

12 *M. semispinalis thoracis.* o: Transverse processes of T7–12. i: Spinous processes of C6–T6. F: Primarily dorsiflexion. A

13 *M. semispinalis cervicis.* o: Transverse processes of T1–6. i: Spinous processes of C2–5. F: Mainly dorsiflexion. A

14 *M. semispinalis capitis.* o: Transverse processes of C4–T6. i: Occipital bone between superior and inferior nuchal lines. F: Dorsiflexion of head and rotation, depending upon starting position. A

15 **Mm. multifidi.** Portion of the transversospinal system spanning 2–4 vertebrae. F: Dorsolateral flexion and slight rotation. B

16 **Mm. rotatores.** Deepest layer of the transversospinal system with short fibers taking an especially transverse course and providing thereby a stronger rotation. They attach to an adjacent vertebra or to the one lying above it. A B C

17 *Mm. rotatores cervicis.* o: Inferior articular process. i: Arch or root of spinous process of cervical vertebrae. A

18 *Mm. rotatores thoracis.* o: Transverse process of thoracic vertebrae. i: Spinous process. A C

19 *Mm. rotatores lumborum.* o: Mamillary process. i: Roots of spinous process of lumbar vertebrae. A C

20 **Thoracolumbar fascia.** Fascia thoracolumbalis. Encasing fascia of the erector spinae muscle. It is attached to the spinous processes with a superficial layer, to the transverse processes with a deep layer, both layers being united laterally. Associated muscles: transversus abdominis, serrati posteriores, latissimus dorsi. F

21 **Nuchal fascia.** Fascia nuchae (nuchalis). Dorsal continuation of the superficial layer of the cervical fascia. (Investing fascia of the true neck musculature.)

22 HEAD MUSCLES. MUSCULI CAPITIS.

23 **Mm. suboccipitales.** The following seven muscles:

24 **M. rectus capitis anterior.** o: Lateral mass of the atlas. i: Basilar part of occipital bone. F: Forward flexion of head. I: Ventral rami of spinal nerves. E

25 **M. rectus capitis posterior major.** o: Spinous process of axis. i: Middle of inferior nuchal line. F: Outward rotation and dorsiflexion of head. I: Suboccipital nerve. D See 79A

26 **M. rectus capitis posterior minor.** o: Posterior tubercle of atlas. i: Inner third of inferior nuchal line. F: Mainly dorsiflexion of head. I: Suboccipital nerve. D See 79A

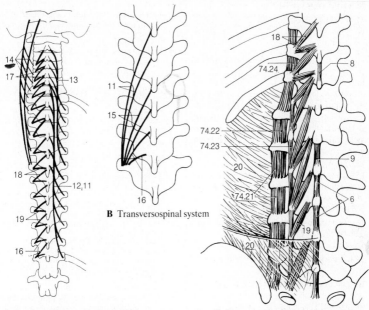

A Systems of Mm. transversospinales

B Transversospinal system

C Short muscles of the vertebral column

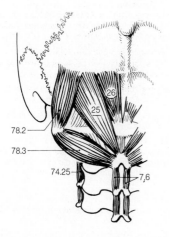

D Short neck muscles

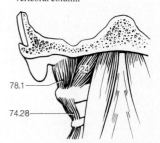

E Deep neck muscles, anterior view

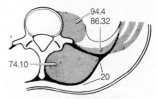

F Thoracolumbar fascia

1 **M. rectus capitis lateralis.** o: Transverse process of atlas. i: Jugular process of occipital bone. F: Lateral flexion of head. I: Ventral rami of spinal nerves C1–2. A B see 77 E

2 **M. obliquus capitis superior.** o: Transverse process of atlas. i: Field above attachment of rectus capitis posterior major. F: Backward and lateral flexion of head. I: Dorsal rami of spinal nerves C1–2. A see 77 D

3 **M. obliquus capitis inferior.** o: Spinous process of axis. i: Transverse process of atlas. F: Lateral rotation of atlas and face toward the same side. I: Dorsal rami of spinal nerves C1–2. A see 77 D

4 **M. longus capitis.** o: Anterior tubercle of transverse processes of C3–6. i: Basal part of occipital bone. F: Forward and lateral flexion of head and cervical vertebral column. I: Ventral rami of spinal nerves C1–2. B

5 **Facial and masticatory muscles.** Musculi faciales et masticatorii.

6 **M. epicranius.** Collective term for the muscles attaching to the galea aponeurotica. I: Facial nerve. C

7 M. occipitofrontalis. Musculature extending into the galea aponeurotica in front and behind. C

8 *Frontal belly.* Venter frontalis. The portion of the occipitofrontalis which passes from the galea aponeurotica to the eyebrows. F: Moves scalp forward and raises the eyebrows. C

9 *Occipital belly.* Venter occipitalis. The portion of the occipitofrontalis which passes from the supreme nuchal line to the galea aponeurotica. F: Moves galea aponeurotica backward. C

10 M. temporoparietalis. o: Region of superior auricular muscle. i: Galea aponeurotica. C

11 Galea aponeurotica (Aponeurosis epicranialis). Displaceable, helmet-like, superficial tendon for the two parts of the epicranius. It lies against the periosteum and is attached to the supreme nuchal line and to the external occipital protuberance. C

12 **M. procerus.** o: Dorsum of nose. i: Skin above the nose. F: Depression of frontal skin. I: Facial nerve. C

13 **M. nasalis.** Common term for the following two nasal muscles: I: Facial nerve. D

14 Transverse part of nasalis. Pars transversa [[Compressor naris]]. o: Field over root of canine tooth. i: Superficial tendon on dorsum of nose. D

15 Alar part of nasalis. Pars alaris [[Dilatator naris]]. o: Over the lateral incisor tooth. i: Margins of the nasal openings and the adjacent region. D

16 **M. depressor septi.** o: Over the medial incisor tooth. i: Cartilaginous nasal septum. F: Depresses tip of nose. I: Facial nerve. D

17 **M. orbicularis oculi.** Circular sphincter muscle of the eye. Comprises three segments. It closes the eyelids and assists the flow of tears into the lacrimal sac and into the nose. I: Facial nerve. C D

18 Palpebral part. Pars palpebralis. Fibers situated in the eyelids passing from the medial palpebral ligament and the adjacent bones to the lateral palpebral ligament. C

19 Orbital part. Pars orbitalis. Arising from the medial palpebral ligament and adjacent bones, this part encircles the eye. C

20 Lacrimal part. Pars lacrimalis. o: Posterior lacrimal crest. It curves around the lacrimal canaliculus, lies partially behind the lacrimal sac and radiates into the palpebral part below the medial palpebral ligament. D

21 **M. corrugator supercilii.** o: Nasal part of frontal bone. i: Skin over the middle of the eyebrow. It lies below the orbicularis oculi muscle. I: Facial nerve. D

22 **M. depressor supercilii.** It lies medial to the corrugator supercilii and radiates from the orbicular oculi into the skin of the medial part of the eyebrow. I: Facial nerve. D

23 **M. auricularis anterior.** It lies in front of the ear. o: Temporal fascia. i: Spine of helix. I: Facial nerve. C

24 **M. auricularis superior.** o: Galea aponeurotica. i: Root of pinna. I: Facial nerve. C

25 **M. auricularis posterior.** o: Mastoid process. i: Root of pinna. I: Facial nerve. C

26 **M. orbicularis oris.** Encircles the mouth opening and consists of the following two parts: It assists in closing the lips and helps to empty the vestibule of the mouth. I: Facial nerve. C D E

27 Marginal part. Pars marginalis. The peripheral margin radiating into the neighboring muscles. D

28 Labial part. Pars labialis. The main part of the orbicularis oris including the portion which takes a hook-like bend externally below the red portion of the lips. C D E

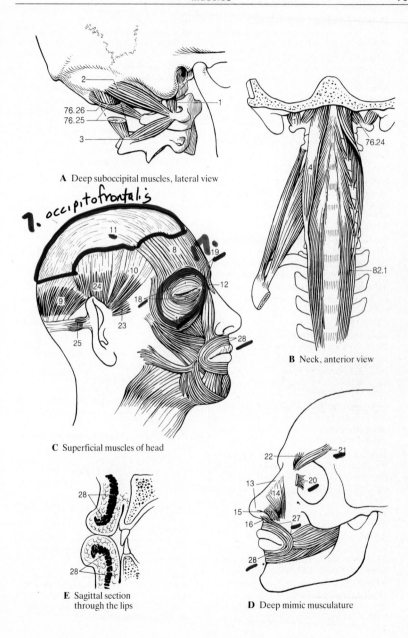

A Deep suboccipital muscles, lateral view

7. occipitofrontalis

B Neck, anterior view

C Superficial muscles of head

E Sagittal section through the lips

D Deep mimic musculature

80 **Muscles**

1 **M. depressor anguli oris.** [[Triangularis]]. o: Anterior and lateral part of mandible. i: Angle of mouth. I: Facial nerve. A

2 **M. transversus menti.** Transverse muscular connection between the right and left depressor anguli oris muscles below the chin. I: Facial nerve. A

3 **M. risorius.** o: Parotid fascia and buccal skin. i: Angle of mouth. I: Facial nerve. A

4 **M. zygomaticus major.** o: Lateral side of zygomatic bone. i: Angle of mouth. I: Facial nerve. A

5 **M. zygomaticus minor.** o: Anterior side of zygomatic bone. i: Upper lip. I: Facial nerve. A

6 **M. levator labii superioris** [[Quadratus labii sup., M. levator nasi et labii maxillaris lat.]]. o: Above the infra-orbital foramen. Radiates into orbicularis oris. I: Facial nerve. A

7 **M. levator labii superioris alaeque nasi** [[Quadratus labii sup., M. lev. nasi et labii maxillaris med]]. o: Medial to orbit. i: Nasal ala and upper lip. I: Facial nerve. A

8 **M. depressor labii inferioris** [[Quadr. labii inf.]]. Located below the depressor anguli oris. o: Platysma and mandible. i: Lower lip. I: Facial nerve. A

9 **M. levator anguli oris** [[Caninus]]. o: Canine fossa. i: angle of mouth. I: Facial nerve. A

9 a **Modiolus.** Palpable muscular point lateral to the angle of the mouth. Point of convergence of adjacent muscles radiating into the orbicularis oris.

10 **M. buccinator.** Cheek muscle. o: Pterygomandibular raphe and adjoining parts of upper and lower jaw. i: Angle of mouth and orbicularis oris. I: Facial nerve. A B

11 **M. mentalis.** Over the roots of the lower incisors. i: Skin of chin (chin dimple). I: Facial nerve. A

12 **M. masseter.** External masticatory muscle. It closes the rows of teeth and is important for masticatory pressure. It consists of the following two parts: I: Mandibular nerve. A C

13 Superficial part. *Pars superficialis*. o: Anterior two-thirds of zygomatic arch. i: Angle of mandible. It courses obliquely backward and downward. It also draws the mandible somewhat forward. C

14 Deep part. *Pars profunda*. o: Posterior two-thirds of zygomatic arch. i: Mandible. It courses obliquely forward and downward. C

15 **M. temporalis.** o: Temporal fossa. i: Coronoid process of mandible and from there downward as far as the level of the occlusal plane. F: Elevates and draws mandible backward. I: Mandibular nerve. B

16 **Lateral pterygoid muscle.** M. pterygoideus lateralis. o: Lateral surface of lateral pterygoid plate and lower surface of greater wing of sphenoid. i: Two-headed: at the articular disc of mandible and into pterygoid fovea on condylar process of the mandible. F: It pulls the articular disc and mandible forward. The upper head controls the velocity of disc backward movement. I: Mandibular nerve. B

17 **Medial pterygoid muscle.** M. pterygoideus medialis. o: Pterygoid fossa and tuber of maxilla. i: Pterygoid tuberosity and inner aspect of angle of mandible. It courses obliquely downward and backward and is a synergist to the temporalis and masseter muscles. I: Mandibular nerve. B

18 **Buccopharyngeal fascia.** Fascia buccopharyngea. It lies on the buccinator muscle and extends from the angle of the mouth deeply as far as the pharyngeal constrictor muscle. C

19 **Masseteric fascia.** Fascia masseterica. Fascia covering the masseter muscle, partly attached below to the parotid, above to the zygomatic arch. D

20 **Parotid fascia.** Fascia parotidea. Fascial covering of the parotid, partly identical with the masseteric fascia. D

21 **Temporal fascia.** Fascia temporalis. External connective tissue investment of the temporalis muscle between the superior temporal line and the zygomatic arch. It consists of the following two layers. D

22 Superficial layer. Lamina superficialis. Layer of the temporal fascia attached to the outer margin of the zygomatic arch. D

23 Deep layer. Lamina profunda. Layer of the temporal fascia attached to the inner margin of the zygomatic arch. D

24 NECK MUSCLES. MUSCULI COLLI (CERVICIS). A C

25 **Platysma.** Cutaneous muscle occupying an extensive area in the neck. It extends from the lower part of the face to the upper thorax. I: Facial nerve. A D

26 **Sternocleidomastoid muscle.** M. sternocleidomastoideus. o: Sternum and clavicle. i: Mastoid process and superior nuchal line. It elevates the chin and rotates it to the opposite side. I: Accessory nerve. C

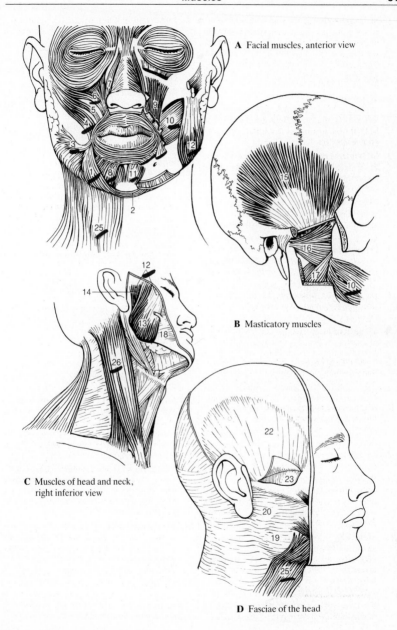

A Facial muscles, anterior view

B Masticatory muscles

C Muscles of head and neck, right inferior view

D Fasciae of the head

1 **M. longus colli.** Connects, arch-like, the vertebral bodies of C2–5 with those of the lower cervical and upper thoracic. Fibers also extend from the vertebral bodies to the transverse processes with the C6 transverse process as the central point. F: Lateral and forward flexion of the neck. I: Ventral ramus of spinal nerve. D

2 **M. scalenus anterior.** o: Transverse processes of C3–6. i: Scalene tubercle on 1st rib. F: Elevation of 1st rib, lateral flexion and rotation of neck. It separates the anterior from the posterior scalenus gaps. I: See 1.D

3 **M. scalenus medius.** o: Transverse processes of C2–7. i: 1st rib behind groove for subclavian artery. F: Elevation of 1st rib and lateral flexion of neck. I: See 1.D

4 **M. scalenus posterior.** o: Transverse processes of C4–6. i: Upper margin of 2nd rib. F: Elevates the rib, laterally flexes the neck. I: See 1.D

5 **[M. scalenus minimus].** Extra muscle occasionally present between scalenus anterior and medius. o: Transverse process of C6 or 7. i: 1st rib and pleural cupola.

6 **Suprahyoid muscles.** M. suprahyoidei. The following muscles above the hyoid bone. A

M. digastricus. o: Notch medial to the mastoid process. i: Inner side of mandible. It has an intermediate tendon which acts on the lesser horn of the hyoid bone by means of a connective tissue sling. F: Elevation of hyoid. A

8 Anterior belly. Venter anterior. It extends from the mandible to the intermediate tendon. F: Pulls mandible forward and depresses it. I: Mylohyoid nerve. A E

9 Posterior belly. Venter posterior. It passes from the mastoid process to the intermediate tendon. F: It draws back the hyoid bone. I: Facial nerve. A E

10 **M. stylohyoideus.** o: Styloid process. i: Lesser horn of hyoid bone. It accompanies the posterior belly of the digastric and can pass through it via a fissure. F: It pulls the hyoid backward and upward. I: Facial nerve. A E

11 **M. mylohyoideus.** Muscle of the floor of the mouth. o: Mylohyoid line of mandible. i: Body of hyoid bone. F: Draws the hyoid forward and upward and forms the diaphragma oris. I: Mylohyoid nerve. A B

12 **M. ~~geniohyoideus~~ hyoglossus** o: Mental spine. i: Body of hyoid bone. F: Draws the hyoid forward and upward. I: C1 via the hypoglossal nerve. B

13 **Infrahyoid muscles.** Mm. infrahyoidei. The muscles below the hyoid bone (infrahyale M.). I: Ansa cervicalis. A

14 **M. sternohyoideus.** o: Posterior surface of manubrium sterni. i: Body of hyoid bone. F: Draws the hyoid downward. I: See 13. A

15 **M. omohyoideus.** o: Upper margin of scapula medial to scapular notch. i: Body of hyoid bone. An intermediate tendon situated above the jugular vein divides it into two bellies. F: It draws the hyoid downward and tenses the cervical fascia. I: See 13. A C

16 Superior belly. Venter superior. Upper segment of omohyoid between the hyoid and intermediate tendon. A

17 Inferior belly. Venter inferior. Lower half of omohyoid from the intermediate tendon to the scapular notch. A

18 **M. sternothyroideus.** o: Posterior surface of manubrium and 1st rib. i: Oblique line of thyroid cartilage. F: Draws larynx downward. I: See 13. A

19 **M. thyrohyoideus.** o: Oblique line of thyroid cartilage. i: Greater horn of hyoid bone. F: Brings hyoid and thyroid cartilage closer together. I: C1 via hypoglossal nerve. A

20 **[M. levator glandulae thyroideae].** A splitting off of the thyrohyoid muscle to the thyroid gland.

21 **Cervical fascia.** Fascia cervicalis. Collective term for the connective tissue layers of the neck.

22 Superficial (investing) layer. Lamina superficialis. Superficial layer of cervical fascia. It surrounds the sternocleidomastoid and trapezius muscles. It is attached to the anterior margin of the manubrium, the clavicle and the mandible. C

23 Pretracheal layer. Lamina pretrachealis. It lies spread out between the two omohyoid muscles and is attached to the posterior margin of the manubrium and clavicle. It surrounds the infrahyoid muscles. C

24 Prevertebral layer. Lamina prevertebralis. It lies between the vertebral column and pharyngeal constrictors as well as the esophagus, covers the scaleni muscles and contains the sympathetic trunk and phrenic nerve. C

25 Carotid sheath. Vagina carotica. Connective tissue investing the neurovascular bundle (carotid artery, jugular vein and vagus nerve) and continuous with the pretracheal layer. C

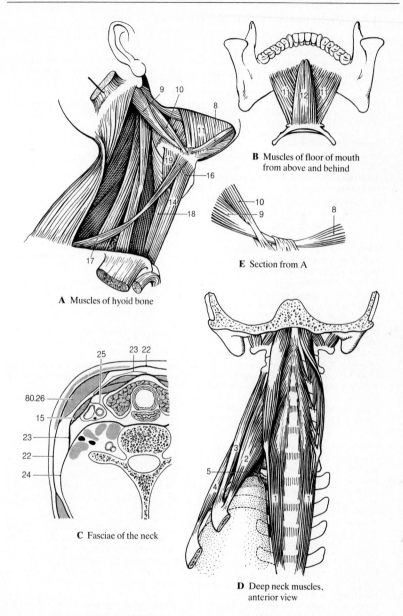

A Muscles of hyoid bone

B Muscles of floor of mouth from above and behind

E Section from A

C Fasciae of the neck

D Deep neck muscles, anterior view

1   MUSCLES OF THORAX. MUSCULI THORA-
CIS. A–F

2   [M. sternalis]. Variable (4%). It crosses the pectoralis major muscle parallel to and near the sternum. A

3   M. pectoralis major. It consists of the following
three parts (4–6). o: Clavicle, sternum, first 4–6
costal cartilages and rectus sheath. i: Crest of greater tubercle of humerus. F: Adduction and medial
rotation of arm. I: Medial and lateral pectoral
nerves. A

4   Clavicular part. Pars clavicularis. The portion
originating from the clavicle. A

5   Sternocostal part. Pars sternocostalis. The portion arising from the sternum and ribs. A

6   Abdominal part. Pars abdominalis. The portion
arising from the rectus sheath. A

7   M. pectoralis minor. It lies beneath the pectoralis
major. o: Ribs 3–5. i: Coracoid process. F: Draws
scapula forward and downward and ribs upward.
Accessory respiratory muscle. I: See 3. A

8   M. subclavius. o: 1st costal cartilage. i: Lower
surface of clavicle. F: Stabilizes sternoclavicular
joint against tension. I: Nerve to subclavius. A

9   Pectoral fascia. Fascia pectoralis. It covers the
pectoralis major muscle, is attached to the clavicle
and sternum and is continuous with the axillary
fascia.

10 Clavipectoral fascia. Fascia clavipectoralis. It is
attached to the coracoid process and the clavicle;
it covers the pectoralis minor and subclavius
muscles. A

11 M. serratus anterior. o: Ribs 1–9. i: Medial margin of scapula. F: Fixes, lowers and rotates scapula and draws it forward. It assists in raising the arm
high above the horizontal plane. I: Long thoracic
nerve. A

12 Mm. levatores costarum. They lie behind and below the long back muscles. o: Thoracic transverse
processes. i: Ribs. I: Dorsal rami of spinal nerves.
B

13 Mm. levatores costarum longi. o: Transverse processes. i: A rib is passed over to insert on
the next lower rib. F: Elevates rib. B

14 Mm. levatores costarum breves. o: Transverse process. i: Next lower rib. B

15 External intercostal muscles. Mm. intercostales
externi. They extend obliquely forward and
downward between the ribs. F: Inspiration.
Bracing of the ribs. I: Intercostal nerves. A E F

16 External intercostal membrane. Membrana intercostalis externa. Membranous continuation of
the external intercostal muscles anteriorly between the costal cartilages. A

17 Internal intercostal muscles. Mm. intercostales
interni. They pass between the ribs obliquely
backward and downward. F: Partially expiratory.
Bracing of the ribs. I: Intercostal nerves. E F

18 Internal intercostal membrane. Membrana intercostalis interna. Continuation of the internal intercostal muscles from the rib angle to the vertebral body. E

19 Innermost intercostal muscles. Mm. intercostales intimi. Internally separated portion of the internal intercostal muscles caused by the intercostal
vessels. F

20 Subcostal muscles. Mm. subcostales. Internal intercostal muscles that pass over 1–2 ribs. I: See
17.E

21 M. transversus thoracis. Situated on the inner
surface of the anterior thoracic wall, it radiates obliquely upward from the sternum to costal cartilages 2–6. I: See 17.C

22 Thoracic fascia. Fascia thoracica. Epimysium of
the thoracic inner musculature.

23 Diaphragm. Diaphragma [thoraco-abdominale].
Dome-shaped, muscular partition between the
thoracic and abdominal cavities. I: Phrenic nerve.
C D

24 Lumbar part of diaphragm. Pars lumbalis diaphragmatis. Medial part of the diaphragm arising
from the lumbar vertebral bodies, intervertebral
discs and fibrous arches. D

25 Right crus of lumbar part. Crus dextrum. o:
L1–3(4). D

26 Left crus of lumbar part. Crus sinistrum. o:
L1–2(3). D

27 Costal part of diaphragm. Pars costalis diaphragmatis. The part of the diaphragm originating
from ribs 7–12. C D

28 Sternal part of diaphragm. Pars sternalis diaphragmatis. The part of the diaphragm arising
from the sternum. C D

29 Aortic (opening) hiatus. Hiatus aorticus. Passageway for the aorta between the right and left crus
of the lumbar part. D

30 Esophageal (opening) hiatus. Hiatus oesophage-
us. Passageway for the esophagus and the vagus
nerves above the aortic opening. D

31 Central tendon. Centrum tendineum. Cloverleaf-
shaped, tendinous central area of the diaphragm. D

32 Foramen for the inferior vena cava. Foramen
venae cavae. Opening in the central tendon for the
inferior vena cava. D

33 Medial arcuate ligament. Lig. arcuatum mediale. Tendinous arch between the body and transverse process of L1 or L2 forming the passageway
for the psoas muscle. D

34 Lateral arcuate ligament. Lig. arcuatum laterale.
Tendinous arch over the quadratus lumborum
muscle between the transverse process of L1 and
the 12th rib. D

35 Median arcuate ligament. Lig. arcuatum medianum. Tendinous arch over the aortic hiatus. D

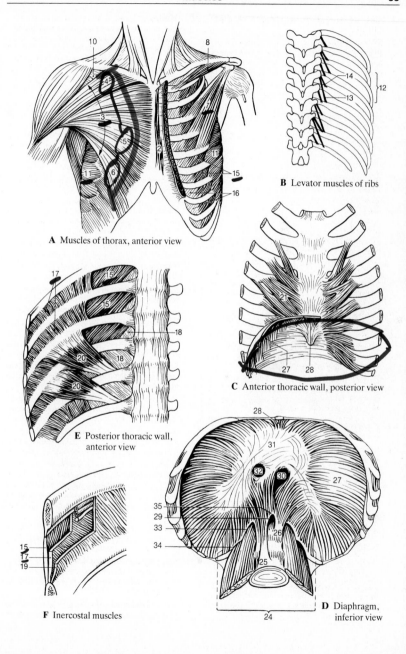

A Muscles of thorax, anterior view

B Levator muscles of ribs

C Anterior thoracic wall, posterior view

E Posterior thoracic wall, anterior view

F Intercostal muscles

D Diaphragm, inferior view

1 ABDOMINAL MUSCLES. MUSCULI ABDO-
MINIS.

2 **M. rectus abdominis.** o: Costal cartilages 5–7. i:
Pubis and symphysis. F: Forward flexion of trunk.
Lowering of thorax. Elevation of pelvis. I: Inter-
costal nerves 7–12. A E

3 Tendinous intersections. Intersectiones tendineae. The 3–4 intermediate tendons of the rectus
abdominis muscle. They fuse with the anterior
wall of the rectus sheath. A

4 Rectus sheath. Vagina m. recti abdominis.
Covering of the rectus abdominis muscle formed
by the aponeuroses of the flat abdominal muscles.
A

5 *Anterior layer of rectus sheath.* Lamina anterior. A

6 *Posterior layer of rectus sheath.* Lamina posterior.
A

7 *Arcuate line.* Linea arcuata. Caudal end of the
posterior layer of the rectus sheath. A

8 **M. pyramidalis.** It is enclosed within the split anterior layer of the rectus sheath and passes from the
pubis and symphysis to the linea alba. I: Subcostal
nerve. A

9 **External abdominal oblique muscle.** M. obliquus externus abdominis. o: Outer surface of ribs
5–12. i: Iliac crest, rectus sheath, linea alba. F:
Lowering of thorax, rotation of trunk, lateral flexion. I: Intercostal nerves 5–12. A B D

10 Inguinal ligament. Lig. inguinale (Arcus in-
~ guinalis). The lower edge of the external oblique
aponeurosis. It passes from anterior superior iliac
spine to the pubic tubercle. D E

11 *Lacunar ligament.* Lig. lacunare. Connective tissue fibers extending arch-like downward to the pubis at the medial attachment of inguinal ligament.
D

12 *Pectineal ligament.* Lig. pectineale. Continuation
of the lacunar ligament to the pecten pubis. D

13 *Reflected ligament.* Lig. reflexum. Bow-shaped
band of fibers passing upward from the medial
attachment of the inguinal ligament and forming
the medial lining of the superficial inguinal ring. D

14 Superficial inguinal ring. Anulus inguinalis
~ superficialis. External opening of the inguinal canal. A D

15 *Medial crus.* Crus mediale. Group of fibers of the
external oblique aponeurosis ascending obliquely
medial to the superficial inguinal ring. D

16 *Lateral crus.* Crus laterale. Group of fibers of the
external oblique aponeurosis ascending lateral to
the superficial inguinal ring. D

17 *Intercrural fibers.* Fibrae intercrurales. Bow-
shaped fibers between the medial and lateral
crura. D

18 **Internal abdominal oblique muscle.** M. obliquus internus abdominis. o: Thoracolumbar fascia, iliac crest, inguinal ligament. i: Ribs 10–12
and rectus sheath. F: Lowering of ribs, forward
and lateral flexion. I: Intercostal nerves 8–12, iliohypogastric and ilio-inguinal nerves. A B

19 M. cremaster. Muscle fibers derived primarily
from the internal abdominal oblique. It invests the
spermatic cord and elevates the testis. A

20 **M. transversus abdominis.** o: Inner surface of
ribs 7–12, thoracolumbar fascia, iliac crest, inguinal ligament. i: Rectus sheath. I: Intercostal nerves
7–12, iliohypogastric, ilio-inguinal, genitofemoral nerves. A

21 Conjoined tendon. Falx inguinalis (Tendo con-
junctivus). Fibers radiating arch-like from the
aponeurosis of the transversus into the pectineal ligament. A E

22 **Linea alba.** The white tendinous stripe (Raphe) of
the abdominal aponeuroses situated between the
right and left rectus abdominis muscles. A E

23 Umbilical ring. Anulus umbilicalis. Fibrous
ring around the umbilicus in the linea alba. A

24 Adminiculum lineae albae. Inferior attachment of the linea alba at the symphysis. A E

25 **Suspensory ligament of penis (clitoris).** Lig. suspensorium penis/clitoridis. It radiates from the pubis into the deep fascia of the penis (clitoris). A

26 **Fundiform ligament of penis.** Lig. fundiforme
penis. Elastic band arising from the abdominal
fascia and linea alba and extending sling-like
onto the penis. A

27 **Lumbar triangle.** Trigonum lumbale. Weak area
at the back bordered by the latissimus dorsi, external abdominal oblique and iliac crest. B

28 **Transversalis fascia.** Fascia transversalis. Fascia
between the peritoneum and abdominal musculature. A E

29 Deep inguinal ring. Anulus inguinalis profundus. Inner inguinal ring at the transition of the
transversalis fascia into the internal spermatic
fascia. A E

30 **Inguinal canal.** Canalis inguinalis. Walls: Inguinal ligament, external oblique aponeurosis, internal oblique and transversus abdominis muscles,
interfoveolar ligament. It contains the spermatic
cord. E

31 **Interfoveolar ligament.** Lig. interfoveolare.
Thickened portion of the transversalis fascia behind the inguinal canal. A E

32 **M. quadratus lumborum.** o: Iliac crest and processes of lumbar vertebrae. i: 12th rib, transverse
processes of lumbar vertebrae. F: Lower ribs, lateral flexion. I: See 20. C

33 **Linea semilunaris.** Bow-shaped musculotendi-
nous margin of the transversus abdominis muscle.

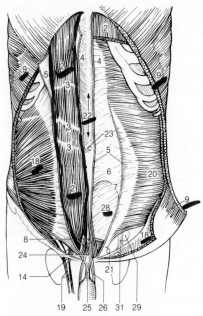

A Abdominal muscles, anterior view

19 25 26 31 29

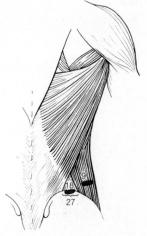

B Lumbar triangle

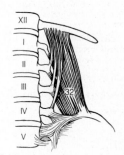

C Musculus quadratus lumborum, anterior view

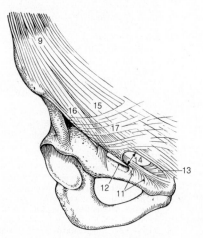

D Inguinal region, anterior view

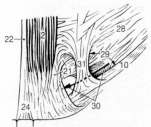

E Inguinal region, posterior view

1 COCCYGEAL MUSCLES. MUSCULI COCCYGEI.

2 **M. coccygeus.** o: Ischial spine. i: Coccyx and adjoining sacrum. It lies medial to the sacrospinous ligament. I: Spinal nerve. A See also 174.13.

3 [[**Ventral (anterior) sacrococcygeus muscle**]]. M. sacrococcygeus ventralis. Occasional rudiment of the primitive coccygeal musculature passing anteriorly from the sacrum to the coccyx. A

4 [[**Dorsal (posterior) sacrococcygeus muscle**]]. M. sacrococcygeus dorsalis. Rudimentary remnant of coccygeal musculature passing posteriorly from the sacrum to the coccyx. A

5 MUSCLES OF THE UPPER LIMB. MUSCULI MEMBRI SUPERIORIS.

6 **M. deltoideus.** o: Spine of scapula, acromion, clavicle. i: Deltoid tuberosity of humerus. F: Lateral and medial rotation, abduction, adduction, forward and backward flexion. I: Axillary nerve. B E F G

7 **M. supraspinatus.** o: Supraspinous fossa. i: Greater tubercle of humerus. F: Abduction, medial and lateral rotation. I: Suprascapular nerve. B E F G

8 **M. infraspinatus.** o: Infraspinous fossa. i: Greater tubercle of humerus. F: Lateral rotation. I: Suprascapular nerve. B F G

9 **M. teres minor.** o: Beside the infraspinatus muscle. i: Greater tubercle. F: Lateral rotation and weak adduction. I: Axillary nerve. B F G

10 **M. teres major.** o: Lateral margin of scapula. i: Crest of lesser tubercle. F: Medial rotation and adduction with dorsiflexion of arm. I: Subscapular nerve. B D E G

11 **M. subscapularis.** o: Subscapular fossa. i: Lesser tubercle. Medial rotation of arm. I: Subscapular nerve. C D E

12 **M. biceps brachii.** Two headed upper arm muscle with the following parts (13–15). i: Radial tuberosity and ulna via the bicipital aponeurosis. F: Flexion and supination at the elbow joint. I: Musculocutaneous nerve. D

13 Long head of biceps. Caput longum. o: Supraglenoid tubercle. i: Radial tuberosity and ulna. F: Flexion at the elbow joint and supination, weak abduction at the shoulder joint. C D

14 *Intertubercular tendon sheath.* Vagina tendinis intertubercularis. Synovial sheath for the tendon of the long head of the biceps in the intertubercular groove. D

15 Short head of biceps. Caput breve. o: Coracoid process. i: Radial tuberosity of ulna. F: Flexion at the elbow joint and supination. Moreover, forward flexion of the arm at the shoulder joint. C D

16 Bicipital aponeurosis. Aponeurosis m. bicipitis brachii (Aponeurosis bicipitalis) [[Lacertus fibrosus]]. Aponeurotic expansion of the biceps tendon medially into the forearm fascia. F: Transmits the pull of the biceps to the ulna when the arm is supinated. D

17 **M. coracobrachialis.** o: Coracoid process. i: Middle third of humerus anteriorly. F: Forward flexion, weak adduction and medial rotation of the arm. I: Musculocutaneous nerve. C D E

18 **M. brachialis.** o: Lower 2/3 of anterior surface of humerus. i: Ulnar tuberosity. F: Flexor at the elbow joint. I: Musculocutaneous nerve. D E F

19 **M. triceps brachii.** Three-headed upper arm muscle with common attachment to the olecranon. G

20 Long head of triceps. Caput longum. o: Infraglenoid tubercle. i: Olecranon. F: Extension at the elbow joint, adduction at the shoulder joint. It separates the medial (triangular) from the lateral (quadrangular) space. B C D G

21 Lateral head of triceps. Caput laterale. o: Posterior surface of humerus lateral and proximal to groove for radial nerve. i: Olecranon. F: Extension at the elbow joint. F G

22 Medial head of triceps. Caput mediale. o: Medial and distal to groove for radial nerve. i: Olecranon. F: Extension at the elbow joint. F G

23 **Superior and inferior apertures.** [[Aperturae superior et inferior]]. Medial and lateral ends of the fascial cone for the large neurovascular bundles in the axilla.

24 **M. anconaeus.** o: Lateral humeral epicondyle. Continuation of medial head of triceps. i: Lateral margin of olecranon and posterior surface of ulna. F: Extension at the elbow joint. I: Radial nerve. G

25 **M. articularis cubiti.** Articular muscle of elbow. Fibers passing from the triceps brachii to the articular capsule. F: Tenses the capsule. I: Radial nerve.

26 **M. pronator teres.** o: Medial epicondyle of humerus and coronoid process of ulna. i: Middle of lateral surface of radius. F: Pronation and flexion at the elbow joint. I: Median nerve. D

27 Humeral head of pronator teres. Caput humerale. The portion arising from the medial epicondyle. D E

28 Ulnar head of pronator teres. Caput ulnare. The part arising from the coronoid process. D

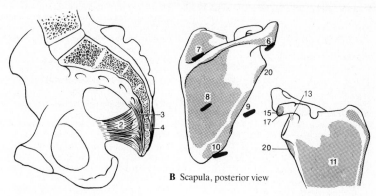

A Right half of pelvis, medial view

B Scapula, posterior view

C Scapula, anterior view

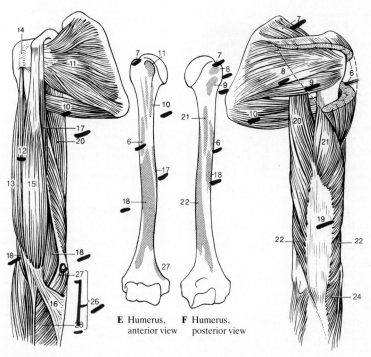

D Upper arm, anterior view

E Humerus, anterior view

F Humerus, posterior view

G Upper arm, posterior view

1 **M. flexor carpi radialis.** o: Medial epicondyle of humerus. i: Base of 2nd metacarpal bone. F: Pronation, flexion and radial abduction at the wrist joint. I: Median nerve. A

2 **M. palmaris longus.** o: Medial epicondyle of humerus. i: Palmar aponeurosis. F: Tenses aponeurosis and flexes at the wrist joint and fingers 2–5 at the metacarpophalangeal joints. Its tendon lies above the flexor retinaculum. I: Median nerve. A

3 **M. flexor carpi ulnaris.** o: Medial epicondyle of humerus, olecranon and ulna. i: Pisiform bone as well as hamate and 5th metacarpal bones via the pisohamate and pisometacarpal ligaments. F: Ulnar abduction and flexion at the wrist joint. I: Ulnar nerve. A

4 Humeral head of flexor carpi ulnaris. Caput humerale. The part arising from the epicondyle of the humerus.

5 Ulnar head of flexor carpi ulnaris. Caput ulnare. The portion originating from the ulna. E

6 **M. flexor digitorum superficialis.** o: Medial epicondyle of humerus, coronoid process of ulna and anterior surface of radius. i: Middle phalanx of fingers 2–5. F: Flexion at all joints it crosses. Each tendon is perforated by the corresponding tendon from the flexor digitorum profundus. I: Median nerve. A B

7 Humeroulnar head of flexor digitorum superficialis. Caput humeroulnare. The portion arising from the humerus and ulna. A E F

8 Radial head of flexor digitorum superficialis. Caput radiale. The portion arising from the radius. A E

9 **M. flexor digitorum profundus.** o: Upper half of ulna. i: Base of distal phalanges of fingers 2–5. F: Flexion of all joints crossed. The tendon perforates the corresponding superficial flexor tendon. I: Median and ulnar nerves. B E F

10 **M. flexor pollicis longus.** o: Middle of anterior surface of radius and usually the medial epicondyle. i: Distal phalanx of thumb. F: Flexion of joints crossed. I: Median nerve. B E

11 **M. pronator quadratus.** o: Lower fourth of anterior surface of ulna. i: Lower fourth of anterior surface of radius. F: Pronation. I: Median nerve. A B E

12 **M. brachioradialis.** o: Intermuscular septum and lateral margin of humerus. i: Styloid process of radius. F: Flexion at the elbow joint. It brings the arm from the extreme pronation and supination position to the intermediate position. I: Radial nerve. A C E

13 **M. extensor carpi radialis longus.** o: Lateral intermuscular septum, lateral epicondyle. i: Extensor side of metacarpal 2. F: Radial abduction and dorsiflexion at the wrist joint. Flexion at the elbow joint. I: Radial nerve. A C

14 **M. extensor carpi radialis brevis.** o: Lateral epicondyle of humerus. i: Proximal extensor side of metacarpal 3. F: Extension and radial abduction of wrist joint. I: Radial nerve. C

15 **M. extensor digitorum.** o: Lateral epicondyle of humerus. i: Distal phalanges 2–5 via their dorsal aponeuroses. F: Extension of fingers and dorsiflexion at the wrist joint. I: Radial nerve. C

16 Intertendinous connections. Connexus intertendineus [[Juncturae tendineum]]. Oblique tendinous connections between the extensor tendons of the fingers on the dorsum of the hand. C

17 **M. extensor digiti minimi.** o: Lateral epicondyle of humerus. i: Dorsal aponeurosis of 5th finger. F: Extension of little finger, abduction and dorsiflexion at the wrist joint. I: Radial nerve. C

18 **M. extensor carpi ulnaris.** o: Lateral epicondyle of humerus, radial collateral ligament, posterior surface of ulna. i: Base of 5th metacarpal. F: Dorsiflexion, ulnar abduction. I: Radial nerve. C D

19 Humeral head of extensor carpi ulnaris. Caput humerale. The part arising from the humerus.

20 Ulnar head of extensor carpi ulnaris. Caput ulnare. The portion arising from the ulna. F

21 **M. supinator.** o: Lateral epicondyle, radial collateral ligament, supinator crest of ulna. i: Anterior surface of radius. F: Supination. I: Radial nerve. D E F

22 **M. abductor pollicis longus.** o: Dorsal side of interosseous membrane and adjacent surfaces of radius and ulna. i: Base of 1st metacarpal. F: Radial abduction and dorsiflexion at the metacarpophalangeal joint of the thumb. Supination. I: Radial nerve. C D F

23 **M. extensor pollicis brevis.** o: Radius (extensor side) and interosseous membrane. i: Base of proximal phalanx of thumb. F: Abduction and extension of thumb at the metacarpophalangeal joint. I: Radial nerve. C D F

24 **M. extensor pollicis longus.** o: Interosseous membrane and dorsal surface of ulna. i: Distal phalanx of thumb. F: Adducts and extends the thumb. Supinator. I: Radial nerve. C D F

25 **M. extensor indicis.** o: Interosseous membrane and dorsal surface of ulna. i: Dorsal aponeurosis of index finger. F: Extends the index finger and wrist joint. I: Radial nerve. D F

26 **M. palmaris brevis.** o: Ulnar side of palmar aponeurosis. i: Skin of ulnar aspect of hand. I: Ulnar nerve. A

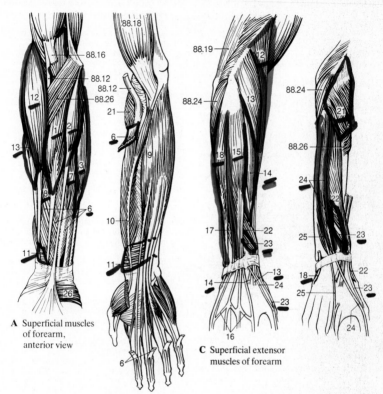

A Superficial muscles
of forearm,
anterior view

B Deep muscles of forearm,
anterior view

C Superficial extensor
muscles of forearm

D Deep extensor muscles
of forearm

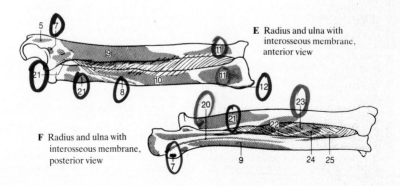

E Radius and ulna with
interosseous membrane,
anterior view

F Radius and ulna with
interosseous membrane,
posterior view

1   **M. abductor pollicis brevis.** o: Scaphoid bone and flexor retinaculum. i: Lateral sesamoid bone and radially at the proximal phalanx of the thumb. F: Abduction and flexion of the thumb. I: Median nerve. B

2   **M. flexor pollicis brevis.** o: Carpal bones, base of 1st metacarpal and flexor retinaculum. i: Lateral sesamoid bone, radial aspect of proximal phalanx of thumb. F: Adducts and flexes thumb. B

3   Superficial head of flexor pollicis brevis. Caput superficiale. The portion situated on the tendon of the flexor pollicis longus and innervated by the median nerve. B

4   Deep head of flexor pollicis brevis. Caput profundum. The portion situated below the tendon of the flexor pollicis longus and supplied by the ulnar nerve. B

5   **M. opponens pollicis.** o: Trapezium and flexor retinaculum. i: First metacarpal. F: Adduction and opposition of thumb. I: Median nerve. B

6   **M. adductor pollicis.** o: Capitate, radiate carpal ligament, metacarpal bone 3. i: Medial sesamoid bone, ulnar aspect of base of proximal phalanx of thumb. F: Adduction and opposition of thumb. I: Ulnar nerve. B

7   Oblique head of adductor pollicis. Caput obliquum. The portion arising from the capitate and radiate carpal ligament. B

8   Transverse head of adductor pollicis. Caput transversum. The portion originating from the 3rd metacarpal bone. B

9   **M. abductor digiti minimi.** o: Pisiform and flexor retinaculum. i: Base of proximal phalanx of little finger and dorsal aponeurosis. F: Abduction, flexion and extension of the little finger. I: Ulnar nerve. B

10 **M. flexor digiti minimi brevis.** o: Hook of hamate and flexor retinaculum. i: Base of proximal phalanx of little finger. F: Flexion at the metacarpophalangeal joint. I: Ulnar nerve. B

11 **M. opponens digiti minimi.** o: Hook of hamulus and flexor retinaculum. i: head and shaft of 5th metacarpal. F: Draws the little finger in the direction of the palm of the hand. I: Ulnar nerve. B

12 **Mm. lumbricales.** o: Tendons of flexor digitorum profundus. i: Dorsal aponeuroses of fingers 2–5. Flexion at the metacarpophalangeal joints, extension at the interphalangeal joints. I: Ulnar and median nerves. B C

13 **Mm. interossei dorsales.** o: Double headed from the metacarpals. i: Dorsal aponeurosis of fingers 2–4. F: Spreading of fingers 2–4 away from axis of middle finger, radial and ulnar abduction of middle finger, flexion at the metacarpophalangeal joint and extension of the interphalangeal joints. I: Ulnar nerve. C D E

14 **Mm. interossei palmares.** o: Metacarpal bones 2, 4 and 5. i: Dorsal aponeuroses of fingers 2, 4 and 5. F: Adduction of index, ring and little fingers toward the middle finger, flexion at the metacarpo-

phalangeal joints, extension at the interphalangeal joints. I: Ulnar nerve. B D

15 **Axillary fascia.** Fascia axillaris. Situated on the axillary fat body, it unites the lateral margins of the pectoral and latissimus dorsi muscles. G

16 **Deltoid fascia.** Fascia deltoidea. Strongly fused investing fascia of the deltoid muscle.

17 **Brachial fascia.** Fascia brachii (brachialis). Fascia enclosing the upper arm muscles. F

18 **Medial intermuscular septum of the arm.** Septum intermusculare brachii mediale. Tendinous sheet for muscle origin between the medial margin of the humerus and the brachial fascia. F

19 **Lateral intermuscular septum of the arm.** Septum intermusculare brachii laterale. Tendinous sheet for muscle origin between the lateral margin of the humerus and the brachial fascia. F

20 **Antebrachial fascia.** Fascia antebrachii. Fascia enveloping the forearm musculature. A

21 **Fascia of the dorsum of the hand.** Fascia dorsalis manus. Fascia situated on the dorsal tendons of the hand. E

22 **Extensor retinaculum.** Retinaculum extensorum [[Lig. carpi dors.]]. Transverse fascial fibers over the 6 conduction canals of the 10 extensor tendons. E

23 **Superficial transverse metacarpal ligament.** Lig. metacarpale transversum superficiale. Transverse reinforcement of the palmar fascia of the hand at the level of the heads of the metacarpals. A

24 **Palmar aponeurosis.** Aponeurosis palmaris. Membranous expansion of the tendon of the palmaris longus muscle. A

25 Transverse fasciculi. Fasciculi transversi. Transversely oriented fibrous bundles of the palmar aponeurosis. A

26 **Flexor retinaculum.** Retinaculum flexorum [[Lig. carpi transversum]]. Stout fibrous band between the scaphoid and trapezium as well as pisiform and hook of hamate. It binds the flexor tendons. B

27 **Fibrous sheaths of fingers.** Vaginae fibrosae digitorum manus. Connective tissue, synovial canal for the flexor tendons to the fingers. B

28 **Annular part of fibrous sheath.** Pars anularis vaginae fibrosae. Very compact circular fibers of the fibrous sheath located between the joints. B

29 Cruciate part of fibrous sheath. Pars cruciformis vaginae fibrosae. Crossed, reinforcement fibers at the joints. B

30 **Synovial sheaths of the fingers.** Vaginae synoviales digitorum manus. Tendon sheaths of the flexor of the fingers.

31 Vincula tendinum. Connective tissue fasciculi (mesotendons) transporting vessels to the tendons. C

32 Vinculum longum. Longer fasciculus at the level of the proximal phalanx. C

33 Vinculum breve. Shorter fasciculus near the insertions of the tendons. C

34 **Chiasma tendinum.** Crossing of the tendons of the flexor digitorum superficialis and profundus. C

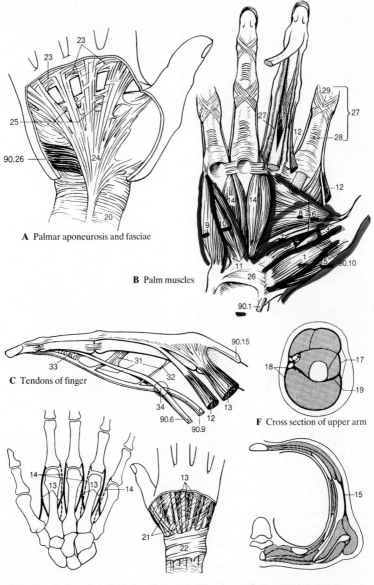

A Palmar aponeurosis and fasciae

B Palm muscles

C Tendons of finger

F Cross section of upper arm

D Interosseous muscles, schematic **E** Dorsum of hand **G** Cross section of thorax

1 MUSCLES OF LOWER LIMB. MUSCULI MEMBRI INFERIORIS.

2 **M. iliopsoas.** Comprised of two muscles: psoas major and iliacus. o: Lesser trochanter. F: Flexion, medial and lateral rotation at the hip joint. B C D

3 *M. iliacus.* o: Iliac fossa. i: Lesser trochanter. F: Flexion, medial and lateral rotation at the hip joint. I: Femoral nerve and lumbar plexus. C

4 *M. psoas major.* o: Bodies and transverse processes of L1–4. i: Lesser trochanter. F: Flexion, medial and lateral rotation at the hip joint. I: Lumbar plexus. C

5 **[M. psoas minor].** o: Bodies of T12, L1. i: Iliac fascia. I: Lumbar plexus. C

6 **M. gluteus maximus.** o: Posterior, external surface of ilium, sacrum, coccyx, sacrotuberous ligament. i: Iliotibial tract, gluteal tuberosity, lateral intermuscular septum, linea aspera. F: Extension, lateral rotation, abduction and adduction at the hip joint. I: Inferior gluteal nerve. A D E

7 **M. gluteus medius.** o: External surface of ilium. i: Greater trochanter. F: Abduction, medial and lateral rotation, flexion and extension at the hip joint. I: Superior gluteal nerve. A D E

8 **M. gluteus minimus.** o: External surface of ilium between anterior and inferior gluteal lines. i: Greater trochanter. F: Abduction, medial-lateral rotation, flexion and extension of the thigh at the hip joint. I: Superior gluteal nerve. A D E

8 a **Gluteal aponeurosis.** Aponeurosis glutealis. Deep, sheet-like tendon of origin of the gluteus maximus lying on the gluteus medius.

9 **M. tensor fasciae latae.** o: Near the anterior superior iliac spine. i: Above the iliotibial tract lateral to the tibial tuberosity. F: Flexor, abductor and medial rotator at the hip joint. Flexion, extension and final rotation at the knee joint. I: Superior gluteal nerve. C E

10 **M. piriformis.** o: Anterior surface of sacrum. i: Greater trochanter, inner side of apex. F: Abductor, extender and lateral rotator at the hip joint. I: Sacral plexus. A D

11 **M. obturator internus.** o: Inner surface of obturator membrane and environs. i: Trochanteric fossa. F: Lateral rotation, abduction and adduction. I: Sacral plexus. A D

12 **M. gemellus superior.** o: Ischial spine. i: Tendon of obturator internus and trochanteric fossa. F: Lateral rotator, adductor and abductor. I: Sacral plexus. A D E

13 **M. gemellus inferior.** o: Ischial tuberosity. i: Tendon of obturator internus, trochanteric fossa. F: Lateral rotator, adductor and abductor. I: Sacral plexus. A D E

14 **M. quadratus femoris.** o: Ischial tuberosity. i: Intertrochanteric crest. F: Lateral rotator and adductor. I: Sacral plexus. A D E

15 **M. sartorius.** o: Anterior superior iliac spine. i: Medial to tibial tuberosity. F: Flexor, abductor, lateral rotator at the hip joint. Flexor and medial rotator at the knee joint. I: Femoral nerve. C E

16 **M. quadriceps femoris.** The muscle group comprising the three vasti muscles and the rectus femoris. I: Femoral nerve.

17 *M. rectus femoris.* o: Anterior inferior iliac spine = straight head and upper margin of acetabulum = reflected head. i: Tibial tuberosity. F: Flexor at the hip joint, extensor at the knee joint. B C E

18 *M. vastus lateralis.* o: Greater trochanter, lateral lip of linea aspera. i: Quadriceps tendon. F: Extension at the knee joint. B C D

19 *M. vastus intermedius.* o: Anterior surface of femur. i: Quadriceps tendon. F: Knee joint extensor. B D

20 *M. vastus medialis.* o: Distal to intertrochanteric line, medial lip of linea aspera. i: Quadriceps tendon. F: Knee joint extensor. C D

21 **M. articularis genus.** o: Anterior surface of femur. i: Knee joint capsule. F: Tenses capsule. I: Femoral nerve. D

22 **M. pectineus.** o: Pecten pubis. i: Pectineal line below the lesser trochanter. F: Flexion, adduction and lateral rotation at the hip joint. I: Femoral and obturator nerves. B C D E

23 **M. adductor longus.** o: Near the symphysis. i: Medial lip of linea aspera. F: Adduction and flexion at the hip joint. I: Obturator nerve. B C D E

24 **M. adductor brevis.** o: Inferior ramus of pubis. i: Medial lip of linea aspera. F: Adduction, flexion, extension and lateral rotation at the hip joint. I: Obturator nerve. B D E

25 **M. adductor magnus.** o: Ischial tuberosity, ischial ramus. i: Medial lip of linea aspera and with a long tendon to the medial epicondyle. F: Adduction and extension at the hip joint. I: Obturator and sciatic nerves. B C D E

25 a **M. adductor minimus.** Small, proximal, anterior part of adductor magnus.

26 **M. gracilis.** o: Inferior ramus of pubis medial to adductor magnus. i: Medial to tibial tuberosity. F: Adduction, flexion and extension at the hip joint. Flexion and medial rotation at the knee joint. I: Obturator nerve. A C E

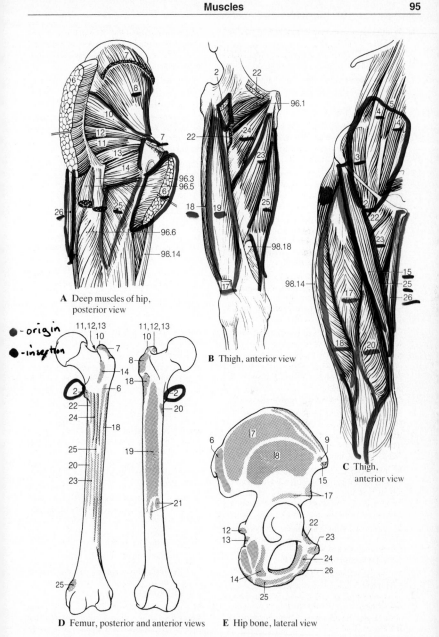

A Deep muscles of hip, posterior view

B Thigh, anterior view

C Thigh, anterior view

● - origin
● - insertion

D Femur, posterior and anterior views

E Hip bone, lateral view

1 **M. obturator externus.** o: External surface of obturator membrane and environs. i: Trochanteric fossa. F: Lateral rotation and adduction at the hip joint. I: Obturator nerve. A

2 **M. biceps femoris.** o: pelvis and femur via two heads. i: Head of fibula. I: Sciatic nerve, tibial part. A B E F

3 Long head of biceps femoris. Caput longum. o: Ischial tuberosity. i: Head of fibula. F: Extension, adduction and lateral rotation at the hip joint; Flexion and lateral rotation at the knee joint. I: Tibial nerve. A B

4 Short head of biceps femoris. Caput breve. o: Lateral lip of linea aspera. i: Head of fibula. F: Flexion and lateral rotation at the knee joint. I: Common peroneal nerve. A B

5 **M. semitendinosus.** o: Ischial tuberosity. i: Medial to tibial tuberosity [pes anserinus]. F: Extension, medial rotation and adduction at the hip joint; Flexion and medial rotation at the knee joint. I: Tibial nerve. A D E

6 **M. semimembranosus.** i: Ischial tuberosity. i: Medial condyle of tibia and oblique popliteal ligament. It is partially covered by the semitendinosus. F: Extension, adduction and medial rotation at the hip joint; Flexion and medial rotation at the knee joint. Tenses knee joint capsule. I: Tibial nerve. A B F

7 **M. tibialis anterior.** o: Lateral surface of tibia, interosseous membrane, fascia of leg (crural fascia). i: Medial aspect of medial cuneiform bone and 1st metatarsal. F: Dorsiflexion and supination of foot. I: Deep peroneal nerve. D E

8 **M. extensor digitorum longus.** o: Lateral tibial condyle, interosseous membrane, fibula. i: Dorsal aponeurosis of toes 2–5. F: Dorsiflexion and pronation of foot, extension of toes. I: Deep peroneal nerve. D E

9 **M. peroneus tertius (M. fibularis tertius).** Muscle split off from the extensor digitorum longus with insertion into the base of the 5th metacarpal. F: Dorsiflexion and pronation. I: Deep peroneal nerve. D

10 **M. extensor hallucis longus.** o: Interosseous membrane and fibula. i: Distal phalanx of big toe. F: Dorsiflexion of foot, extension of big toe. I: Deep peroneal nerve. D E

11 **M. peroneus longus [[M. fibularis longus]].** o: Fibula and crural fascia. i: Medial cuneiform bone and 1st metatarsal after an oblique course below the dorsum of the foot. F: Plantar flexor and pronator. I: Superficial peroneal nerve. C D E F

12 **M. peroneus brevis [[M. fibularis brevis]].** o: Distal 2/3 of fibula. i: Tuberosity of 5th metatarsal. F: Plantar flexion and pronation. I: Superficial peroneal nerve. C D E F

13 **M. triceps surae.** Muscle group consisting of gastrocnemius and soleus; it forms the Achilles tendon (Tendo calcaneus). I: Tibial nerve.

14 *M. gastrocnemius.* The superficial calf muscle formed by the following two heads. F: Flexor at the knee joint, plantar flexor and supinator at the ankle joint. A B C D

15 Lateral head of gastrocnemius. Caput laterale. o: Proximal to the lateral femoral condyle. i: Achilles tendon. A B C

16 Medial head of gastrocnemius. Caput mediale. o: Proximal to the medial femoral condyle. i: Achilles tendon. A B C D

17 *M. soleus.* o: Proximal ends of fibula and tibia. i: Achilles tendon. F: Plantar flexor and supinator. B F

18 *Tendinous arch of soleus muscle.* Arcus tendineus musculi solei. Tendinous arch above the interosseous membrane. Passageway for the tibial nerve and posterior tibial artery and vein. B

19 *Tendo calcaneus [[Achilles tendon]].* The tendon of the triceps surae inserting at the tuber of the calcaneus. B C

20 **M. plantaris.** o: Above the lateral femoral condyle. i: Achilles tendon. I: Tibial nerve. B C

21 **M. popliteus.** o: Lateral femoral condyle. i: Posterior surface of tibia. F: Flexor at knee joint and medial rotator of leg. B C F

22 **M. tibialis posterior.** o: Tibia, fibula, interosseous membrane. i: Navicular, cuneiforms, cuboid and metatarsals 2–4. A tendinous band courses retrograde to the sustentaculum tali of the calcaneus. F: Plantar flexor and supinator. I: Tibial nerve. C F

23 **M. flexor digitorum longus.** o: Tibia. i: Distal phalanges of toes 2–5. F: Plantar flexion, supination, flexor of toes. I: Tibial nerve. C F

24 **M. flexor hallucis longus.** o: Fibula. i: Distal phalanx of big toe. F: Plantar flexion, supination, flexion of big toe. I: Tibial nerve. C F

25 **M. extensor hallucis brevis.** o: Dorsal surface of calcaneus. i: Proximal phalanx of big toe. F: Extends the big toe. I: See 26. D

26 **M. extensor digitorum brevis.** o: Dorsal surface of calcaneus. i: Dorsal aponeuroses of toes 2–4. F: Extends toes. I: Deep peroneal nerve. D

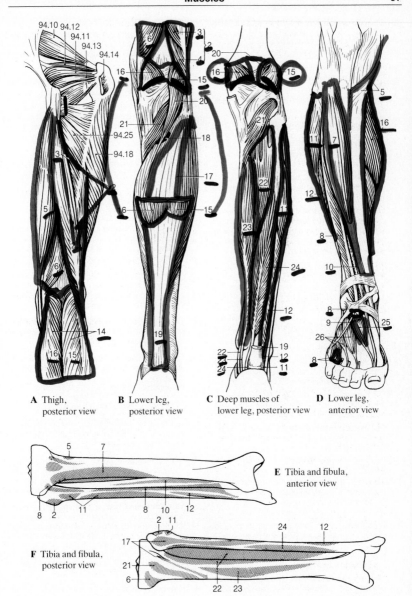

A Thigh, posterior view

B Lower leg, posterior view

C Deep muscles of lower leg, posterior view

D Lower leg, anterior view

E Tibia and fibula, anterior view

F Tibia and fibula, posterior view

1 **M. abductor hallucis.** o: Medial process of tuber
~ calcanei. i: Medial sesamoid and proximal phalanx of big toe. F: Medial abduction, supports the
longitudinal arch. I: See 2. A B

1 a **Medial head.** Caput mediale. The portion of abductor hallucis emanating from the retinaculum of
the flexor muscles.

1 b **Lateral head.** Caput laterale. The remaining portion of the abductor hallucis.

2 **M. flexor hallucis brevis.** o: Cuboid bone, long
plantar ligament among others. i: Both sesamoid
bones and proximal phalanx. F: Flexes big toe,
supports longitudinal arch. I: Medial and lateral
plantar nerves. A B

3 **M. adductor hallucis.** Important muscle for the
transverse arch of the foot consisting of the following two heads.

4 Oblique head. Caput obliquum. o: Metatarsals
2–4, lateral cuneiform and cuboid. i: Lateral sesamoid bone and proximal phalanx of big toe together with the transverse head. F: Important sup-
porter of transverse and longitudinal arches. B

5 Transverse head. Caput transversum. o: Capsules of metatarsophalangeal joints 3–5. i: Lateral
sesamoid bone. F: Primary function is support of
the transverse arch of the foot. A B

6 **M. abductor digiti minimi.** o: Calcaneus and
plantar aponeurosis. i: Laterally on proximal phalanx of 5th toe. F: Plantar flexion and abduction of
the 5th toe. I: Lateral plantar nerve. A B

7 **M. flexor digiti minimi brevis.** o: Base of 5th metatarsal, long plantar ligament. i: Proximal phalanx of little toe. F: Flexor and abductor of little
toe. I: Lateral plantar nerve. A B

7 a **[M. opponens digiti minimi].** Muscle occasionally split off from the flexor digiti minimi brevis.
o: Distal half of 5th metatarsal.

8 **M. flexor digitorum brevis.** o: Tuber calcanei and
plantar aponeurosis. i: Middle phalanges of toes
2–5 via divided tendons. F: Flexes toes and supports the longitudinal arch of the foot. I: Medial
plantar nerve. A B

9 **M. quadratus plantae (M. flexor accessorius).**
o: Calcaneus. i: Lateral border of tendon of flexor
digitorum longus. F: Flexes toes and supports longitudinal arch of foot. I: Lateral plantar nerve. B

10 **Lumbricals.** Mm. lumbricales. o: Tendons of
flexor digitorum longus. i: Bases of proximal phalanges 2–5. F: Flexion at the metatarsophalangeal
joint. Brings toes closer to the big toe. I: Medial
and lateral plantar nerves. A B

11 **Mm. interossei dorsales.** o: Two-headed from adjacent metatarsal bones. i: Dorsal aponeurosis of
toes. F: Abduction, flexion at the metatarsophalangeal joints and extension at the interphalangeal
joints. I: Lateral plantar nerve. C

12 **Mm. interossei plantares.** o: Single-headed from
metatarsal bones 3–5. i: Base of proximal phalanges. F: Adduction and flexion at the metatarsophalangeal joints, extension at the interphalangeal joints. I: See 11. C

13 **Fascia lata.** Fascia of thigh which envelops the
entire thigh musculature. D

14 Iliotibial tract. Tractus iliotibialis. Vertical
reinforcement band of the fascia lata from the anterior segment of the iliac crest to the lateral tibial
condyle into which radiate the tensor fasciae latae
and gluteus maximus. D

15 **Lateral intermuscular septum of thigh.** Septum
intermusculare femoris laterale. Firm connective
tissue layer from the fascia lata to the lateral lip of
the linea aspera between the biceps femoris and
vastus lateralis muscles.

16 **Medial intermuscular septum of thigh.** Septum
intermusculare femoris mediale. Stout connective
tissue layer from the fascia lata to the medial lip of
the linea aspera between the vastus medialis, sartorius and adductor muscles.

17 **Adductor canal.** Canalis adductorius. Channel
between adductors, vastus medialis and [Vasto-
adductor membrane]. It ends with the hiatus tendineus within the adductor magnus. D

18 **Hiatus tendineus (adductorius).** Opening at the
attachment of the adductor magnus at the level of
the inferior margin of the adductor longus.

19 **Iliac fascia.** Fascia iliaca. Fascia over the iliacus
and inferior portion of the psoas muscles. It attaches to the iliac crest and arcuate line as well as
the inguinal ligament. D

20 **Muscular lacuna.** Lacuna musculorum. Compartment for the passage of the iliopsoas muscle
and the femoral and lateral femoral cutaneous
nerves between the ilium, inguinal ligament and
iliopectineal arch. E

21 **Iliopectineal arch.** Arcus iliopectineus. Portion
of the iliac fascia between the inguinal ligament
and the iliopubic [iliopectineal] eminence. It separates the vascular from the muscular lacuna. E

22 **Vascular lacuna.** Lacuna vasorum. Compartment
between the pubis, inguinal ligament and iliopectineal arch for the passage of the femoral artery and
the femoral branch of the genitofemoral nerve. E

23 **Femoral triangle.** Trigonum femorale. Triangle
between the sartorius and adductor longus muscles and the inguinal ligament. D

24 **Femoral canal.** Canalis femoralis. It lies within
the medial segment of the vascular lacuna and extends from the inguinal ligament to the saphenous
opening. E

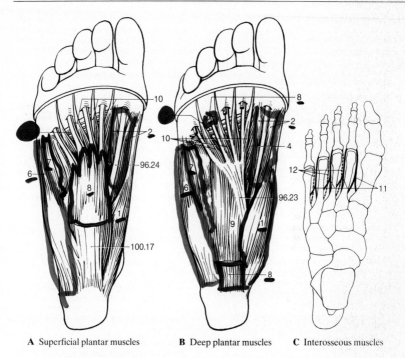

A Superficial plantar muscles   **B** Deep plantar muscles   **C** Interosseous muscles

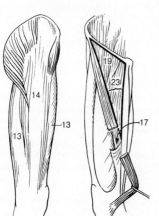

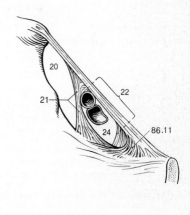

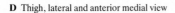

D Thigh, lateral and anterior medial view   **E** Vascular lacuna

1 **Femoral ring.** Anulus femoralis. Entrance into the femoral canal bordered by the femoral vein, inguinal ligament, falx inguinalis and pectineal ligament. A

2 **Femoral septum.** Septum femorale. Connective tissue closure at the entrance of the femoral canal. A

3 **Saphenous opening.** Hiatus saphenus. Large opening in the fascia lata directly below the inguinal ligament for the passage of the great saphenous vein. B

4 **Falciform margin.** Margo falciformis. Bow-shaped, principal lateral margin of the saphenous opening. B

5 *Superior horn.* Cornu superius. Upper, curved portion of the falciform margin. B

6 *Inferior horn.* Cornu inferius. Lower, curved portion of the falciform margin. B

7 **Cribriform fascia.** Fascia cribrosa. Loose, perforated connective tissue lamina covering the saphenous opening. B

8 **Fascia of the leg (Crural fascia).** Fascia cruris. Superficial fascial covering of the leg which serves partially as a muscle origin and is attached to the free bony margins of the tibia. C D F

9 **Anterior intermuscular septum of leg.** Septum intermusculare cruris anterius. Connective tissue septum between the peroneal and extensor compartments. F

10 **Posterior intermuscular septum of leg.** Septum intermusculare cruris posterius. Connective tissue septum between the peroneal and flexor compartments. F

11 **Superior extensor retinaculum.** Retinaculum mm. extensorum superius. Transverse thickening (about two finger widths) of the crural fascia for the support of the extensor tendons. C D

12 **Flexor retinaculum.** Retinaculum mm. flexorum. Fibrous band situated on the long flexor tendons and extending from the medial malleolus to the calcaneus. It bridges over the main route for vessels, nerves and tendons passing to the sole of the foot (tibial nerve, posterior tibial artery and vein, tibialis posterior, flexor digitorum longus, and flexor hallucis longus muscles). D

13 **Inferior extensor retinaculum.** Retinaculum mm. extensorum inferius. Supporting band for the extensor tendons, usually cruciate, extending from booth malleoli to the foot margins of the opposite side, especially to the calcaneus. C D

14 **Superior peroneal (fibular) retinaculum.** Retinaculum mm. peroneorum (fibularium) superius. Upper supporting band for the peroneal tendons extending from the lateral malleolus to the calcaneus. C

15 **Inferior (fibular) peroneal retinaculum.** Retinaculum mm. peroneorum (fibularium) inferius. Lower supporting band for the peroneal tendons. It passes from the extensor retinaculum to the outer surface of the calcaneus. A fibrous tract goes to the peroneal trochlea and separates the upper lying peroneus brevis from the preoneus longus muscle. C

16 **Fascia dorsalis pedis.** Thin fascia on the dorsum of the foot connected above with the inferior extensor retinaculum. C D

17 **Plantar aponeurosis.** Aponeurosis plantaris. Tough, tendinous sheet on the sole of the foot extending from the tuber calcanei to as far as the middle phalanges. It braces the longitudinal arch of the foot. E

18 **Transverse fasciculi.** Fasciculi transversi. Transverse fibrous sheets in the distal plantar aponeurosis. E

19 **Superficial transverse metatarsal ligament.** Lig. metatarsale transversum superficiale. Transverse fibrous tract in the vicinity of the distal transverse fibers of the plantar aponeurosis. E G

20 **Synovial sheaths of the digits of the foot.** Vaginae synoviales tendinum digitorum pedis. Synovial portion of the tendon sheaths for the flexors of the toes. G

21 **Vincula tendinum.** Connective tissue tract passing obliquely through the tendon sheaths bearing blood vessels. G

22 **Fibrous sheaths of the digits of the foot.** Vaginae fibrosae tendinum digitorum pedis. Tough connective tissue reinforcement of the tendon sheaths on the flexor side of the toes. G

23 **Annular part of fibrous sheath.** Pars anularis vaginae fibrosae. Circular tracts in the fibrous sheaths between the joints. G

24 **Cruciate part of fibrous sheath.** Pars cruciformis vaginae fibrosae. Cruciate connective tissue tracts in the fibrous sheaths over the joints. G

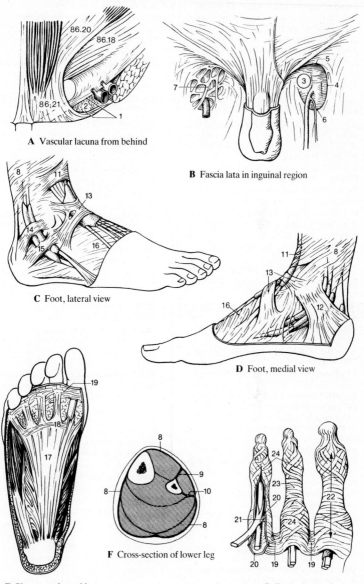

A Vascular lacuna from behind

B Fascia lata in inguinal region

C Foot, lateral view

D Foot, medial view

E Plantar surface of foot

F Cross-section of lower leg

G Toes, plantar view

BURSAE AND SYNOVIAL SHEATHS.

1 **Tendon sheath of superior oblique muscle.** Vagina tendinis m. obliqui superioris. Tendon sheath at the trochlea for the tendon of the superior oblique muscle of the eyeball. See p. 364.12

2 **Synovial bursa of tensor veli palatini.** B. m. tensoris veli palatini. Synovial bursa between the pterygoid hamulus and the tendon of the tensor veli palatini muscle. See pp. 116.20, 117.C

3 **Subcutaneous bursa of the laryngeal prominence.** B. subcutanea prominentiae laryngealis. Synovial bursa between the skin and the laryngeal prominence of the thyroid cartilage. A

4 **Retrohyoid bursa.** B. retrohyoidea. Synovial bursa between the body of the hyoid and the thyrohyoid membrane. A

5 **Infrahyoid bursa.** B. infrahyoidea. Synovial bursa between the upper end of the sternohyoid muscle and the thyrohyoid membrane. A B

5 a **Synovial bursae of upper limb.** Bursae membri superioris.

6 **Subtendinous bursa of trapezius.** B. subtendinea m. trapezii. Synovial bursa between the trapezius muscle (ascending part) and the spine of the scapula. C

7 **[B. subcutanea acromialis]. Synovial bursa between acromion and the skin.** D

8 **Subacromial bursa.** B. subacromialis. Synovial bursa beneath the acromion and the deltoid muscle. It lies on the joint capsule with its tendons. D E

9 **Subdeltoid bursa.** B. subdeltoidea. Synovial bursa between the deltoid muscle and the capsule of the shoulder joint. It occasionally communicates with the subacromial bursa. D

10 **Coracobrachial bursa.** [B. m. coracobrachialis]. Synovial bursa between the tendons of the subscapularis and coracobrachialis muscles below the apex of the coracoid process. D

11 **Subtendinous bursa of infraspinatus muscle.** B. subtendinea m. infraspinati. Synovial bursa between the tendon of insertion of the infraspinatus and the capsule of the shoulder joint. E

12 **Subtendinous bursa of subscapularis muscle.** B. subtendinea m. subscapularis. Synovial bursa between the tendon of insertion of the subscapularis and the capsule of the shoulder joint. It communicates with the joint cavity. D

13 **Subtendinous bursa of teres major muscle.** B. subtendinea m. teretis majoris. Synovial bursa between the tendon of insertion of the teres major and the humerus. D

14 **Subtendinous bursa of latissimus dorsi muscle.** B. subtendinea m. latissimi dorsi. Synovial bursa between the tendons of insertion of the teres major and latissimus dorsi. D

15 **Subcutaneous bursa of olecranon.** B. subcutanea olecrani. Synovial bursa between the olecranon and the skin. F

16 **Intratendinous bursa of olecranon.** [B. intratendinea olecrani]. Synovial bursa within the triceps tendon near the olecranon. F

17 **Subtendinous bursa of triceps brachii.** B. subtendinea m. tricipitis brachii. Synovial bursa between the triceps tendon and the olecranon. F

18 **Bicipitoradial bursa.** B. bicipitoradialis. Synovial bursa between the insertion tendon of the biceps and the anterior part of the radial tuberosity. F

19 **[B. cubitalis interossea].** Synovial bursa between the biceps tendon and the ulna or oblique cord. F

20 **Tendon sheath of abductor pollicis longus and extensor pollicis brevis muscles.** Vag. tendinum mm. abductoris longi et extensoris brevis pollicis. Common tendon sheath forming the first tendon compartment on the dorsum of the hand. G

21 **Tendon sheath of extensor carpi radialis longus and brevis muscles.** Vag. tendinum mm. extensorum carpi radialium. Common tendon sheath forming the second tendon compartment on the dorsum of the hand. G

22 **Tendon sheath of extensor pollicis longus muscle.** Vag. tendinis m. extensoris pollicis longi. Forms the third tendon compartment. G

23 **Tendon sheath of extensor digitorum and extensor indicis muscles.** Vag. tendinum mm. extensoris digitorum et extensoris indicis. Tendon sheath forming the fourth tendon compartment on the dorsum of the hand. G

24 **Tendon sheath of extensor digiti minimi muscle.** Vag. tendinis m. extensoris digiti minimi. Forms the fifth tendon compartment on the dorsum of the hand. G

25 **Tendon sheath of extensor carpi ulnaris muscle.** Vag. tendinis m. extensoris carpi ulnaris. Forms the sixth tendon compartment on the dorsum of the hand. G

26 **Sheath of extensor carpi radialis brevis muscle.** Vag. m. extensoris carpi radialis brevis. Synovial bursa at the attachment between the tendon and base of the 3rd metacarpal.

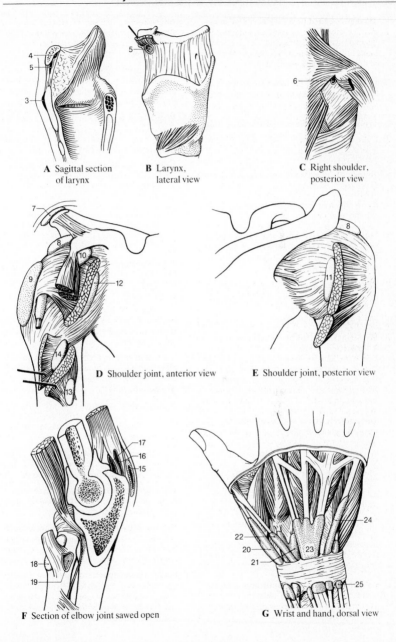

A Sagittal section of larynx

B Larynx, lateral view

C Right shoulder, posterior view

D Shoulder joint, anterior view

E Shoulder joint, posterior view

F Section of elbow joint sawed open

G Wrist and hand, dorsal view

1 **Tendon sheath of flexor carpi radialis muscle.** Vag. tendinis m. flexoris carpi radialis. Individual tendon sheath for the flexor carpi radialis at the insertion of the tendon to the base of the 2nd metacarpal bone. A

2 **Common sheath of flexor muscles.** Vag. communis mm. flexorum. Common tendon sheath for the two long flexors of the fingers. A

3 **Tendon sheath of flexor pollicis longus muscle.** Vag. tendinis m. flexoris pollicis longi. Separate synovial sheath for the long flexor of the thumb. A

4 **Tendon sheaths for flexors in region of fingers.** Vagg. tendinum digitorum manus. A

4a **Synovial bursae of lower limb.** Bursae membri inferioris.

5 **Subcutaneous trochanteric bursa.** Bursa subcutanea trochanterica. Synovial bursa on the tendon of the gluteus maximus between the skin and greater trochanter. B

6 **Trochanteric bursa of gluteus maximus.** B. trochanterica m. glutei maximi. Synovial bursa between the tendon of the gluteus maximus and the greater trochanter. B

7 **Trochanteric bursae of gluteus medius.** Bb. trochantericae m. glutei medii. This designation comprises two synovial bursae, an anterior one between the tendon of insertion of the gluteus medius and the greater trochanter and a posterior one between this tendon and the piriformis muscle. B C

8 **Trochanteric bursa of gluteus minimus.** B. troch. m. glutei minimi. Synovial bursa between the tendon of insertion of the gluteus minimus and the greater trochanter. B C

9 **Bursa of piriformis muscle.** B. m. piriformis. Synovial bursa between the tendon of attachment of the piriformis and the greater trochanter. B

10 **Ischial bursa of obturator internus muscle.** B. ischiadica (sciatica) m. obturatoris interni. Synovial bursa between the cartilage covered surface of the lesser sciatic notch and the tendon of the obturator internus. B

11 **Subtendinous bursa of obturator internus muscle.** B. subtendinea m. obturatoris interni. Synovial bursa below the insertion of the obturator internus. B

12 **Intermuscular bursae of gluteal muscles.** Bb. intermusculares mm. gluteorum. 2–3 synovial bursae below the attachment of the gluteus maximus to the linea aspera. B

13 **Ischial bursa of gluteus maximus muscle.** B. ischiadica (sciatica) m. glutei maximi. Synovial bursa between the ischial tuberosity and the inferior surface of the gluteus maximus. B

14 **Iliopectineal bursa.** [B. iliopectinea]. Synovial bursa between the iliopsoas muscle and the pelvic bone. It lies above the hip joint with which it often communicates. C

15 **Subtendinous iliac bursa.** B. subtendinea iliaca. Synovial bursa between the lesser trochanter and the tendon of insertion of the iliopsoas muscle. C

16 **Superior bursa of biceps femoris muscle.** B. m. bicipitis femoris superior. Synovial bursa between the origins of the biceps femoris and semimembranosus muscles. B

17 **Subcutaneous prepatellar bursa.** B. subcutanea prepatellaris. Synovial bursa directly between the skin and the fascia in front of the knee. D

18 **Subfascial prepatellar bursa.** [B. subfascialis prepatellaris]. Synovial bursa between the fascia and the tendon fibers of the quadratus femoris muscle. D

19 **Subtendinous prepatellar bursa.** [B. subtendinea prepatellaris]. Synovial bursa directly on the knee joint below the tendon fibers of the quadratus femoris. D

20 **Suprapatellar bursa.** B. suprapatellaris. Synovial bursa between the quadriceps tendon and the femur. It almost always communicates with the joint cavity. D

21 **Subcutaneous infrapatellar bursa.** B. subcutanea infrapatellaris. Synovial bursa between the ligamentum patellae and the skin. D

22 **Deep infrapatellar bursa.** B. infrapatellaris profunda. Synovial bursa between the ligamentum patellae and the tibia. D

23 **Subcutaneous bursa of tibial tuberosity.** B. subcutanea tuberositas tibiae. Synovial bursa between the tibial tuberosity and the skin. It is involved mostly when kneeling. D

24 **Subtendinous bursae of sartorius muscle.** Bb. subtendineae m. sartorii. Synovial bursae between the tendon of attachment of the sartorius and the tendons of the gracilis and semitendinosus situated below it. E

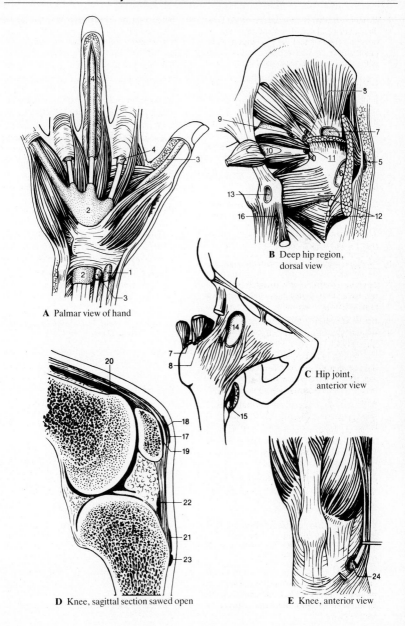

A Palmar view of hand

B Deep hip region, dorsal view

C Hip joint, anterior view

D Knee, sagittal section sawed open

E Knee, anterior view

1   **Anserine bursa.** B. anserina. Synovial bursa
on the tibial collateral ligament below the tendons of the semitendinosus, gracilis and sartorius muscles. It occasionally communicates
with the subtendinous bursa of the sartorius. A

2   **Inferior subtendinous bursa of biceps femoris muscle.** B. subtendinea m. bicipitis femoris
inferior. Synovial bursa located partially on the
fibular collateral ligament below the tendon of
insertion of the biceps femoris. B

3   **Subpopliteal recess.** Recessus subpopliteus
[Bursa m. poplitei]. Synovial bursa on the
lateral femoral condyle below the tendon of
origin of the popliteus muscle. It always communicates with the knee joint cavity, more
rarely with the tibiofibular joint. B

4   **Lateral subtendinous bursa of gastrocnemius muscle.** B. subtendinea m. gastrocnemii
lateralis. Synovial bursa between the lateral
condyle of the femur and the lateral tendon of
origin of the gastrocnemius. B

5   **Medial subtendinous bursa of gastrocnemius muscle.** B. subtendinea m. gastrocnemii
medialis. Synovial bursa between the medial
condyle of the femur and the medial tendon of
origin of the gastrocnemius. A B

6   **Bursa of semimembranosus muscle.** B. m.
semimembranosi. Synovial bursa between the
tendon of attachment of the semimembranosus
and the upper margin of the tibia. A

7   **Subcutaneous bursa of lateral malleolus.** B.
subcutanea malleoli lateralis. Synovial bursa
between the skin and the lateral malleolus. C

8   **Subcutaneous bursa of medial malleolus.** B.
subcutanea malleoli medialis. Synovial bursa
between the skin and the medial malleolus. D

9   **Tendon sheath of tibialis anterior muscle.**
Vag. tendinis m. tibialis anterioris. It begins already below the extensor retinaculum. D

10   **Tendon sheath of extensor hallucis longus
muscle.** Vag. tendinis m. extensoris hallucis
longi. It extends below the extensor retinaculum and farther distally. C D

11   **Tendon sheath of extensor digitorum longus
muscle.** Vag. tendinum m. extensoris digitorum pedis longi. It lies below the extensor
retinaculum and further distally. C

12   **Tendon sheath of flexor digitorum longus
muscle.** Vag. tendinum m. flexoris digitorum
pedis longi. It lies behind and below the medial malleolus covered by the flexor retinaculum.
D

13   **Tendon sheath of tibialis posterior muscle.**
Vag. tendinis m. tibialis posterioris. It resides
below the flexor retinaculum and begins at the
point where it is crossed over by the flexor
digitorum longus. D

14   **Tendon sheath of flexor hallucis longus muscle.** Vag. tendinis m. flexoris hallucis longi. It
extends up to the proximal end of the sole where it crosses under the tendon of the flexor digitorum longus. D

15   **Common tendon sheath for peroneal muscles.** Vag. tendinum mm. peroneorum (fibularium) communis. It lies below the peroneal retinaculum as far as the cuboid bone. C

16   **Subtendinous bursa of tibialis anterior muscle.** B. subtendinea m. tibialis anterioris. Synovial bursa at the attachment between the tendon and the medial cuneiform bone. D

17   **Subcutaneous calcaneal bursa.** B. sucutanea
calcanea. Synovial bursa between the skin and
the posterior surface of the calcaneus. D

18   **Bursa of calcaneal [[Achilles]] tendon.** B. tendinis calcanei [Achilles]. Synovial bursa between the calcaneus and the Achilles tendon. D

19   **Tendon sheath of peroneus longus muscle at
the sole of the foot.** Vag. tendinis m. peronei
(fibularis) longi plantaris. D

20   **Tendon sheaths for the flexors of the toes.**
Vagg. tendinum digitorum pedis. D

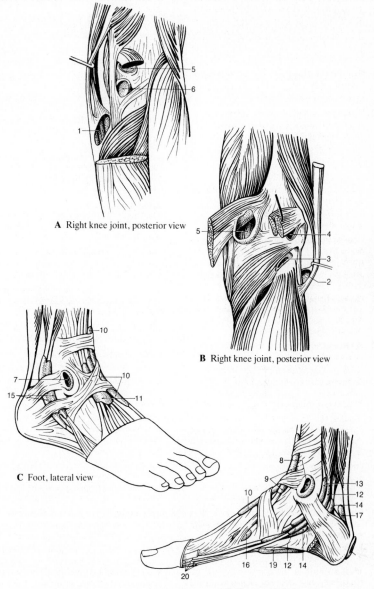

A Right knee joint, posterior view

B Right knee joint, posterior view

C Foot, lateral view

D Foot, medial view

1 DIGESTIVE SYSTEM. APPARATUS DIGE-
STORIUS (SYSTEMA ALIMENTARIUM).

2 ORAL CAVITY. CAVITAS ORIS.

3 **Vestibule of mouth.** Vestibulum oris. Space between the rows of teeth and the lips or cheeks. B C

4 **Oral fissure.** Rima oris. Mouth opening between the lips. A

5 **Lips.** Labia oris.

6 Upper lip. Labium superius. A B C

7 *Philtrum.* Groove extending from nasal septum to upper lip. A

8 *Tuberculum.* Small eminence on upper lip at end of philtrum. A

9 Lower lip. Labium inferius. A B C

10 *Commissure of lips.* Commissura labiorum. Transition of upper lip into lower lip at the angle of the mouth. A B

11 **Angle of mouth.** Angulus oris. A

12 **Cheek.** Bucca. Lateral wall of vestibule of mouth. A

13 Buccal fat pad. Corpus adiposum buccae. [[Bichat]]. Encapsulated body of fat between the buccinator and masseter muscles. A

14 **Oral cavity proper.** Cavitas oris propria. True
~ oral cavity enclosed anteriorly and laterally by the teeth and extending as far as the faucial (oropharyngeal) isthmus. C

15 **Palate.** Palatum. Partition between oral and nasal cavities.

16 Hard palate. Palatum durum. Hard, bony part of the palate. C D

17 Soft palate. Palatum molle (Velum palatinum). Soft, posteriorly situated part of the palate. C D

18 Palatine raphe. Raphe palati. Median mucosal ridge at the junction of the right and left bony palatal processes. D

19 **Oral mucosa.** Tunica mucosa oris. Mucous membrane of oral cavity consisting throughout of stratified squamous, nonkeratinized epithelium with underlying mixed glands.

20 **Frenulum of upper lip.** Frenulum labii superioris. Median mucosal fold between the gums and upper lip. B

21 **Frenulum of lower lip.** Frenulum labii inferioris. Median mucosal fold between the gums and lower lip. B

22 **Gums.** Gingivae. Mucous membrane united firmly with the teeth and jaw bones. B D

23 Gingival (gum) margin. Margo gingivalis. B D

24 Gingival (interdental) papilla. Papilla gingivalis (interdentalis). B D

25 Gingival sulcus. Sulcus gingivalis. Shallow furrow between the gum margin and the tooth. Its deepening leads to cavity formation. See p. 113. A

26 **Sublingual papilla.** Caruncula sublingualis. A small mucosal eminence on the right and left side of the frenulum. It receives the opening of the submandibular duct and the major sublingual duct. B

27 **Sublingual fold.** Plica sublingualis. Mucosal fold overlying the sublingual gland and extending posterolaterally from the sublingual papilla. B

28 **Parotid papilla.** Papilla ductus parotidei. Small mucosal elevation at the opening of the parotid duct lateral to the second upper molar tooth. B

29 **Transverse palatine folds.** Plicae palatinae transversae. Mucosal folds running transversely on the anterior part of the hard palate. D

30 **Incisive papilla.** Papilla incisiva. Small mucosal elevation over the incisive foramen at the anterior end of the palatine raphe. D

31 SMALL GLANDS OF THE ORAL CAVITY.
~ GLANDULAE SALIVARIAE MINORES.

32 **Labial glands.** Gll. labiales. Small salivary glands at the inner aspect of the lips. B

33 **Buccal glands.** Gll. buccales. Small mucous salivary glands at the inner aspect of the cheeks. B

34 **Molar glands.** Gll. molares. Salivary glands corresponding to the buccal glands situated beneath the mucosa at the level of the molar teeth. B

35 **Palatine glands.** Gll. palatinae. Salivary glands situated beneath the mucosa of the palate. (Two large groups right and left of the midline.) D

36 **Lingual glands.** Gll. linguales. Numerous mucous, serous and mixed glands primarily in the lateral and posterior areas of the tongue. B

37 Anterior lingual glands. Gl. lingualis anterior [[gl. apicis linguae, Nuhn' glands]]. Mixed glands in the apex of the tongue with several excretory ducts on the undersurface of the tongue. B

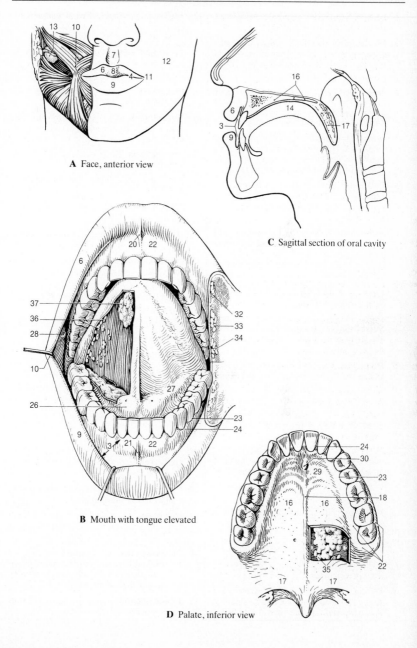

A Face, anterior view

C Sagittal section of oral cavity

B Mouth with tongue elevated

D Palate, inferior view

1   LARGE SALIVARY GLANDS. GLANDU-
    LAE SALIVARIAE MAJORES.

2   **Sublingual gland.** Glandula sublingualis.
    Predominantly mucous gland situated on the
    mylohyoid muscle (diaphragma oris). It pos-
    sesses several excretory ducts. D

3   **Major sublingual duct.** Ductus sublingulis
    major. Main excretory duct of the sublingual
    gland. It opens on the sublingual papilla next to
    the submandibular duct. D

4   **Minor sublingual ducts.** Ductus sublinguales
    minores. About 40 small excretory ducts of the
    sublingual gland with openings on the sublin-
    gual fold and the sublingual papilla. D

5   **Submandibular gland.** Glandula sub-
    mandibularis. Predominantly serous salivary
    gland located almost entirely below the mylo-
    hyoid. D F

6   **Submandibular duct.** Ductus submandibula-
    ris. Excretory durct of the submandibular
    gland. It loops around the posterior margin of
    the mylohyoid accompanied by glandular tis-
    sue and opens on the sublingual papilla. D

7   **Parotid gland.** Glandula parotidea. Sali-
~   vary gland located behind and on the mandibu-
    lar ramus. F

8   **Superficial part.** Pars superficialis. Superfici-
    al lobules located on the branches of the facial
    nerve. F

9   **Deep part.** Pars profunda. Deeper lobules
    situated below the branches of the facial nerve.
    F

10 **Accessory parotid gland.** Glandula parotidea
    accessoria. Additional glandular lobules on the
    masseter muscle near the parotid excretory
    duct. F

11 **Parotid duct.** Ductus parotideus. Excretory
    duct of the parotid gland. Its passes around the
    anterior margin of the masseter and opens near
    the second upper molar tooth. F

12 TEETH. DENTES. A B C D E G

13 **Crown of tooth.** Corona dentis. Portion of the
    tooth covered by enamel. E

14 Cusp of tooth. Cuspis dentis [[Tuberculum]].
    1–5 protuberances on the occlusal surface of
    tooth (with the exception of the incisors). E

15 *Apex of cusp.* Apex cuspidis. E

16 Dental tubercle. Tuberculum dentis. Dis-
~   tinctly pronounced eminence on the side of the
    crown especially in canine and incisor teeth. A

17 Transverse ridge. Crista transversalis.
    Transverse connecting ridge between adjacent
    cusps. B

18 Triangular ridge. Crista triangularis. Trian-
    gular connecting ridge between the cusps of the
    molars. B

19 **Clinical crown.** Corona clinica. Portion of the
    tooth projecting above the gum. C

20 **Neck of tooth.** Cervix [[Collum]] dentis. Por-
~   tion of the tooth at the enamel-cementum bor-
    der. E

21 **Root of tooth.** Radix dentis. Portion of the
    tooth covered by cementum. E

22 Apex of root of tooth. Apex radicis dentis.
    E

23 **Clinical root.** Radix clinica. Portion of the
    tooth situated below the gum. C

24 **Occlusal (masticatory) surface.** Facies
    occlusalis (masticatoria). B E

25 **Vestibular (facial) surface.** Facies vestibula-
    ris (facialis). Crown surface facing the vestibu-
    le. D G

25 a **Buccal surface.** Facies buccalis. Crown sur-
    face facing the cheek.

25 b **Labial surface.** Facies labialis. Crown surface
    facing the lips.

26 **Lingual, palatine surface.** Facies lingualis,
    palatalis. Crown surface facing the tongue, the
    palate, respectively. A G

27 **Approximal surface.** Facies approximalis.
    Crown surface facing the adjacent tooth. G

28 Mesial surface. Facies mesialis. Vertical
    contact surface of a tooth turned away from the
    last molar. G

29 Distal surface. Facies distalis. Vertical
    contact surface of a tooth facing away from the
    first incisor. G

29 a Contingent area. Area contingens. Direct
    contact surface of adjacent teeth.

30 **Cingulum.** Ridge near the neck of a tooth
    connecting both marginal crests at the lingual
    surface of incisor and canine teeth. A

31 **Marginal crest.** Crista marginalis. Lateral
    marginal ridge on the lingual surface of the in-
    cisor and canine teeth which goes over into the
    cingulum at the neck region. A

32 **Incisal margin.** Margo incisalis. Occlusal
    edge of incisor and canine teeth. A

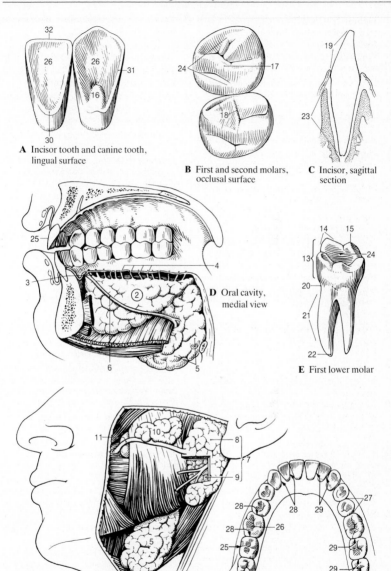

A Incisor tooth and canine tooth, lingual surface

B First and second molars, occlusal surface

C Incisor, sagittal section

D Oral cavity, medial view

E First lower molar

F Salivary glands, lateral view

G Teeth of lower jaw

1 **Pulp cavity of tooth.** Cavitas dentis (pulparis).
~ Cavity in the dentine. Towards the root, it is
continuous with the root canal. A

2 Pulp chamber in the crown. Cavitas coro-
~ nae. Crown portion of the pulp cavity. A

3 Root canal of tooth. Canalis radicis dentis.
Canal between the pulp cavity and the apical
foramen. A

4 *Apical foramen of root of tooth.* Foramen apicis radicis dentalis. The opening of the root canal at the apex of the root. A

5 **Pulp of tooth.** Pulpa dentis. Contents of the
pulp cavity consisting of loose, finely fibered
connective tissue, blood vessels and nerves.

6 Crown pulp. Pulpa coronalis. Pulp within the
crown portion of the pulp cavity.

7 Root pulp. Pulpa radicularis. Pulp within the
root canal portion of the pulp cavity.

8 **Dental papilla.** Papilla dentis. A mass of
mesenchyme contained in the bell stage of
tooth development. B

9 **Dentine.** Dentinum [[Substantia eburnea]].
Predominant mass of a tooth consisting of in-
organic and organic material (especially collagenous fibers). A C

10 **Enamel.** Enamelum [[Substantia adamanti-
na]]. The extremely hard substance surrounding the crown of the tooth like a mantle. A C

11 **Gomphosis.** Type of fibrous joint in which a
conical process, e.g., a tooth, is inserted into a
socket, e.g., alveolus of the jaw (Dentoalveolar
articulation).

12 **Periodontium.** Tissues surrounding and supporting the tooth within the alveolus. It consists
of the following parts: A

13 Periodontium protectoris [[Gingiva]].
The outer part of the periodontium with the external border epithelium. A

14 Periodontium insertionis. Portion of the
periodonium touching the tooth. It consists of
the inner border epithelium and the periodontal ligament. A

15 *Periodontal ligament.* Desmodontium. All
connective tissue fibers which are anchored in
the cementum and with their vessels and nerves
extend partly into the gum and partly into the
alveolar wall. A

16 Cementum. Substance similar to bone. It surrounds the tooth from the enamel border to the
apex of the root and receives the fibers of the
periodontal ligament. A

17 Alveolar bone. Os alveolare. Bony wall of
the alveolus. A

18 **Superior dental arch.** Arcus dentalis superior.
Curved row of teeth of the maxilla.

19 **Inferior dental arch.** Arcus dentalis inferior.
Curved row of teeth of the mandible.

20 **Incisor teeth.** Dentes incisivi. Cutting teeth located on both sides of the midline at the 1st and
2nd positions of the dental arch. D

21 **Canine teeth.** Dentes canini. Tooth located at
the 3rd position of the dental arch. D

22 **Premolar teeth.** Dentes premolares. Teeth occupying the 4th and 5th position of the dental
arch. D

23 **Molar teeth.** Dentes molares. Teeth located at
the 6th, 7th and 8th positions of the dental arch.
D

24 Wisdom tooth. Dens serotinus [Molaris ter-
~ tius]. Tooth located at the 8th position of the
dental arch. D

25 **Deciduous (milk) teeth.** Dentes decidui.

26 **Permanent teeth.** Dentes permanentes. Teeth
developing after the deciduous teeth.

27 **Diastema.** Space between adjacent teeth.

28 TONGUE. LINGUA. D E

29 **Body of tongue.** Corpus linguae. Portion of the
tongue situated between the apex and root. E

30 **Root of tongue.** Radix linguae. Anchoring region of the tongue at the mandible and hyoid
bone. Also the posterior, vertical segment of
the tongue. E

31 **Dorsum of tongue.** Dorsum linguae. E

32 Anterior, oral portion of tongue. Pars
presulcalis (anterior). The part of the dorsum of
the tongue situated anterior to the sulcus terminalis. 115 B

33 Posterior, pharyngeal part of tongue.
Pars postsulcalis (posterior). The vertical portion of the dorsum of the tongue between the
sulcus terminalis and the epiglottis. 115 B

34 **Inferior surface of tongue.** Facies inferior linguae. D E

35 Fimbriated fold. Plica fimbriata. Serrated
fold lateral to the frenulum. It is a remnant of
the inferior tongue. D

36 **Lateral margin of tongue bordering the
teeth.** Margo linguae. D

37 **Apex of tongue.** Apex linguae. D E

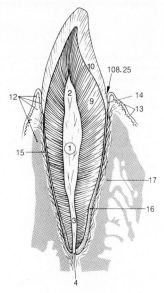

A Longitudinal section of tooth

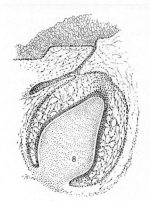

B Tooth development

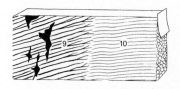

C Enamel-dentin border

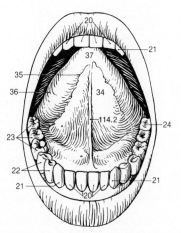

D Mouth with tongue elevated

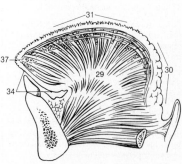

E Tongue, sagittal section

1 **Mucous membrane of tongue.** Tunica mucosa linguae. C

2 **Frenulum of tongue.** Frenulum linguae. Mucosal fold extending from the floor of the mouth to the inferior side of the tongue. D see also 113 D

3 **Lingual papillae.** Papillae linguales. Collective term for the following five different types of mucosal formations: A B

4 Filiform papillae. Papillae filiformes. Fine, almost thread-like epithelial elevations residing on a connective tissue core and possessing tips that are often clefted. A

5 Conical papillae. Papillae conicae. Special form of filiform papilla. They are somewhat larger, longer and exhibit conical apices which bend backwards. A

6 Fungiform papillae. Papillae fungiformes. Mushroom-like papillae which are not pointed above but terminate with a small plateau. A B

7 Vallate (circumvallate) papillae. Papillae vallatae. 7–12 large papillae located in front of the sulcus terminalis. They are circular in cross-section and are surrounded by a moat the wall of which contains taste buds. A B

8 Lenticular papillae. Papilla lentiformes. Short fungiform papillae. A

9 Foliate papilla. Papillae foliatae. Several parallel oriented folds containing taste buds at the posterolateral margin of the tongue. B D

10 **Median groove of tongue.** Sulcus medianus linguae. Shallow, median longitudinal groove situated above the lingual septum. B C

11 **Sulcus terminalis** [["V" linguae]]. Bilateral groove passing obliquely forward from the foramen caecum. It lies behind the row of vallate papillae which run parallel to it. B

12 **Foramen caecum linguae.** Pit situated at the apex of the sulcus terminalis. It is the embryological remains of the thyroglossal duct. B

13 **Thyroglossal duct.** Ductus thyroglossalis. Embryological connection between thyroid gland and tongue. At the site of the future foramen caecum, it grows downward from the base of the tongue as an epithelial cone.

14 **Lingual tonsil.** Tonsilla lingualis. Accumulation of lymphatic tissue (lingual follicles) which is irregularly distributed over the base of the tongue. B D

15 Lingual follicles. Folliculi linguales. Dome-shaped protrusions of the mucosa, 1–5 mm in diameter, caused by the lymphatic tissue formations located below it. Each has a crypt in its center. A

16 **Lingual septum.** Septum lingualis. Connective tissue plate with a special fibrous architecture located in the midsagittal plane. C

17 **Lingual aponeurosis.** Aponeurosis lingualis. Stout connective tissue framework of the tongue between the musculature and the mucosa. C

18 **Tongue musculature.** Musculi linguae (linguales). The following eight tongue muscles are innervated by the hypoglossal nerve (XII).

19 M. genioglossus. o: Mental spine of mandible. i: Fan-shaped distribution within the tongue from the apex to the base. F: It pulls the tongue forward or towards the chin. I: Hypoglossal nerve. C D

20 M. hyoglossus. o: Body and greater horn of hyoid bone. i: Coming from below, it radiates into the lateral parts of the tongue and penetrates up to the mucosa. F: It draws the base of the tongue backward and downward. I: Hypoglossal nerve. D

21 M. chondroglossus. o: Lesser horn of hyoid. i: Same as hyoglossus. I: Hypoglossal nerve. D

22 M. styloglossus. o: Styloid process. i: Coming from behind and above, it radiates to the lateral parts of the tongue and interweaves with the hyoglossus. F: It draws the tongue backward and upward. I: Hypoglossal nerve. D

23 Superior longitudinal muscle of tongue. M. longitudinalis superior. Longitudinal bundles of muscle lying just below the mucosa and extending from the apex of tongue to the region of the hyoid bone. I: Hypoglossal nerve. C

24 Inferior longitudinal muscle of tongue. M. longitudinalis inferior. Longitudinal fibrous system situated close to the inferior surface of the tongue. It passes from the base to the apex of the tongue. I: Hypoglossal nerve. C

25 Transverse muscle of tongue. M. transversus linguae. Transversely oriented muscle fibers extending between the longitudinal system of fibers. o: Lingual septum. i: Mucous membrane along lateral margins of tongue. F: Extension of tongue together with the vertical muscle of the tongue. I: Hypoglossal nerve. C

26 Vertical muscle of tongue. M. verticalis linguae. Vertical muscle fibers coursing from the back of the tongue to the inferior surface. I: Hypoglossal nerve. C

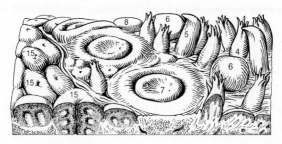

A Surface of tongue, enlarged

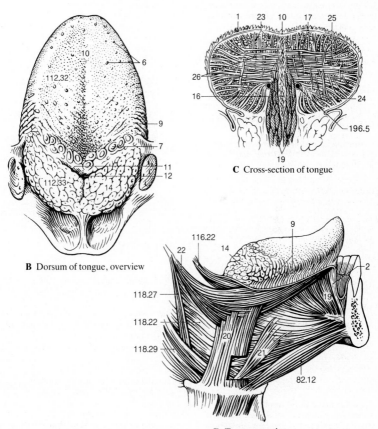

B Dorsum of tongue, overview

C Cross-section of tongue

D Tongue muscles

1 **Pharynx.** Passageway for air and food. 14–16 cm long, it reaches from the fornix to the beginning of the esophagus in front of the 6th cervical vertebra. E

2 FAUCES. Space between soft palate and base of tongue. E

3 **Faucial isthmus.** Isthmus faucium. Space between right and left palatoglossal and palatopharyngeal arches.

4 **Soft palate.** Palatum molle (Velum palatinum). Its dorsal portion projects downward in front of the posterior pharyngeal wall and assists swallowing by closing off the nasopharyngeal space, valve-like, from the oral cavity. A D E

5 Uvula. Uvula palatina. Conical process projecting downward from the posterior margin of the soft palate. A D E

6 Palatoglossal arch. Arcus palatoglossus. Mucosal fold overlying the same-named muscle and extending from the palate to the tongue in front of the tonsillar fossa. A

7 Palatopharyngeal arch. Arcus palatopharyngeus. Mucosal fold overlying the same-named muscle and extending between the palate and pharyngeal wall behind the tonsillar fossa. A

8 **Salpingopalatine fold.** Plica salpingopalatina [[Plica palatotubalis]]. Fold extending from the anterior lip of the auditory tube to the soft palate in front of the tubal elevation. A

9 **Palatine tonsil.** Tonsilla palatina. Tonsil situated between the palatoglossal and palatopharyngeal arches. A

10 Tonsillar pits. Fossulae tonsillae. Pit-like openings of the tonsillar crypts visible on the surface. B

11 *Tonsillar crypts.* Cryptae tonsillares. Epithelial invaginations extending into the tonsil from the tonsillar pits. B

12 *Capsule of tonsil.* Capsula tonsillaris. Connective tissue capsule of the organ.

13 Triangular fold. Plica triangularis. Triangular fold emanating from the palatoglossal arch in front of the tonsil. A

14 **Semilunar fold.** Plica semilunaris. Arched fold between the palatoglossal and palatopharyngeal arches. It borders the tonsillar fossa superiorly. A

15 **Tonsillar fossa.** Fossa tonsillaris. Recess for the tonsil bordered by the palatoglossal and palatopharyngeal arches as well as by the triangular and semilunar folds. D

16 **Supratonsillar fossa.** Fossa supratonsillaris. Superior portion of tonsillar fossa not occupied by the tonsil. A

17 **Muscles of palate and fauces.** Musculi palati et faucium.

18 **Palatine aponeurosis.** Aponeurosis palatina. It is formed primarily by the tendon of the tensor veli palatini muscle. C

19 **M. levator veli palatini.** o: Petrous temporal bone in front of lower opening of the carotid canal. i: Palatine aponeurosis. It passes through the pharyngeal wall above the superior constrictor muscle and moves the soft palate backward and upward thereby taking along the dorsomedial part of the auditory tube cartilage below the pharyngeal opening of the auditory tube. I: Vagus (X) nerve. C

20 **M. tensor veli palatini.** o: Spine of sphenoid, scaphoid fossa and anterior (lateral) lip of cartilaginous auditory tube. i: After looping around the pterygoid hamulus, it radiates into the palatine aponeurosis, stiffens the anterior (lateral) membranous wall of the auditory tube and tenses the soft palate. I: Mandibular nerve. C

21 **M. uvulae.** o: Palatine aponeurosis. i: Connective tissue of uvulae. I: Vagus nerve. C

22 **M. palatoglossus.** o: Transversus linguae muscle. i: Palatine aponeurosis. F: Elevates the base of the tongue, depresses the palate and narrows the faucial isthmus. I: Vagus nerve. D

23 **M. palatopharyngeus** *[[M. pharyngopalatinus]].* o: Palatine aponeurosis, pterygoid hamulus and medial plate of pterygoid process. i: Lateral wall of pharynx and thyroid cartilage. F: It lowers the palate and constricts the faucial isthmus. I: Vagus nerve. D

24 **PHARYNGEAL CAVITY.** CAVITAS
~ PHARYNGIS. Space enclosed by the pharyngeal walls.

25 **Pharyngeal fornix.** Fornix pharyngis. Roof of the pharyngeal cavity beneath the sphenoid bone. E

26 **Nasopharynx.** Pars nasalis pharyngis. The portion of the pharyngeal cavity located behind the choanae. E

27 **Nasopharyngeal tonsil (adenoids).** Tonsilla pharyngealis (adenoidea). It lies at the pharyngeal fornix. E

28 Tonsillar pits. Fossulae tonsillares. Openings of crypts visible on surface of tonsil. See also 116.10. B

29 *Tonsillar crypts.* Cryptae tonsillares. Epithelial invaginations emanating from the tonsillar pits. See also 116.11. B

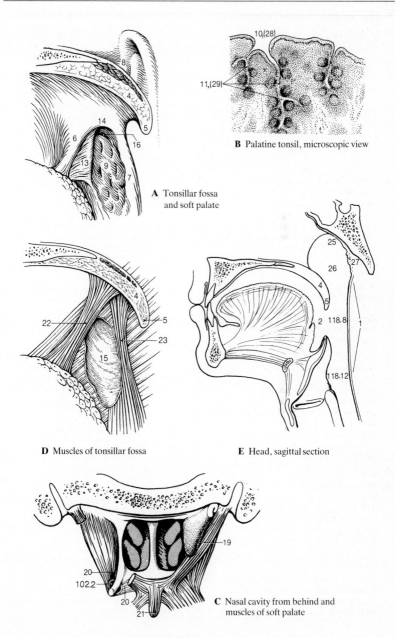

A Tonsillar fossa and soft palate

B Palatine tonsil, microscopic view

D Muscles of tonsillar fossa

E Head, sagittal section

C Nasal cavity from behind and muscles of soft palate

1 **Pharyngeal bursa.** [Bursa pharyngealis]. Blind
~ pouch in the roof of the pharynx; it is more frequently present in children, less often in adults. A

2 **Pharyngeal opening of auditory tube.** Ostium
pharyngeum tubae auditivae (auditoriae). It is
found in the nasopharynx. A

3 *Torus tubarius.* Elevation produced by the dorsomedial cartilage of the auditory tube behind its
opening. A

4 *Salpingopharyngeal fold.* Plica salpingopharyn-
gea. Mucosal fold overlying the salpingopharyngeus muscle and extending obliquely downward
from the dorsomedial lip of the auditory tube cartilage. A

5 *Torus levatorius.* Elevation situated in front of the
dorsomedial lip of the cartilage of the auditory
tube and below its opening. It overlies the levator
veli palatini muscle. A

6 Tubal tonsil. Tonsilla tubaria. Submucosal lymphatic tissue near the opening of the auditory tube.

7 Pharyngeal recess. Recessus pharyngeus [[Ro-
senmüller's]]. Lateral recess of the nasopharyngeal space behind the auditory tube. A

8 **Oropharynx.** Pars oralis pharyngis. The portion of the pharyngeal cavity located behind the
oral cavity. 117. E

9 **Vallecula epiglottica.** Fossa between the median
and lateral glossoepiglottic folds. B

10 Median glossoepiglottic fold. Plica glos-
soepiglottica mediana. Unpaired mucosal fold located in the median plane between the base of the
tongue and the epiglottis. B

11 Lateral glossoepiglottic fold. Plica glos-
soepiglottica lateralis. Bilateral mucosal fold between the base of the tongue and the epiglottis. B

12 **Laryngopharynx.** Pars laryngea pharyngis.
The portion of the pharyngeal cavity situated behind the larynx. See p. 117 E

13 **Piriform recess.** Recessus piriformis. Channel
between the aryepiglottic fold and the thyrohyoid
membrane or thyroid cartilage. B

14 Plica nervi laryngei. Mucosal fold in the piriform recess produced by the underlying internal
branch of the superior laryngeal nerve and the superior laryngeal artery. B

15 **Pharyngobasilar fascia.** Fascia pharyngobasila-
ris. Membranous wall of the uppermost muscular-
free portion of the pharynx. C D E

16 **Submucosa.** Tela submucosa. Connective tissue
layer between the mucosa and muscularis. A

17 **Mucosa.** Tunica mucosa. Pharyngeal mucous
membrane lined by stratified squamous or pseudostratified ciliated columnar (nasopharynx)
epithelium.

18 Pharyngeal glands. Gll. pharyngis. Small sub-
epithelial mixed salivary glands.

19 **Muscularis of pharynx.** Tunica muscularis
pharyngis. Muscular layer of pharyngeal wall. A

20 **Pharyngeal raphe.** Raphe pharyngis. Connective
tissue seam between the right and left pharyngeal
musculature extending posteriorly in the midline.
C

21 **Pterygomandibular raphe.** Raphe pterygoman-
dibularis. Tendinous seam between the buccinator
muscle and the superior pharyngeal constrictor. It
extends from the pterygoid hamulus to the mandible. D

22 **Superior pharyngeal constrictor muscle.** M.
constrictor pharyngis superior. Uppermost constrictor of the pharynx consisting of the following
four parts which attach to the pharyngeal raphe. I:
Pharyngeal plexus. C D

23 Pterygopharyngeal part. Pars pterygo-
pharynea. o: Medial plate of pterygoid process and
ptergoid hamulus. D

24 Buccopharyngeal part. Pars buccopharyngea.
o: Pterygomandibular raphe. D

25 Mylopharyngeal part. Pars mylopharyngea.
o: Posterior end of mylohyoid line of mandible. D

26 Glossopharyngeal part. Pars glossopharyn-
gea. o: Intrinsic muscles of tongue. D

27 **M. stylopharyngeus.** o: Styloid process. i: Between superior and middle pharyngeal constrictors radiating into the pharyngeal wall, thyroid
cartilage and epiglottis. I: Glossopharyngeal (IX).
nerve C

28 **M. salpingopharyngeus.** o: Dorsomedial lip of
auditory tube cartilage and part of longitudinal
musculature of pharyngeal wall. i: Lateral wall of
pharynx. F: Prevents backward sliding of levator
veli palatini muscle. I: Pharyngeal plexus. A

29 **Middle pharyngeal constrictor muscle.** M. constrictor pharyngis medius. More centrally located
pharyngeal constrictor coming from the hyoid
bone. o: Pharyngeal raphe. I: Pharyngeal plexus. C

30 Chondropharyngeal part. Pars chondro-
pharyngea. o: Lesser horn of hyoid. D

31 Ceratopharyngeal part. Pars ceratopharyn-
gea. o: Greater horn of hyoid. D

32 **Inferior pharyngeal constrictor muscle.** M.
constrictor pharyngis inferior. o: Larynx. I:
Pharyngeal plexus. C D

33 Thyropharyngeal part. Pars thyropharyngea.
o: Oblique line of thyroid cartilage. D

34 Cricopharyngeal part. Pars circopharyngea.
o: Cricoid cartilage. D

34 a **Buccopharyngeal fascia.** Fascia buccopharynge-
alis. Investing fascia of the entire system.

35 **Peripharyngeal space.** Spatium peripharynge-
um. Connective tissue space associated with the
pharynx.

36 Retropharyngeal space. Spatium retro-
pharyngeum. The portion of the peripharyngeal
space between the pharynx and the prevertebral
layer of the cervical fascia. A

37 Lateropharyngeal space. Spatium latero-
pharyngeum. Portion of the peripharyngeal space
lateral to the pharynx.

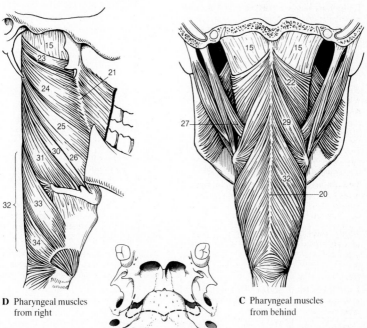

A Pharyngeal opening of auditory tube

B Base of tongue and laryngeal opening

D Pharyngeal muscles from right

E Attachment of the pharyngobasilar fascia

C Pharyngeal muscles from behind

1 DIGESTIVE TRACT (ALIMENTARY CANAL). [[[CANALIS ALIMENTARIUS].

2 ESOPHAGUS. OESOPHAGUS. 23–26 cm
~ long from below the cricoid cartilage at the level of C6 to the cardiac part of the stomach. A B

3 **Cervical part.** Pars cervicalis. The segment of the esophagus situated in front of the cervical vertebral column (from C6–T1). A

4 **Thoracic part.** Pars thoracica. The portion of the esophagus extending from T1 to the passageway through the diaphragm (about T11). A

5 **Abdominal part.** Pars abdominalis. The short esophageal segment between the diaphragm and the stomach. A

6 **Tunica adventitia.** Loose connective tissue investment which binds the esophagus to the surrounding tissues and permits its movement. C

7 **Tunica muscularis.** Two layers of muscle, inner circular and outer longitudinal, occupying the esophageal wall and consisting of skeletal muscle in the upper third, smooth muscle in the lower third. C

8 Cricoesophageal tendon. Tendo cricoesophageus. Tendinous attachment of the esophageal longitudinal musculature to the posterior wall of the cricoid cartilage. B

9 **Bronchoesophageal muscle.** M. bronchoesophageus. Smooth muscle fibers from the left main bronchus to the esophagus. B

10 **Pleuroesophageal muscle.** M. pleuroesophageus. Smooth muscle tract between the esophagus and the left mediastinal pleura. B

11 **Tela submucosa.** Movable layer between the muscularis and mucosa consisting predominantly of collagenous connective tissue with blood vessels, nerves and glands. C

12 **Tunica mucosa.** Mucous membrane lining of the esophagus consisting of stratified squamous, nonkeratinized epithelium, lamina propria (connective tissue) and muscularis mucosae. C

13 *Lamina muscularis mucosae.* Distinct layer of smooth muscle between the submucosa and lamina propria. C

14 **Esophageal glands.** Gll. esophageae. Discrete mixed glands scattered within the submucosa. C

15 *STOMACH.* GASTER (VENTRICULUS). It extends from the end of the esophagus to the pylorus. A D

16 **Anterior surface of stomach.** Paries anterior. D

17 **Posterior surface of stomach.** Paries posterior. D

18 **Greater curvature of stomach.** Curvatura gastrica (ventricularis) major. Large curvature of the stomach profile directed toward the left and downward. D

19 **Lesser curvature of stomach.** Curvatura gastrica (ventricularis) minor. Small curvature of stomach directed toward the right and upward. D

20 Angular notch. Incisura angularis. Radiographically evident notch at the deepest point of the lesser curvature. D

21 **Cardiac part of stomach.** Pars cardiaca. The portion of the stomach into which the esophagus opens. D

22 Cardiac orifice. Ostium cardiacum (Cardia). Opening of the esophagus into the cardiac stomach. D

23 **Fundic stomach.** Fundus gastricus (ventricu-
~ laris). Fundus (dome) of the stomach lying beneath the diaphragm. D

23a **Fornix of stomach.** Fornix gastricus (ventricularis).

24 Cardiac notch. Incisura cardiaca. Acute angle between the esophagus and the stomach wall. D

25 **Body of stomach.** Corpus gastricum (ventriculare). Portion of stomach situated between the cardiac and fundic portions above and the pyloric portion below. D

26 Gastric canal. Canalis gastricus (ventricularis). Stomach route along the lesser curvature produced by the orientation of the longitudinal mucosal folds located there. D

27 **Pyloric part of stomach.** Pars pyloricum. Distal segment of the stomach beginning with the angular notch and ending with the pylorus. D

28 Pyloric antrum. Antrum pyloricum. Initial segment of the pyloric stomach beginning at the angular notch and capable of being completely closed off from the remaining gastric lumen by the passage of a peristaltic contraction. D

29 Pyloric canal. Canalis pyloricus. Lower terminal segment, about 2–3 cm long. D

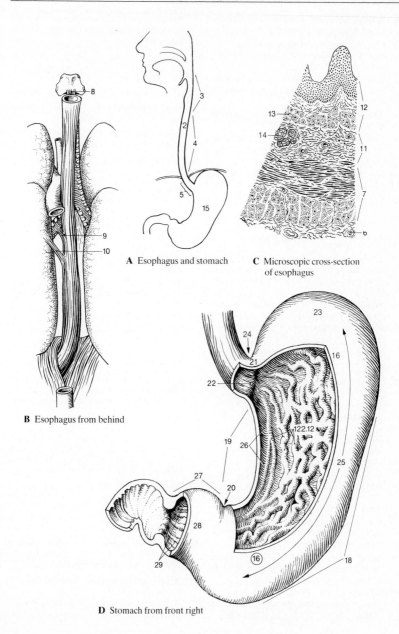

A Esophagus and stomach

C Microscopic cross-section
of esophagus

B Esophagus from behind

D Stomach from front right

1 **Pylorus.** Distal end of the stomach provided with reinforced circular muscle. A

2 Pyloric opening. Ostium pyloricum. Lumen of the pylorus connecting the stomach with the duodenum. A

3 **Serous membrane.** Tunica serosa. Serous, peritoneal covering containing simple squamous epithelium. B

4 **Tela subserosa.** Connective tissue component of the serosa underlying the epithelium. B

5 **Tunica muscularis.** Muscularis of the stomach exhibiting fibers oriented in three directions. A B

6 Longitudinal layer. Stratum longitudinale. External layer of longitudinal muscle fibers situated primarily along the greater and lesser curvatures. A B

7 Circular layer. Stratum circulare. Middle layer of circular muscle. A B

8 *Pyloric sphincter.* M. sphincter pyloricus. Thick layer of circular muscle at the pylorus. A

9 Oblique fibers. Fibrae obliquae. Obliquely directed fibers occupying the innermost muscular layer. A B

10 **Tela submucosa.** Displaceable layer situated between the muscularis mucosae and the muscularis and composed primarily of collagenous connective tissue bearing vessels and nerves. B

11 **Tunica mucosa.** Gastric mucous membrane consisting of simple columnar epithelium, connective tissue (lamina propria) and muscularis mucosae. B

12 Gastric folds. Plicae gastricae. Mucosal folds extending primarily in a longitudinal direction. See p. 121 D

13 *Lamina muscularis mucosae.* Layer of smooth muscle between the lamina propria and the submucosa. Its contraction produces folds in the mucosa. B

14 Gastric (mamillated) areas. Areae gastricae. Hump-like fields of the mucosal surface bordered by shallow grooves and having a diameter of 1–6 mm. B

15 Villous folds. Plicae villosae. Epithelial ridges invisible to the naked eye between the openings of glands. B C D

16 Gastric pits (foveolae). Foveolae gastri-
~ cae. Openings of the gastric glands between the villous folds. B C D

17 Gastric glands proper. Glandula gastrica
~ propria. Tubular glands in the fundus and body of the stomach made up of 4 cell types. B C

18 Pyloric glands. Glandula pylorica. Mucoid
~ glands in the pyloric part of the stomach consisting of two cell types. D

19 Lymphatic nodules (follicles). [[Folliculi lymphatici gastrici]]. Small aggregations of lymphatic tissue in the lamina propria. C D

20 SMALL INTESTINE. INTESTINUM TENUE. It comprises the duodenum, jejunum and ileum.

21 **Tunica serosa.** Peritoneal covering containing simple squamous epithelium. F

22 **Tela subserosa.** Connective tissue underlying the serosa. F

23 **Tunica muscularis.** Two principal muscle layers occupy the intestinal wall. F

24 Longitudinal layer. Stratum longitudinale. External, longitudinally oriented muscle layer. F

25 Circular layer. Stratum circulare. Internal, circularly arranged muscle layer. F

26 **Tela sumucosa.** Displaceable layer between the muscularis mucosae and the muscularis consisting primarily of collagenous connective tissue bearing blood vessels and nerves. F

27 **Tunica mucosa.** Intestinal mucous membrane consisting of simple columnar epithelium, connective tissue (lamina propria) and muscularis mucosae.

28 *Lamina muscularis mucosae.* Layer of smooth muscle between the lamina propria and submucosa. Its action produces folds in the mucosa. F

29 Circular folds [Valves of Kerckring]. Plicae circulares. Permanent folds of mucosa and submucosa spanning about 2/3 around the intestinal lumen and projecting up to 8 mm high, perpendicular to the intestinal axis. E F

30 Intestinal villi. Villi intestinales. Finger-like projections about 0.5–1.5 mm in length. F

31 Intestinal glands. Gll. intestinales. Crypt-like glands. F

32 Solitary lymphatic follicles. Folliculi lymphatici solitarii. Solitary lymphatic nodules in the lamina propria (401.42) F

33 **Aggregated lymphatic follicles** *[[Peyer's patches]].* Folliculi lymphatici aggregati. Aggregation of several lymphatic nodules in the ileum.

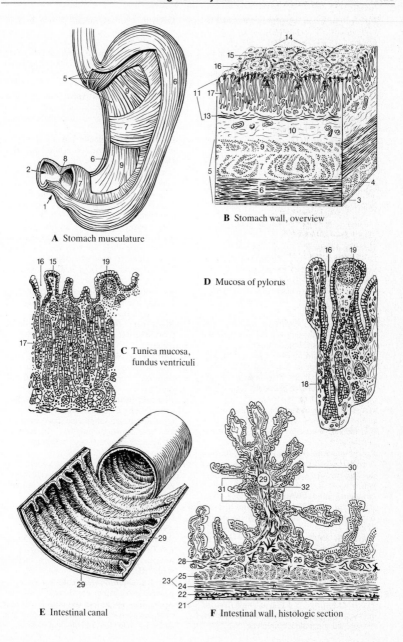

A Stomach musculature

B Stomach wall, overview

C Tunica mucosa, fundus ventriculi

D Mucosa of pylorus

E Intestinal canal

F Intestinal wall, histologic section

1 **Duodenum.** Initial segment of the small intestine, about 25–30 mm long, between the pylorus and the duodenojejunal flexure. A

2 **Superior part.** Pars superior. Horizontal beginning part of the duodenum. A

3 **Ampulla** [[Bulbus duodeni]]. Functional dilatation at the beginning of the duodenum. It is briefly visible in radiograms. A

4 **Descending part.** Pars descendens. Lateral, vertical segment. A

5 **Horizontal (inferior) part.** Pars horizontalis (inferior). Horizontal segment below the head of the pancreas. A

6 **Ascending part.** Pars ascendens. Segment of duodenum lying to the left of the head of the pancreas and ascending up to the duodenojejunal flexure. A

7 **Superior duodenal flexure.** Flexura duodeni superior. Flexure between the superior and horizontal parts of the duodenum medial to the gallbladder. A

8 **Inferior duodenal flexure.** Flexura duodeni inferior. Flexure between the descending and horizontal parts of the duodenum. A

9 **Duodenojejunal flexure.** Flexura duodenojejunalis. Flexure between the duodenum and jejunum. A

10 **Suspensory muscle of duodenum.** M. suspensorius duodeni. Bundle of smooth muscle which fixes the duodenojejunal flexure to the diaphragm or to the celiac trunk. A

11 **Longitudinal folds of duodenum.** Plicae longitudinales duodeni. Longitudinal mucosal folds on the medial aspect of the posterior wall of the descending part produced by the pancreatic and bile ducts. A

12 **Greater duodenal papilla.** Papilla duodeni major. Projection at the end of the longitudinal fold with the openings of the bile and pancreatic ducts. A

13 **Lesser duodenal papilla.** Papilla duodeni minor. Projection located superior to the greater duodenal papilla. The opening of the accessory pancreatic duct is usually present here. A

14 **Duodenal glands** [[Brunner's glands]]. Glandulae duodenales. Mucous glands located predominantly in the submucosa of the duodenum. A

15 **Jejunum.** Middle segment of the small intestine. It extends about 2.5 meters from the duodenojejunal flexure. A C

16 **Ileum.** Terminal segment of small intestine, about 3.5 mm long. C

17 LARGE INTESTINE. INTESTINUM CRASSUM. Measuring 1.5–1.8 m in length from the cecum to the anus, it is characterized by tenia, haustra and appendices epiploicae.

18 **Cecum.** Caecum. Initial portion of large
~ intestine, about 7 cm long below the ileal opening. C D

19 **Ileocecal valve.** Valva ileocaecalis (Valva ilealis). Twolipped valve at the entrance of the ileum into the large intestine. D

19 a **Papilla ilealis.** B

20 **Opening of ileocecal valve.** Ostium valvae ilealis. Transverse, slit-like aperture of ileum at entrance into the large intestine in the cadaver. D

21 **Frenulum valvae ilealis.** Fold formed by the union of the lips of the ileocecal valve. D B

21 a **Ostium papillae ilealis.** B

22 **Vermiform appendix.** Appendix vermiformis. Appendage of the cecum, usually 9 cm long, with abundant lymphatic tissue. B C D

23 *Ostium appendicis vermiformis.* Opening of vermiform appendix into the cecum. D

24 Aggregated lymphatic nodules of vermiform appendix. Folliculi lymphatici aggregati appendicis vermiformis. Lymphatic tissue within the wall of the appendix.

25 **Colon.** Portion of large intestine extending from the ileocecal valve to the rectum.

26 **Ascending colon.** Colon ascendens. Segment of large intestine ascending retroperitoneally on the right side. C

27 **Right colic flexure.** Flexura coli dextra. Flexure between the ascending and transverse colon. C

28 **Transverse colon.** Colon transversum. Transverse segment of large intestine situated intraperitoneally between the right and left colic flexures. C

29 **Left colic flexure.** Flexura coli sinistra. Flexure between the transverse and descending colon below the left subphrenic space. In its vicinity lies Cannon-Böhm's ring, the boundary between the cranial (vagus nerve) and sacral parasympathetics. C

30 **Descending colon.** Colon descendens. Segment of large intestine extending retroperitoneally on the left side between the left colic flexure and sigmoid colon. C

31 **Sigmoid colon.** Colon sigmoideum. Portion of colon lying intraperitoneally between the descending colon and the rectum. C

32 **Semilunar folds of colon.** Plicae semilunares coli. Crescentic contraction folds between two haustra. It contains all layers of the intestinal wall. C D

33 **Haustra (sacculationes) coli.** Outpocketings between two semilunar folds. C D

34 **Appendices epiploicae (omentales).** Serosa-covered appendages containing adipose tissue and lying on the free and omental tenia. C

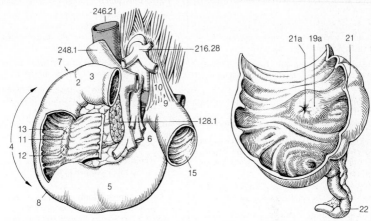

A Portal vein, inferior vena cava, aorta and duodenum

B Cecum in the living organism [91]

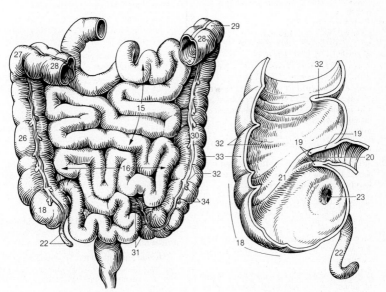

C Small and large intestines, anterior view

D Cecum in the cadaver

1 **Tunica muscularis.** Bilayered muscle wall of colon. B

2 Longitudinal layer. Stratum longitudinale. Distinct outer layer of longitudinally oriented muscle of variable thickness. B

3 *Taenia coli.* Taeniae coli. About 1 cm wide thickened bands of the longitudinal musculature. B

4 Taenia mesocolica. Tenia located at the attachment of the mesocolon. At the ascending and descending colon it lies posteromedially. A

5 Taenia omentalis. Tenia of transverse colon located at the attachment of the greater omentum. At the ascending and descending colon it lies posteromedially. A

6 *Taenia libera.* Free tenia located between the tenia mesocolica and tenia omentalis. A

7 Circular layer. Stratum circulare. Inner muscular layer of colon. B

8 **Tela submucosa.** Displaceable layer lying between the muscularis mucosa and the muscularis and consisting mainly of collagenous connective tissue with nerves and blood vessels. B

9 **Tunica mucosa.** Villus-free mucous membrane of colon consisting of simple columnar epithelium with abundant goblet cells, connective tissue (lamina propria) and muscularis mucosae. B

10 Lamina muscularis mucosae. Layer of smooth muscle cells between the lamina propria and submucosa. Its contraction produces a wrinkling of the mucosa. B

11 *Intestinal glands.* Glandulae intestinales. Tubular glands of the colonic mucosa. B

12 Solitary lymphatic nodules. Nodi lymphatici solitarii. Individual lymphatic nodules dispersed in the lamina propria. B

13 **Rectum.** Tenia-free segment, about 15 cm long, located between the sigmoid colon and the anus. C

14 **Sacral flexure.** Flexura sacralis. Rectal curvature, concave anteriorly, in conformity to the sacrum. C

15 **Perineal flexure.** Flexura perinealis. Rectal curvature, convex anteriorly, just above the anus. C

16 **Ampulla recti.** Expansion of the rectum above the anal canal. C

17 **Tunica muscularis.** Muscular wall of rectum. C

18 *Longitudinal layer.* Stratum longitudinale. It is distributed uniformly over the entire circumference. C

19 Circular layer. Stratum circulare. Situated internally, it forms no semilunar folds. C

20 **Internal anal sphincter.** M. sphincter ani internus. Reinforced, 1–2 cm high, muscular ring of the circular layer at the anus. C

21 **M. rectococcygeus.** Thin plate of smooth muscle extending from coccygeal vertebrae 2 and 3 to the rectum. C

22 **M. rectourethralis.** Smooth muscle fibers from the membranous part of the urethra to the rectum. C

23 **Transverse rectal folds.** Plicae transversae recti. Usually three lateral transverse folds. The middle is the largest (*Kohlrausch*) and projects about 6 mm above the anus from the right side, the others from the left. C

24 **Anal canal.** Canalis analis. Terminal segment of the digestive tube beginning with the anal columns. D

25 **Anal columns.** Columnae anales. Six to ten longitudinal folds provided with abundant venous plexuses. D

26 **Anal sinuses.** Sinus anales. Recesses between the anal columns. D

27 **Anal valves.** Valvulae anales. Small transverse folds bordering the anal sinuses distally. D

28 **Anorectal line.** Linea anorectalis. Upper border of anal canal at the level of the levator sling formed by the puborectalis muscle. It lies just above the anal columns. D

29 **Anal pecten.** [[Pecten analis]]. A lighter stripe between the anal valves and the anocutaneous line. It is firmly connected with the underlying tissues by longitudinal muscles radiating like connective tissue. D

30 **Anocutaneous line.** [[Linea anocutanea]]. Lower border of anal pecten at the level of the lower margin of the internal anal sphincter. D

31 **External anal sphincter.** M. sphincter ani externus. Circular layer of skeletal muscle lying on the internal anal sphincter. C D See 174.14–17

32 **Anus.** Lower opening of anal canal surrounded by the subcutaneous and superficial parts of the external anal sphincter. C D

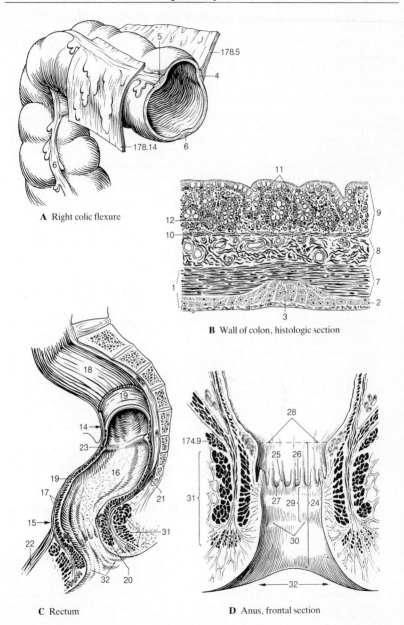

A Right colic flexure

B Wall of colon, histologic section

C Rectum

D Anus, frontal section

1 **PANCREAS.** It is 13–15 cm in length and lies partly in the duodenal loop, partly behind the omental bursa at the level of L1–2. A B

2 **Head of pancreas.** Caput pancreatis. It is nestled within the loop of the duodenum. A

3 Uncinate process. Processus uncinatus. Hook-shaped process passing behind the superior mesenteric vessels. A B

4 Pancreatic notch. Incisura pancreatis. Groove between the uncinate process and the remaining part of the head of the pancreas. A B

5 **Body of pancreas.** Corpus pancreatis. Part of the pancreas lying mainly in front of the vertebral column. It arises from the dorsal anlage of the pancreas. A B

6 Anterior surface. Facies anterior. Surface directed anterosuperiorly. A

7 Posterior surface. Facies posterior. Surface directed posteriorly. B

8 Inferior surface. Facies inferior. Surface directed anteroinferiorly. It is bordered above by the root of the transverse mesocolon. A

9 Superior margin. Margo superior. Upper border between the anterior and posterior surfaces. A B

10 Anterior margin. Margo anterior. It corresponds to the line of attachment of the transverse mesocolon (178.5) and also forms the lower boundary line of the omental bursa at the posterior abdominal wall. A

11 Inferior margin. Margo inferior. Inferior boder situated between the lower anterior and posterior surfaces. A

12 Tuber omentale. Prominence on the body of pancreas near the head. It projects into the omental bursa and is caused by the vertebral column. A B

13 **Tail of pancreas.** Cauda pancreatis. Lying on the left side and above, it borders on the spleen. A B

14 **Capsule of pancreas.** Capsula pancreatis.

15 **Exocrine pancreas.** Pars exocrina pancreatis. The main mass of the gland producing pancreatic juice.

16 **Pancreatic lobule.** Lobulus pancreaticus. The macroscopically demonstrable lobule of the pancreas. A

17 **Pancreatic duct.** Ductus pancreaticus. Main excretory duct of the pancreas opening on the greater duodenal papilla together with the bile duct. B

18 Sphincter muscle of pancreatic duct. Musculus sphincter ductus pancreatici. Circular muscle before the duct opening. See 135 A

19 **Accessory pancreatic duct.** Ductus pancreaticus accessorius. Additional excretory duct usually present. It opens on the lesser duodenal papilla (124.13) above the greater duodenal papilla. B

20 **Accessory pancreas.** (Pancreas accessorium). Pancreatic tissue dispersed within the wall of the stomach or duodenum.

21 **Endocrine pancreas.** Pars endocrina pancreatis. Islets of Langerhans, about 1 million, producing glucagon and insulin.

22 LIVER. HEPAR. It is divided into segments on the basis of the branchings of its blood vessels and biliary ducts. The individual segments, however, are not represented uniformly in the literature. The International Nomenclature Committee has adopted Hjortsjö's classification. C

23 **Diaphragmatic surface.** Facies diaphragmatica. Surface of liver facing the diaphragm. C

24 **Superior part.** Pars superior. Part of the diaphragmatic surface facing cranially. C

25 Cardiac impression. Impressio cardiaca. Flat indentation produced by the heart on the left side in front of the inferior vena cava. C

26 **Anterior part.** Pars anterior. Segment of diaphragmatic surface directed anteriorly. C

27 **Right part.** Pars dextra. Segment of diaphragmatic surface directed toward the right side. C

28 **Posterior part.** Pars posterior. Segment of diaphragmatic surface directed posteriorly. C

29 **Bare area.** Area nuda [[Pars affixa]]. Part of diaphragmatic surface not covered by peritoneum. C

30 Groove for vena cava. Sulcus venae cavae. Deep groove for reception of the inferior vena cava. C

31 Groove for ligamentum venosum. Fissura lig. venosi. Groove from the liver hilum to the inferior vena cava between the caudate and left lobes. C

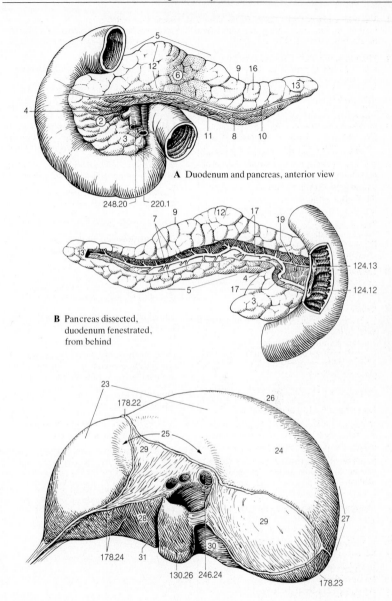

A Duodenum and pancreas, anterior view

B Pancreas dissected,
duodenum fenestrated,
from behind

C Liver, superior view

1   **Visceral surface.** Facies visceralis. Postero-inferior, partially concave surface of liver facing the viscera.

2   **Fossa of gallbladder.** Fossa vesicae biliaris. It occupies the visceral surface. A

3   **Fissure for round ligament.** Fissura lig. teretis. Groove on the visceral surface for the round ligament of liver. A

4   Round ligament of liver. Lig. teres hepatis. The connective tissue remains of the umbilical vein. B

5   **Ligamentum venosum.** Lig. venosum [[Arantii]]. The connective tissue remains of the ductus venosus. B

6   **Hilum of liver.** Porta hepatis. Fissure between the caudate and quadrate lobes in which run the hepatic artery proper, portal vein and hepatic duct. A B

7   **Tuber omentale.** Bulge on the visceral surface of the left lobe to the left of the ligamentum venosum. A B

8   **Esophageal impression.** Impressio oesophagea. Groove on the left lobe indented by the esophagus. A

9   **Gastric impression.** Impressio gastrica. Impression of the stomach on the visceral surface of the left lobe. A

10 **Duodenal impression.** Impressio duodenalis. Impression of the duodenum on the right side of the visceral surface next to the neck of the gallbladder. A B

11 **Colic impression.** Impressio colica. Impression of the colon on the visceral surface of the right lobe to the right of the gallbladder. A

12 **Renal impression.** Impressio renalis. Impression of the right kidney on the visceral surface of the right lobe. It overlaps the bare area. A

13 **Suprarenal impression.** Impressio suprarenalis. Impression of the right suprarenal gland in the bare area on the right side near the inferior vena cava. A

14 **[Appendix fibrosa hepatis].** Connective tissue band occasionally present at the upper end of the left lobe of the liver. A

15 Inferior margin. Margo inferior. Border between the diaphragmatic and visceral surfaces of the liver. A

16 **Incisura lig. teretis.** Notch for round ligament at the lower border of the liver. A B

17 **Lobes of liver.** Lobi hepatis. Four lobes are macroscopically evident:

18 **Right lobe of liver.** Lobus hepatis dexter. Its border to the left lobe corresponds to the line connecting the inferior vena cava and fundus of the gallbladder. A B C

19 Anterior segment of liver. Segmentum anterius. C D

20 Posterior segment of liver. Segmentum posterius. C D

21 **Left lobe of liver.** Lobus hepatis sinister. Its right border corresponds to a line connecting the inferior vena cava and fundus of gallbladder. A B C

22 Medial segment. Segmentum mediale. C D

23 *Quadrate part*. Pars quadrata. Part belonging to the quadrate lobe. D

24 Lateral segment. Segmentum laterale. C D

25 **Quadrate lobe.** Lobus quadratus. Liver lobe situated between the gallbladder, round ligament and hilum. A B

26 **Caudate lobe.** Lobus caudatus. Liver lobe situated between the inferior vena cava, hilum and ligamentum venosum. A B

27 Papillary process. Processus papillaris. Portion of caudate lobe projecting caudally. A B

28 Caudate process. Processus caudatus. Parenchymal connection between the caudate and right lobes cranial to the hilum. A B

29 **Tunica serosa.** Peritoneal covering containing simple squamous epithelium.

30 **Tela subserosa.** Connective tissue layer beneath the serosa.

31 **Tunica fibrosa.** Immovable connective tissue capsule of liver, well developed especially in the bare area not covered by peritoneum.

32 **Ligament of vena cava.** [[Lig. venae cavae]]. Connective tissue bridging over the inferior vena cava.

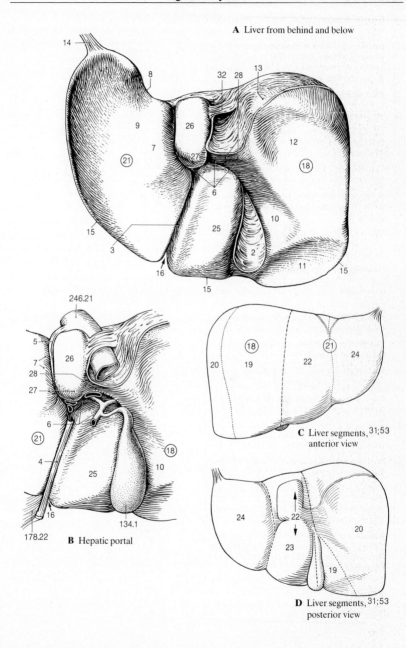

A Liver from behind and below

B Hepatic portal

C Liver segments, 31;53 anterior view

D Liver segments, 31;53 posterior view

1 **Hepatic lobules.** Lobuli hepatis. They measure 1–2 mm in size. A

2 **Perivascular fibrous capsule.** Capsula fibrosa perivascularis. Connective tissue accompanying the liver vessels and biliary ducts until their terminal branches. A

3 **Interlobular arteries.** Arteriae interlobulares. Branches of the hepatic artery proper between the liver lobules. A

4 **Interlobular veins.** Venae interlobulares. Branches of the portal veins between the liver lobules: A

5 **Central veins.** Venae centrales. Efferent veins in the center of the liver lobule. A

6 **Interlobular ductules.** Ductuli interlobulares. Biliary ductules situated between the liver lobules. A

7 **Ductuli biliferi.** Biliary excretory ductules which connect the interlobular ductules with the right and left hepatic ducts.

8 **Common hepatic duct.** Ductus hepaticus communis. Biliary duct between the cystic duct and the junction of right and left hepatic ducts. B

9 Right hepatic duct. Ductus hepaticus dexter. Biliary duct from the right lobe of liver. B

10 *Anterior branch.* Ramus anterior. Branch from the anterior segment. B

11 Posterior branch. Ramus posterior. Branch from the posterior segment. B

12 Left hepatic duct. Ductus hepaticus sinister. Biliary duct from the left lobe of the liver. B

13 *Lateral branch.* Ramus lateralis. Branch from the lateral segment. B

14 *Medial branch.* Ramus medialis. Branch from the medial segment. B

15 **Right duct of caudate lobe.** Ductus lobi caudati dexter. Branch coming from the right half of the caudate lobe and usually leading into right hepatic duct. B

16 **Left duct of caudate lobe.** Ductus lobi caudati sinister. Branch coming from the left half of the caudate lobe and emptying usually into the left hepatic duct. B

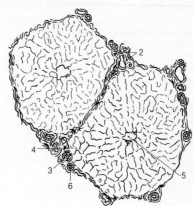

A Two liver lobules

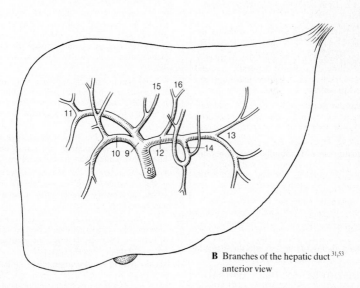

B Branches of the hepatic duct [31,53]
anterior view

1 **Gallbladder.** Vesica biliaris (fellea). 8–12
~ cm long and pear-shaped. A

2 **Fundus of gallbladder.** Fundus ves. biliaris. Rounded end of gallbladder directed caudally. A

3 **Body of gallbladder.** Corpus ves. biliaris. Portion of gallbladder between the fundus and neck. A

4 **Neck of gallbladder.** Collum ves. biliaris. It is continuous with the cystic duct. A

5 **Tunica serosa.** Peritoneal covering of gallbladder. B

6 **Tela subserosa.** Connective tissue underlying the peritoneum. B

7 **Tunica muscularis.** Muscle layer in the wall of the gallbladder. B

8 **Tunica mucosa.** Mucous membrane of gallbladder with simple, tall columnar epithelium. B

9 *Plicae mucosae.* Mucosal folds projecting into the lumen and producing a chambered embossment. A B

10 **Cystic duct.** Ductus cysticus. Excretory duct of the gallbladder. It joins the common hepatic duct to form the bile duct (ductus choledochus). A

11 Spiral fold. Plica spiralis. It occupies the neck of the gallbladder and the cystic duct. A

12 **Bile duct.** Ductus choledochus (biliaris). Formed by the union of the cystic duct and common hepatic duct, it passes into the greater duodenal papilla. A

13 **Sphincter muscle of bile duct.** M. sphincter ductus choledochi. Circular muscle reinforced into a sphincter directly before the hepatopancreatic ampulla. A

14 **Hepatopancreatic ampulla.** Ampulla hepatopancreatica. Dilatation in the wall of the duodenum immediately after the opening of the pancreatic duct into the bile duct. A

15 *M. sphincter ampullae hepatopancreaticae (sphincter ampullae).* Reinforced circular musculature around the ampulla (*Sphincter of Oddi*). A

16 **Biliary glands.** Gll. biliares. Mucous glands in the wall of the biliary excretory ducts.

17 RESPIRATORY SYSTEM. APPARATUS RESPIRATORIUS (SYSTEMA RESPIRATORIUM).

18 EXTERNAL NOSE. NASUS EXTERNUS. E

19 **Root of nose.** Radix nasi (nasalis). It lies superiorly between the two orbits. D E

20 **Dorsum (bridge) of nose.** Dorsum nasi. E

21 **Tip of nose.** Apex nasi. E

22 **Alae (wings) of nose.** Alae nasi. They form the lateral border of the nares. E

23 **Nasal cartilages.** Cartilagines nasi (nasalis). Pieces of cartilage which form the non-osseous supporting skeleton of the nose. E

24 **Lateral nasal cartilage.** [Cartilago nasi lateralis]. No longer perceived as independent left and right plates of cartilage, but as part of the nasal septum with which each is partially fused. C

25 Greater alar cartilage. Cartilago alaris major. Hook-shaped cartilage surrounding the naris and forming the tip of the nose. C

26 *Medial crus.* Crus mediale. It forms the anterior and lower part of the cartilaginous wall of the nasal septum. C D

27 *Lateral crus.* Crus laterale. It curves around the naris laterally. C

28 Lesser alar cartilages. Cartilagines alares minores. Single, small cartilage plates which supplement the greater alar cartilage. C

29 Accessory nasal cartilages. Cartilagines nasales accessoriae. Small pieces of cartilage occasionally present between the cartilaginous nasal septum and greater alar cartilage for supplementation of the cartilaginous nasal skeleton.

30 Cartilaginous nasal septum. Cartilago septi nasi. Large independent piece of cartilage in the wall of the nasal septum between the perpendicular plate of the ethmoid and the vomer. D

30a **Lateral process.** Processus lateralis. Dorsolateral cartilaginous ridge of the nasal septum fused above with the lateral nasal cartilage. D

31 *Posterior process.* Processus posterior (sphenoidalis). Variable long process between the vomer and the perpendicular plate; it can extend as far as the sphenoid. D

32 Vomeronasal cartilage. Cartilago vomeronasalis [[Jacobson's cartilage]]. Narrow strip of cartilage inferiorly between the cartilaginous nasal septum and the vomer. D

33 **Mobile part of nasal septum.** [[Pars mobilis septi nasi]]. Anterior, inferior, very mobile part of the nasal septum which contains the medial crus of the greater alar cartilage.

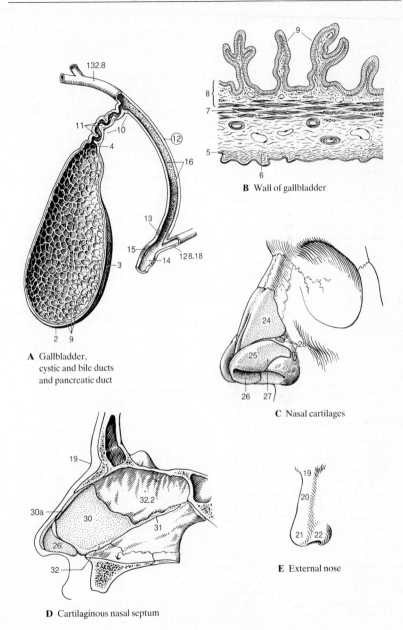

A Gallbladder,
cystic and bile ducts
and pancreatic duct

B Wall of gallbladder

C Nasal cartilages

D Cartilaginous nasal septum

E External nose

1 NASAL CAVITY. CAVITAS NASALIS. A B
~ C

2 **Nasal openings (nostrils).** Nares. They are surrounded by the nasal alae and nasal septum. B C

3 **Choanae.** Posterior openings of nasal cavity. C

4 **Nasal septum.** Septum nasale. It comprises bony, cartilaginous and connective tissue (membranous) segments. C

5 Membranous part. Pars membranacea. Connective tissue portion of nasal septum at the tip of the nose. C

6 Bony part of nasal septum. Pars ossea. Perpendicular plate of ethmoid and vomer. C

7 Vomeronasal (Jacobson's) organ. Organum vomeronasale. Blind sac occasionally present above the incisive canal. It is a vestige of a phylogenetically earlier accessory organ of smell. A C

8 **Vestibule of nose.** Vestibulum nasi (nasale). Anterior segment of nasal cavity extending up to the limen nasi. It is covered by squamous epithelium which changes to ciliary epithelium at the limen. A B

9 **Limen nasi.** Ridge at the end of the vestibule produced by the margin of the alar cartilage. A B

10 **Olfactory sulcus.** Sulcus olfactorius. Groove on the olfactory area passing between the root of the middle nasal concha and the bridge of the nose. A B

11 **Superior nasal concha (turbinate).** Concha nasalis superior. Small, upper concha situated in front of the sphenoidal sinus. A B

12 **Middle nasal concha (turbinate).** Concha nasalis media. Below it lies most of the openings of the paranasal sinuses. A B

13 **Inferior nasal concha (turbinate).** Concha nasalis inferior. Lowest and longest of the nasal conchae. It covers the opening of the nasolacrimal duct. A B

14 [[**Tunica mucosa nasi**]]. Nasal mucous membrane consisting primarily of pseudostratified ciliated columnar epithelium with goblet cells.

15 Respiratory region. Regio respiratoria. Part of the nasal mucosa with ciliated epithelium. It begins in the vestibule and lines the entire nasal cavity except for the olfactory region.

16 Olfactory region. Regio olfactoria. Area about the size of a nickel containing olfactory cells and located superiorly on the nasal septum and on the lateral nasal wall below the cribriform plate. A

16 a **Nasal (olfactory) glands.** Glandulae nasales. Predominantly serous, tubular glands. Their thin secretions cleanse the olfactory epithelium and can enhance the odorous substances.

17 **Cavernous plexus of concha.** Plexus cavernosi concharum. Venous plexuses especially in the region of the inferior concha and posterior nasal cavity.

18 **Agger nasi.** Ridge-like elevated remains of an earlier accessory concha directly in front of the middle nasal concha. A

19 **Sphenoethmoidal recess.** Recessus sphenoethmoidalis. Recess above the superior nasal concha between the anterior wall of the sphenoidal sinus and the roof of the nasal cavity. A

20 **Superior nasal meatus.** Meatus nasi superior. Nasal passage above the middle nasal concha. A

21 **Middle nasal meatus.** Meatus nasi medius. Nasal passage between the middle and inferior nasal concha. A

22 Atrium of middle meatus. Atrium meatus medii. Area at the beginning of the middle meatus in front of the middle and above the inferior concha. A

23 **Inferior nasal meatus.** Meatus nasi inferior. Lower nasal passage between the inferior nasal concha and the floor of the nasal cavity. A

23 a **Aperture of nasolacrimal duct.** Apertum ductus nasolacrimalis. Opening of the nasolacrimal duct provided with a flap-like mucosal fold. See 364.23

24 **Nasopharyngeal meatus.** Meatus nasopharyngeus. Junction of the three nasal passages behind the conchae. A

25 **Incisive duct.** [Ductus incisivus]. Blind sac occasionally present on the floor of the nasal cavity near the septum, about 2 cm behind the external nasal opening. A

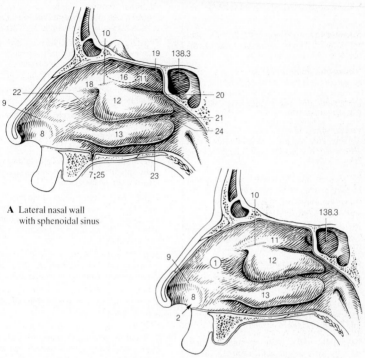

A Lateral nasal wall
with sphenoidal sinus

B Lateral nasal wall

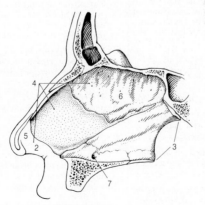

C Nasal septum

1 PARANASAL SINUSES. SINUS PARANA-SALES. A B

2 **Maxillary sinus.** Sinus maxillaris. Situated below the orbit and lateral to the nose, it opens below the middle nasal concha. A

3 **Sphenoidal sinus.** Sinus sphenoidalis. Situated within the sphenoid bone behind the sphenoethmoidal recess and above the nasopharyngeal cavity, this paired sinus opens into the sphenoethmoidal recess. B

4 **Frontal sinus.** Sinus frontalis. Situated in the squama of the frontal bone and often also in the orbital part, it opens below the middle concha. A B

5 **Ethmoidal sinus.** Sinus ethmoidales. System of cavities with about pea-sized air cells between the nasal cavity and orbit. It is divided into the following groups. A

6 Anterior sinus. Sinus anteriores. Anterior group of ethmoidal air cells which opens below the middle nasal concha. A

7 Middle sinus. Sinus medii. Middle group of ethmoidal air cells which opens below the middle nasal concha. A

8 Posterior sinus. Sinus posteriores. Posterior group of ethmoidal air cells which opens below the superior nasal concha. A

9 **Ethmoidal bulla.** Bulla ethmoidalis. Rudimentary nasal concha in the form of a vesicular-like, bulging ethmoidal air cell located below the middle nasal concha. B

10 **Infundibulum ethmoidale.** Recess in front of the ethmoidal bulla in the middle nasal meatus. It receives the openings of the maxillary and frontal sinuses. B

11 Hiatus semilunaris. Semilunar fissure between the ethmoidal bulla and the uncinate process. B

12 LARYNX. It lies between the pharynx and trachea. C

13 **Laryngeal cartilages and joints.** Cartilagines et articulationes laryngeales.

14 **Thyroid cartilage.** Cartilago thyroidea. Largest laryngeal cartilage. It partially encloses the others. C D

15 **Laryngeal prominence.** Prominentia laryngea. Prominence in the midline of the neck produced by the thyroid cartilage. It is more pronounced in males (Adam's apple). C D

16 **Right/left lamina.** Lamina dextra/sinistra. Lateral plates of the thyroid cartilage meeting in the midline like the bow of a ship. C D

17 **Superior thyroid notch.** Incisura thyroidea superior. Deep, median notch superiorly between the right and left thyroid laminae. C D

18 **Inferior thyroid notch.** Incisura thyroidea inferius. Shallow median notch at the lower margin of the thyroid cartilage. D

19 **Superior thyroid tubercle.** Tuberculum thyroideum superior. Small lateral prominence on the outside of the thyroid lamina at the upper end of the oblique line. C D

20 **Inferior thyroid tubercle.** Tuberculum thyroideum inferius. Small lateral prominence at the lower end of the oblique line. C D

21 **Oblique line.** Linea obliqua. Oblique ridge on the outside of the thyroid cartilage for the attachment of the sternothyroid and thyrohyoid muscles and the inferior constrictor muscle of the pharynx. C D

22 **Superior horn (cornu).** Cornu superius. Superior process of thyroid cartilage. It serves for the attachment of the thyrohyoid ligament. C D

23 **Inferior horn (cornu).** Cornu inferius. Inferior process of posterior margin of thyroid cartilage for articular connection with the cricoid cartilage. C D

24 **Thyroid foramen.** [Foramen thyroideum]. Hole occasionally present laterally below the superior tubercle simetimes for the passage of the superior laryngeal artery and vein. C

25 **Thyrohyoid membrane.** Membrana thyrohyoidea. Membrane rich in elastic fibers between the upper posterior margin of the hyoid bone and the thyroid cartilage. C

26 Median thyrohyoid membrane. Lig. thyrohyoideum medianum. Median reinforcement of the thyrohyoid membrane with abundant elastic fibers. C

26a **Pre-epiglottic fat body.** Corpus adiposum prae-epiglotticum. Space-filling fat body between epiglottis, thyronhyoid membrane and hyo-epiglottic ligament. C See 143 C

27 Lateral thyrohyoid ligament. Ligamentum thyrohyoideum laterale. Ligament extending from the superior horn to the posterior end of the greater horn of the hyoid bone. It provides lateral strengthening for the thyrohyoid membrane. C

28 *Cartilago triticea*. Elastic cartilage, the size of a grain of wheat, in the thyrohyoid ligament. C

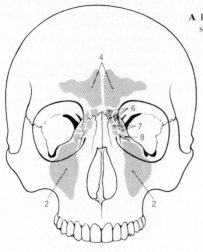

A Paranasal sinuses without sphenoidal sinus

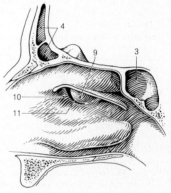

B Lateral nasal wall without middle nasal concha

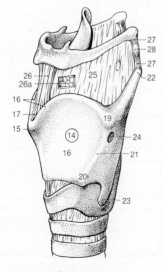

C Larynx

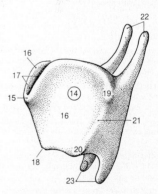

D Thyroid cartilage

1 **Cricoid cartilage.** Cartilago cricoidea. Ring of cartilage lying at the upper end of the trachea and articulating with the thyroid cartilage. A B D

2 **Arch of cricoid cartilage.** Arcus cartilaginis cricoideae. Anterior and lateral parts of cricoid cartilage. A B

3 **Lamina of cricoid cartilage.** Lamina cartilaginis cricoideae. Tall posterior plate of the cricoid cartilage. A B

4 Articular surface for arytenoid cartilage. Facies articularis arytenoidea. Obliquely placed, oval articular facet for the arytenoid cartilage located laterally at the upper margin of the cricoid lamina. A

5 Articular surface for thyroid cartilage. Facies articularis thyroidea. Somewhat prominent articular facet for the thyroid cartilage situated inferiorly on the lateral margin of the lamina. A

6 **Cricothyroid joint.** Articulatio cricothyroidea. Articulation between the thyroid and cricoid cartilages. It permits tilting movements as well as horizontal and vertical gliding movements. B

7 Cricothyroid joint capsule. Capsula articularis cricothyroidea. Thin articular capsule. B

7a Ceratocricoid ligament. Lig ceratocricoideum. Capsular reinforcement for limitation of shearing movements. B

8 Median cricothyroid ligament. Lig. cricothyroideum medianum. Strong vertical ligament in the midline between the thyroid and cricoid cartilages. B D

9 Cricotracheal ligament. Lig. cricotracheale. Elastic membrane between the cricoid cartilage and the first tracheal cartilage. B D

10 **Arytenoid cartilage.** Cartilago arytenoidea. Pyramid-like cartilage sitting on the cricoid cartilage. C D

11 **Articular surface.** Facies articularis. Cylindrical, concave joint surface below the muscular process for articulation with the cricoid. C

12 **Base of arytenoid.** Basis cartilaginis arytenoideae. Under surface of arytenoid cartilage. C

13 **Anterolateral surface.** Facies anterolateralis. Surface directed anterolaterally for muscular insertion and origin. C

14 **Vocal process.** Processus vocalis. Process directed anteriorly for the attachment of the vocal ligament. C

15 *Arcuate crest.* Crista arcuata. Cartilaginous ridge which begins between the oblong and triangular foveae, arches around the triangular fovea and ends at the colliculus. C

16 *Colliculus.* Small projection at the end of the arcuate crest. C D

17 *Oblong fovea.* Fovea oblonga. Depression antero-inferiorly for the attachment of the thyroarytenoid muscle. C

18 *Triangular fovea.* Fovea triangularis. Depression above the oblong fovea. It is filled with glands. C

19 **Medial surface.** Facies medialis. C

20 **Posterior surface.** Facies posterior. C

21 *Apex of arytenoid.* Apex cartilaginis arytenoideae. It is arched posteriorly. C D

22 *Muscular process.* Processus muscularis. Short process posterolaterally for attachment of the posterior and lateral cricoarytenoid muscles. C

23 **Cricoarytenoid joint.** Articulatio cricoarytenoidea. Cylindrical joint between the cricoid and arytenoid cartilages. It permits oscillating movements around an obliquely placed cylindrical axis and gliding movements parallel to the axis. D

24 Articular capsule of cricoarytenoid joint. Capsula articularis cricoarytenoidea. Thin-walled, flaccid capsule of joint between cricoid and arytenoid cartilages. D

25 Cricoarytenoid ligament. Lig. cricoarytenoideum. Important elastic ligament for the closure of the rima glottidis. It passes posteriorly from the cricoid lamina to the medial part of the arytenoid. D

26 **Cricopharyngeal ligament.** Lig. cricopharyngeum. Fiber tract beginning at the corniculate cartilage. After attachment to the posterior side of the cricoid, it passes beneath the pharyngeal mucosa lying on this surface. D

27 **Sesamoid cartilage.** [Cartilago sesamoidea]. Piece of elastic cartilage occasionally present in the anterior end of the vocal ligament and near the arytenoid cartilage. D

28 **Corniculate cartilage.** Cartilago corniculata [[Santorini]]. Small elastic cartilage at the apex of the arytenoid cartilage. It produces the corniculate tubercle. C D

29 **Corniculate tubercle.** Tuberculum corniculatum. Mucosal covered prominence over the same named cartilage directly above the apex of the arytenoid cartilage. See 142.9

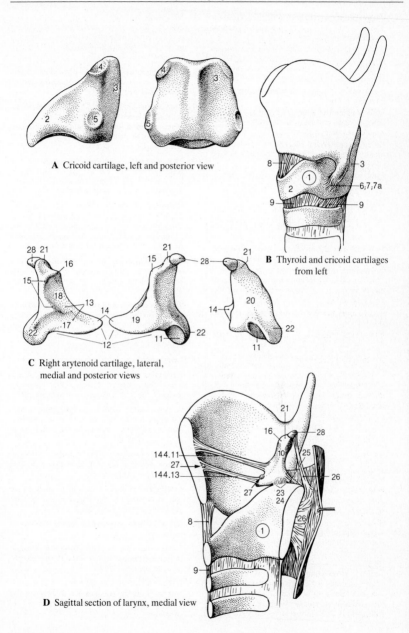

A Cricoid cartilage, left and posterior view

B Thyroid and cricoid cartilages from left

C Right arytenoid cartilage, lateral, medial and posterior views

D Sagittal section of larynx, medial view

1 **Cuneiform cartilage.** Cartilago cuneiformis. Variable small cartilage beneath a small group of glands in the aryepiglottic fold. D

2 **Cuneiform tubercle.** Tuberculum cuneiforme. Prominence in the aryepiglottic fold caused by the cuneiform cartilage. If the cartilage is absent, it can also be caused by glands. B D

3 **Epiglottis.** Elastic cartilage shaped like a shoe-horn. B C E

4 **Stalk of epiglottis.** Petiolus epiglottidis. Directed downward, it is attached to the thyroid cartilage by connective tissue. A D

5 **Epiglottic tubercle.** Tuberculum epiglotticum. Small prominence at the posterior surface of the mucosa above the stalk. B

6 **Epiglottic cartilage.** Cartilago epiglottica. Skeleton of epiglottis consisting of elastic cartilage. A C D

7 **Thyroepiglottic ligament.** Lig. thyroepiglotticum. Ligament attaching the stalk of the epiglottis to the posterior surface of the thyroid cartilage. A D

8 **Hyoepiglottic ligament.** Lig. hyoepiglotticum. Ligament between the hyoid and epiglottis. C

9 **Corniculate tubercle.** Tuberculum corniculatum. Mucosal covered prominence over the same named cartilage just above the apex of the arytenoid. B D

10 **Laryngeal musculature.** Musculi laryngis. B C D E

11 **[[M. aryepiglotticus]].** Now the aryepiglottic part of the arytenoid muscle. See 21a. B D

12 **M. cricothyroideus.** o: Anterolateral aspect of cricoid cartilage. i: Inferiorly at outer and inner surface of the thyroid cartilage lamina. F: Tenses vocal ligament by depressing and pulling the thyroid cartilage forward. I: Superior laryngeal nerve (different innervation than other intrinsic laryngeal muscles). C E

13 **Straight part.** Pars recta. Anterior, somewhat steeper coursing fibers. C

14 **Oblique part.** Pars obliqua. Posterior, more horizontally coursing fibers. C

15 **Posterior Cricoarytenoid muscle.** M. cricoarytenoideus posterior. o: Posterior surface of cricoid. i: Muscular process of arytenoid. F: By swinging the vocal process upward and outward, it opens the rima glottidis. It is the only abductor of the vocal folds. I: Recurrent laryngeal nerve. B D

16 **Ceratocricoid muscle.** [M. ceratocricoideus]. Variant. o: Inferior horn of thyroid cartilage. i: Inferior margin of cricoid. I: Recurrent laryngeal nerve. B

17 **Lateral cricoarytenoid muscle.** M. cricoarytenoideus lateralis. o: Upper part of lateral margin of cricoid. i: Anteriorly at muscular process of arytenoid and adjacent area. F: Synergist in closing of rima glottidis. I: Recurrent laryngeal nerve. D

18 **M. vocalis.** o: Inner surface of thyroid cartilage near the midline. i: Vocal process and oblong fovea of arytenoid. F: By its tension it alters the intrinsic vibrations of the vocal cord. I: Recurrent laryngeal nerve. E

19 **Thyroepiglottic muscle.** [[M. thyroepiglotticus]]. Now is the thyroepiglottic part of the thyroarytenoid muscle. See 20a.

20 **Thyroarytenoid muscle.** M. thyroarytenoideus. o: Anterior inner surface of thyroid cartilage. i: Muscular process and lateral surface of arytenoid. F: Synergist in closure of rima glottidis. I: Recurrent laryngeal nerve. D E

20a **Thyroepiglottic part.** Pars thyroepiglottica. o: Anterior, inner surface of thyroid cartilage. i: Epiglottis and quadrangular membrane. I: Recurrent laryngeal nerve. D See 19.

21 **Oblique arytenoid muscle.** M. arytenoideus obliquus. o: Posterior surface of muscular process. i: Apex of contralateral arytenoid. F: Draws the arytenoids closer together. Synergist in closure of rima glottidis. I: Recurrent laryngeal nerve. B

21a **Aryepiglottic part.** Pars aryepiglottica. o: Apex of arytenoid. i: Margin of epiglottis. Foundation for aryepiglottic fold. F: Depresses the epiglottis. See 11.

22 **Transverse arytenoid muscle.** M. arytenoideus transversus. o: Posterior surface of arytenoid. i: Same surface of contralateral arytenoid. F: Approximates arytenoids. Synergist in closure of rima glottidis. I: Recurrent laryngeal nerve. B

23 **Laryngeal cavity.** Cavitas laryngis. E

24 **Laryngeal inlet (aditus).** Aditus laryngis. Entrance into larynx between the epiglottis, aryepiglottic folds and interarytenoid notch. B E

25 **Aryepiglottic fold.** Plica aryepiglottica. Mucosal fold over the same named muscle. It extends from the apex of the arytenoid to the lateral margin of the epiglottis. B D

26 **Interarytenoid notch.** Incisura interarytenoidea. Mucosal covered slit between the two apices of the arytenoids. B

27 **Vestibule of larynx.** Vestibulum laryngis. Upper part of laryngeal cavity extending as far as the vestibular [ventricular] folds. E

28 **Rima vestibuli.** Interval between the two vestibular folds. E

29 **Vestibular (ventricular) fold.** Plica vestibularis [ventricularis]. Fold produced by the vestibular ligament. It lies between the laryngeal ventricle and vestibule. E

29a **Intermediate laryngeal cavity.** Cavitas laryngis intermedia. Space between the vestibular and vocal folds.

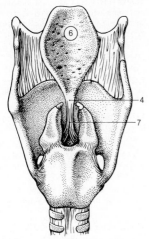

A Laryngeal cartilages, posterior view

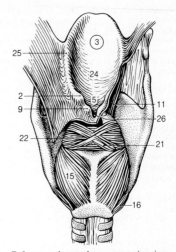

B Laryngeal musculature, posterior view

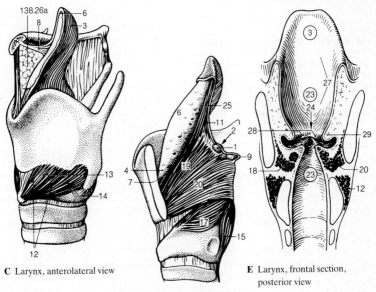

C Larynx, anterolateral view

D Larynx, left lamina of thyroid
cartilage removed

E Larynx, frontal section,
posterior view

1 **Ventricle of larynx.** Ventriculus laryngis [[Morgagni]]. Lateral outpocketings between the vocal and vestibular folds. B C D

2 **Saccule (appendix) of larynx.** Sacculus laryngis [[appendix ventriculi laryngis]]. Small blind sac directed upward from the ventricle. B

3 **Glottis.** Voice-producing part of the larynx consisting of the two vocal folds and the interval (Rima glottidis) between them. A

4 **Rima glottidis.** Space between the two arytenoid cartilages and the vocal cords. A

5 Vocal fold. Plica vocalis. Mucosal fold supported by the underlying vocal ligament and laterally by the vocalis muscle. A

6 Intermembranous part. Pars intermembranacea. Portion of the rima glottidis extending from the thyroid cartilage to the apex of the vocal process. A

7 Intercartilaginous part. Pars intercartilaginea. Portion of rima glottidis between the arytenoid cartilages. A

7 a **Interarytenoid fold.** Plica interarytenoidea. Mucosal fold between the arytenoid cartilages. A

8 **Infraglottic cavity.** Cavitas infraglottica.
~ Lowest portion of laryngeal cavity. It is enclosed by the conus elasticus and extends from the rima glottidis to the trachea. C

9 **Fibroelastic membrane of larynx.** Membrana fibroelastica laryngis [[Membrana elastica laryngis]]. Submucosa of laryngeal wall provided with abundant elastic fibers. It begins at the quadrangular membrane and ends at the lower margin of the conus elasticus. B

10 Quadrangular membrane. Membrana quadrangularis. Membrane spread out between the epiglottis, aryepiglottic fold and vestibular fold. C D

11 *Vestibular ligament.* Lig. vestibulare. It strengthens the lower margin of the quadrangular membrane. C

12 *Conus elasticus (Membrana cricovocalis).* Reinforced fibroelastic membrane between the vocal ligament and cricoid. D

13 Vocal ligament. Lig. vocale. It spreads out between the vocal process of the arytenoid and the thyroid cartilage and forms the upper end of the conus elasticus. C

14 **Tunica mucosa.** Laryngeal mucous membrane provided with nonkeratinized, stratified squamous epithelium only on the upper part of the posterior surface of the epiglottis and on the vocal folds, the rest of the larynx being lined by pseudostratified, ciliated columnar epithelium with goblet cells. B

15 **Laryngeal glands.** Gll. laryngeales. Mixed glands occupying the submucosa of the laryngeal wall. B

16 **Lymph nodes of larynx.** [[Nodi lymphatici laryngis]]. Lymphatic nodules are especially found in the submucosa of the ventricle. B

17 **TRACHEA.** Airway characterized by its cartilage-containing wall and its branches, the bronchi. E

18 **Cervical part.** Pars cervicalis. The cervical segment of the trachea extending from C6 to C7.

19 **Thoracic part.** Pars thoracica. The thoracic segment reaching from T1 to T4 inclusively.

20 **Tracheal cartilages.** Cartilagines tracheales. Horseshoe-shaped cartilages of the tracheal wall. E F H

21 **Tracheal muscle.** Musculus trachealis. Smooth muscle between the free ends of the horseshoe-shaped tracheal cartilages. H

22 **Annular ligaments of trachea.** Ligg. anularia, trachealia. Connective tissue bridges between the tracheal cartilages. E F

23 **Membranous wall.** Paries membranaceus. Posterior wall of trachea. F

24 **Bifurcation of trachea.** Bifurcatio tracheae [trachealis]. Asymmetrical division of trachea at level of T4. E G

25 Carina tracheae. Ridge projecting into the lumen of the trachea at its bifurcation and providing an aerodynamic effect. G

26 **Tunica mucosa.** Tracheal mucosa lined by pseudostratified ciliated columnar epithelium with goblet cells. H

27 Tracheal glands. Gll. tracheales. Mixed glands in the submucosa. H

28 **BRONCHI.** Branches of trachea.

29 **Bronchial tree.** Arbor bronchialis. The entire branching system of the bronchi.

30 **Main bronchus (right and left).** Bronchus principalis (dexter et sinister). Right and left stem bronchi arising directly from the trachea. E

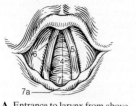

A Entrance to larynx from above

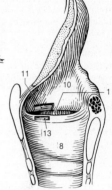

B Laryngeal ventricle

C Sagittal section
of larynx

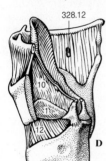

D Larynx, posterolateral view,
left lamina of thyroid cartilage removed

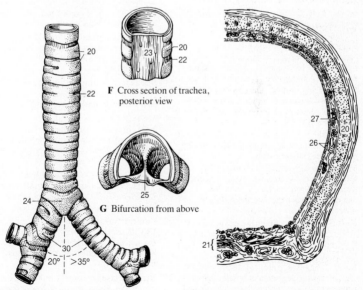

F Cross section of trachea,
posterior view

G Bifurcation from above

E Trachea and bronchi from front

H Cross section of trachea, histologic view

1 **Lobar and segmental bronchi.** Bronchi lobares et segmentales. Bronchi for the five lobes of the lung and their 20 segments. A B

2 **Right superior lobar bronchus.** Bronchus lobaris superior dexter. Bronchus for the superior lobe of the right lung. It is given off just after the tracheal bifurcation. A B

3 Apical segmental bronchus (B I). Bronchus segmentalis apicalis. Bronchus for the apical segment extending inferiorly as far as the 3rd rib. A B

4 Posterior segmental bronchus (B II). Bronchus segmentalis posterior. Bronchus for the posterior segment extending forward about as far as the midaxillary line. A B

5 Anterior segmental bronchus (B III). Bronchus segmentalis anterior. Bronchus for the anterior segment reaching backward about as far as the midaxillary line. A B

6 **Right middle lobar bronchus.** Bronchus lobaris medius dexter. Lobar bronchus for the middle lobe of the right lung. A

7 Lateral segmental bronchus (B IV). Bronchus segmentalis lateralis. Bronchus for the lateral segment located dorsally in the middle lobe. A B

8 Medial segmental bronchus (B V). Bronchus segmentalis medialis. Segmental bronchus situated anteromedially in the middle lobe. A B

9 **Right inferior lobar bronchus.** Bronchus lobaris inferior dexter. Lobar bronchus for the right inferior lobe reaching posteriorly up to the 4th rib. A B

10 Superior segmental bronchus (B VI). Bronchus segmentalis superior. Bronchus for the apical segment which borders only on the upper lobe. B

11 Subapical segmental bronchus. [[Bronchus segmentalis subapicalis]]. Occasionally present accessory bronchus.

12 Medial basal segmental bronchus (B VII). Bronchus segmentalis basalis medialis (cardiacus). Bronchus for the medial segment that does not reach the external surface of the lower lobe. A B

13 Anterior basal segmental bronchus (B VIII). Bronchus segmentalis basalis anterior. Bronchus for the wedge-shaped anterior end of the lower lobe. A B

14 Lateral basal segmental bronchus (B IX). Bronchus segmentalis basalis lateralis. Bronchus for the small lateral segment situated between the anterior and posterior segments. A B

15 Posterior basal segmental bronchus (B X). Bronchus segmentalis basalis posterior. Bronchus for the segment extending posteriorly up to the vertebral column. A B

16 **Left inferior lobar bronchus.** Bronchus lobaris superior sinister. Lobar bronchus for the left upper lobe. A B

17 Apicoposterior segmental bronchus (B I + II). Bronchus segmentalis apicoposterior. Bronchus for the left apical segment located posterosuperiorly. A B

18 Anterior segmental bronchus (B III). Bronchus segmentalis anterior. Bronchus for the anterior segment of the left upper lobe situated in front of the apical segment. A B

19 Superior lingular bronchus (B IV). Bronchus lingularis superior. Bronchus for the second lowermost segment of the left upper lobe extending posteriorly as far as the border of the lower lobe. A B

20 Inferior lingular bronchus (B V). Bronchus lingularis inferior. Bronchus for the lowest segment of the upper lobe situated mainly anteriorly. A B

21 **Left inferior lobar bronchus.** Bronchus lobaris inferior sinister. Lobar bronchus for the left lower lobe extending dorsally up to the 4th thoracic vertebra. A B

22 Superior segmental bronchus (B VI). Bronchus segmentalis superior. Bronchus for the apical segment located posterosuperiorly in the lower lobe. B

23 Subapical segmental bronchus. [[Bronchus segmentalis subapicalis]]. Bronchus for an occasionally-present accessory segment.

24 Medial basal segmental bronchus (B VII). Bronchus segmentalis basalis medialis (cardiacus). Bronchus for the medial basal segment which does not reach the lateral lung surface. A

25 Anterior basal segmental bronchus (B VIII). Bronchus segmentalis basalis anterior. Bronchus for the anterior basal segment adjoining the lower anterior border. A B

26 Lateral basal segmental bronchus (B IX). Bronchus segmentalis basalis lateralis. Bronchus for the basal middle segment located between the anterior and posterior basal segments. A B

27 Bronchus segmentalis basalis posterior (B X). Bronchus for the posterior basal segment of the lower lobe situated below the apical segment. A B

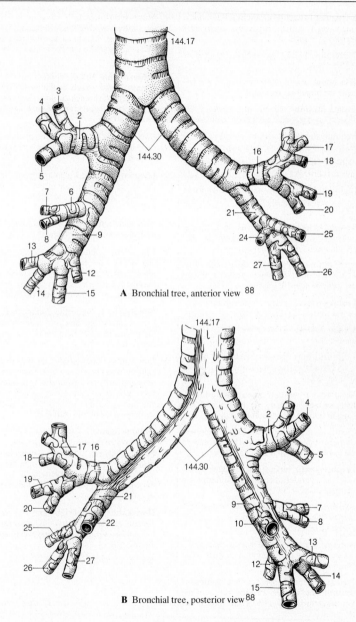

A Bronchial tree, anterior view [88]

B Bronchial tree, posterior view [88]

1 **Segmental bronchial branches.** Rami bronchiales segmentorum. Branches of individual segmental bronchi.

2 **Tunica muscularis.** Muscle layer in the wall of the bronchus.

3 **Tela submucosa.** Connective tissue layer beneath the bronchial mucosa.

4 **Tunica mucosa.** Mucous membrane of the bronchi lined by ciliated columnar epithelium.

5 Bronchial glands. Gll. bronchiales. Mixed glands located below the mucosa.

6 LUNGS. PULMONES. They occupy the
~ greatest portion of the thoracic space. A B C D

7 **Right/left lungs.** Pulmo dexter/sinister. Right lobes are larger; left lobes smaller (10%). A B C D

8 **Base of lung.** Basis pulmonis (pulmonalis). Lower lung segment bordering on the diaphragm. A B C D

9 **Apex of lung.** Apex pulmonis (pulmonalis). Apical portion of the lung partially occupying the superior thoracic aperture. A B C D

10 **Costal surface.** [[Facies costalis]]. Lung surface bordering the ribs. A C

11 **Medial surface.** [[Facies medialis]]. Medial lung surface facing the mediastinum. B D

12 Vertebral part. Pars vertebralis. Dorsal portion of medial surface applied to the vertebral column. B D

13 Mediastinal surface. Facies mediastinalis. Lung surface bordering the mediastinum and lying in front of the vertebral part. B D

14 Cardiac impression of lung. Impressio cardiaca. Indentation produced by the heart on the medial surface of both lungs. B D

15 **Diaphragmatic surface.** Facies diaphragmatica. Concave inferior surface of the lung facing the diaphragm. A B C D

16 **Interlobar surface.** Facies interlobaris. Surface of lung tissue found in the spaces between the lobes.

17 **Anterior margin.** Margo anterior. Sharp border anteriorly at the junction of the medial and costal surfaces. A B C D

18 Cardiac notch. Incisura cardiaca [pulmonis sinistri]. Notch on the anterior margin of the left upper lobe produced by the cardiac impression. C D

19 **Margo inferior.** Sharp border at the junction of the costal and diaphragmatic surfaces. The margin is less sharp at the transition of the diaphragmatic surface into the medial surface. A B C D

20 **Hilum of lung.** Hilum pulmonis. Site of entry
~ of bronchi and vessels on the medial surface. Essentially, the bronchi lie posteriorly, the pulmonary artery craniad and the pulmonary veins caudad. B D

21 **Root of lung.** Radix [pediculus] pulmonis. It consists of the pulmonary vessels and bronchi of the hilum. B

22 **Lingula of left lung.** Lingula pulmonis sinistri. Portion of the upper lobe of the left lung between the cardiac notch and the oblique fissure. C D

22 a **Culmen of left lung.** Culmen pulmonis sinistri. Upper lobe without lingula.

23 **Upper lobe.** Lobus superior. Extends posteriorly as far as the 4th rib. On the right side its lower border runs anteriorly somewhat along the 4th rib. On the left side it passes as far as the cartilage-bone border of the 6th rib. A B C D

24 **Middle lobe.** Lobus medius (pulmonis dextri). Present only in the right lung, it lies in front of the midaxillary line between the 4th and 6th ribs. A B

25 **Lower lobe.** Lobus inferior. It has its main expansion dorsally. Its superior border courses obliquely from posterosuperiorly to antero-inferiorly. It begins paravertebrally at the 4th rib and ends at the intersection of the midclavicular line and the 6th rib. A B C D

26 **Oblique fissure.** Fissura obliqua. Oblique fissure between the lower and upper lobes of the left lung, between the lower and upper lobes, as well as the middle lobe, of the right lung. Accordingly, it passes paravertebrally from the 4th rib up to the 6th rib in the midclavicular line. A B C D

27 **Horizontal fissure of right lung.** Fissura horizontalis (pulmonis dextri). Fissure separating the middle and upper lobes. Its level is near the 4th rib. A B

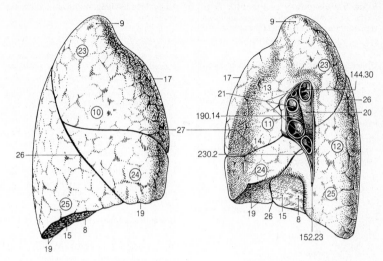

A Right lung, lateral view   **B** Right lung, medial view

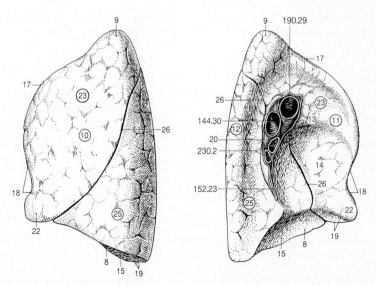

C Left lung, lateral view   **D** Left lung, medial view

1 **Bronchopulmonary segments.** Segmenta bronchopulmonalia. Lung segments supplied by individual bronchi and arteries and separated by veins and connective tissue septa. A B

2 **Upper lobe, right lung.** Pulmo dexter, lobus superior. A

3 Apical segment of upper lobe of right lung. Segmentum apicale (S I). It is inserted wedge-shaped between the anterior and posterior segments. A

4 Posterior segment of upper lobe of right lung. Segmentum posterius (S II). It lies between the apical segment and the lower lobe. A

5 Anterior segment of upper lobe of right lung. Segmentum anterius (S III). It lies between the apical segment and the middle lobe. A

6 **Middle lobe, right lung.** Pulmo dexter, lobus medius. A

7 Lateral segment of middle lobe. Segmentum laterale (S IV). It occupies the dorsal portion of the middle lobe and does not reach the hilum. A

8 Medial segment of middle lobe. Segmentum mediale (S V). It forms the medial and diaphragmatic surfaces of the middle lobe. A

9 **Lower lobe, right lung.** Pulmo dexter, lobus inferior. A

10 Superior segment. Segmentum superius (S VI). Apical portion of lower lobe situated posterosuperiorly. A

11 Subapical segment. [[Segmentum subapicale]]. An accessory segment occasionally present below the superior segment.

12 Medial basal (cardiac) segment (S VII). Segmentum basale mediale (cardiacum). It does not reach the lateral surface of the lung and is only seen from the medial and inferior surfaces. A

13 Anterior basal segment (S VIII). Segmentum basale anterius. It lies between the middle lobe and diaphragm. A

14 Lateral basal segment (S IX). Segmentum basale laterale. It lies between the posterior and anterior basal segments. A

15 Posterior basal segment (S X). Segmentum basale posterius. It is between the vertebral column and lateral basal segment. A

16 **Upper lobe, left lung.** Pulmo sinister, lobus superior. B

17 Apicoposterior segment (S I + II). Segmentum apicoposterius. It comprises two segments (apical and posterior) which lie wedge-shaped between the oblique fissure and the anterior segment of the upper lobe. B

18 Anterior segment (S III) of upper lobe. Segmentum anterius. It lies between the superior lingular and apicoposterior segments. B

19 Superior lingular segment (S IV). Segmentum lingulare superius. It lies predominantly on the inferior lingular segment. B

20 Inferior lingular segment (S V). Segmentum lingulare inferius. It lies between the superior lingular segment and the oblique fissure. B

21 **Lower lobe, left lung.** Pulmo sinister, lobus inferior. B

22 Superior segment (S VI). Segmentum superius. Apical portion of lower lobe situated posterosuperiorly near the vertebral column. B

23 Subapical segment. [[Segmentum subapicale]]. Accessory segment occasionally present below the superior segment of the lower lobe.

24 Medial basal (cardiac) segment (S VII). Segmentum basale mediale (cardiacum). It is often an inseparable part of the anterior basal segment. B

25 Anterior basal segment (S VIII). Segmentum basale anterius. It lies between the oblique fissure and the lateral basal segment. B

26 Lateral basal segment (S IX). Segmentum basale laterale. It lies between the anterior and posterior basal segments. B

27 Posterior basal segment (S X). Segmentum basale posterius. It lies beside the vertebral column below the superior segment of the lower lobe. B

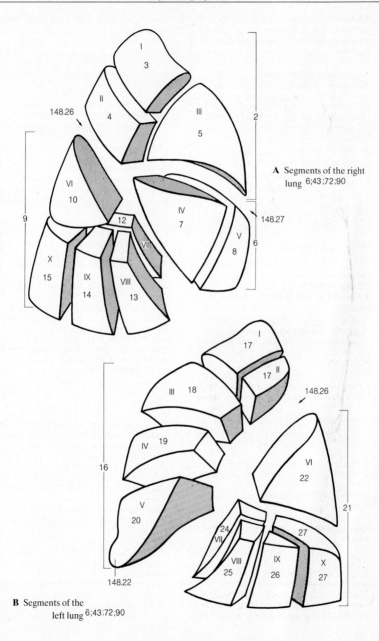

A Segments of the right lung 6;43;72;90

B Segments of the left lung 6;43;72;90

1 **Bronchioles.** Bronchioli. Noncartilaginous segment of the respiratory tree directly following the bronchi. They are lined initially by pseudostratified, ciliated, columnar epithelium which subsequently becomes replaced by simple cuboidal epithelium. A

2 **Respiratory bronchioles.** Bronchioli respiratorii. Last bronchiolar segment the wall of which already consists partially of alveoli. A

3 Alveolar ducts. Ductuli alveolares. Terminal branches of the respiratory bronchioles the walls of which contain only alveoli. A

4 Alveolar sacs. Sacculi alveolares. Blind, expanded ends of the alveolar ducts. A

5 Pulmonary alveoli. Alveoli pulmonis. Smallest outpocketings, 0.1–0.9 mm. in diameter, the thin walls of which permit gaseous exchange. A

6 THORACIC CAVITY. CAVITAS THORA-
~ CIS (THORACICA). Internal thoracic space enclosed by the ribs and limited inferiorly by the diaphragm. B C

7 **Pleuropulmonary regions.** Regiones pleuropulmonales. Relations between pleura and lungs.

8 **Endothoracic fascia.** Fascia endothoracica.
~ Displaceable layer of loose connective tissue between the parietal pleura and chest wall. B

9 Suprapleural membrane. Membrana suprapleuralis [[Sibson]]. Thickened portion of the endothoracic fascia in the region of the pleural cupola. B

10 Phrenicopleural fascia. Fascia phrenicopleuralis. Portion of the endothoracic fascia which connects the parietal pleura with the diaphragm. B

11 **Pleural cavity.** Cavitas pleuralis. Capillary,
~ fissure-shaped space between the parietal and visceral pleura containing a little serous fluid. B C

12 **Pleura.** Serous membrane consisting of simple squamous epithelium and underlying connective tissue. It comprises two portions (visceral and parietal pleura) which become continuous at the hilum. The visceral (pulmonary) pleura covers the lungs whereas the parietal pleura lines the chest wall, diaphragm and mediastinum. B

13 Cupula (dome) of pleura. Cupula pleurae.
~ It covers the apex of the lung at the superior thoracic aperture and forms the boundary between the neck and thorax. B

14 Visceral (pulmonary) pleura. Pleura vis-
~ ceralis (pulmonalis). Portion of the pleura that envelops the lung and passes into the interlobar spaces. B C

15 Parietal pleura. Pleura parietalis. Serous lining of the space in which the lungs have become lodged. B C

16 Mediastinal part of parietal pleura (mediastinal pleura). Pars mediastinalis. Portion of the parietal pleura lining the mediastinum. B C

17 Costal part of parietal pleura (costal pleura). Pars costalis. It lines the ribs. B C

18 Diaphragmatic part of parietal pleura (diaphragmatic pleura). Pars diaphragmatica. It covers the diaphragm. B

19 **Pleural recesses.** Recessus pleurales. Fissure-shaped spaces formed by the parietal pleura for the reception of the lungs during inspiration.

20 Costodiaphragmatic recess. Recessus costodiaphragmaticus. Pleural recess between the descending sides of the diaphragm and the lateral wall of the thorax. B

21 Costomediastinal recess. Recessus costomediastinalis. Pleural space anteriorly between the costal and mediastinal pleura, more extensive on the left than on the right. C

22 Phrenicomediastinal recess. Recessus phrenicomediastinalis. Pleural recess situated dorsally between the diaphragm and the mediastinum.

23 **Pulmonary ligament.** Lig. pulmonale. Doubled reflective fold of the visceral pleura onto the mediastinal pleura extending downward from the hilum. Between both folds the lung abuts against the mediastinal connective tissue free of pleura. B See 149 B D

24 **Mediastinum.** Thoracic area between both pleural sacs. It extends from the anterior surface of the vertebral column to the posterior surface of the sternum. B

25 Superior mediastinum. Mediastinum superius. Portion of the mediastinum above the heart. It contains the arch of the aorta together with its branches, as well as the brachiocephalic veins, superior vena cava, trachea, esophagus, vagus nerves, thoracic duct, thymus, etc. B

26 Inferior mediastinum. Mediastinum inferius. Collective term for the following three divisions.

27 Anterior mediastinum. Mediastinum anterius. Area between the pericardium and sternum. C

28 Middle mediastinum. Mediastinum medium. Area occupied by the heart, pericardium and phrenic nerves with their accompanying vessels. C

29 Posterior mediastinum. Mediastinum posterius. Area between the pericardium and the vertebral column. It contains the esophagus, vagus nerves, descending aorta, thoracic duct, azygos and hemiazygos veins. C

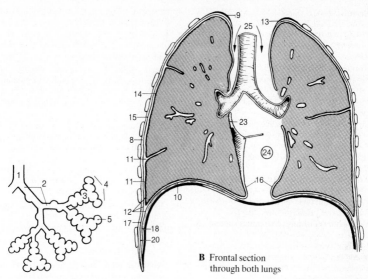

A Bronchiole and alveolar ducts

B Frontal section through both lungs

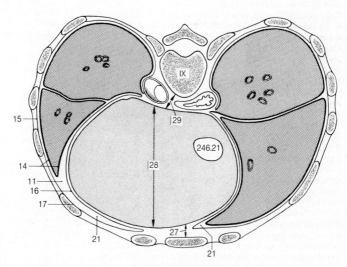

C Horizontal section at level of the ninth thoracic vertebra. View from below

1 UROGENITAL SYSTEM. APPARATUS UROGENITALIS (SYSTEMA UROGENITALE). Urinary and genital organs.

2 URINARY ORGANS. ORGANA URINARIA.

3 **Kidney.** Ren (nephros). A B F

4 **Lateral margin.** Margo lateralis. Convex lateral border of kidney. A

5 **Medial margin.** Margo medialis. Concave at the hilum. A

6 Renal hilum. Hilum renale. Site of entry and
~ exit of renal blood vessels and ureter. A

7 Renal sinus. Sinus renalis. Strongly concave cavity at the medial border for the renal hilum. B D

8 **Anterior surface.** Facies anterior. Strongly curved anterior surface of the kidney. A D

9 **Posterior surface.** Facies posterior. Nearly flat posterior surface of the kidney. D

10 **Upper pole of kidney.** Extremitas superior. A B

11 **Lower pole of kidney.** Extremitas inferior. B

12 **Renal fascia.** Fascia renalis. Doubling of the subperitoneal fascia. It curves around the fatty capsule with the kidney. D

13 Pararenal fat body. Corpus adiposum pararenale. Fat pad between the posterior layer of the renal fascia and the transversalis fascia. D

14 **Fatty capsule.** Capsula adiposa. Fatty capsule of the kidney more prominent posteriorly and medially. D

15 **Fibrous capsule.** Capsula fibrosa. Tough organ capsule fused with the surface of the kidney, but removable. D F

16 **Renal segments.** Segmenta renalia. Five segments of the kidney corresponding to the blood supply regions of the branches of the renal artery.

17 **Superior segment.** Segm. superius. Upper segment extending up to the posterior surface. A B

18 **Upper anterior segment.** Segm. anterius superius. A

19 **Lower anterior segment.** Segm. anterius inferius. A

20 **Inferior segment.** Segm. inferius. It reaches as far as the posterior and anterior surfaces. A B

21 **Posterior segment.** Segm. posterius. B

22 **Renal (uriniferous) tubule (nephron).** Tubulus renalis. Tubular system representing the structural unit of the kidney in which filtration and selective reabsorption take place. C

23 Convoluted uriniferous tubules. [[Tubuli renales contorti]]. Tortuous parts of the renal tubules. C

24 Straight segments of renal tubules. [[Tubuli renales recti]]. C

25 **Renal lobes.** Lobi renales. Still preserved in the newborn, they correspond to renal pyramids with cortical caps.

26 **Renal cortex.** Cortex renalis. About 6 mm
~ thick, it consists of glomeruli and predominantly convoluted uriniferous tubules. It extends up to the wall of the renal pelvis as renal columns. F

27 Convoluted part (cortical labyrinth). Pars convoluta. Cortical region consisting of glomeruli and convoluted uriniferous tubules. F

28 Radiating part (medullary rays). Pars radiata. Collecting tubules coursing radially into the cortex from the medulla. F

29 Cortical lobules. Lobuli corticales. Areas delimited by interlobular arteries.

29 a **Medullary rays.** Radii medullares. Consisting of pale-appearing collecting tubules which project into the cortex. F

30 **Renal medulla.** Medulla renalis. Medullary
~ tissue in the shape of renal pyramids and consisting of the straight portions of the uriniferous tubules and the collecting ducts. F

31 Renal pyramids. Pyramides renales. Six to 20 pyramidal areas separated by renal columns. They form the medullary substance. F

32 *Base of pyramid.* Basis pyramidis. It lies at the corticomedullary border. F

33 *Renal papillae.* Papillae renales. Rounded apical portion of the renal pyramid projecting into the renal calyx. F

34 *Area cribrosa.* Surface of renal papillae perforated sieve-like by openings of the uriniferous tubules. F

35 *Papillary foramina.* Foramina papillaria. Holes in the area cribrosa produced by the openings of the uriniferous tubules.

36 Renal columns. Columnae renales. Cortical substance which extends toward the hilum between the renal pyramids. F

37 **Renal corpuscle.** Corpusculum renale. Com-
~ posed of a glomerulus and its capsule, it lies in the convoluted part of the cortex. E

38 **Glomerulus.** Capillary tuft within a renal cor-
~ puscle. E

39 Glomerular [[Bowman's]] capsule. Capsula glomerularis [[Bowman's]]. The capsule around a capillary tuft (glomerulus) of a renal corpuscle. It is continuous with a convoluted tubule. E

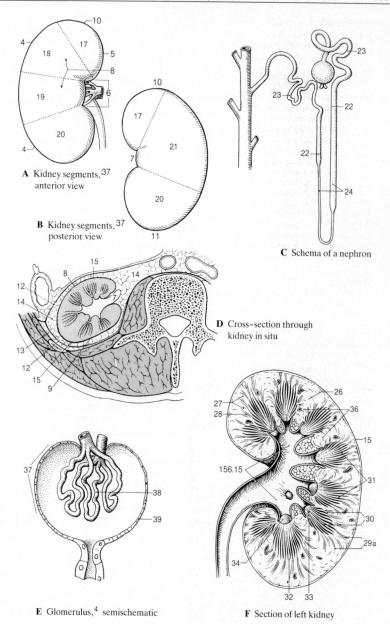

A Kidney segments, 37 anterior view

B Kidney segments, 37 posterior view

C Schema of a nephron

D Cross-section through kidney in situ

E Glomerulus, 4 semischematic

F Section of left kidney

1 **Renal arteries.** Arteriae renales.

2 **Interlobar arteries.** Arteriae interlobares. They run between the pyramids. B

3 **Arcuate arteries.** Arteriae arcuatae. Arising from the interlobar arteries, they take an arched course along the medullo-cortical border. B

4 Interlobular arteries. Arteriae interlobulares. Radially oriented branches of the arcuate arteries lying between two medullary rays. B

5 *Afferent glomerular arteriole.* Arteriola glomerularis afferens (Vas afferens). Arteriole arising from an interlobular artery and entering a renal corpuscle where it subdivides to form the capillary tuft (glomerulus). B

6 *Efferent glomerular arteriole.* Arteriola glomerularis efferens (Vas efferens). Arteriole leaving the glomerulus and forming a capillary network between the convoluted tubules. B

7 *Capsular branches.* Rami capsulares. Small arteries passing from the cortex to the capsule. B

8 *Straight arterioles.* Arteriolae rectae (Vasa recta). Straight vessels coursing from the efferent glomerular arterioles to the capillary network of the tubules or coming from the arcuate arteries into the medulla. B

9 **Renal veins.** Venae renales.

10 **Interlobar veins.** Venae interlobares. Veins coming from the periphery between the renal pyramids. B

11 **Arcuate veins.** Venae arcuatae. Veins taking an arched course along the corticomedullary border. B

12 Interlobular veins. Venae interlobulares. Lobular veins corresponding to the interlobular arteries. B

13 *Straight venules.* Venulae rectae. Fine veins in the medullary substance which open into the arcuate veins. B

14 *Stellate venules.* Venulae stellatae. Veins forming a stellate network beneath the capsule and emptying into the interlobular veins. B

15 **Renal pelvis.** Pelvis renalis. Funnel-shaped beginning of the ureter occupying the renal hilum. A

16 **Renal calices.** Calices renales. More or less long tubular-like processes of the renal pelvis for the drainage of the renal papillae. A

17 Major calices of kidney. Calices renales majores. Two to three primary tube-like diverticula of the renal pelvis. A

18 Minor calices of kidney. Calices renales minores. Seven to 13 calices formed by further divisions of the major calices. Each receives a renal papilla. A

19 **URETER.** Excretory duct of the kidney situated retroperitoneally. It connects the renal pelvis with the urinary bladder. A C

20 **Abdominal part of ureter.** Pars abdominalis. It extends from the renal pelvis to the terminal line of the pelvis.

21 **Pelvic part of ureter.** Pars pelvica. It extends from the terminal line to the urinary bladder.

22 **Tunica adventitia.** Superficial connective tissue of the ureter. It unites it with the surrounding tissues and permits its mobility. C

23 **Tunica muscularis.** Muscular layer in the wall of the ureter. C

24 **Tunica mucosa.** Mucous membrane lined by transitional epithelium with underlying connective tissue. C

25 URINARY BLADDER. VESICA URINARIA. Receptacle for about 350–500 ml or more of urine. D

26 **Apex of urinary bladder.** Apex vesicae (vesicalis). Apical portion of urinary bladder directed anterosuperiorly. D

27 **Body of urinary bladder.** Corpus vesicae. Portion of the urinary bladder situated between the fundus and apex. D

28 **Fundus of urinary bladder.** Fundus vesicae. Posterior wall of the urinary bladder lying opposite to the apex, specifically in its lower segment between the ureters. D

29 **Cervix (neck) of urinary bladder.** Cervix vesicae. It gives rise to the urethra. D

30 **Median umbilical ligament.** Lig. umbilicale medianum. Fibrous cord derived from the urachus and passing from the apex of the bladder to the umbilicus. D

31 **Urachus.** Connecting passage between the cloaca and allantois present only during embryonic development.

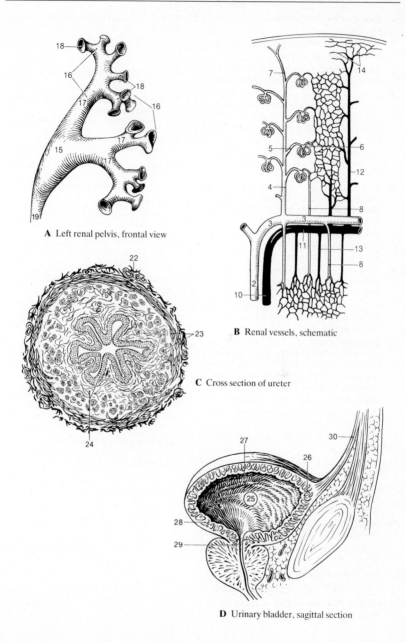

A Left renal pelvis, frontal view

B Renal vessels, schematic

C Cross section of ureter

D Urinary bladder, sagittal section

1 **Tunica serosa.** Peritoneal covering of the urinary bladder. C

2 **Tela subserosa.** Connective tissue layer beneath the serosa of the urinary bladder. C

3 **Tunica muscularis.** Entire musculature of the urinary bladder with the following four parts.

4 **Detrusor urinae muscle.** Musculus detrusor vesicae. True musculature of the wall of the bladder. It consists of an inner and outer longitudinal layer as well as a middle circular layer. B C

5 **M. pubovesicalis.** Smooth muscle extending from the lower portion of the pubic symphysis to the neck of the bladder. A

6 **M. rectovesicalis.** Smooth muscle passing from the longitudinal musculature of the rectum to the lateral base (fundus) of the bladder. A

7 **M. rectourethralis.** Smooth muscle extending from the longitudinal musculature of the rectum to the male urethra. A

8 **Tela submucosa.** Connective tissue layer beneath the mucosa of the bladder. It is absent in the trigone. C

9 **Tunica mucosa.** Mucous membrane of the urinary bladder. It is lined by transitional epithelium. C

10 **Trigone of bladder.** Trigonum vesicae. Triangular region between the openings of the ureters and the exit site of the urethra. Here the mucosa is firmly united with the muscularis and consequently exhibits no folds. B

11 **Interureteric ridge.** Plica interureterica. Transverse mucosal fold between the two ureteric openings. B

12 **Ostium ureteris.** Slit-like opening of the ureter. B

13 **Ostium urethrae internum.** Initial portion of the urethra at the anterior apex of the trigone. B

14 **Uvula of bladder.** Uvula vesicae. Sagittal ridge located behind the urethral opening and above the middle lobe of the prostate. B

15 INTERNAL MALE GENITALIA. ORGANA
~ GENITALIA MASCULINA INTERNA.

16 **Testis (Orchis).** It measures about 5 cm in length. D E

17 **Superior end of testis.** Extremitas superior. D

18 **Inferior end of testis.** Extremitas inferior. D

19 **Lateral, flattened surface of testis.** Facies lateralis. D

20 **Medial, flattened surface of testis.** Facies medialis. D

21 **Anterior, free margin of testis.** Margo anterior. D

22 **Posterior margin of testis.** Margo posterior. attached to a serous reflected fold. D

23 **Tunica vaginalis testis.** Serous covering of the testis formed developmentally by the vaginal process of the peritoneum. See also 162.1–6

24 **Tunica albuginea.** Tough connective tissue capsule of the testis. D

25 **Mediastinum testis.** Connective tissue mass projecting into the interior of the testis from the posterior margin of the tunica albuginea. D

26 **Septa of testis.** Septula testis. Connective tissue partitions radiating out from the mediastinum to the tunica albuginea. D E

27 **Lobules of testis.** Lobuli testis. Compartmentalized lobules of testicular parenchyma formed by the septa. D E

28 **Parenchyma testis.** Specific testicular tissue made up of seminiferous tubules. D

29 **Convoluted seminiferous tubules.** Tubuli seminiferi contorti. Tortuous testicular tubules which occupy the lobules of the testis. E

30 **Straight seminiferous tubules.** Tubuli seminiferi recti. Short straight tubules extending from the convoluted seminiferous tubules to the rete testis. E

31 **Rete testis.** Network of canals within the mediastinum testis. Lined by simple cuboidal epithelium, they connect the straight seminiferous tubules with the efferent ductules. E

32 **Efferent ductules of testis.** Ductuli efferentes testis. 10–12 ductules between the rete testis and the duct of the epididymis. D E

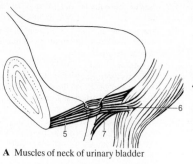

A Muscles of neck of urinary bladder

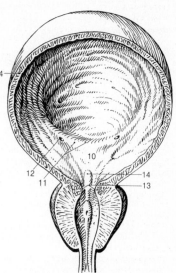

B Urinary bladder and prostate, opened, frontal view

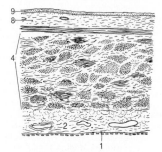

C Wall of urinary bladder

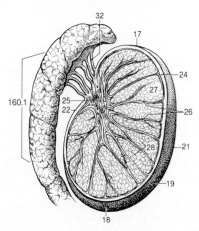

D Testicle and epididymis

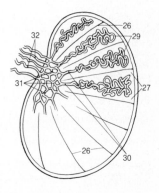

E Testicle, schematic

1 **Epididymis.** Lying on the posteromedial surface of the testis, it serves as a storage receptacle for sperm. A

2 **Head of epididymis.** Caput epididymidis. It is occupied by the efferent ductules. A

3 **Body of epididymis.** Corpus epididymidis. Middle segment of the epididymis consisting of the convolutions of the duct of the epididymis. A

4 **Tail of epididymis.** Cauda epididymidis. Inferior, terminal portion of the epididymis consisting of the convolutions of the duct of the epididymis. A

5 **Lobules (cones) of epididymis.** Lobuli coni epididymidis. Wedge-shaped lobules in the head of the epididymis separated by connective tissue and formed by one or two efferent ductules. A

6 **Duct of epididymis.** Ductus epididymidis. Coiled duct, 5–6 meters long, beginning at the end of the head of the epididymis where it receives the efferent ductules and terminating at the end of the tail where it is continuous with the ductus deferens. A

7 **Aberrant ductules.** Ductuli aberrantes. Blind branches of the efferent ductules and duct of the epididymis representing vestiges of the caudal mesonephric tubules.

8 *[Ductulus aberrans superior].* Superior aberrant ductule in the head of the epididymis.

9 *[Ductulus aberrans inferior].* Inferior aberrant ductule in the tail of the epididymis. A

10 *Appendix testis.* Vesicular appendage superior to the testis (vestige of the paramesonephric duct). A

11 *[Appendix epididymidis].* Appendix of epididymis. Pedunculate appendage at the head of the epididymis (vestige of the mesonephros). A

12 **Paradidymis.** Bilateral blind ductules superior to the head of the epididymis and in front of the spermatic cord (remnant of mesonephric tubules). A

13 **Ductus deferens.** Sperm duct, about 60 cm long, between the epididymis and the seminal vesicle. It is initially coiled and then becomes straight. A B D E

14 **Ampulla of ductus deferens.** Ampulla ductus deferentis. Oval enlargement of ductus deferens just prior to joining the duct of the seminal vesicle. B

15 **Diverticula of ampulla.** Diverticula ampullae. Lateral sacculations in the wall of the ampulla of the ductus deferens. B

16 **Tunica adventitia.** Connective tissue covering of the ductus deferens. E

17 **Tunica muscularis.** Relatively very thick muscle layer of the ductus deferens. E

18 **Tunica mucosa.** Mucous membrane of ductus deferens lined by pseudostratified, stereociliated, columnar epithelium. E

19 **Ejaculatory duct.** Ductus ejaculatorius. Sperm duct formed by the union of the ductus deferens and the duct of the seminal vesicle. It traverses the prostate and empties into the prostatic urethra. B

20 **Seminal vesicle.** Vesicula seminalis. Erroneously designated as a receptacle for sperm, this organ is a vesicular gland which consists of a coiled tube, about 12 cm in length. B C

21 **Tunica adventitia.** Connective tissue covering of the seminal vesicle. C

22 **Tunica muscularis.** Muscular layer in the wall of the seminal vesicle. C

23 **Tunica mucosa.** Multichambered mucous membrane of the seminal vesicle lined by a simple secretory epithelium. C

24 **Excretory duct.** Ductus excretorius. Efferent duct of the seminal vesicle. It unites with the ductus deferens to form the ejaculatory duct. B

25 **Spermatic cord.** [[Funiculus spermaticus]]. It consists of the ductus deferens, accompanying vessels, nerves and connective tissue, together with its coverings. D

26 **Tunicae funiculi spermatici.** Coverings of the spermatic cord and the testis are as follows: D

27 **External spermatic fascia.** Fascia spermatica externa. Continuation of the external oblique fascia forming the superficial covering of the spermatic cord. It also envelops the testis together with its remaining coverings. D

28 **M. cremaster.** Elevator of the testis. It is derived mainly from internal abdominal oblique muscle. D

29 **Cremasteric fascia.** Fascia cremasterica. Connective tissue on and between the cremaster muscle fibers. D

30 **Internal spermatic fascia.** Fascia spermatica interna [[Tunica vaginalis communis]]. Continuation of the transversalis fascia which protrudes like the fingers of a glove. It lies beneath the cremaster muscle and surrounds the testis, epididymis and ductus deferens together with blood vessels and nerves. D

31 **Vestige of vaginal process.** [Vestigium processus vaginalis]. Remnant of the embryological vaginal process of the peritoneum which has not completely disappeared. D

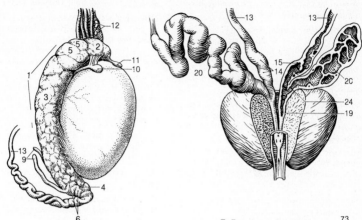

A Testicle and epididymis

B Prostate and seminal vesicle,[73] opened, frontal view

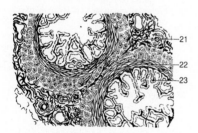

C Seminal vesicle, histologic section

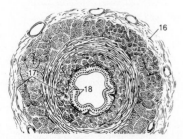

E Sperm duct (ductus deferens), cross section

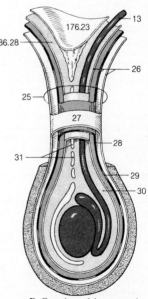

D Coverings of the spermatic cord and the testis

1 **Tunica vaginalis testis.** Double-layered serous covering of the testis remaining from the vaginal process of the peritoneum. A

2 Parietal layer. Lamina parietalis [[Periorchium]]. External layer of the serous tunica vaginalis testis. A

3 Visceral layer. Lamina visceralis [[Eporchium]]. Layer of serous covering lying on the testis. A

4 Superior ligament of epididymis. Lig. epididymidis superius. Reflected fold of the tunica vaginalis testis located superiorly at the head of the epididymis. A

5 Inferior ligament of epididymis. Lig. epididymidis inferius. Reflected fold of the tunica vaginalis testis situated inferiorly at the tail of the epididymis. A

6 Sinus of epididymis. Sinus epididymidis. Serous cleft between the testis and epididymis. It is accessible laterally and is bordered above and below by the superior and inferior ligaments of the epididymis, respectively. A

7 **Descent of testis.** [[Descensus testis]]. Downward migration of the testis during the last fetal weeks of pregnancy. It descends from the peritoneal cavity into the scrotal sac via the inguinal canal.

8 [[**Gubernaculum testis**]]. Fetal connective tissue band which arises from the caudal gonadal fold and guides the testis during its descent.

9 **Genitoinguinal ligament.** [[Lig. genitoinguinale]]. Embryonic precursor of the gubernaculum testis.

10 **Prostate.** Prostata (Glandula prostatica). Chestnut-sized organ consisting of 30–50 tubulo-alveolar glands. Situated below the urinary bladder, it is penetrated by the urethra. B C D

11 **Base of prostate.** Basis prostatae. Part of the prostate fused with the urinary bladder. B

12 **Apex of prostate.** Apex prostatae. Portion of prostate directed downward and forward and containing the urethra. B

13 **Anterior surface.** Facies anterior. Surface of the prostate facing the symphysis. B D

14 **Posterior surface.** Facies posterior. Surface of the prostate facing the rectum. B

15 **Inferolateral surface.** Facies inferolateralis. Surface of the prostate directed downward and lateral. D

16 **Right/left lobe.** Lobus (dexter/sinister). Part of the prostate arising from the caudal anlage. B D

17 **Isthmus of prostate.** Isthmus prostatae. Median part of the prostate in front of the urethra and connecting the right and left lobes. It is devoid of glands and possesses a fibromuscular stroma. D

18 **Middle lobe.** [Lobus medius]. Prostatic lobe situated between the ejaculatory duct and the urethra. It tends to undergo hormone-induced hypertrophy in the elderly which can close the urethral canal valve-like. B D

19 **Capsule of prostate.** Capsula prostatica. Provided with smooth muscle fibers, it is firmly fused to the prostate. D

20 **Parenchyma.** Glandular component of the prostate.

21 **Prostatic ductules.** Ductuli prostatici. 15–30 glandular excretory ductules which open into the prostatic urethra. C

22 **Substantia muscularis.** Smooth muscle situated between the glandular alveoli. C

23 **M. puboprostaticus.** Tracts of smooth muscle contained within the puboprostatic (pubovesical) ligament extending from the pubic symphysis to the prostate.

24 **Bulbourethral [[Cowper's]] gland.** Glandula bulbourethralis [[Cowper's]]. Pea-sized mucous gland located in the urogenital diaphragm. E

25 **Duct of bulbourethral gland.** Ductus gl. bulbourethralis. Excretory duct of the bulbourethral gland, 3–4 cm long. E

26 EXTERNAL MALE GENITALIA. ORGANA GENITALIA MASCULINA EXTERNA. E

27 **Penis.** Male copulatory organ consisting of cavernous bodies and the urethra. E

28 **Root of penis.** Radix penis. Portion of the penis that is attached to the pubis. E

29 **Body (shaft) of penis.** Corpus penis. Portion of the penis situated between the root and the glans. E

30 **Crus penis.** Cavernous body attached to the inferior ramus of the pubis. E

31 **Dorsum penis.** Flattened upper surface of penis.

32 **Urethral surface.** Facies urethralis. Underside of penis. It bears the urethra within the corpus spongiosum. E

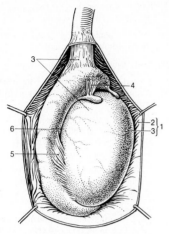

A Right testicle with epididymis and investing layers, lateral view

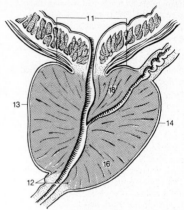

B Prostate, sagittal section

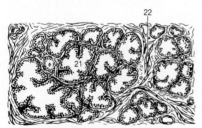

C Prostate, histologic view

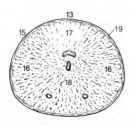

D Prostate, horizontal section

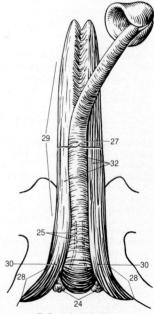

E Penis from below

1   **Glans penis.** Expanded end of the corpus spongiosum penis. A D

2   *Corona glandis.* Raised posterior margin of the glans. A D

3   *Septum glandis.* Median partition in the glans. C

4   *Collum glandis.* Neck of glans. Constriction behind the corona. A

5   **Prepuce (foreskin) of penis.** Preputium penis. Double layer of skin over the glans. A

6   **Frenulum of prepuce.** Frenulum preputii. Reflected fold passing from the prepuce to the underside of the glans. A

7   **Raphe penis.** Developmentally produced skin suture on the underside of the penis. B

8   **Corpus cavernosum penis.** Cavernous body divided into two halves by the septum of the penis. A B D

9   **Corpus spongiosum penis.** Cavernous body surrounding the urethra. A B D

10 **Bulb of penis.** Bulbus penis. Posterior thickened end of the corpus spongiosum. D

11 **Tunica albuginea of corpora cavernosa.** Tunica albuginea corporum cavernosorum. Tough connective tissue covering of the corpora cavernosa. B

12 **Tunica albuginea of corpus spongiosum.** Tunica albuginea corporis spongiosi. Less firm connective tissue covering of the corpus spongiosum. B

13 **Septum of penis.** Septum penis ⟦Septum pectiniforme⟧. Pectinate partition between the right and left corpus cavernosum. Gaps are present. B

14 **Trabeculae corporum cavernosorum.** Connective tissue tracts within the corpora cavernosa interspersed with smooth muscle. A B D

15 **Trabeculae corporis spongiosi.** Connective tissue tracts within the corpus spongiosum interspersed with smooth muscle. B

16 **Cavernae corporum cavernosorum.** Broad-
~   ly-meshed, blood-filled spaces within the corpora cavernosa. B D

17 **Cavernae corporis spongiosi.** Blood-filled,
~   finely meshed spongy network within the corpus spongiosum. B

18 **Helicine arteries.** Arteriae helicinae. Coiled branches of the deep artery of the penis. D

19 **Cavernous veins.** Venae cavernosae. Dilated veins in the cavernous bodies.

20 **Superficial fascia of penis.** Fascia penis superficialis. Quite delicate subcutaneous fascia with individual smooth muscle fibers. It corresponds to the dartos of the scrotum. B

21 **Deep fascia of penis.** Fascia penis profunda. Deeper, somewhat tougher fascia surrounding the three cavernous bodies. B

22 **Preputial glands.** Gll. preputiales. Sebaceous glands, mainly on the corona of the glans.

23 **Male urethra.** Urethra masculina. D

24 **Prostatic part of urethra.** Pars prostatica. Portion of male urethra passing through the prostate. D

25 **Urethral crest.** Crista urethralis. Mucosal fold in the dorsal wall of the prostatic urethra continuous with the uvula of the urinary bladder. D

26 **Colliculus seminalis.** Elevated portion (verumontanum) of the urethral crest containing the openings of the ejaculatory duct. D

27 **Prostatic utricle.** Utriculus prostaticus. Blind sac in the colliculus seminalis measuring up to 1 cm in length and representing a rudiment of the paramesonephric duct. D

28 **Prostatic sinus.** Sinus prostaticus. Furrow on both sides of the colliculus seminalis containing the openings of the prostatic ductules. D

29 **Membranous part of urethra.** Pars membranacea. Portion of the male urethra passing through the urogenital diaphragm. D

30 **Spongy part of urethra.** Pars spongiosa. Portion of male urethra surrounded by the corpus spongiosum. D

31 **Navicular fossa of urethra.** Fossa navicularis urethrae. Oval dilatation of the male urethra before its external opening. A D

32 **Valve of navicular fossa.** [Valvula fossae navicularis]. Mucosal fold on the upper wall of the navicular fossa.

33 **External urethral orifice.** Ostium urethrae externum. D

34 **Urethral lacunae.** Lacunae urethrales. Numerous outpocketings in the urethral mucosa with the openings of the urethral glands. D

35 **Urethral glands.** Gll. urethrales. Small mucous glands opening into the urethral lacunae.

36 **Ductus (canales) paraurethrales.** Inconstant excretory ducts of laterally-situated urethral glands with openings in the vicinity of the external urethral orifice.

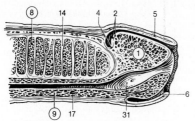

A End of penis, longitudinal section

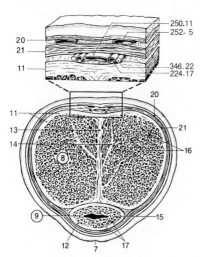

B Penis, cross section

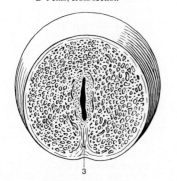

C Glans, cross-section

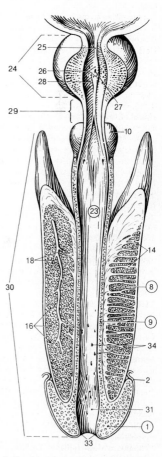

D Penis with prostate and base of bladder opened from dorsal up to the urethra

1 **Scrotum.** The scrotal sac containing the two testes. A

2 **Raphe of scrotum.** Raphe scroti (scrotalis). Developmental median skin suture on the scrotum. A

3 **Septum of scrotum.** Septum scroti (scrotale). Median connective tissue partition in the scrotum. A

4 **Dartos.** Tunica, musculus dartos. Layer of
~ smooth muscle with elastic fibers in the dermis. It wrinkles the skin of the scrotum. A

5 INTERNAL FEMALE GENITALIA. ORGA-
~ NA GENITALIA FEMININA INTERNA. B C
  D

6 **Ovary.** Ovarium. Intraperitoneal, almond-shaped gonad, about 2.5–4.5 cm long and 0.5–1 cm thick. C D

7 **Hilum of ovary.** Hilum ovarii. Place of entry
~ and exit of the ovarian vessels, as well as the attachment site of the mesovarium. C

8 **Medial surface.** Facies medialis. Surface of the ovary directed medial to the intrapelvic space. D

9 **Lateral surface.** Facies lateralis. Surface of the ovary adjoining the wall of the pelvis. D

10 **Free margin.** Margo liber. Free margin of the ovary lying opposite the hilum of the ovary. C D

11 **Mesovarian border.** Margo mesovaricus. Margin of attachment of the mesovarian lying opposite the free margin. D

12 **Tubal end.** Extremitas tubaria (tubalis). Upper pole of the ovary turned toward the uterine tube. D

13 **Uterine end.** Extremitas uterina. Lower pole of the ovary facing the uterus. D

14 **Tunica albuginea.** Thin organ capsule beneath the epithelial covering of the ovary, the alleged "germinal epithelium." C

15 **Stroma of ovary.** Stroma ovarii. Particularly nucleus-rich connective tissue framework of the ovary. C

16 **Cortex of ovary.** Cortex ovarii. Cortical region of the ovary with follicles of variable maturity. C

17 **Medulla of ovary.** Medulla ovarii. Vascular-rich central area. C

18 **Primary ovarian follicles.** Folliculi ovarici primarii. Units of egg development consisting of the ovum surrounded by a single layer of follicular epithelial cells and the absence of a lumen. C

19 **Vesicular ovarian [[Graafian]] follicles.** Folliculi ovarici vesiculosi. More mature follicles with a liquor-filled cavity (antrum). B C

20 [[Thecae folliculi]]. Specific connective tis-
~ sue investments of the follicles. B

21 *Theca externa.* External, fibrous layer of the
~ theca folliculi. B

22 *Theca interna.* Internal, cellular- and vascular-
~ rich layer of the theca folliculi. When the follicle is mature, it produces estradiol. B

23 Follicular epithelium. Epithelium folliculare (stratum granulosum). Nuclear-rich, stratified layer of follicular epithelial cells. B

24 Cumulus oophorus (ovifer). Mass of follicular epithelial cells projecting into the antrum of the follicle. It surrounds the ovum. B C

25 *Ovum (oocyte, egg).* Ovocytus. B
~

26 **Corpus luteum.** Endocrine gland arising from the follicular and thecal cells of the ruptured follicle. C

27 **Corpus albicans.** Connective tissue replacement of the degenerated corpus luteum. C

28 **Ovarian ligament.** Lig. ovarii proprium [[Chorda utero-ovarica]]. Ligament between the uterine end of the ovary and the tubal angle. It arises from the caudal gonadal fold. D

29 **Uterine (Fallopian) tube, oviduct.**
~ Tuba uterina (Salpinx). Thin connecting tube from the region of the ovary to the uterus. It is about 10 cm long. D

30 **Abdominal opening of uterine tube.** Ostium abdominale tubae uterinae. It is at the base of the infundibulum and communicates with the peritoneal cavity. D

31 **Infundibulum of uterine tube.** Infundibulum tubae uterinae. Funnel-shaped beginning of the uterine tube at the ovary. D

32 **Fimbriae of uterine tube.** Fimbriae tubae. Fringe-like processes of the infundibulum. D

33 Ovarian fimbria. Fimbria ovarica. An especially long fimbria projecting from the base of the infundibulum to the ovary where it is attached. D

34 **Ampulla of uterine tube.** Ampulla tubae uterinae. Lateral 2/3 of the tube. Its lumen tapers toward the isthmus. D

35 **Isthmus of uterine tube.** Isthmus tubae uterinae. Narrow medial 1/3 of the tube. D

36 **Uterine part of uterine tube.** Pars uterina. Portion of the tube within the wall of the uterus. D

37 **Uterine opening of uterine tube.** Ostium uterinum tubae. Opening of the tube into the uterine cavity. D

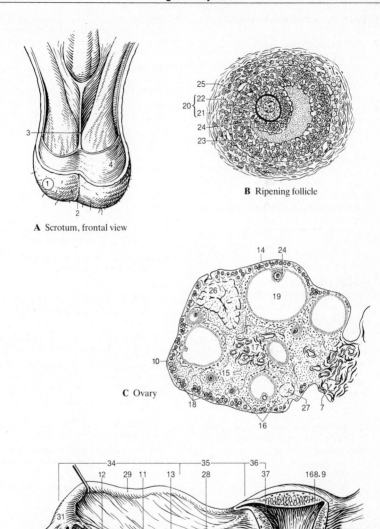

A Scrotum, frontal view

B Ripening follicle

C Ovary

D Uterine tube, ovary and uterus, posterior view

1 **Tunica serosa.** Peritoneal covering of the uterine tube. B

2 **Tela subserosa.** Connective tissue layer beneath the peritoneal covering of the uterine tube. B

3 **Tunica muscularis.** Layer of muscle in the wall of the uterine tube. B

4 **Tunica mucosa.** Mucous membrane lined by ciliated columnar epithelium with glandular cells and thrown into abundantly branched folds. B

5 **Tubal folds.** Plicae tubariae (tubales). Extensively branched mucosal folds which in some areas fill up the entire lumen of the uterine tube. B

6 **Uterus [[Metra]].** It measures about 7.5 cm
~ in length. A C

7 **Body of uterus.** Corpus uteri. Portion of the uterus situated between the cervix and fundus and possessing a lumen which is flattened from anterior to posterior. C

8 **Fundus of uterus.** Fundus uteri. Dome of the uterus lying above the entrance of the uterine tube. C

9 **Right/left horn of uterus.** Cornu uteri dextrum/sinistrum. Pointed extension of the uterus at the entrance of the uterine tube owing to the incomplete union of both paramesonephric ducts. See 167 D

10 **Right/left margin of uterus.** Margo uteri dexter/sinister. Blunt lateral border of uterus to which the broad ligament of the uterus is attached. A

11 **Intestinal surface.** Facies intestinalis. Surface of uterus facing posterosuperiorly and bordering on the intestine. C

12 **Cavity of uterus.** Cavitas uteri. It is lined by a
~ mucosa. A C

13 **Vesical surface.** Facies vesicalis. Uterine surface directed antero-inferiorly and facing the urinary bladder. C

14 **Isthmus uteri.** Portion of the uterus between the body and cervix. It is about 1 cm long. C

15 **Cervix uteri.** More tube-shaped, lower third of the uterus adjacent to the isthmus and about 2.5 cm long. C

16 **Supravaginal part of cervix.** Portio supravaginalis cervicis. Portion of the cervix surrounded on all sides by connective tissue. C

17 **Vaginal part of cervix.** Portio vaginalis cervicis. Cone-shaped portion of the cervix that projects into the vagina and is covered on all sides by vaginal epithelium. C

18 **Opening between uterus and vagina.** Ostium uteri. It is pit-like in the nullipara and becomes slit-like after parturition. C

19 **Anterior lip.** Labium anterius. Anterior border of uterine ostium. C

20 **Posterior lip.** Labium posterius. Posterior border of uterine ostium. C

21 **Cervical canal.** Canalis cervicis uteri. Tube-shaped canal of the cervix. C

22 **Palmate folds.** Plicae palmatae. Mucosal folds in the cervix organized like leaves of a palm tree. C

23 **Cervical glands.** Gll. cervicales (uteri). Branched, tubular mucous glands in the mucosa of the cervix.

24 **Parametrium.** Connective tissue between the two layers of the broad ligament. A

25 **Paracervix.** Continuation of the parametrium
~ into the cervical region.

26 **Tunica serosa (perimetrium).** Peritoneal covering of the uterus. A

27 **Tela subserosa.** Connective tissue layer beneath the peritoneal covering of the uterus. A

28 **Tunica muscularis (myometrium).** Very thick muscular layer of the wall of the uterus. Its fibers are arranged in a spiral system. A

29 **Tunica mucosa (endometrium).** Mucous membrane of uterus lined by simple columnar epithelium and glands. It undergoes changes corresponding to the menstrual cycle. A

30 **Uterine glands.** Gll. uterinae. Simple, branched, tubular glands within the endometrium. A

31 **M. recto-uterinus.** Smooth muscle within the rectouterine fold. C

32 **Round ligament of uterus.** Lig. teres uteri. Derived from the caudal gonadal fold, it extends from the tube angle to the labium majus by way of the broad ligament and the inguinal canal. C

33 **[[Processus vaginalis peritonei]].** Transient developmental diverticulum of the peritoneum extending through the inguinal canal. In rare cases it is the site of a congenital inguinal hernia in the female.

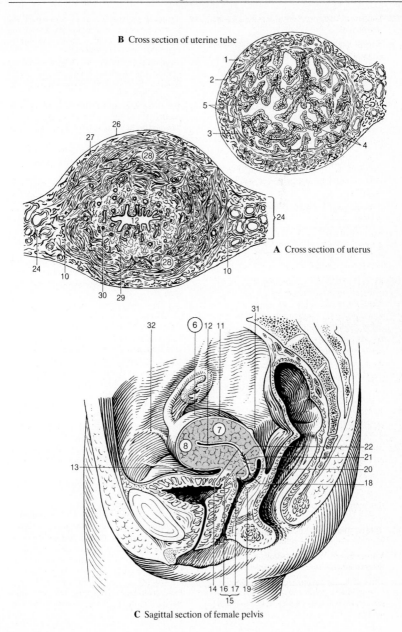

B Cross section of uterine tube

A Cross section of uterus

C Sagittal section of female pelvis

1   **Vagina.** Flat canal, about 10 cm long, leading into the uterus. A

2   **Fornix vaginae.** Recess between the vaginal part of the cervix and the wall of the vagina. A

3   Anterior part. Pars anterior. Anterior, shallower fornix of the vagina. A

4   Posterior part. Pars posterior. Posterior fornix of the vagina with its clinically very significant relationship to the peritoneal cavity. A

5   Lateral part. Pars lateralis. Lateral connection between the anterior and posterior fornices.

6   **Anterior wall of vagina.** Paries anterior. A

7   **Posterior wall of vagina.** Paries posterior. A

8   **Hymen.** Cutaneous fold emanating especially from the posterior wall of the vagina and, as a virginal membrane, partially closing off the entrance (introitus) into the vagina. C

9   Hymenal caruncle. Carunculae hymenales. Fleshy remains of the hymen in the wall of the vagina after parturition. A D

10 **Tunica muscularis.** Relatively thin layer of muscle in the vagina. A

11 **Tunica mucosa.** Mucous membrane of the vagina lined by glycogen-rich, stratified squamous, nonkeratinized epithelium. A

12 Rugae vaginales. Transverse folds (rugae) in the vaginal mucosa. A

13 Columns of rugae. Columnae rugarum. Two longitudinal ridges in the anterior and posterior walls of the vagina produced by underlying venous plexuses.

14 *Posterior column of rugae*. Columna rugarum posterior. It lies in the posterior wall of the vagina. A D

15 *Anterior column of rugae*. Columna rugarum anterior. It lies in the anterior wall of the vagina. A D

16 *Urethral carina of vagina*. Carina urethralis vaginae. Longitudinal ridge produced by the urethra in the lower part of the anterior column of the rugae. A C D

16 a **Tunica spongiosa.** Layer of spongy vascular plexuses outside of the tunica muscularis. A

17 **Epo-ophoron.** Developmental derivative of the mesonephros within the mesosalpinx. B

18 **Duct of epoophoron.** Ductus epoophorontis longitudinalis. Remnant of the mesonephric duct and some of its tubules. It lies in the mesosalpinx. B

19 Transverse ductules of epoophoron. Ductuli transversi. Remains of 10–20 transversely-running mesonephric tubules opening into the duct of the epoophoron. B

20 **Appendices vesiculosae.** Dispersed remains of mesonephric tubules in the vicinity of the infundibulum of the uterine tube. They terminate in vesicles. B

21 **Paro-ophoron.** Tubules derived from the caudal part of the mesonephros and situated between the lowermost branches of the ovarian artery. B

22 Vestigial ductus deferens. [Ductus deferens vestigialis]. Remains of the embryonic mesonephric duct in the female.

23 FEMALE EXTERNAL SEX ORGANS. ORGANA GENITALIA FEMININA EXTERNA. C D

24 **Female pudendum.** Pudendum femininum. External female genitalia. C D

25 **Mons pubis.** Fat pad situated in front of and above the pubic symphysis. C

26 **Labium majus pudendi.** Cutaneous fold covered with hair externally. The internal lining is smooth and hairless resembling a mucosa. C

27 Anterior labial commissure. Commissura labiorum anterior. Anterior union between right and left labium majus. C

28 Posterior labial commissure. Commissura labiorum posterior. Posterior union between right and left labium majus. C

29 Pudendal fissure. Rima pudendi. Fissure between right and left labium majus. C

30 **Labium minus pudendi.** Thinner cutaneous fold devoid of hair and provided with abundant sebaceous glands. C

31 Frenulum of pudendal labia. Frenulum labiorum pudendi. Sharply bordered cutaneous fold in front of the posterior labial commissure representing the union of the labia minora. C

32 **Vestibule of vagina.** Vestibulum vaginae. Space enclosed by the labia minora. C

33 Fossa of vestibule of vagina. Fossa vestibuli vaginae. Part of the vestibule between the frenulum and the vaginal opening. C

34 **Bulb of vestibule.** Bulbus vestibuli. Erectile tissue corresponding to the male corpus spongiosum, particularly at the root of the labia majora. C

35 Intermediate part of bulb of vestibule. Pars intermedia [Commissura] bulborum. Bridge between right and left bulb at the clitoris.

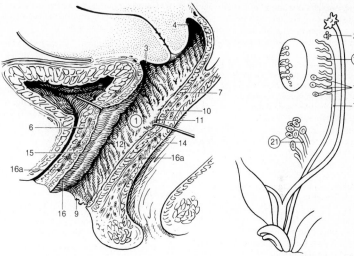

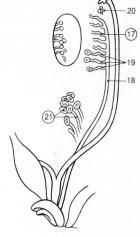

A Urinary bladder, urethra, vagina, uterus and rectum, sagittal section

B Development of the female urogenital system

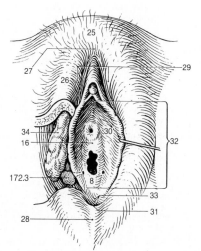

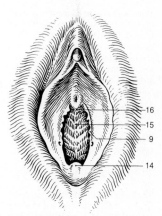

C External female virginal genitalia

D External female genitalia

1 **Orifice (introitus) of vagina.** Ostium vaginae. Opening of vagina into vestibule. A

2 **Lesser vestibular glands.** Gll. vestibulares minores. Simple, tubular mucosal glands near the urethra.

3 **Greater vestibular [[Bartholin's]] gland.** Gl. vestibularis major [[Bartholini]]. Pea-sized mucous gland situated posteriorly in the urogenital diaphragm. It opens into the lower third of the vestibule between the labium minus and hymen or hymenal caruncle. A

4 **Clitoris.** Rudimentary penis at the anterior end of the labia minora. It lacks a urethra and corpus spongiosum. A

5 **Crus of clitoris.** Crus clitoridis. It is attached to the inferior pubic ramus. A

6 **Body of clitoris.** Corpus clitoridis. Shaft of clitoris formed by the two crura. A

7 **Glans of clitoris.** Glans clitoridis. Acorn-shaped cap of the clitoris connected with the bulb of the vestibule by a thin cord. A

8 **Frenulum of clitoris.** Frenulum clitoridis. Double fold approaching the clitoris inferiorly from the labia minora. A

9 **Prepuce of clitoris.** Preputium clitoridis. Union of the two folds of the labia minora above the clitoris. A

10 RIGHT AND LEFT CORPUS CAVERNOSUM OF CLITORIS. Corpus cavernosum clitoridis (dextrum/sinistrum). Right and left cavernous bodies joined with the shaft of the clitoris. A

11 **Septum of corpus cavernosum.** Septum corporum cavernosorum. Incomplete connective tissue partition between the right and left corpus cavernosum.

12 **Fascia clitoridis.** Connective tissue layer covering the clitoris.

13 **Urethra feminina.** 2.5 to 4 cm long female urethra. D

14 **External opening of urethra.** Ostium urethrae externum. It is situated 2–3 cm below the clitoris. A

15 **Tunica muscularis.** Layer in female urethra consisting primarily of circular smooth muscle fibers. D

16 **Tunica spongiosa.** Submucosal, venous, erectile tissue. D

17 **Tunica mucosa.** Mucous membrane of female urethra lined by transitional epithelium as it leaves the bladder and subsequently by stratified columnar epithelium. D

18 Urethral glands. Gll. urethrales. Small mucous glands opening into the urethra. D

19 Urethral lacunae. Lacunae urethrales. Outpocketings in the urethral mucosa into which the urethral glands open. D

20 **Paraurethral duct.** [Ductus paraurethrales]. Glandular duct, 1–2 cm long, which opens into the female urethra near the urethral orifice. D

21 **Urethral crest.** Crista urethralis. Well-developed longitudinal fold in the posterior wall of the female urethra. D

22 EMBRYOLOGICAL TERMINOLOGY. NOMINA ONTOGENETICA.

23 **Decidual membranes.** [[Membranae deciduae]]. Mucous membranes of the pregnant uterus. C

24 Decidua parietalis. Mucosa lining the uterine wall not occupied by the embryo. C

25 Decidua capsularis. Uterine mucosa between the embryo and the uterine cavity. C

26 Decidua basalis. Mucous membrane between the embryo and the uterine wall. C

27 **Placenta.** Organ of metabolic interchange between mother and fetus and consisting of trophoblast and uterine mucosa (endometrium). E

28 Uterine part. [[Pars uterina]]. Part of the placenta consisting of the basal plate (decidua basalis) and placental septa. E

29 Fetal part. [[Pars fetalis]]. Part of the placenta consisting of the chorion and amnion. E

30 **Umbilical cord.** Funiculus umbilicalis. It is derived from the body stalk. E

31 **Embryonic excretory organ.** Mesonephros. Phylogenetically, it appears after the pronephros and is involved in the development of the permanent metanephros. B

32 **Mesonephric [*Wolffian*] duct.** Ductus mesonephricus. Excretory duct formed by the pronephros. It forms the ductus deferens in the male. B

33 **Paramesonephric [[*Müllerian*]] duct.** Ductus paramesonephricus. Duct formed by an epithelial invagination lateral to the mesonephric duct. It gives rise to the uterus, uterine tube and a part of the vagina. B

34 **Primitive urogenital sinus.** Sinus urogenitalis primitivus. Anterior portion of the cloaca separated off by the embryonic urorectal septum. It gives rise to the inferior pole of the urinary bladder, urethra and vestibule of the vagina. B

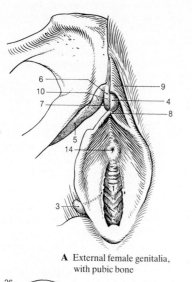

A External female genitalia,
with pubic bone

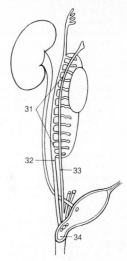

B Development of the
female urogenital system

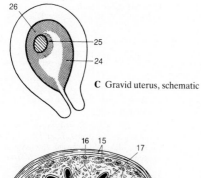

C Gravid uterus, schematic

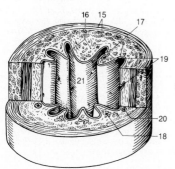

D Female urethra

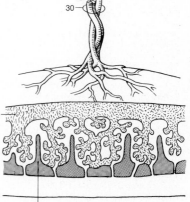

E Placenta, schematic

1 **PERINEUM.** Segment between anus and genitalia.

2 **Perineal raphe.** Raphe perinealis. Developmentally produced median cutaneous suture at the perineum. It is a continuation of the scrotal raphe.

3 Muscles of perineum. Musculi perinei (perineales).

4 Perineal body. Centrum tendineum perinei. Tough fibromuscular mass in the median plane at the union of the muscles of the perineum between the rectum and vagina, or urethra. A

5 **Pelvic diaphragm.** Diaphragma pelvis. Muscular floor of pelvis formed mainly by the levator ani muscle.

6 **M. levator ani.** Muscle passing funnel-shaped from the pubis and obturator fascia to the anus and the anococcygeal ligament. I: Pudendal nerve and S3–4. A B

7 M. pubococcygeus. Fibers of the levator ani passing from the pubis to the perineal body, sphincter ani muscle and coccyx. A B

8 M. levator prostatae (m. pubovaginalis). Fibers of the pubococcygeus muscle radiating into the fascia of the prostate or the wall of the vagina. A

9 M. puborectalis. Muscle running posteriorly from the pubis and looping around the perineal flexure of the rectum. A

10 M. iliococcygeus. Muscle passing from the tendinous arch of the levator ani to the coccyx and the anococcygeal ligament. A B

11 **Tendinous arch of levator ani muscle.** [Arcus tendineus m. levatoris ani]. Arched tendinous thickening of the obturator fascia at the origin of the levator ani. A B

12 **Anococcygeal ligament.** Lig. anococcygeum. Tough connective tissue tract between the anus and coccyx. A C

13 **M. coccygeus.** Muscle fibers passing fan-shaped from the ischial spine to the lateral surfaces of the sacrum and coccyx. They are fused with the sacrospinous ligament. I: S4–5. A

14 **M. sphincter ani externus.** External anal sphincter. Composed of skeletal muscle, it consists of the following three parts. I: Pudendal nerve. B C

15 Subcutaneous part. Pars subcutanea. More superficial portion of the external anal sphincter radiating into the dermis in front of and behind the anus. B C See p. 177 B

16 Superficial part. Pars superficialis. Fibers of external anal sphincter which spread out between the perineal body and the anococcygeal ligament. B C

17 Deep part. Pars profunda. Purely circular portion of the external anal sphincter which attains a height of 3–4 cm. B C

18 **Pelvic fascia.** Fascia pelvis. Connective tissue covering of the pelvic viscera and the pelvic wall. It is the caudal continuation of the transversalis fascia.

19 Parietal pelvic fascia. F. pelvis parietalis. Portion of the pelvic fascia lining the pelvic wall. A B

20 Obturator fascia. Fascia obturatoria. Especially strong portion of the pelvic fascia situated on the obturator internus muscle. A B

21 Visceral pelvic (endopelvic) fascia. Fascia pelvis visceralis [[F. endopelvina]]. Portion of the pelvic fascia ensheathing the pelvic viscera. B

22 *Prostatic fascia.* Fascia prostatae. Fascia of prostate which fuses with the surrounding tissues. C

23 *Peritoneoperineal fascia.* Fascia peritoneoperinealis. Collective term for 24 and 25.

24 *Rectovesical septum.* Septum rectovesicale. Connective tissue partition between the rectum and urinary bladder. It is a part of the pelvic and prostatic fascia. C

25 *Rectovaginal septum.* Septum rectovaginale. Connective tissue partition between the rectum and vagina. It is a part of the pelvic fascia.

26 Superior fascia of pelvic diaphragm. Fascia diaphragmatis pelvis superior. Fascial covering on the superior surface of the pelvic diaphragm (facing the pelvis). B

27 Tendinous arch of pelvic fascia. Arcus tendineus fasciae pelvis. Tendinous reinforcement of the pelvic fascia extending bow-shaped from the symphysis downward to the ischial spine. It corresponds to a band where the visceral vessels and nerves leave the lateral wall of the pelvis and where the pelvic connective tissue is especially firmly united with the pelvic wall. A

28 Puboprostatic (pubovesical) ligament. Lig. puboprostaticum (pubovesicale). Reinforced connective tissue permeated with smooth muscle passing from the pubic symphysis to the prostate (to the neck of the bladder in females). C

29 Inferior fascia of pelvic diaphragm. Fascia diaphragmatis pelvis inferior. Fascia covering the levator ani muscle on the side of the ischio-anal fossa. B

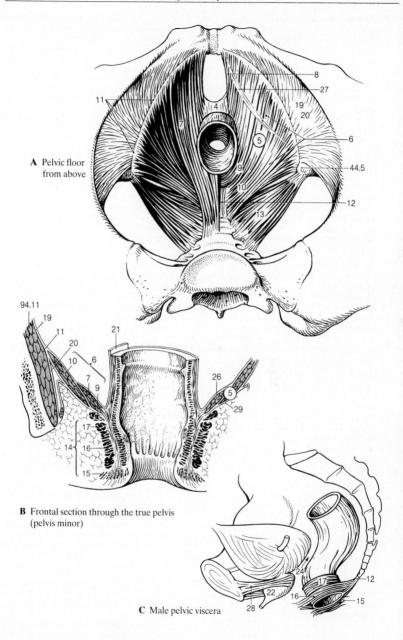

A Pelvic floor from above

B Frontal section through the true pelvis (pelvis minor)

C Male pelvic viscera

1　**Urogenital diaphragm.** [[Diaphragm urogenitale]]. Fibromuscular wall spread out between the right and left inferior rami of the pubis. A B E

2　**Deep perineal space.** Spatium perinei profundum. Space between the inferior and superior fascia of the urogenital diaphragm. Contents: Deep transversus perinei and sphincter urethrae muscles; bulbo-urethral glands; nerves and vessels for the penis. A

3　**M. transversus perinei profundus.** Trapezoid-shaped muscular plate stretched out in the pubic arch. I: Pudendal nerve. A B E

4　**M. sphincter urethrae.** Muscular fibers surrounding the membranous part of the urethra. I: Pudendal nerve. A E

4a　**M. compressor urethrae.** Fibers continuing distally from the M. sphincter urethrae and passing to the ramus of the ischium. F

4b　**M. sphincter urethrovaginalis.** Fibers continuing distally from the M. compressor urethrae and passing to the bulb of the vestibule. F

5　**Superior fascia of urogenital diaphragm.** Fascia diaphragmatis urogenitalis superior. Fascia of the deep transverse perinei muscle located on the side of the ischio-anal fossa. A

6　**Perineal membrane [Inferior fascia of urogenital diaphragm].** Membrana perinei [fascia diaphragmatis urogenitalis inferior]. Fascia on the deep transverse perinei muscle anteriorly and inferiorly. A

7　**Transverse perineal ligament.** Lig. transversum perinei. Thickened fusion of both fasciae of the urogenital diaphragm at the anterior, upper margin of the deep transverse perinei muscle. E

8　**Superficial perineal space.** Spatium perinei superficiale. Space between the superficial perineal fascia and the inferior fascia of the urogenital diaphragm. It contains the root of the penis. A

9　**M. transversus perinei superficialis.** Inconstant separated portion of the deep transverse perineal muscle. It radiates out into the perineal body. I: Pudendal nerve. B

10　**M. ischiocavernosus.** It arises from the ramus of the ischium, lies on the crus of the penis and attaches to its tunica albuginea. I: Pudendal nerve. B

11　**M. bulbospongiosus** [[m. bulbocavernosus]]. It arises from the perineal body and at a median raphe on the corpus spongiosum and passing lateral to them, extends to the inferior fascia of the urogenital diaphragm and the dorsum of the penis. In the female it curves around the bulb of the vestibule. I: Pudendal nerve. A B, 225 D

12　**Superficial perineal fascia.** Fascia perinei superficialis. Fascia bordering the superficial perineal space anteroinferiorly. A

13　**Ischioanal fossa.** Fossa ischioanalis. Space between the levator ani and obturator internus muscles. It is bordered anteroinferiorly by the urogenital diaphragm. A B

14　Fat pad of ischioanal fossa. Corpus adiposum fossae ischioanalis. Structural fat in the ischioanal fossa.

15　**Pudendal [[Alcock's]] canal.** Canalis pudendalis [[Alcock]]. Splitting of the obturator fascia in the lateral wall of the ischioanal fossa to form a tunnel for the passage of the pudendal vessels and nerves. A

16　**Retropubic space.** Spatium retropubicum [[spatium praevesicale; cavum Retzii]]. Space between the urinary bladder and the pubis filled with loose connective tissue and bordered inferiorly by the puboprostatic ligament. C

17　**PERITONEUM.** Serous lining of peritoneal cavity.

18　**Abdominal cavity.** [[Cavitas abdominalis]] without peritoneum.

19　**Peritoneal cavity.** Cavitas peritonealis. Space enclosed by the peritoneum.

19a　**Extraperitoneal space.** Spatium extraperitoneale. Space in connective tissue with no relationship to the peritoneum.

20　**Retroperitoneal space.** Spatium retroperitoneale. Space between the peritoneum and the transversalis fascia.

21　*Extraperitoneal fascia.* Fascia extraperitonealis. Connective tissue layer of varying thickness beneath the peritoneum.

22　*Extraperitoneal organ.* Organum extraperitoneale. Organ in extraperitoneal space.

23　*Parietal peritoneum.* Peritoneum parietale. Peritoneum of abdominal wall. D

24　*Tunica serosa.* Serous membrane lined by smooth, simple peritoneal epithelium.

25　*Tela subserosa.* Connective tissue layer beneath the serosa.

26　**Visceral peritoneum.** Peritoneum viscerale. Peritoneum covering the abdominal viscera. D

27　*Tunica serosa.* See 24.

28　*Tela subserosa.* See 25.

29　**Epiploic foramen [[of Winslow]].** Foramen omentale (epiploicum). Opening into the lesser sac behind the hepatoduodenal ligament. D

30　**Omental bursa [[lesser sac of peritoneum]].** Bursa omentalis. Space situated mainly behind the stomach and lined by peritoneum. D

31　*Vestibule of omental bursa.* Vestibulum bursae omentalis. Portion of the omental bursa situated at the caudate lobe of the liver and bordered toward the left side by the gastropancreatic folds. D

32　*Upper omental recess.* Recessus superior omentalis. Upward directed recess between the inferior vena cava and the esophagus. D

33　*Lower omental recess.* Recessus inferior omentalis. Lower portion between the stomach and transverse colon or, in a given case, between the anterior and posterior layers of the greater omentum. D

34　*Splenic recess.* Recessus splenicus (lienalis). Left portion of lower omental recess bordered by splenic ligaments. D

35　*Gastropancreatic folds.* Plicae gastropancreaticae. Folds in the posterior wall of the lesser sac formed by the left gastric and common hepatic arteries. D

35a　**Hepatopancreatic fold.** Plica hepatopancreatica. Synonym for Plica gastropancreatica dextra. Encloses the common hepatic artery.

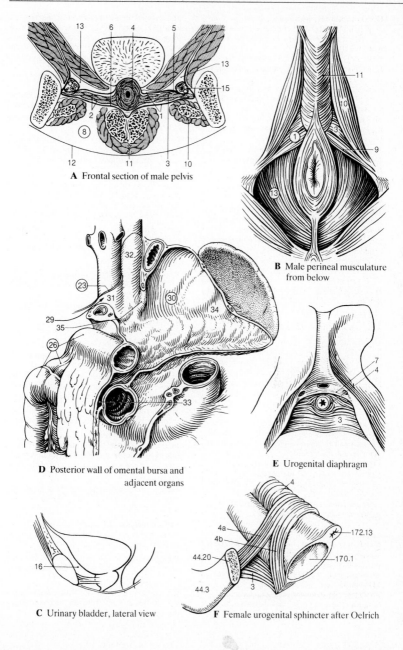

A Frontal section of male pelvis

B Male perineal musculature from below

D Posterior wall of omental bursa and adjacent organs

E Urogenital diaphragm

C Urinary bladder, lateral view

F Female urogenital sphincter after Oelrich

178 Peritoneum

1 **Dorsal mesentery.** [[Mesenterium dorsale commune]]. Embryologically original, common, dorsal suspensory ligament of the still undifferentiated intestinal tube.

2 **Mesentery.** Mesenterium. Dorsal peritoneal fold for the fixation of the intraperitoneal small intestine. It transports blood vessels and nerves. B

3 Root of mesentery. Radix mesenterii. Located at the posterior wall of the abdominal cavity, it extends from L2 to the right iliac fossa. A

4 **Mesocolon.** Peritoneal fold bearing vessels and nerves for the fixation and maintenance of the colon.

5 Transverse mesocolon. Mesocolon transversum. Suspensory ligament of the transverse colon. A B

6 Mesocolon of ascending colon. Mesocolon ascendens. It fuses with the posterior abdominal wall in the 4th embryonic month.

7 Mesocolon of descending colon. Mesocolon descendens. It fuses with the posterior abdominal wall in the 4th embryonic month.

8 Sigmoid mesocolon. Mesocolon sigmoideum. Suspensory ligament of sigmoid colon. B

9 Mes-oappendix [[Mesenteriolum]]. Suspensory ligament of vermiform appendix. B

10 **Lesser omentum.** Omentum minus. Peritoneal sheet extending mainly between the stomach and liver.

11 **Hepatogastric ligament.** Lig. hepatogastricum. Part of the lesser omentum between the stomach and liver. B

12 **Hepatoduodenal ligament.** Lig. hepatoduodenale. Part of lesser omentum between the duodenum and liver. It contains the hepatic artery proper, bile duct and the portal vein. B

13 **Hepatocolic ligament.** [Lig. hepatocolicum]. Inconstant continuation of the hepatoduodenal ligament toward the right at the right colic flexure or at the transverse colon. B

14 Greater omentum. Omentum majus. Doubled peritoneal apron hanging down from the stomach and transverse colon and containing a variable amount of fat. B

15 **Gastrophrenic ligament.** Lig. gastrophrenicum. Upper continuation of the phrenicosplenic and gastrosplenic ligaments between the stomach and diaphragm. A B

16 **Gastrosplenic (gastrolienal) ligament.** Lig. gastrosplenicum (gastrolienale). Peritoneal connection from the lesser curvature of the stomach to the hilum of the spleen. B

17 **Gastrocolic ligament.** Lig. gastrocolicum. Peritoneal connection between the lesser curvature of the stomach and the omental tenia of the transverse colon. It is attached to the gastrosplenic ligament. B

18 **Phrenicocolic ligament.** Lig. phrenicocolicum. Peritoneal fold on the left side between the diaphragm and the descending colon. B

19 **Splenorenal (lienorenal, phrenicosplenic) ligament.** Lig. splenorenale (lienorenale, phrenicosplenicum). Peritoneal fold from the diaphragm, kidney and pancreas to the hilum of the spleen; on the right side it is continuous with the transverse mesocolon. B

20 **Hepatic ligaments.** Ligg. hepatis.

21 Coronary ligament. Lig. coronarium. Reflection of the parietal peritoneum of the diaphragm to the visceral peritoneum of the liver at the margin of the bare area. A

22 Falciform ligament of liver. Lig. falciforme (hepatis). Peritoneal fold from the anterior and inferior sides of the liver to the anterior abdominal wall. B

23 Right triangular ligament. Lig. triangulare dextrum. Triangular peritoneal fold between the right lobe of the liver and the diaphragm. It is the right end of the coronary ligament. A

24 Left triangular ligament. Lig. triangulare sinistrum. Triangular peritoneal fold between the liver and diaphragm. It is the left end of the coronary ligament. A

25 Hepatorenal ligament. Lig. hepatorenale. Extension of the coronary ligament attached to the right kidney. A

26 **Folds and recesses.** Plicae et fossae (recessus).

27 **Fascia retinens rostralis.** Band passing upward at the duodenojejunal flexure, perhaps with the suspensory muscle of the duodenum. See 124.9. A

28 **Superior duodenal fold (duodenojejunal fold).** Plica duodenalis superior (plica duodenojejunalis). Peritoneal fold on the left side of the duodenojejunal flexure in front of the superior duodenal recess. It contains the inferior mesenteric vein. A

29 **Superior duodenal recess.** Recessus duodenalis superior. Peritoneal recess behind the superior duodenal fold. A

30 **Inferior duodenal fold (duodenomesocolic fold).** Plica duodenalis inferior (plica duodenomesocolica). Peritoneal fold just in front of duodenojejunal flexure. A

31 **Inferior duodenal recess.** Recessus duodenalis inferior. Peritoneal recess behind the inferior duodenal fold. A

32 **Paraduodenal fold.** [Plica paraduodenalis]. Peritoneal fold located on the left side of the duodenum. A

33 **Paraduodenal recess.** [Recessus paraduodenalis]. Peritoneal recess behind the paraduodenal fold with its opening toward the right. A

34 **Retroduodenal recess.** [Recessus retroduodenalis]. Peritoneal recess between the aorta and the duodenum with its opening toward the left. A

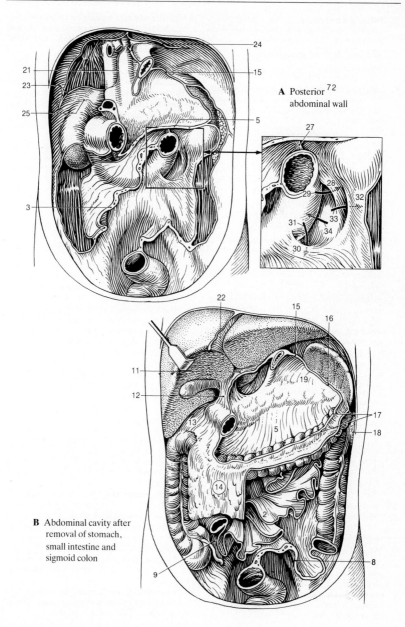

A Posterior [72] abdominal wall

B Abdominal cavity after removal of stomach, small intestine and sigmoid colon

1 **Intersigmoid recess.** Recessus intersigmoideus. Peritoneal recess on the left side below the root of the sigmoid mesocolon. A

2 **Superior ileocecal recess.** Recessus ileocaecalis superior. Peritoneal recess above the opening of the ileum into the cecum. A

3 **Vascular cecal fold.** Plica caecalis vascularis. Peritoneal fold in front of the superior ileocecal recess containing a branch of the ileocolic artery. A

4 **Inferior ileocecal recess.** Recessus ileocaecalis inferior. Peritoneal recess below the opening of the ileum into the cecum. A

5 **Ileocecal fold.** Plica ileocaecalis. Peritoneal fold in front of inferior ileocecal recess and extending inferiorly up to the appendix. A

6 **Retrocecal recess.** Recessus retrocaecalis. Peritoneal fold often present on the right side behind the cecum or ascending colon. A

7 **Cecal folds.** Plicae caecales. Peritoneal folds on the outside of the cecum. They correspond to the semilunar folds in the colon. A

8 **Paracolic sulci.** Sulci paracolici. Occasional pockets left of the descending colon. A

9 **Subphrenic recess.** Recessus subphrenici. Peritoneal recess between the diaphragm and both liver lobes, right and left of the falciform ligament, and bordered posterosuperiorly by the coronary ligament. C

10 **Subhepatic recess.** Recessus subhepatici. Recess between the liver and transverse colon or adjoining viscera. C

11 **Hepatorenal recess.** Recessus hepatorenalis. Portion of the subhepatic recess bordered by the kidney and suprarenal gland. C

12 **Anterior parietal peritoneum.** Peritoneum parietale anterius.

13 **Median umbilical fold.** Plica umbilicalis mediana [[Plica umbilicalis media]]. Fold passing from the apex of the urinary bladder to the umbilicus. It contains the remains of the urachus. A B

14 **Supravesical fossa.** Fossa supravesicalis. Shallow depression in front of the urinary bladder between the median and medial umbilical folds. B

15 **Medial umbilical fold**. Plica umbilicalis medialis [[Plica umbilicalis lateralis]]. Fold corresponding to the obliterated umbilical artery. It is located in the anterior abdominal wall between the median umbilical (obliterated urachus) and lateral umbilical (inferior epigastric artery) folds. A B

16 **Medial inguinal fossa.** Fossa inguinalis medialis. Depression lying opposite the external inguinal ring between the medial and lateral umbilical folds. B

17 **Inguinal trigone.** Trigonum inguinale. Triangular area between the lateral margin of the rectus abdominis, inguinal ligament and lateral umbilical fold (inferior epigastric artery). B

18 **Lateral umbilical fold [epigastric fold].** Plica umbilicalis lateralis [[Plica epigastrica]]. Peritoneal fold produced by the inferior epigastric artery. A B

19 **Lateral inguinal fossa.** Fossa inguinalis lateralis. Depression lateral to the lateral umbilical fold corresponding to the deep inguinal ring. B

20 **Transverse vesical fold.** Plica vesicalis transversa. Peritoneal fold extending transversely over the moderately filled bladder. It is obliterated when the bladder is full. A

21 **Paravesical fossa.** Fossa paravesicalis. Shallow depression lateral to the bladder. It is bordered laterally by the ductus deferens. B

22 **Urogenital peritoneum.** Peritoneum urogenitale. Peritoneum of the reproductive organs.

23 **Vaginal process of peritoneum.** [[Processus vaginalis peritonei]]. Finger-like diverticulum of the peritoneum through the inguinal canal preceding the descent of the testis.

24 **Broad ligament of uterus.** Lig. latum uteri. Peritoneal duplication between the uterus and lateral pelvic wall carrying vessels and nerves. A

25 **Mesometrium.** Portion of the broad ligament passing to the uterus. A

26 **Mesosalpinx.** Mesentery of uterine tube. A

27 **Mesovarium.** Mesentery of ovary. A

28 **Suspensory ligament of ovary.** Lig. suspensorium ovarii. Derived from the cranial gonadal fold, it suspends the ovary superiorly and carries its vessels. A

29 **Ovarian fossa.** Fossa ovarica. Depression at the origin of the internal and external iliac arteries.

30 **Rectouterine fold.** Plica rectouterina. Peritoneal fold between the rectum and uterus. A

31 **Rectouterine pouch [[of Douglas]].** Excavatio rectouterina. Deepest part of abdominal cavity between the rectum, uterus and the two rectouterine folds. A

32 **Vesicouterine pouch.** Excavatio vesicouterina. Peritoneal space between the uterus and bladder. A

33 **Rectovesical pouch.** Excavatio rectovesicalis. Deepest part of the abdominal cavity between the rectum and bladder in the male.

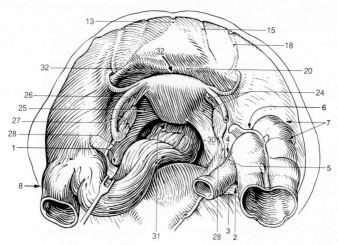

A View of the female true pelvis (pelvis minor) from above

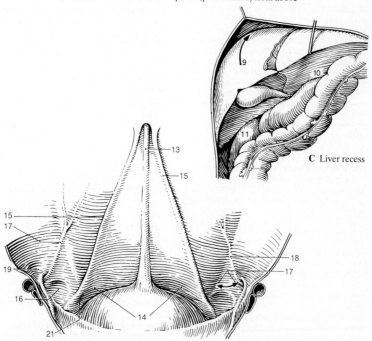

C Liver recess

B Anterior abdominal wall, posterior view

1 ENDOCRINE GLANDS. GLANDULAE ENDOCRINAE. Ductless glands.

2 **Thyroid gland.** Glandula thyroidea. It produces the metabolic-stimulating hormones, thyroxine and tri-iodothyronine. It can become enlarged pathologically to form a goiter. A B

3 **Right and left lobe.** Lobus (dexter/sinister). Situated beside the trachea. A

4 **Isthmus of thyroid gland.** Isthmus gl. thyroideae. Portion connecting the right and left lobes. A

5 **Pyramidal lobe.** [Lobus pyramidalis]. Developmental remnant occasionally present in the form of a median cord of thyroid tissue. A

6 **Accessory thyroid glands.** Glandulae thyroideae accessoriae. Dispersed islands of thyroid glandular tissue, e.g., at the base of the tongue. A

7 **Fibrous capsule.** Capsula fibrosa. Double connective tissue capsule of thyroid gland.

8 **Stroma.** Connective tissue framework of thyroid gland. C

9 **Parenchyma.** Specific glandular cells of thyroid. C

10 **Lobules.** Lobuli. Segments of thyroid parenchyma partitioned by connective tissue.

11 **Superior parathyroid gland.** Glandula parathyroidea superior. Superior lentil-sized epithelial body located behind the thyroid. It produces parathormone which regulates calcium and phosphorus metabolism. B

12 **Inferior parathyroid gland.** Glandula parathyroidea inferior. Inferior lentil-shaped epithelial body located behind the thyroid. Its hormone, parathormone, regulates calcium and phosphorus metabolism. B

13 **Hypophysis (pituitary gland).** Hypophysis (glandula pituitaria). Located within the sella turcica, it is the most versatile functioning endocrine gland. D

14 **Adenohypophysis (anterior lobe).** Large anterior lobe of pituitary derived from stomodeal ectoderm (Rathke's pouch). Its parenchyma contains functionally and histochemically different cell types. D

15 *Pars tuberalis*. Portion of adenohypophysis covering the hypophyseal stalk. D

16 *Pars intermedia*. Narrow middle part of adenohypophysis containing colloidal cysts. D

17 *Pars distalis*. Anterior, largest segment of the adenohypophysis. D

18 *[[Pars pharyngea]]*. Remains of Rathke's pouch beneath the pharyngeal mucosa in the form of adenohypophyseal tissue.

19 **Neurohypophysis (posterior lobe).** Smaller posterior portion of the pituitary gland derived from the diencephalon. It serves only as a storage depot for hormones. D

20 **Infundibulum.** Funnel-like stalk of the pituitary. D

21 **Neural lobe.** Lobus nervosus. True posterior lobe. It is a hormon storage area. D

22 **Pineal body (gland).** Corpus pineale (Glandula pinealis). Derived from the diencephalon, it lies above the quadrigeminal plate (lamina tecti). D

23 **Thymus.** Lymphatic organ situated behind the sternum. It undergoes regression at puberty. E

24 **Right/left lobe of thymus.** Lobus (dexter/sinister). E

25 Accessory thymic nodules. [Noduli thymici accessorii]. Scattered islands of thymic tissue.

26 **Thymic lobules.** Lobuli thymi. Lobules of thymus formed by connective tissue trabeculae. E

27 **Cortex of thymus.** Cortex thymi. Lymphocyte-rich cortical area.

28 **Medulla of thymus.** Medulla thymi. Lymphocyte-poor medullary region containing Hassell's (thymic) corpuscles.

29 **Suprarenal (adrenal) gland.** Glandula suprarenalis (adrenalis). Sitting like a cap medially on the upper pole of the kidney, it develops from two sources. F

30 **Anterior surface of suprarenal.** Facies anterior. F

31 **Posterior surface of suprarenal.** Facies posterior.

32 **Renal surface.** Facies renalis. Concave surface facing the kidney and directed inferolaterally. F

33 **Superior margin.** Margo superior. Upper margin between the anterior and posterior surfaces. F

34 **Medial margin.** Margo medialis. Between the anterior and posterior surface. F

35 **Hilum.** Site of exit of central vein. It is directed forward, downward or upward. F

36 Central vein. Vena centralis. Principal vein of the suprarenal. It exits anterosuperiorly or antero-inferiorly. F

37 **Cortex.** Arising developmentally from the coelomic epithelium, the suprarenal cortex is divided into three zones. G

38 **Medulla.** Arising from the neural crest, the suprarenal medulla consists of chromaffin cells, sympathetic ganglion cells and venous sinuses. G

39 **Accessory suprarenal glands.** Glandulae suprarenales accessoriae. Scattered suprarenal tissue.

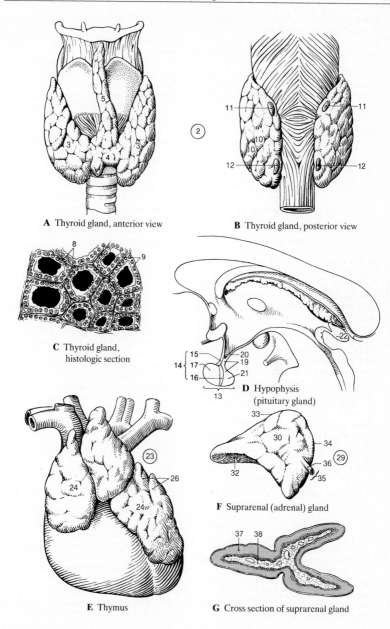

A Thyroid gland, anterior view

B Thyroid gland, posterior view

C Thyroid gland, histologic section

D Hypophysis (pituitary gland)

E Thymus

F Suprarenal (adrenal) gland

G Cross section of suprarenal gland

1 **PERICARDIUM.** Enveloping and gliding system of the heart comprising a fibrous and a bilayered serous pericardium. A

2 **Fibrous pericardium.** Pericardium fibrosum. Tough, external, connective tissue portion of the pericardium. It is partially fused with the diaphragm.

3 Sternopericardiac ligaments. Ligg. sternopericardiaca. Connective tissue reinforcement of the pericardium at the sternum.

4 **Serous pericardium.** Pericardium serosum. It represents the simple squamous epithelium (mesothelium) which lines the fibrous pericardium (parietal layer) and covers the surface of the heart (visceral layer). Visceral and parietal layers become continuous in the region of the great vessels.

5 Parietal layer. Lamina parietalis. Serous portion of pericardium. It lines the fibrous pericardium.

6 Visceral layer. Lamina visceralis [epicardium]. Serous covering of the surface of the heart (epicardium). It consists of mesothelium and a fiber-rich lamina propria.

7 **Pericardial cavity.** Cavitas pericardialis.
~ Space between the parietal and visceral layers of the serous pericardium. It contains a film of serous fluid.

8 Transverse sinus of pericardium. Sinus transversus pericardii. Narrow passage in pericardial space behind the aorta and pulmonary trunk and in front of the veins. A

9 Oblique sinus of pericardium. Sinus obliquus pericardii. Recess in the pericardial space between the right pulmonary veins and inferior cava on the one side and the left pulmonary veins on the other. A

10 HEART. COR.

11 **Base of heart.** Basis cordis. Upper, broad surface of the nearly cone-shaped heart lying opposite to the apex and directed dorsally. It is formed mainly by the posterior wall of the left atrium.

12 **Sternocostal surface.** Facies sternocostalis
~ [anterior]. Convex surface of heart directed anteriorly. B D

13 **Diaphragmatic surface.** Facies diaphragmatica [inferior]. Inferior surface of heart
~ touching the diaphragm. D

14 **Pulmonary surface.** Facies pulmonalis. Lateral surface of heart contacted by the lungs. D
~

15 **Right margin.** Margo dexter. It often displays
~ a sharp odge in the cadaver. B

16 Apex cordis. Apex of heart directed forward, toward the left side and downward. B

17 Incisure of apex of heart. Incisura apicis cordis. Notch on the right side near the apex of the heart lying in the prolongation of the longitudinal interventricular grooves. B

18 **Anterior interventricular groove.** Sulcus interventricularis anterior. Longitudinal groove located on the anterior surface above the interventricular septum and containing the anterior interventricular branch. B D

19 **Posterior interventricular groove.** Sulcus interventricularis posterior. Longitudinal groove
~ on the diaphragmatic surface corresponding to the interventricular septum and containing the posterior interventricular branch. D

20 **Coronary (atrioventricular) groove.** Sulcus coronarius. It courses around the heart corresponding to the atrioventricular boundary. B C

21 **Right/left ventricle of heart.** Ventriculus [dexter/sinister] cordis. As a result of functional requirements, the left ventricular wall is thicker than the right. C

22 **Interventricular septum.** Septum interventriculare. Partition between the right and left ventricle recognizable externally by the anterior and posterior interventricular grooves.

23 Pars muscularis. Muscular part of interventricular septum, by far the largest and thickest part. C

24 Pars membranacea. Membranous part of interventricular septum. Located superiorly at the exit of the aorta, it is the shortest, thinnest and most fibrous part of the interventricular septum and arises from the endocardium. C

25 **Atrioventricular septum.** Septum atrioventriculare. Portion of the membranous part of the interventricular septum between the right atrium and left ventricle above the root of the septal cusp. C

26 **Right/left atrium of heart.** Atrium [dextrum/sinistrum] cordis. Thin-walled chambers. C

27 Auricle of atrium. Auricula atrialis. Finger-
~ like diverticulum of the right and left atrium. B C

28 **Interatrial septum.** Septum interatriale. Partition between the right and left atrium.

29 **Ostium atrioventriculare (dext. et sin.).** Atrioventricular opening (right/left) between the atrium and ventricle. D

30 **Ostium of pulmonary trunk.** Ostium trunci pulmonalis. Opening between the right ventricle and the pulmonary trunk. D

31 **Ostium of aorta.** Ostium aortae. Opening between the left ventricle and aorta. C D

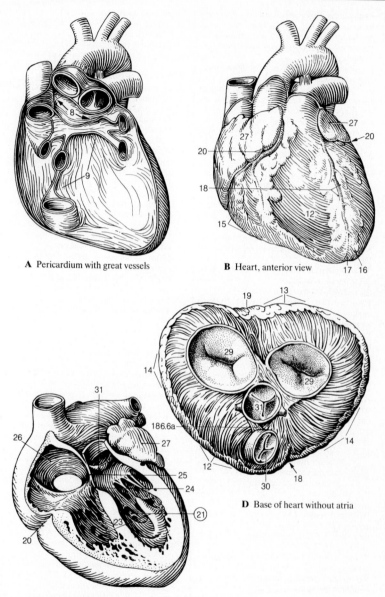

A Pericardium with great vessels

B Heart, anterior view

C Opened heart, left anterior view

D Base of heart without atria

1 **Trabeculae carneae.** Muscular cords projecting into the lumen of the heart. A

2 **Vortex of heart.** Vortex cordis. Whorled arrangement of the heart muscle cells at the apex of the heart. B

3 **Papillary muscles.** Musculi papillares. Cone-shaped muscles projecting into the lumen of the heart. They are connected to the valvular cusps via chordae tendineae and regulate the position of the cusps. A D

4 **Chordae tendineae.** Tendinous filaments between the papillary muscles and the atrioventricular valve. A D

5 **Right/left fibrous trigone.** Trigonum fibro-
~ sum dextrum/sinistrum. Connective tissue wedge between the aorta and the atrioventricular opening anteriorly and posteriorly. C

6 **Right/left fibrous ring.** Anulus fibrosus dex-
~ ter/sinister. Rings of connective tissue between the atria and ventricles giving rise to the atrioventricular valves. C

6 a **Tendon of infundibulum.** Tendo infundibuli. Vestige of the embryonic spiral septum. C, 185 D

7 **Myocardium.** Transversely striated heart musculature with intercalated discs including the impulse-conducting system. A D

7 a **Conducting system of heart.** Systema conducens cordis. D

8 **Sinu-atrial (SA) node.** Nodus sinu-atrialis [[Keith-Flack sinus node]]. Ribbon-like specialized cardiac muscle situated in front of the entrance of the superior vena cava. It represents the primary impulse formation center (pacemaker) which determines the rhythm of the heart. D

9 **Atrioventricular (AV) node.** Nodus atrioventricularis [[Node of Aschoff-Tawara]]. Small complex of specialized cardiac muscle fibers in the interatrial septum below the fossa ovalis and in front of the opening of the coronary sinus. After a latency period, the impulse transmitted to it myogenically from the SA node is conducted further into the ventricle via the bundle of His and its crura. In case of failure of the SA node, the AV node can take over the control of heart rhythm as the secondary pacemaker. D

10 **Atrioventricular (AV) bundle.** Fasciculus atrioventricularis. Bundle of impulse-conducting fibers between the AV node and the papillary muscles. D

11 Trunk [[bundle of His]]. [[Truncus]] [[His' bundle]]. Initial segment of the AV bundle up to the division into a right and left crus at the membranous part of the septum. D

12 *Crus (dextrum/sinistrum).* Right/left crus of the impulse-conducting system passing right and left, respectively, into the interventricular septum as far as the papillary muscles into which each then ramifies. D

12 a **Subendocardial rami.** Rami subendocardiales. Superficial branchings of the impulse-conducting system (Purkinje fibers). D

13 **Endocardium.** Internal serous lining of the heart containing simple squamous epithelium (endothelium).

14 **Right atrium.** Atrium dextrum. A D

15 **Pectinate muscles.** Mm. pectinati. Muscular bundles in the right atrium emanating from the terminal crest. They resemble the teeth of a comb. A

16 **Sulcus terminalis.** Terminal groove. Visible at the border between the embryonic sinus venosus and the atrium proper. It surrounds the opening regions of both venae cavae. D

17 **Terminal crest.** Crista terminalis. Curved muscular ridge in the interior of the right atrium at the border between the atrium proper and the embryonic sinus venosus. It corresponds to the course of the sulcus terminalis. A

18 **Sinus venarum cavarum.** Smooth-walled space for the blood from both venae cavae. It is bordered by the terminal crest. A

19 **Fossa ovalis.** Depression in the interatrial septum caused by the fetal foramen ovale. A

20 **Limbus fossae ovalis.** Slightly raised margin of the fossa ovalis. A

21 **[Foramen ovale].** Embryological opening in the interatrial septum that is present until birth.

22 **Right auricle.** Auricula dextra. Diverticulum of right atrium. A

23 **Opening of superior vena cava.** Ostium venae cavae superioris. A

24 **Opening of inferior vena cava.** Ostium venae cavae inferioris. A

25 **Intervenous tubercle.** Tuberculum intervenosum. Small elevation on the lateral wall of the right atrium between the openings of the venae cavae. A

26 **Valve of inferior vena cava.** Valvula venae cavae inferioris [[Valvula Eustachii]]. Semilunar fold at the opening of the inferior vena cava. During fetal life it directs the blood into the foramen ovale. A

27 **Valve of coronary sinus.** Valvula sinus coronarii [[Valvula Thebesii]]. Semilunar fold at the opening of the coronary sinus. A

27 a **Opening of the coronary sinus.** Ostium sinus coronarii. A

28 **Foramina venarum minimarum.** Numerous openings of small veins [Vv. Thebesii minimae] which convey blood from the tissues of the heart directly into the right atrium or other heart spaces. A

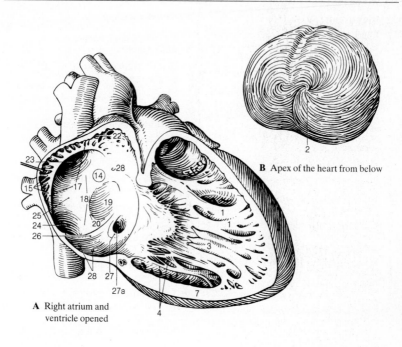

B Apex of the heart from below

A Right atrium and
ventricle opened

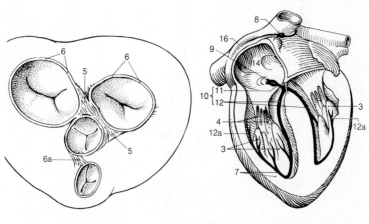

C Valves of the heart from above

D Internal conduction system of heart

1 **Right ventricle.** Ventriculus dexter. C

2 **Right atrioventricular opening.** Ostium atrioventriculare dextrum. Opening between the right atrium and the right ventricle. A

3 **Right atrioventricular (tricuspid) valve.** Valva atrioventricularis dextra (v. tricuspidalis). Valvular apparatus between the right atrium and right ventricle comprised of three parts which arise from the fibrous ring and, by means of the chordae tendineae, are attached to the papillary muscles of the right ventricle. A

4 Anterior cusp. Cuspis anterior. A C

5 Posterior cusp. Cuspis posterior. A

6 Septal cusp. Cuspis septalis. It arises from the septum. A

7 **Supraventricular crest.** Crista supraventricularis. Muscular ridge which separates the conus arteriosus from the rest of the ventricle. C

8 **Conus arteriosus [infundibulum].** Funnel-shaped, smooth-walled outflowing tract in front of the opening into the pulmonary trunk. It represents the embryonic bulbus cordis. C

9 **Opening of pulmonary trunk.** Ostium trunci pulmonalis. Beginning of the pulmonary trunk flanked by the pulmonary valve. A

10 **Valve of pulmonary trunk.** Valve trunci pul-
~ monalis. It is made up of three parts. A

11 Anterior semilunar cusp of pulmonary valve. Valvula semilunarsi anterior. A

12 Right semilunar cusp of pulmonary valve. Valvula semilunaris dextra. A

13 Left semilunar cusp of pulmonary valve. Valvula semilunaris sinistra. A

14 Nodules of semilunar cusps. Noduli valvularum semilunarium. Small thickening in the middle of each free margin of the semilunar cusps for sealing of the wedge-like space between the three cusps during closing. C

15 Lunules of semilunar cusps. Lunulae valvularum semilunarium. Thin, crescentic area on both side of the nodules at the margin of the cusps. C

16 Anterior papillary muscle. Musculus papillaris anterior. Large papillary muscle situated anteriorly. C

17 Posterior papillary muscle. Musculus papillaris posterior. C

18 Septal papillary muscles. [[Musculi papillares septales]]. Short papillary muscles sometimes present, arising from the interventricular septum. C

19 Septomarginal trabecula. Trabecula septomarginalis. Muscular bundle extending from the interventricular septum to the base of the anterior papillary muscle and containing the right crus of the bundle of His. C

20 **Left atrium.** Atrium sinistrum. B

21 **Left auricle.** Auricula sinistra. Hollow finger-like diverticulum of the left atrium to the left of the pulmonary trunk. B

21 a **Musculi pectinati.** Muscular trabeculae in the left atrium similar to the teeth of a comb.

22 **Valve of foramen ovale.** Valvula foraminis ovalis [Falx septi]. Floor of the fossa ovalis derived from the septum primum. In the fetus it is pushed into the left atrium by the flow of blood. B

23 **Ostia venarum pulmonalium.** Openings of pulmonary veins into the left atrium. B

24 **Left ventricle.** Ventriculus sinister. B

25 **Ostium atrioventriculare sinistrum.** Left atrioventicular opening. Opening between the left atrium and left ventricle. A

26 **Left atrioventricular (mitral) valve.** Valva atrioventricularis sinistra (V. mitralis) [[Valvula bicuspidalis]]. Valvular apparatus between the left atrium and left ventricle. It consists of two parts which arise from the fibrous ring and are united with the papillary muscles of the left ventricle by means of chordae tendineae. A

27 Anterior cusp. Cuspis anterior. Cusp situated anterior to the interventricular septum. A B

28 Posterior cusp. Cuspis posterior. Cusp situated posterior to the lateral wall. A B

28 a *Cuspides commissurales.* Annot. p. 409

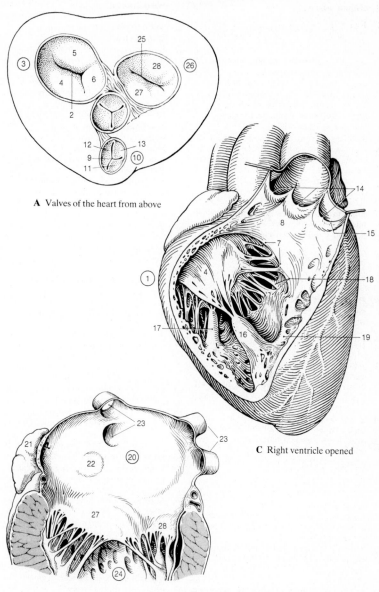

A Valves of the heart from above

C Right ventricle opened

B Left atrium opened

1   **Ostium aortae.** Opening of left ventricle
~   leading into the aorta. A

1 a **Trabeculae carneae.** Muscle bundles projecting into the lumen of the heart. A

2   **Aortic valve.** Valva aortae. Tripartite valvular
~   apparatus lying at the beginning of the aorta. A

3   Posterior semilunar cusp of aortic valve. Valvula semilunaris posterior. A

4   Right semilunar cusp of aortic valve. Valvula semilunaris dextra. A

5   Left semilunar cusp of aortic valve. Valvula semilunaris sinistra. A

6   Nodules of semilunar cusps. Noduli valvularum semilunarium. Thickening in the middle of each free margin of a semilunar cusp for sealing the wedge-shaped space between the three cusps during closing. A

7   Lunules of semilunar cusps. Lunulae valvularum semilunarium. Thin, crescentic area at the margin of a semilunar cusp on both sides of their nodules. A

8   **Anterior papillary muscle.** Musculus papillaris anterior. A

9   Posterior papillary muscle. Musculus papillaris posterior. A

10 ARTERIES. ARTERIA. Blood vessels which transport blood away from the heart.

11 PULMONARY TRUNK. TRUNCUS PULMONALIS. Arterial trunk between the right ventricle and the beginning of the left and right pulmonary artery. B

12 **Sinuses of pulmonary trunk.** Sinus trunci pulmonalis. Three dilatations of the wall of the pulmonary trunk, each at the root of a semilunar valve. B

13 **Bifurcation of pulmonary trunk.** Bifurcatio trunci pulmonalis. Division of the pulmonary trunk into its two branches. B

14 **Right pulmonary artery.** A. pulmonalis dextra. It lies behind the ascending aorta. B

14 a **Branches to superior lobe.** Rami lobi superioris.

15 Apical branch. Ramus apicalis. Branch to the apical segment. B

16 Posterior descending branch. Ramus posterior descendens. Branch to the lower part of the posterior segment. B

17 Anterior descending branch. Ramus anterior descendens. Branch to the lower part of the anterior segment. B

18 Anterior ascending branch. Ramus anterior ascendens. Branch to the upper part of the anterior segment. B

19 Posterior ascending branch. Ramus posterior ascendens. Branch to the upper part of the posterior segment. B

20 **Main branches for middle lobe.** Rami lobi medii. B

21 *Lateral branch.* Ramus lateralis. Branch to the lateral segment. B

22 *Branch to medial segment.* Ramus medialis. B

22 a **Branches to inferior lobe.** Rami lobi inferioris.

23 *Superior (apical) branch to inferior lobe.* Ramus superior (apicalis) lobi inferioris. Branch to superior (apical) segment of right lower lobe. B

24 **Basal part.** Pars basalis. Branches for basal segments of lower lobe. B

25 Medial [cardiac] basal branch. Ramus basalis medialis [[cardiacus]]. Branch to medial basal segment. B

26 Anterior basal branch. Ramus basalis anterior. Branch to anterior basal segment. B

27 Lateral basal branch. Ramus basalis lateralis. Branch to lateral basal segment. B

28 Posterior basal branch. Ramus basalis posterior. Branch to posterior basal segment. B

29 **Left pulmonary artery.** A. pulmonalis sinistra. B

29 a Branches to upper lobe. Rami lobi superioris.

30 Apical branch. Ramus apicalis. Branch to upper part of apicoposterior segment. B

31 Anterior descending branch. Ramus anterior descendens. Branch to lower part of anterior segment. B

32 Posterior branch. Ramus posterior. Branch to lower part of apicoposterior segment. B

33 Anterior ascending branch. Ramus anterior ascendens. Branch to upper part of anterior segment. B

34 Lingular branch. Ramus lingularis. Branch for the two lingular segments. B

35 *Upper lingular branch.* Ramus lingularis superior. Branch to superior lingular segment. B

36 *Lower lingular branch.* Ramus lingularis inferior. Branch to inferior lingular segment. B

36 a **Lower lobe branches.** Rami lobi inferioris.

37 Upper branch to lower lobe. Ramus superior lobi inferioris. Branch to apical (superior) segment of left lower lobe. B

38 **Basal part.** Pars basalis. Branches to basal part of left lower lobe. B

39 Medial basal branch. Ramus basalis medialis. Branch to medial basal segment. B

40 Anterior basal branch. Ramus basalis anterior. Branch to anterior basal segment. B

41 Lateral basal branch. Ramus basalis lateralis. Branch to lateral basal segment. B

42 Posterior basal branch. Ramus basalis posterior. Branch to posterior basal segment. B

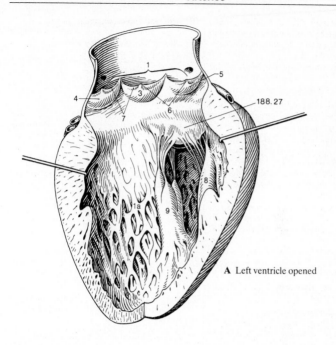

A Left ventricle opened

188.27

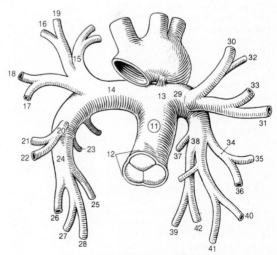

B Pulmonary arteries [6; 43; 81]

1 **Ductus arteriosus** [[*Botalli*]]. Short arterial duct in the fetus between the division of the pulmonary trunk and the arch of the aorta. It is patent until birth. A

2 **Ligamentum arteriosum.** Connective-tissue remains of the ductus arteriosus. B

3 **AORTA.** Principal artery of the body. B

4 ASCENDING AORTA. PARS ASCENDENS
~ AORTAE. Proximal ascending part of the aorta up to the loss of its pericardium. B

5 **Bulb of aorta.** Bulbus aortae. Bulbous enlargement of the aorta caused by the aortic sinus. It lies distal to the root of the aorta. C

6 **Aortic sinus.** Sinus aortae. Dilatation of the aortic lumen at the level of each of the three aortic valvular cusps. C

7 **Right coronary artery.** A. coronaria dextra. It arises in the region of the right aortic sinus and courses in the right coronary groove. C D

7a **Atrioventricular branches.** Rami atrioventriculares. Occupying the atrioventricular groove, they also supply the AV node. D

8 **Branch to conus arteriosus.** Ramus coni arteriosi. Inferior branch. C

9 **Branch to sinuatrial node.** Ramus nodi sinuatrialis. Most frequent branch (55%) to a vascular plexus at the entrance of the superior vena cava and then to the SA node. C

9a **Atrial branches.** Rami atriales. Branches to right atrium. C

10 **Right marginal branch.** Ramus marginalis dexter. Inferior branch to outer margin of the right ventricle. C D

11 **Intermediate atrial branch.** Ramus atrialis intermedius. Superior branch on posterior side of right atrium. D

12 **Posterior interventricular branch.** Ramus interventricularis posterior. Terminal branch of right coronary artery lying in posterior interventricular groove. D

13 Septal interventricular branches. Rami interventriculares septales. Branches in interventricular septum. D

14 Branch to atrioventricular node. Ramus nodi atrioventricularis. Branch at beginning of interventricular branch to AV node. D

15 Right posterolateral branch. [Ramus posterolateralis dexter]. Occasional branch at posterior wall of left ventricle. D

16 **Left coronary artery.** A. coronaria sinistra. Short artery arising in region of left aortic sinus. C

17 **Anterior interventricular branch.** Ramus interventricularis anterior. Branch coursing in anterior interventricular groove. C

18 Branch to conus arteriosus. Ramus coni arteriosi. Right branch. C

19 Lateral branch. Ramus lateralis. Left branch at anterior wall of left ventricle. C

20 Septal interventricular branches. Rami interventriculares septales. Perforating branches for anterior $\frac{2}{3}$ of interventricular septum. C

21 **Circumflex branch.** Ramus circumflexus. Branch coursing in left coronary groove as a continuation of left coronary artery. C D

22 Anastomotic atrial branch. Ramus atrialis anastomoticus. It passes from left atrium to right atrium via interatrial septum and anastomoses directly with right coronary artery or indirectly with one of its branches. C

22a **Atrioventricular branches.** Rami atrioventriculares. Distal portion of circumflex branch in atrioventricular groove. D

23 Left marginal branch. Ramus marginalis sinister. Branch at outer margin of left ventricle. C

24 Intermediate atrial branch. Ramus atrialis intermedius. Atrial branch on posterior side. D

25 Left posterior ventricular branch. Ramus posterior ventriculi sinistri. Occasional branch at posterior side of left ventricle. D

26 Sinuatrial node branch. [Ramus nodi sinuatrialis]. Frequent branch (45%) from beginning of left coronary artery to SA node. C

27 Atrioventricular node branch. [Ramus nodi atrioventricularis]. Occasional branch for AV node. D

27a **Atrial branches.** Rami atriales. Branches to left atrium.

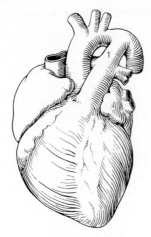

A Fetal heart

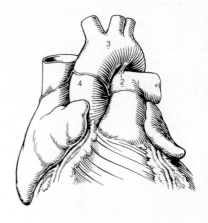

B Aorta and pulmonary trunk,
anterior view

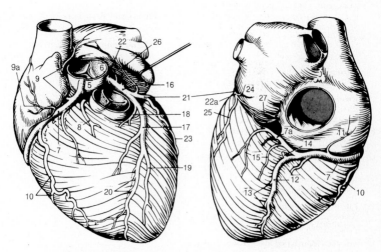

C Cardiovascular system,[62]
anterior view

D Cardiovascular system,[62]
posterior view

1 ARCH OF AORTA. ARCUS AORTAE. Part of aorta situated between ascending and descending aortae. A

2 **Isthmus aortae.** Narrowing of aorta between left subclavian artery and ligamentum arteriosum. A

3 **Para-aortic bodies.** Corpora para-aortica. Irregular islands of chromaffin tissue scattered beside the aorta.

4 **Brachiocephalic trunk.** Truncus brachiocephalicus. First branch of arch of aorta. It divides into subclavian and right common carotid arteries. A

5 **(A. thyroidea ima).** Inconstant (10%) unpaired artery for thyroid gland arising from the brachiocephalic trunk or directly from the aorta. A

6 **Common carotid artery.** A. carotis communis. Devoid of branches, it runs on each side of trachea and larynx below the sternocleidomastoid muscle. A

7 **Carotid body.** Glomus caroticum. Chemoreceptor at the bifurcation of the common carotid. It contains capillary tufts, epithelioid cells and abundant nerve endings. It responds predominantly to the oxygen content of the blood, less strongly to carbon dioxide changes. A

8 **Carotid sinus.** Sinus caroticus. Slight dilatation at the division of the common carotid. It contains baroreceptors. A

8a **Carotid bifurcation.** Bifurcatio carotica. Site of division of the common carotid artery. A

9 **External carotid artery.** A. carotis externa. It extends from the bifurcation of the carotid to its terminal division into the superficial temporal and maxillary arteries at the neck of the mandible. A

10 **Superior thyroid artery.** A. thyroidea superior. First branch of external carotid artery. It supplies, among others, parts of the larynx and thyroid gland. A

11 **Infrahyoid branch.** Ramus infrahyoideus. It courses on the hyoid bone and anastomoses with the branch of the opposite side. A

12 **Sternocleidomastoid branch.** Ramus sternocleidomastoideus. It supplies this muscle. A

13 **Superior laryngeal artery.** A. laryngea superior. It penetrates the thyrohyoid membrane and lies beneath the mucosa of the piriform recess. A

14 **Cricothyroid branch.** Ramus cricothyroideus. Branch for the cricothyroid muscle and the interior of the larynx. It anastomoses with the branch of the opposite side. A

15 **Anterior glandular branch.** Ramus glandularis anterior. It supplies mainly the anterior portion of the thyroid gland. A

16 **Posterior glandular branch.** Ramus glandularis posterior. It supplies mainly the upper portion of the thyroid gland and to a lesser degree the posterior portion also. A

16a **Lateral glandular branch.** Ramus glandularis lateralis. It supplies mainly the lateral portion of the thyroid gland. A

17 **Ascending pharyngeal artery.** A. pharyngea ascendens. It arises from the postero-inferior aspect of the external carotid artery and passes between the pharynx and the musculature of the styloid process up to the base of the skull. A

18 **Posterior meningeal artery.** A. meningea posterior. It lies first of all lateral to the internal carotid artery, then passes through the jugular foramen and supplies the dura of the posterior cranial fossa. A

19 **Pharyngeal branches.** Rami pharyngeales. Branches for the wall of the pharynx. A

20 **Inferior tympanic artery.** A. tympanica inferior. It reaches the tympanic cavity through the tympanic canaliculus. A

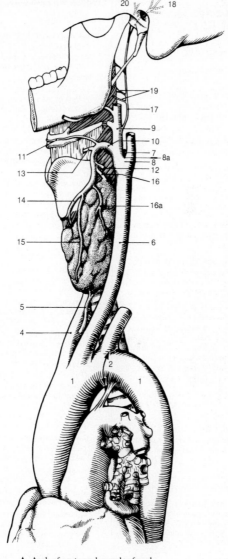

A Arch of aorta and vessels of neck

1 **Lingual artery.** A. lingualis. Second anterior branch of external carotid artery. Covered by the hyoglossus muscle, it passes laterally into the tongue. A B C

2 **Suprahyoid branch of lingual artery.** Ramus suprahyoideus. It anastomoses at the hyoid bone with the infrahyoid branch and the branch from the opposite side. B

3 **Sublingual artery.** A. sublingualis. Arising at the anterior margin of the hyoglossus, it passes between the mylohyoid and the sublingual gland up to the gingiva. B

4 **Rami dorsales linguae.** Dorsal lingual branches of lingual artery for base of the tongue. B

5 **Deep lingual artery.** A. profunda linguae. As the main branch of the lingual artery, it passes between the genioglossus and inferior longitudinal muscles of the tongue to the apex of the tongue and anastomoses with the artery of the opposite side. B

6 **Linguofacial trunk.** [Truncus linguofacialis]. Occasionally present common trunk of lingual and facial arteries. A

7 **Facial artery.** A. facialis. Third anterior branch of external carotid artery. It runs below the styloyoid muscle, first upward, then laterad, and crosses the mandible at the anterior margin of the masseter. A B C

8 **Ascending palatine artery.** A. palatina ascendens. Arising from the proximal portion of the facial artery, it passes medial to the styloglossus muscle at the lateral wall of the pharynx to supply the palatal arches and adjacent musculature, often also the tonsils from above. It and the ascending pharyngeal artery can be reciprocally replaced. C

9 **Tonsillar branch.** Ramus tonsillaris. Branch frequently arising from the ascending palatine artery and supplying the palatine tonsils. C

10 **Submental artery.** A. submentalis. It lies caudal to the mylohyoid muscle and supplies mainly this muscle and the submandibular gland. It anastomoses with the sublingual artery. C

11 **Glandular branches.** Rami glandulares. Direct branches for the submandibular gland. C

12 **Inferior labial artery.** A. labialis inferior. Artery for the lower lip between the musculature and the mucosa. It anastomoses with the submental and mental arteries as well as the artery of the opposite side. C

13 **Superior labial artery.** A. labialis superior. Artery for the upper lip between the musculature and mucosa. It anastomoses with the transverse facial and infra-orbital arteries as well as the artery of the opposite side. C

13 a **Nasal septum branch.** Ramus septi nasi. Branch to cavernous body of septum (Kiesselbach's area). C

13 b **Lateral nasal branch.** Ramus lateralis nasi. Branch to base of the nasal ala. C

14 **Angular artery.** A. angularis. Terminal branch of facial artery. It anastomoses with the ophthalmic artery. C

15 **Occipital artery.** A. occipitalis. Second dorsal branch of external carotid artery. It passes medial to the mastoid process at the occiput and anastomoses with the superficial temporal, vertebral, deep cervical and posterior auricular arteries. C D

16 **Mastoid branch of occipital artery.** Ramus mastoideus. It passes through the mastoid foramen to the diploë and dura. It also supplies mastoid cells. C

17 **Auricular branch of occipital artery.** Ramus auricularis. It passes beneath the sternocleidomastoid obliquely behind the pinna. C

18 **Sternocleidomastoid branch.** Ramus sternocleidomastoidei. Small branches for the muscle. C

19 **Meningeal branch.** [Ramus meningeus]. Artery occasionally present passing through the parietal foramen to the dura. C

20 **Occipital branches.** Rami occipitales. Usually very tortuous, they penetrate the trapezius and supply the occiput. C

21 **Descending branch of occipital artery.** Ramus descendens. It passes beneath the splenius capitis to supply the musculature situated there. C

22 **Posterior auricular artery.** A. auricularis posterior. Third dorsal branch of external carotid artery. It lies under the parotid gland on the styloid process between the mastoid process and the ear. C D

23 **Stylomastoid artery.** A. stylomastoidea. Slender companion artery of facial nerve. It courses with it through the stylomastoid foramen to the hiatus of the canal for the greater petrosal nerve, and then into the middle and inner ear. D

24 **Posterior tympanic artery.** A. tympanica posterior. It passes with the chorda tympani from the facial canal to the tympanic membrane. D

25 **Mastoid branches.** Rami mastoidei. Branches of posterior tympanic artery to mastoid air cells. D

26 **Stapedial branch.** [Ramus stapedialis]. Slender branch for the stapedial muscle.
~

27 **Auricular branch.** Ramus auricularis. It supplies the posterior side of the pinna with perforating branches as well as the anterior side and the small auricular muscles. D

28 **Occipital branch.** Ramus occipitalis. Branch courses above the mastoid process and anastomoses with the occipital artery. D

28 a **Parotid branch.** Ramus parotideus. It supplies the parotid gland. D

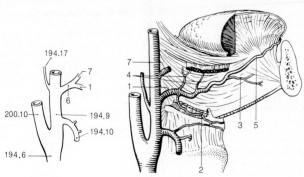

A Linguofacial trunk

B Branches of external carotid artery

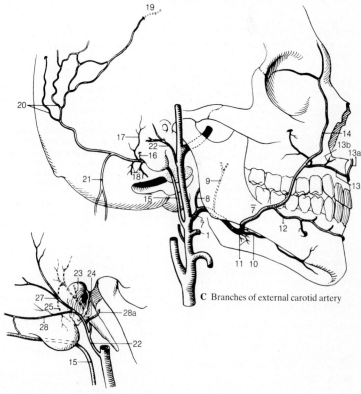

C Branches of external carotid artery

D Branches of external carotid artery

1 **Superficial temporal artery.** A. temporalis superficialis. One of two terminal branches of the external carotid artery. It ascends upward in front of the pinna in company with the auriculotemporal nerve. A B

2 **Parotid branch.** Ramus parotideus. It supplies the parotid gland. A

3 **Transverse facial artery.** A. transversa faciei (facialis). Under cover of the parotid gland, it passes below the zygomatic arch to the cheek. A

4 **Anterior auricular branches.** Rami auriculares anteriores. Several small branches to the pinna and the external acoustic meatus. A

5 **Zygomatico-orbital artery.** A. zygomatico-orbitalis. It passes above the zygomatic arch to the lateral margin of the orbit. A

6 **Middle temporal artery.** A. temporalis media. It passes above the zygomatic arch beneath the temporalis muscle. A

7 **Frontal branch.** Ramus frontalis. Anterior branch of superficial temporal artery. It anastomoses with its fellow of the opposite side as well as with the supra-orbital and supratrochlear arteries from the internal carotid. A

8 **Parietal branch.** Ramus parietalis. Posterior branch of superficial temporal artery. It anastomoses with its fellow of the opposite side as well as with the posterior auricular and occipital arteries. A

9 **Maxillary artery.** A. maxillaris. Larger terminal branch of external carotid artery. It arises beneath the temporomandibular joint, passes lateral or medial to the lateral pterygoid muscle and ramifies in the pterygopalatine fossa. A B

10 **Deep auricular artery.** A. auricularis profunda. It passes backward and upward to the temporomandibular joint, external acoustic meatus and tympanic membrane. B

11 **Anterior tympanic artery.** A. tympanica anterior. In company with the chorda tympani, it passes through the petrotympanic fissure into the tympanic cavity. B

12 **Inferior alveolar artery.** A. alveolaris inferior. It passes between the medial pterygoid muscle and mandibular ramus into the mandibular canal up to the mental foramen. B

13 Dental rami. Rami dentales. Branches to roots of the teeth. B

13 a **Peridental branches.** Rami peridentales.

14 Mylohyoid branch. Ramus mylohyoideus. Exiting in front of the mandibular canal, it accompanies the mylohyoid nerve in the same-named groove and runs anteriorly beneath the mylohyoid muscle. It anastomoses with the submental artery. B

15 Mental branch. Ramus mentalis. Terminal branch of inferior alveolar artery. It supplies the chin. B

16 **Middle meningeal artery.** A. meningea media. It passes medial to the lateral pterygoid muscle and through the foramen spinosum into the middle cranial fossa where it ramifies into its branches. B C

17 Accessory ramus. Ramus accessorius. Accessory branch from the middle meningeal artery or from the maxillary artery to the adjacent muscles, the auditory tube and through the foramen ovale to the dura up to the trigeminal (semilunar) ganglion. B

18 Petrosal branch. Ramus petrosus. It arises as a small branch directly after the entrance of the middle meningeal artery into the cranial cavity and anastomoses with the stylomastoid artery by means of the hiatus of the canal for the greater petrosal nerve. C

19 Superior tympanic artery. A. tympanica superior. It arises close to the petrosal branch and passes into the tympanic cavity with the lesser petrosal nerve. C

20 Frontal branch. Ramus frontalis. Anterior, large terminal branch in the cranium. It lies in a bony groove often closed into a canal. C

21 Parietal branch. Ramus parietalis. Terminal branch passing to the posterior half of the cranium. C

22 Orbital branch. Ramus orbitalis. It runs through the superior orbital fissure in the direction of the lacrimal gland. C

23 Anastomotic branch between the orbital branch and the lacrimal artery. Ramus anastomoticus [[cum a. lacrimalis]]. C

23 a **Pterygomeningeal artery.** A. pterygomeningea. Artery for the pterygoid muscles, the tensor veli palatini, and the auditory tube; it comes out of the maxillary and middle meningeal arteries and passes through the foramen ovale to the semilunar ganglion and the dura mater.

24 **Masseteric artery.** A. masseterica. Artery for the masseter muscle passing laterally through the mandibular notch. B

25 **Anterior deep temporal artery.** A. temporalis profunda anterior. Artery passing upwards into the temporalis muscle. B

25 a **Posterior temporal artery.** A. temporalis posterior. Annot. p. 409

26 **Pterygoid branches.** Rami pterygoidei. Branches for the pterygoid muscles. B

27 **Buccal artery.** A. buccalis. Artery passing downward and forward on the buccinator muscle for the cheek and gingiva. B

28 **Posterior superior alveolar artery.** A. alveolaris superior posterior. It passes posteriorly into the maxilla and the maxillary sinus and supplies the upper molar teeth and their gingiva. B

29 **Dental branches.** Rami dentales. They supply the maxillary molars. B

29 a **Peridental branches.** Rami peridentales.

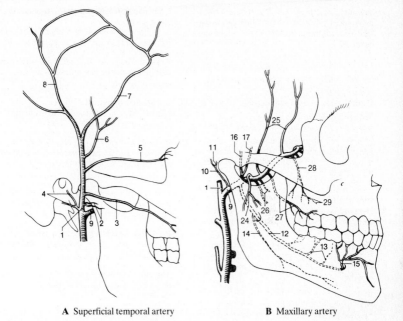

A Superficial temporal artery   **B** Maxillary artery

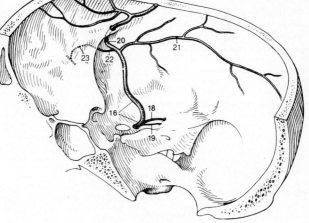

C Middle meningeal artery

1   **Infraorbital artery.** A. infraorbitalis. Terminal branch of maxillary artery. It passes to the face via the inferior orbital fissure, groove and canal. A

2   Anterior superior alveolar arteries. Aa. alveolares superiores anteriores. They leave the infraorbital artery in the infraorbital canal and pass through bone to the anterior teeth. A

3   Dental branches. Rami dentales. Terminal branches passing to the teeth. A

3 a Peridental branches. Rami peridentales.

4   **Artery of pterygoid canal.** A. canalis pterygoidei. It passes through the pterygoid canal posteriorly to the auditory tube and its environs. A B

4 a Pharyngeal branch. Ramus pharyngeus. Branch to the pharyngeal mucosa.

5   **Descending palatine artery.** A. palatina descendens. It descends through the greater palatine canal. A B

6   Greater palatine artery. A. palatina major. It passes through the greater palatine foramen to the anterior palate and the neighboring gingiva. B

7   Lesser palatine arteries. Aa. palatinae minores. They leave the greater palatine artery when in its canal and pass through the lesser palatine foramina to the soft palate. B

7 a **Pharyngeal branch.** Ramus pharyngeus. Branch to the pharyngeal mucosa up to the level of the tonsil and gingiva.

8   **Sphenopalatine artery.** A. sphenopalatina. It passes through the sphenopalatine foramen into the nasal cavity. B

9   **Lateral posterior nasal branches.** Aa. nasales posteriores laterales. As the terminal branches of the sphenopalatine artery, they supply the nasal cavity laterally and posteriorly. B

9 a **Posterior septal branches.** Rami septales posteriores. Branches of the sphenopalatine artery to the postero-inferior part of the nasal septum. B

10   **Internal carotid artery.** Arteria carotis interna. It extends branchless from the bifurcation of the common carotid to the base of the skull where it goes through the carotid canal to its terminal division into the anterior and middle cerebral arteries. B C

11   Cervical part of internal carotid artery. Pars cervicalis. Branchless segment up to its entrance into the carotid canal in the petrous tempo-ral bone. B C

12   **Carotid sinus.** Sinus caroticus. It is occasionally displaced from the end of the common carotid artery (194.8) to the beginning of the internal carotid. Site of baroreceptors. B

13   Petrous part of internal carotid artery. Pars petrosa. Segment coursing in the carotid canal of the petrous temporal. C

14   **Caroticotympanic arteries.** Aa. caroticotym-
~   panicae. Slender arteries passing from the carotid canal to the tympanic cavity. C

15   **Pterygoid branch.** Ramus pterygoideus. Companion artery of the nerve of the pterygoid canal in the lateral wall of the sphenoid sinus. C

16   Cavernous part of internal carotid. Pars cavernosa. Segment in the cavernous sinus up to the vicinity of the optic canal. C

17   **Basal tentorial branch.** Ramus basalis tentorii. Branch to tentorium passing over the petrosal ridge. C

18   **Marginal tentorial branch.** Ramus marginalis tentorii. Branch located near the tentorial notch. C

19   **Meningeal branch.** Ramus meningeus. Branch to dura of the middle cranial fossa. C

20   **Branch to trigeminal ganglion.** Ramus ganglionis trigeminalis. C

21   **Nerve branches.** Rami nervorum.

22   **Cavernous sinus branch.** Ramus sinus cavernosi. Branch in the region of the cavernous sinus. C

23   **Inferior hypophysial artery.** A. hypophysialis inferior. It supplies the posterior lobe of the hypophysis. C

24   Cerebral part of internal carotid artery. Pars cerebralis. As the terminal intradural segment, it reaches from the exit of the ophthalmic artery at the last bend of the carotid up to the terminal branching into the anterior and middle cerebral arteries. C

25   **Superior hypophsial artery.** A. hypophysialis superior. It supplies the hypophysial stalk, infundibulum and part of the lower hypothalamus. C

26   **Clival branch.** Ramus clivi. Branch to clivus. C

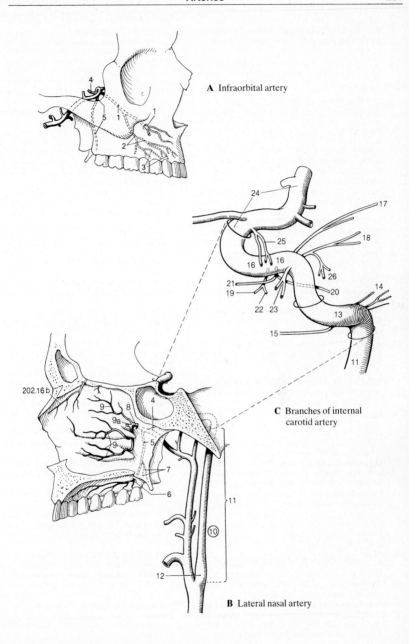

A Infraorbital artery

C Branches of internal carotid artery

B Lateral nasal artery

202.16 b

1 **Ophthalmic artery.** A. ophthalmica. It passes from the anterior convex arch of the internal carotid artery through the optic canal into the orbit with the optic nerve. A

2 **Central retinal artery.** A. centralis retinae. It passes into the optic nerve from below about 1 mm behind the eyeball and is distributed to the internal layers of the retina. A

3 **Lacrimal artery.** A. lacrimalis. Exits lateral to the ophthalmic artery and passes to the lacrimal gland along the upper margin of the lateral rectus muscle. A

4 Anastomotic branch [with the middle meningeal artery].Ramus anastomoticus[cum A. meningea media]. Branch to the orbital branch of the middle meningeal artery. On occasion it can replace the ophthalmic artery. A

5 Lateral palpebral arteries. Aa. palpebrales laterales. They arise from the lacrimal artery and pass laterally to the eyelids. A B

5a Recurrent meningeal branch. Ramus meningeus recurrens. Branch of the lacrimal artery that runs through the superior orbital fissure into the cranial cavity. It anastomoses with the anastomotic branch.

6 **Short posterior ciliary arteries.** Aa. ciliares posteriores breves. 10–15 arteries which penetrate the sclera circumferentially around the optic nerve and supply the choroid. A

7 **Long posterior ciliary arteries.** Aa. ciliares posteriores longae. Lateral and medial artery which pass between the sclera and choroid to the ciliary body. A B

8 **Muscular arteries.** Branches to the eye muscles.

9 Anterior ciliary arteries. Aa. ciliares anteriores. Taking origin from the lacrimal artery or muscle branches, they penetrate the sclera and supply the choroid and ciliary body. A B

10 **Anterior conjunctival arteries.** Aa. conjunctivales anteriores. Branches arising from the anterior ciliary arteries and supplying the conjunctivae. B

11 **Posterior conjunctival arteries.** Aa. conjunctivales posteriores. They arise from the lacrimal and supraorbital arteries. A

12 **Episcleral arteries.** Aa. episclerales. Branchlets of the anterior ciliary arteries situated on the sclera. B

13 **Supraorbital artery.** A. supraorbitalis [[A. frontalis lat.]]. It passes below the roof of the orbit and through the supraorbital notch to the forehead. A B

13a **Diploic branch.** Ramus diploicus. Branch to bone.

14 **Posterior ethmoidal artery.** A. ethmoidalis posterior. It passes below the superior oblique muscle and through the posterior ethmoidal foramen to the posterior ethmoidal air cells and the posterior part of the nasal cavity. A

15 **Anterior ethmoidal artery.** A. ethmoidalis anterior. It passes upward through the anterior ethmoidal foramen into the anterior cranial fossa then through the cribriform plate into the nasal cavity and frontal sinus as well as the anterior ethmoidal cells. A

16 **Anterior meningeal branch.** Ramus meningeus anterior. Branch from the part of the anterior ethmoidal artery lying in the cranial fossa. It supplies the dura. A

16a **Anterior septal branches.** Rami septales anteriores.

Branches from the anterior ethmoidal artery to the upper portion of the nasal septum.

16b **Lateral anterior nasal branches.** Rami nasales anteriores laterales. Branches of the anterior ethmoidal artery to the upper lateral wall of the nasal septum and the anterior upper ethmoidal air cells. See 201 B

17 **Medial palpebral arteries.** Aa. palpebrales mediales. An artery for each eyelid, upper and lower. Arising from the ophthalmic artery, they anastomose with the lateral palpebral artery via the superior and inferior palpebral arches. A B

18 **Superior palpebral arch.** Arcus palpebralis superior. Connection between the medial and lateral palpebral arteries superiorly on the tarsal plate. B

19 **Inferior palpebral arch.** Arcus palpebralis inferior. Connection between the medial and lateral palpebral arteries inferiorly on the tarsal plate. B

20 **Supratrochlear artery.** A. supratrochlearis [[A. frontalis med.]]. Terminal branch of the ophthalmic artery which passes through the frontal notch to the forehead. Anastomoses: Artery of the opposite side, supra-orbital and superficial temporal arteries. A B

21 **Dorsal nasal artery.** A. dorsalis nasi (A. nasi externa). It penetrates the orbicularis oculi and passes downward to the bridge of the nose. Anastomosis: Facial artery. A B

~

22 **Anterior choroidal artery.** Arteria choroidea anterior. Usually arising from the internal carotid artery, it follows the optic tract and enters the choroid plexus of the inferior horn of the lateral ventricle, where it occasionally passes up to the interventricular foramen. C D

23 **Choroidal branches of lateral ventricle.** Rami choroidei ventriculi lateralis. It supplies the choroid plexus of the lateral ventricle. C D

24 **Choroidal branches of third ventricle.** Rami choroidei ventriculi tertii. It supplies the choroid plexus of the third ventricle. C

25 **Branches of anterior perforated substance.** Rami substantiae perforatae anterioris. Branches to the internal capsule. D

26 **Branches of optic tract.** Rami tractus optici. D

27 **Branches of lateral geniculate body.** Rami corporis geniculati lateralis. D

28 **Branches of internal capsule.** Rami capsulae internae. Branches to the posterior part of the internal capsule.

29 **Branches of globus pallidus.** Rami globi pallidi. They come from below.

30 **Branches of tail of caudate nucleus.** Rami caudae nuclei caudati. They come from below.

31 **Branches of tuber cinereum.** Rami tuberis cinerei. D

32 **Branches of hypothalamic nuclei.** Rami nucleorum hypothalamicorum. They come from below.

33 **Branches of substantia nigra.** Rami substantiae nigrae. They pass through the crus cerebri. D

34 **Branches of red nucleus.** Rami nuclei rubri. They pass through the crus cerebri. D

35 **Branches of amygdaloid body.** Rami corporis amygdaloidei. Branches for the medial amygdaloid nucleus. C

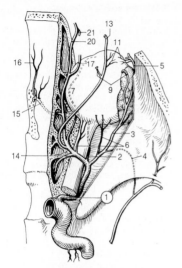

A Ophthalmic artery

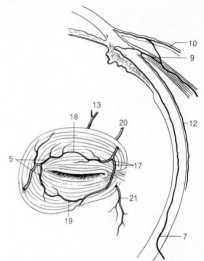

B Facial branches of ophthalmic artery

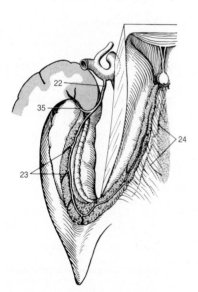

C Anterior choroidal artery from above

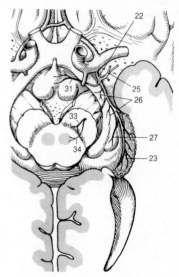

D Anterior choroidal artery from below

1 **Anterior cerebral artery.** A. cerebri anterior. One of the two terminal arteries of the internal carotid. It runs posteriorly above the corpus callosum and supplies the greatest part of the medial surface of the cerebrum. A

2 **Precommunical part.** Pars precommunicalis. Portion of the anterior cerebral artery proximal to the anterior communicating branch. A

3 **Anteromedial central arteries (anteromedial thalamostriate arteries).** Aa. centrales anteromediales (Aa. thalamostriatae anteromediales). Branches arising from the anterior cerebral arteries and passing into the thalamus and corpus striatum from below. A

4 **Short central artery.** A. centralis brevis. Short branch of anterior cerebral artery passing into the cerebrum. A

5 **Long central artery (recurrent artery).** A. centralis longa (A. recurrens) [[Heubner]]. Retrograde branch parallel to the anterior cerebral artery. It penetrates the anterior perforated substance and supplies the middle and lateral parts of the lentiform nucleus, the head of the caudate nucleus and the anterior limb of the internal capsule. A

6 **Anterior communicating artery.** A. communicans anterior. Unpaired connection between the right and left anterior cerebral arteries. A

7 Anteromedial central branches. Rami
~ centrales anteromediales penetrating uniformly into the cerebral substance. A

8 **Postcommunical part of anterior cerebral artery.** Pars postcommunicalis (R. pericallosa). It is the part which is distal to the anterior communicating artery. B

9 **Medial frontobasal artery (medial orbitofrontalis branch).** A. frontobasalis medialis (r. orbitofrontalis medialis). Branch to the lower surface of the frontal lobe. B

10 **Callosomarginal artery.** A. callosomarginalis. Segment running in the sulcus of the corpus callosum. B

11 Anteromedial frontal branch. Ramus frontalis anteromedialis. Branch to lower half of the medial side of the frontal lobe. B

12 Mediomedial frontal branch. Ramus frontalis mediomedialis. Branch to middle portion of the medial side of the frontal lobe. B

13 Posteromedial frontal branch. Ramus frontalis posteromedialis. Branch to posterior portion of the medial surface of the frontal lobe. B

14 Cingular branch. Ramus cingularis. Branch coursing in the cingulate sulcus. B

15 **Paracentral artery.** A. paracentralis. Branch for the field behind the central sulcus. B

16 **Precuneal artery.** A. precunealis. It supplies the region in front of the cuneus. B

17 **Parieto-occipital artery.** A. parieto-occipitalis. Branch in the parieto-occipital sulcus. B

18 **Middle cerebral artery.** A. cerebri media. Second terminal branch of internal carotid artery. It passes in the lateral sulcus between the frontal and temporal lobes and supplies the greatest part of the lateral cerebral surface. A

19 **Sphenoidal part.** Pars sphenoidalis. First part of the middle cerebral artery. It takes a horizontal course somewhat parallel to the lesser wing of the sphenoid bone. A

20 **Anterolateral central arteries.** Aa. centrales anterolaterales (aa. thalamostriatae anterolaterales). They penetrate the anterior perforated substance.

21 Medial branches. Rami mediales. They pass through the lentiform nucleus to the caudate nucleus and internal capsule. A

22 Lateral branches. Rami laterales. They course laterally around the lentiform nucleus to the internal capsule and caudate nucleus. A

23 **Insular part.** Pars insularis. Portion of the middle cerebral artery located on the insula. D

24 **Insular arteries.** Aa. insulares. Branches for the insula. D

25 **Lateral frontobasal artery.** A. frontobasalis lateralis (ramus orbitofrontalis lateralis). Branch passing anterior to the lower and lateral side of the frontal lobe. C D

26 **Anterior temporal artery.** A. temporalis anterior. Anterior branch for the frontal end of the two upper temporal gyri. C D

27 **Middle temporal artery.** A. temporalis media. Branch supplying the middle portion of the temporal lobe. C D

28 **Posterior temporal artery.** A. temporalis posterior. Branch supplying the posterior portion of the temporal lobe. C D

29 **Terminal part.** Pars terminalis (pars corticalis). Terminal ramifications of the middle cerebral artery.

30 **Artery of central sulcus.** A. sulci centralis. C D

31 **Artery of precentral sulcus.** A. sulci precentralis. C D

32 **Artery of postcentral sulcus.** A. sulci postcentralis. C D

33 **Anterior and posterior parietal arteries.** Aa. parietales anterior et posterior. Branches to the parietal lobe. C D

34 **Artery of angular gyrus.** A. gyri angularis. C D

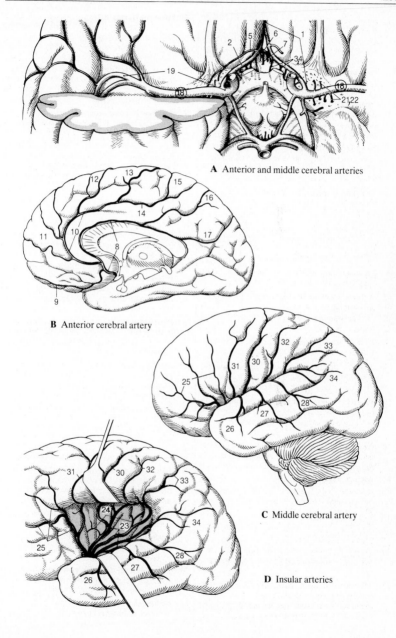

A Anterior and middle cerebral arteries

B Anterior cerebral artery

C Middle cerebral artery

D Insular arteries

1 **Subclavian artery.** Arteria subclavia. It runs between the scalenus anterior and medius in the groove for the subclavian artery on the 1st rib. At the lateral margin of the 1st rib it continues as the axillary artery. A

2 **Vertebral artery.** A. vertebralis. It originates behind the scalenus anterior, passes through the foramina transversaria cranially from C6–C1, and then, after proceeding over the arch of the atlas behind its lateral mass, runs anteriorly through the posterior atlanto-occipital membrane and the foramen magnum into the cranial cavity. A B D

3 **Prevertebral part of vertebral artery.** Pars prevertebralis. This short segment lies in front of the entrance into the foramen transversarium of C6. A

4 **Vertebral part of vertebral artery.** Pars transversaria (cervicalis). It ascends through the foramina transversia of C6 to C1. A

5 **Spinal branches.** Rami spinales (radiculares). Branches passing with the spinal nerves to supply the spinal cord, the meningeal coverings of the spinal cord and the vertebral bodies. A

6 **Muscular branches.** Rami musculares. They supply the surrounding muscles. A

7 **Atlantal (suboccipital) part.** Pars atlantica. Portion of the vertebral artery that winds around the atlas and occupies the suboccipital triangle. A

8 **Intracranial part of vertebral artery.** Pars intracranialis. It lies within the cranium. A

9 **Anterior meningeal branch.** Ramus meningeus [anterior]. Branch at the anterior circumference of the foramen magnum. It supplies bone and dura. A

10 **Posterior meningeal branch.** Ramus meningeus
~ [posterior]. Branch at the posterior circumference of the foramen magnum. It supplies bone and dura. A

11 **Anterior spinal artery.** A. spinalis anterior. Right and left arteries join to form an unpaired vessel in the anterior median fissure of the spinal cord. A B

12 **Posterior inferior cerebellar artery.** A. inferior posterior cerebelli. It supplies, among others, the lower posterior portion of the cerebellum. A B D

13 Choroid branch of fourth ventricle. Ramus choroideus ventriculi quarti. It supplies the choroid plexus of the fourth ventricle.

14 Tonsillar branch of cerebellum. Ramus tonsillae cerebelli. Branch for the tonsil of the cerebellum.

15 Medial and lateral medullary branches. Rami medullares medialis et lateralis. Branches to the medulla oblongata and the inferior cerebellar peduncle.

16 **Posterior spinal artery.** A. spinalis posterior. Slender longitudinal vessel, occasionally paired, behind the spinal cord. It arises intracranially from the posterior inferior cerebellar artery or the vertebral artery. B D

17 **Basilar artery.** A. basilaris. Unpaired, thick trunk between its origin from the right and left vertebral arteries and its termination as the posterior cerebral arteries. A B D

18 **Anterior inferior cerebellar artery.** A. inferior anterior cerebelli. It passes to the anterior part of the inferior surface of the cerebellum. B D

19 Labyrinthine artery [branch of the inter-
~ nal acoustic meatus]. A. labyrinthi [ramus meatus acustici interni]. It accompanies the vestibulocochlear nerve into the inner ear and can also arise from the basilar artery. B D

20 **Pontine arteries.** Aa. pontis. They supply the pons. B D

21 **Mesencephalic arteries.** Aa. mesencephalicae.

22 **Superior cerebellar artery.** A. superior cerebelli. It passes around the mesencephalon and through the cisterna ambiens to the surface of the cerebellum situated below the tentorium. B D

23 **Posterior cerebral artery.** A. cerebri posterior. Terminal branch of basilar artery. It supplies the occipital lobe and $2/3$ of the temporal lobe of the cerebrum. B C D

24 **Precommunical part of posterior cerebral artery.** Pars precommunicalis. Short trunk which extends up to the entrance of the posterior communicating artery. B

25 **Posteromedial central arteries.** Aa. centrales posteromediales. Branches in the posterior perforated substance for the thalamus, lateral wall of third ventricle and globus pallidus. B

26 **Postcommunical part of posterior cerebral artery.** Pars postcommunicalis. It is that portion following the posterior communicating artery. It curves around the mesencephalon and passes through the cisterna ambiens and tentorial notch to the inferior surface of the cerebrum. B

27 **Posterolateral central arteries.** Aa. centrales posterolaterales. Individual branches to posterior portion of thalamus, the quadrigeminal plate, pineal body and medial geniculate body. C

28 **Thalamic branches.** Rami thalamici. Branches to posterior portion of thalamus. C

29 **Posteromedial choroid branches.** Rami choroidei posteriores mediales. Branches in the roof of the third ventricle. C

30 **Posterolateral choroid branches.** Rami cho-
~ roidei posteriores laterales. Branches posteriorly in the plexus of the lateral ventricle. C

31 **Peduncular branches.** Rami pedunculares. Mesencephalic branches. D

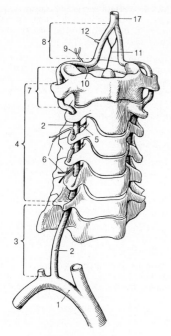

A Vertebral artery

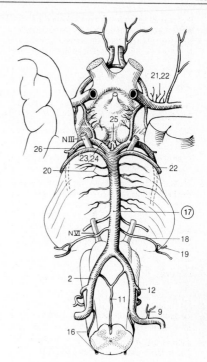

B Arteries of base of the brain

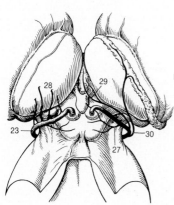

C Posterior cerebral artery

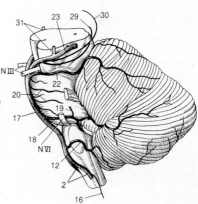

D Basilar artery

1 **Terminal portion of posterior cerebral artery.** Pars terminalis (corticalis). It supplies almost exclusively the posterior cerebral cortex mainly at the base of the brain.

2 **Lateral occipital artery.** A. occipitalis latera-
~ lis. Trunk for the three temporal lobe arteries. A B

3 Anterior temporal lobe branches. Rami
~ temporales anteriores. A B

4 Middle temporal lobe branches. Rami temporales (intermedii mediales). A B

5 Posterior temporal lobe branches. Rami temporales posteriores. A B

6 **Medial occipital artery.** A. occipitalis medialis. Twig for the sagittal surface of the posterior half of the cerebrum. A B

7 Dorsal branch to corpus callosum. Ramus corporis callosi dorsalis. Small, short branch to the splenium of the corpus callosum. A

8 Parietal branch. Ramus parietalis. Anterior branch to posterior portion of the parietal lobe. A

9 Parieto-occipital branch. Ramus parieto-occipitalis. It passes through the parieto-occipital sulcus. A B

10 Calcarine branch. Ramus calcarinus. It passes through the calcarine sulcus. A B

11 Occipitotemporal branch. Ramus occipitotemporalis. Lower branch extending into the temporal lobe. A B

12 **Cerebral arterial circle [[of Willis]].** Circulus arteriosus cerebri [[Willisii]]. Anastomosing arterial circle between the main tributaries of the cerebrum, i.e., between the internal carotid and the posterior cerebral arteries. B C

13 **Internal carotid artery.** A. carotis interna. Main anterior tributary in the cranial cavity. B C

14 **Anterior cerebral artery.** A. cerebri anterior. Anterior terminal branch of internal carotid artery. It supplies chiefly the greatest portion of the medial and orbital surfaces of the cerebrum. C

15 Anterior communicating artery. A. communicans anterior. Anastomosis between right and left anterior cerebral arteries. C

16 *Anteromedial central arteries.* Aa. centrales anteromediales. Short branches penetrating equally into the base of the brain. C

17 **Middle cerebral artery.** A. cerebri media. Lateral terminal branch of internal carotid artery. It frequently gives off the posterior communicating artery. C

18 Posterior communicating artery. A. communicans posterior. Paired anastomoses between the internal carotid or middle cerebral artery and the posterior cerebral artery. A C

19 Chiasmatic branch. Ramus chiasmaticus. Branch to the optic chiasma. C

20 Oculomotor nerve branch. Ramus nervi oculomotorii. C

21 *Thalamic branch.* Ramus thalamicus. Long branch which passes to the thalamus from below. A C

22 *Hypothalamic branch.* Ramus hypothalamicus. Branch to the hypothalamus. A C

23 *Branch to tail of caudate nucleus.* Ramus caudae nuclei caudati. It is located medial to the choroid fissure. C

24 **Posterior cerebral artery.** A. cerebri posterior. Paired terminal branch of basilar artery which, in turn, being formed by the union of the right and left vertebral arteries, thus produces a strong anastomosis of both vertebral arteries. A C

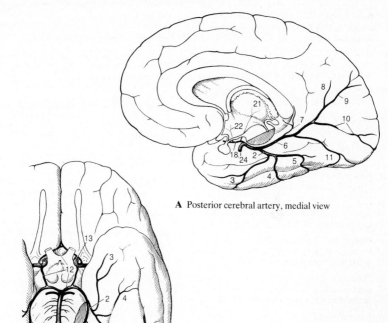

A Posterior cerebral artery, medial view

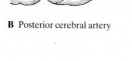

B Posterior cerebral artery

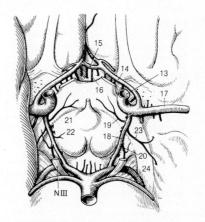

C Cerebral arterial circle (of Willis)

1 **Internal thoracic [[mammary]] artery.** A. thoracica interna [[A. mammaria interna]]. Arising from the subclavian artery, it descends along the anterior, inner surface of the thorax as far as the diaphragm. A B

2 **Mediastinal branches.** Rami mediastinales. Branches for the supply of the mediastinum. B

3 **Thymic branches.** Rami thymici. Branches for the supply of the thymus. B

4 **Bronchial branches.** [Rami bronchiales]. Branches to the bronchi. B

4a **Tracheal branches.** [Rami tracheales]. Branches to the trachea.

5 **Pericardiophrenic artery.** A. pericardiacophrenica. Accompanying the phrenic nerve, it supplies the pericardium and the diaphragm. B

6 **Sternal branches.** Rami sternales. Branches for the sternum. B

7 **Perforating branches.** Rami perforantes. Vessels advancing through intercostal spaces 1–6 to the surface of the thorax. B

8 Medial mammary branches. Rami mammarii mediales. Larger perforating branches to the mammary gland. B

9 **Lateral costal branch.** [Ramus costalis lateralis]. Variant. Arising from the internal thoracic artery, it runs laterally and parallel to it. B

10 **Anterior intercostal branches.** Rami intercostales anteriores. Anterior tributaries of the intercostal spaces. B

11 **Musculophrenic artery.** A. musculophrenica. Passing behind the costal arch, it gives off additional anterior intercostal branches from the 7th intercostal space onward. B

12 **Superior epigastric artery.** A. epigastrica superior. Continuation of the internal thoracic artery after entering the abdominal cavity between the sternal and costal parts of the diaphragm [[Larrey's space = sternocostal triangle]]. B

13 **Thyrocervical trunk.** Truncus thyrocervicalis. Variable common stem of the following arteries: inferior thyroid, transverse cervical, suprascapular. A B

14 **Inferior thyroid artery.** A. thyroidea inferior. It passes along the anterior margin of the scalenus anterior as far as the level of C6 and then behind the common carotid artery to the thyroid gland. A B

15 Inferior laryngeal artery. A. laryngealis inferior. It passes upward behind the trachea, penetrates the inferior pharyngeal constrictor and supplies part of the larynx. A B

16 Glandular branches. Rami glandulares. They supply the inferior and posterior surfaces of the thyroid gland and the parathyroids via inferior and ascending branches. A

17 Pharyngeal branches. Rami pharyngeales. ~ They supply the wall of the pharynx. A B

18 Esophageal branches. Rami oesopha~ geales. A B

19 Tracheal branches. Rami tracheales. A B

20 Ascending cervical artery. A. cervicalis ascendens. Lying medial to the phrenic nerve and the scalenus anterior, it can reach as far as the base of the skull. A B

21 *Spinal branches.* Rami spinales. They pass through the intervertebral foramina to the spinal cord. A B

22 **Transverse cervical (colli) artery.** A. trans~ versa cervicis (colli). The vessel is strongly variable. Here, the second most frequent variant (25%) is represented. Originating usually (75%) from the subclavian artery, it frequently passes through the brachial plexus, supplies the upper part of the trapezius with its branches and ramifies alongside the dorsal scapular nerve. A B

23 Superficial branch. Ramus superficialis. Arising either as a superficial ramus from the transverse cervical artery or as an independent superficial cervical artery from the thyrocervical trunk, it passes beside the accessory nerve to the descending part of the trapezius and the levator scapulae and splenius muscles. A B

23a **Ascending branch.** Ramus ascendens.

23b **Descending branch.** Ramus descendens.

24 Deep branch (dorsal scapular artery). ~ Ramus profundus (A. dorsalis scapulae). This vessel arises either as a deep branch of the transverse cervical artery or directly from the subclavian artery (67%) and accompanies the dorsal scapular nerve. It supplies the medial border of the scapula and adjacent muscles. A B

24a **Dorsal scapular artery.** [A. dorsalis scapulae]. Old designation for the deep branch.

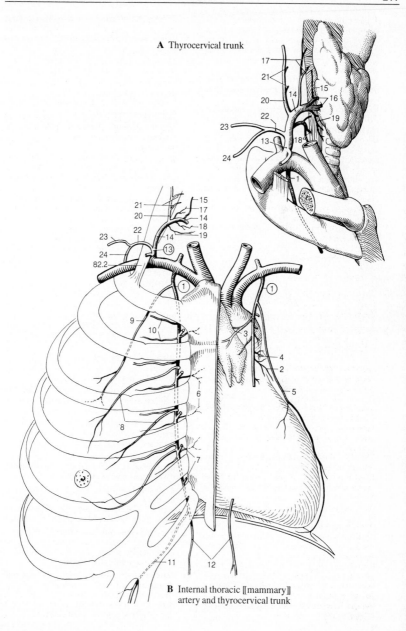

A Thyrocervical trunk

B Internal thoracic [[mammary]] artery and thyrocervical trunk

1 **Suprascapular artery.** A. suprascapularis. Generally arising from the thyrocervical trunk, it crosses over the scalenus anterior and runs above the superior transverse scapular ligament into the supraspinous and infraspinous fossae. It anastomoses with the circumflex scapular artery. A

2 **Acromial branch.** Ramus acromialis. It penetrates the attachment of the trapezius and passes to the acromion. A

3 **Costocervical trunk.** Truncus costocervicalis. Origin: Posterior wall of subclavian artery behind the scalenus anterior. B

4 **Deep cervical artery.** A. cervicalis profunda. It courses posteriorly between the transverse processes of C7 and T1, then upwards on the semispinalis. It supplies the nuchal musculature. B

5 **Highest intercostal artery.** A. intercostalis suprema. Common trunk for the first two intercostal arteries. B

6 First and second posterior intercostal arteries. Aa. intercostalis posterior prima et secunda. They pass in the first two intercostal spaces, respectively. B

7 Dorsal branches. Rami dorsales. Branches for the musculature and skin of the back. B

8 Spinal branches. Rami spinales. Branches to the spinal cord via intervertebral foramina T1–2. B

ARTERIES OF THE UPPER LIMB. ARTERIAE MEMBRI SUPERIORIS.

9 AXILLARY ARTERY. ARTERIA AXILLARIS. Continuation of the subclavian artery as far as the lower margin of the pectoralis major. A B

10 **Subscapular branches.** Rami subscapulares. Individual branches to the subscapularis muscle. A

11 **Superior thoracic artery.** A. thoracica superior.
~ Variable branch to the subclavius, intercostals 1–2 and serratus anterior muscles. A

12 **Thoracoacromial artery.** A. thoracoacromialis. It arises at the upper margin of the pectoralis minor and sends branches in all directions. A

13 Acromial branch. Ramus acromialis. Branch passing superolaterally through the deltoid muscle to the acromion. A

14 Acromial network. Rete acromiale. Arterial network on the acromion. A

15 Clavicular branch. Ramus clavicularis. Small branch to the clavicle and the subclavius muscle. A

16 Deltoid branch. Ramus deltoideus. Branch passing posterolaterally for the deltoid and pectoralis major muscles. A

17 Pectoral branches. Rami pectorales. Branches passing inferiorly for the serratus anterior and pectoral muscles. A

18 **Lateral thoracic artery.** A. thoracica lateralis. It passes downward at the lateral margin of the pectoralis minor to supply the pectoral and serratus anterior muscles. A

19 Lateral mammary branches. Rami mammarii laterales. A

20 **Subscapular artery.** A. subscapularis. Arising at the lateral margin of the subscapularis muscle, it supplies it and the latissimus dorsi and teres major muscles. A

21 Thoracodorsal artery. A. thoracodorsalis. Branch to the latissimus dorsi and teres major. A

22 Circumflex scapular artery. A. circumflexa scapulae. It passes through the triangular space to the infraspinous fossa and anastomoses with the suprascapular artery. A

23 **Anterior circumflex humeral artery.** A. circumflexa anterior humeri. It arises below the latissimus dorsi at the same level or deeper than the posterior circumflex humeral artery and passes in front of the surgical neck of the humerus to the coracobrachialis and biceps. It anastomoses with the posterior circumflex humeral artery. A

24 **Posterior circumflex humeral artery.** A. circumflexa posterior humeri. It passes with the axillary nerve through the quadrangular space to the shoulder joint and the deltoid muscle. It anastomoses with the anterior circumflex humeral, suprascapularis and thoraco-acromial arteries. A

25 **Brachial artery.** A. brachialis. It is a continuation of the axillary artery from the lower margin of the pectoralis major in the medial bicipital groove up to its division into the radial and ulnar arteries. A

26 **Superficial brachial artery.** [A. brachialis superficialis]. Variable appearance, as when the brachial artery lies on the median nerve instead of below it. A

27 **Profunda brachii artery.** A. profunda brachii. Companion artery of the radial nerve in the groove for the radial nerve. A

28 Nutrient arteries of humerus. Aa. nutriciae
~ (nutrientes) humeri. Branches to the bone marrow of the humerus. A

29 Deltoid branch. Ramus deltoideus. Branch coursing laterally behind the humerus, then superiorly and externally to the deltoid muscle. A

30 Middle collateral artery. A. collateralis media. It arises behind the humerus and descends to the articular network of the elbow. A

31 Radial collateral artery. A. collateralis radialis. It passes with the radial nerve to the articular network of the elbow and gives off an anterior branch to the radial recurrent artery. A

32 **Superior ulnar collateral artery.** A. collateralis ulnaris superior. Often arising near the profunda brachii artery, it passes with the ulnar nerve to the articular network of the elbow. A

33 **Inferior ulnar collateral artery.** A. collateralis ulnaris inferior. Originating above the medial epicondyle of the humerus, it passes on the brachialis muscle and through the intermuscular septum to the articular network of the elbow. A

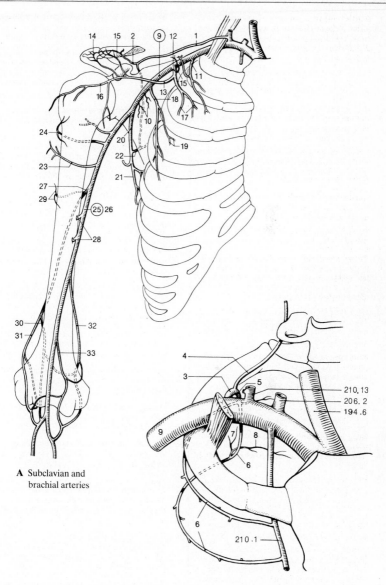

A Subclavian and
brachial arteries

B Subclavian artery

1 **Radial artery.** A. radialis. Beginning at the division of the brachial artery, it courses on the pronator teres and then lateral to the flexor carpi radialis (where its pulsations are readily palpable) up to the hand. B

2 **Radial recurrent artery.** A. recurrens radialis. Retrograde artery ascending medial to the radial nerve to anastomose with the radial collateral artery. B

3 **Palmar carpal branch.** Ramus carpalis palmaris.
~ Small branch at the distal margin of the pronator quadratus. It joins the carpal network. B

4 **Superficial palmar branch.** Ramus palmaris superficialis. Small arterial branch coursing through the thenar eminece to the superficial palmar arch. B

5 **Dorsal carpal branch.** Ramus carpalis dorsalis.
~ Branch passing transversely across the dorsum of the wrist below the long extensor tendons. A

6 Dorsal carpal network. Rete carpale dorsale.
~ Arterial network on the dorsum of the wrist. A

7 *Dorsal metacarpal arteries.* Aa. metacarpales
~ dorsales. Four arteries arising from the dorsal carpal branch or the dorsal carpal network and passing dorsally in the direction of the interdigital spaces. A

8 Dorsal digital arteries. Aa. digitales dorsales. Two short arteries arising from each of the dorsal metacarpal arteries and supplying the dorsum of the individual fingers. A

9 **Princeps pollicis artery.** A. princeps pollicis. It originates from the radial artery after its entrance into the 1st dorsal interosseus muscle and divides at the flexor side of the thumb. B

10 Radialis indicis artery. A. radialis indicis. Frequent branch of the princeps pollicis artery to the radial side of the index finger. B

11 **Deep palmar arch.** Arcus palmaris profundus. Continuation of the radial artery beneath the long flexor tendons. It anastomoses with the ulnar artery. B

12 Palmar metacarpal arteries. Aa. metacar-
~ pales palmares. Small branches of the deep palmar arch passing toward the interdigital spaces. B

13 Perforating branches. Rami perforantes. They anastomose with the dorsal metacarpal arteries at the dorsum of the hand. A B

14 **Ulnar artery.** A. ulnaris. Second terminal branch of brachial artery. It runs beneath the pronator teres, then in company with the flexor carpi ulnaris terminates as the superficial palmar arch. B

15 **Ulnar recurrent artery.** A. recurrens ulnaris. Retrograde branch of the ulnar (or brachial) artery with the following two branches: B

16 Anterior branch. Ramus anterior. It ascends medial to the brachialis muscle to anastomose with the inferior ulnar collateral artery. B

17 Posterior branch. Ramus posterior. In company with the ulnar nerve it ascends behind the medial epicondyle to anastomose with the articular network of the elbow and the superior ulnar collateral artery. B

18 **Articular network of elbow.** Rete articulare cubiti. Arterial plexus around the elbow joint, especially behind it. B

19 **Common interosseous artery.** A. interossea communis. Short segment from its origin from the ulnar artery to its division into the anterior and posterior interosseous arteries. B

20 Posterior interosseous artery. A. interossea posterior. It passes between the interosseous membrane and the oblique cord to the dorsal surface and supplies the extensor muscles of the forearm. A B

21 *Recurrent interosseous artery.* A. interossea recurrens. It passes deep to the anconeus muscle to anastomose with the middle collateral artery. B

22 Anterior interosseous artery. A. interossea anterior. It runs on the interosseous membrane and then beneath the pronator quadratus to anastomose with the dorsal carpal network. B

23 *Accompanying artery of median nerve.* A. comi-
~ tans nervi mediani. Long, slender vessel (median artery) which accompanies the median nerve. B

24 *Palmar carpal branch.* Ramus carpalis palmaris.
~ Branch distal to the pronator quadratus destined for the wrist. B

25 **Dorsal carpal branch.** Ramus carpalis dorsalis.
~ Branch passing laterally around the wrist to the dorsal carpal network. A B

26 **Deep palmar branch.** Ramus palmaris profundus. Weaker ulnar contributor to the deep palmar arch arising at the level of the pisiform bone. B

27 **Superficial palmar arch.** Arcus palmaris superficialis. It lies between the palmar aponeurosis and the long flexor tendons with the main influx from the ulnar artery. It anastomoses with the radial artery. B

28 Common palmar digital arteries. Aa. digitales palmares communes. Three to four arteries running toward the sides of the fingers, being their principal supply. B

29 *Proper palmar digital arteries.* Aa. digitales palmares propriae. Well developed arteries on the ulnar and radial sides of each finger, palmar aspect. B.

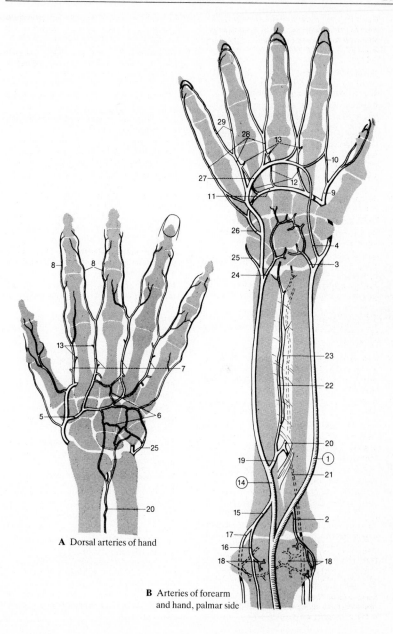

A Dorsal arteries of hand

B Arteries of forearm
and hand, palmar side

1 DESCENDING AORTA. PARS DESCENDENS
~ AORTAE. Descending portion of the aorta beginning at the isthmus of the arch of the aorta and terminating at its bifurcation at the level of the body of L4.

2 THORACIC AORTA. PARS THORACICA
~ AORTAE. Part of the descending aorta extending down to its entrance into the diaphragm. A B

3 **Bronchial branches.** Rami bronchiales. Their origin is very variable but often at the level of the bifurcation of the trachea. They supply the airways up to the respiratory bronchioles including the interlobular connective tissue and the visceral pleura. A

4 **Esophageal branches.** Rami oesophageales.
~ Small branches to the esophagus. A

5 **Pericardial branches.** Rami pericardiaci. Small branches to the posterior wall of the pericardium. A

6 **Mediastinal branches.** Rami mediastinales. Numerous fine branches to the lymph nodes and the connective tissue of the posterior mediastinum. A

7 **Superior phrenic arteries.** Aa. phrenicae superiores. Small branches from the lower thoracic aorta to the adjacent parts of the diaphragm. A

8 **Posterior intercostal arteries.** Aa. intercostales
~ posteriores. Posterior supply of intercostal spaces 3–9. A B

9 Dorsal branch. Ramus dorsalis. Posterior branch for the supply of the musculature and skin of the back. B

10 Spinal branches. Rami spinales. Branches passing through the intervertebral foramina to supply the spinal cord and its membranes. B

10 a *Postcentral branch.* Ramus postcentralis.Annot. 409

10 b *Prelaminar branch.* Ramus praelaminaris. Annot. 409

10 c *Posterior radicular artery.* A. radicularis posterior. Annot. 409

10 d *Anterior radicular artery.* A. radicularis anterior. Annot. 409

10 e *Segmental medullary artery.* A. medullaris segmentalis. Annot. 409

11 *Medial cutaneous branch.* Ramus cutaneus medialis. Branch passing along the spinous process to the skin. B

12 *Lateral cutaneous branch.* Ramus cutaneus lateralis. Branch of the dorsal ramus running beneath the skin further laterally. B

13 Collateral branch [[supracostal branch]]. Ramus collateralis [[Ramus supracostalis]]. Branch arising in the vicinity of the costal angle and running parallel to the intercostal artery. It proceeds anteriorly along the upper margin of the next lowest rib and anastomoses with the internal thoracic artery. A B

14 Lateral cutaneous branch. Ramus cutaneus lateralis. Branch running laterally beneath the skin and ramifying both anteriorly and posteriorly. B

15 *Lateral mammary branches.* Rami mammarii laterales. Branches from the lateral cutaneous branches to the mammary gland. B

16 **Subcostal artery.** A. subcostalis. Segmental arterial branch lying below the 12th rib. It corresponds to an intercostal artery.

17 Dorsal branch. Ramus dorsalis. It passes to the musculature and skin of the back. B

18 Spinal branch. Ramus spinalis. It passes through the 12th intervertebral foramen to supply the spinal cord and its membranes. B

19 ABDOMINAL AORTA. PARS ABDOMINALIS
~ AORTAE. Portion of the aorta extending from its entrance into the diaphragm to its bifurcation at the level of the body of L4. A

20 **Inferior phrenic artery.** A. phrenica inferior. Paired arteries for the supply of the diaphragm which they enter from below. A

21 **Superior suprarenal arteries.** Aa. suprarenales
~ (adrenales) superiores. Uppermost group of three suprarenal arteries. A

22 **Lumbar arteries.** Aa. lumbales. Four segmental arteries which correspond to the intercostal arteries. A

23 **Dorsal branch.** Ramus dorsalis. Branch for the musculature of the back and the medial skin segments. A

24 **Spinal branch.** Ramus spinalis. Branch passing through the intervertebral foramen to supply the spinal cord and its membranes.

25 **Median sacral artery.** A. sacralis mediana. Thin median continuation of the aorta. A

26 **Lowest lumbar arteries.** Aa. lumbales imae. Paired lateral branches of the median sacral artery. They correspond to a 5th lumbar artery. A

26 a **Lateral sacral branches.** Rami sacrales laterales. They anastomose with the lateral sacral arteries of the internal iliac artery.

27 **Coccygeal body.** Glomus coccygeum. Mass containing arteriovenous anastomoses and epithelioid cells located at the end of the median sacral artery in front of the tip of the coccyx. A

28 **Celiac trunk.** Truncus coeliacus. Common
~ stem of the left gastric, common hepatic and splenic arteries at the level of T12. A

29 **Left gastric artery.** A. gastrica sinistra. Artery ascending in the left gastropancreatic fold to the cardiac portion of the stomach and continuing along the lesser curvature. A

30 Esophageal branches. Rami oesophageales.
~ Small branches to the esophageal segment situated above the cardia of the stomach. A

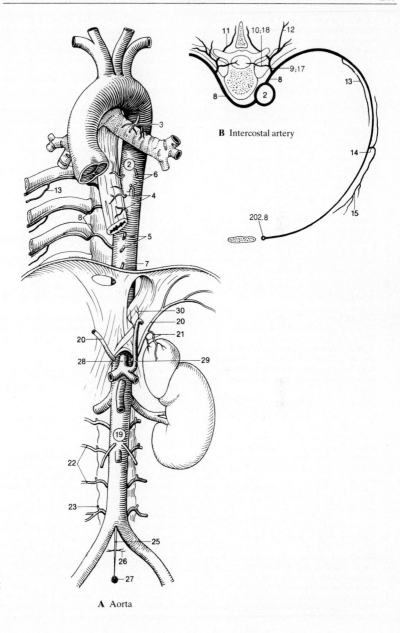

B Intercostal artery

A Aorta

1 **Common hepatic artery.** A. hepatica communis.
Branch of the celiac trunk (occasionally also the
superior mesenteric artery) passing to the right
side toward the liver and dividing into the gastroduodenal artery and the hepatic artery proper. Besides supplying the liver, it also partially supplies
the stomach, duodenum and pancreas. A C

2 Hepatic artery proper. A. hepatica propria.
One of the two terminal branches of the common
hepatic artery. It passes into the liver. B

3 *Right gastric artery.* A. gastrica dextra. It passes to
the upper margin of the pylorus, then along the
lesser curvature of the stomach to anastomose
with the left gastric artery. A

4 *Right branch of hepatic artery proper (right hepatic artery).* Ramus dexter. It passes to the right
side of the hilum of the liver and supplies the
right lobe. It frequently also arises from the
superior mesenteric artery. A B

5 *Cystic artery.* A. cystica. Originating from the
right branch of the hepatic artery proper, it passes
to the anterior and posterior surfaces of the gallbladder. A B

6 *Artery to caudate lobe.* A. lobi caudati. B

7 *Anterior segmental artery.* A. segmenti anterioris.
It supplies the anterior segment of the liver. B

8 *Posterior segmental artery.* A. segmenti posterioris. It supplies the posterior segment of the liver. B

9 *Left branch of hepatic artery proper (left hepatic
artery).* Ramus sinister. It supplies the left lobe of
the liver. A B

10 *Artery to caudate lobe.* A. lobi caudati. B

11 *Medial segmental artery.* A. segmenti medialis. It
supplies the medial segment of the liver. B

12 *Lateral segmental artery.* A. segmenti lateralis. It
supplies the lateral segment of the liver. B

12 a *Intermediate branch.* Ramus intermedius. It supplies the quadrate lobe. B

13 Gastroduodenal artery. A. gastroduodenalis.
Behind the lower margin of the pylorus, it divides
into an anterior supraduodenal artery and the right
gastro-omental artery. A C

14 *Supraduodenal artery.* [A. supraduodenalis]. In-
~ constant first branch. It supplies the anterior $^2/_3$ and
the posterior $^1/_3$ of the duodenum.

15 *Posterior superior pancreaticoduodenal artery.*
A. pacreaticoduodenalis superior posterior. Behind the pancreas it follows the duodenum somewhat and anastomoses with the inferior pancreaticoduodenal artery. C

16 *Pancreatic branches.* Rami pancreatici. Branches
to the head of the pancreas.

17 *Duodenal branches.* Rami duodenales.

18 Retroduodenal arteries. Aa. retroduodenales.
Branches of the gastroduodenal artery to the
posterior surface of the duodenum and the head of
the pancreas. In their course they cross over the
bile duct and supply it with a small vessel.

19 Right gastro-omental [[gastroepiploic]]
artery. A. gastro-omentalis dextra. It originates at
the level of the inferior margin of the pylorus and,

as the continuation of the gastroduodenal artery,
passes in the greater omentum at different distances
from the greater curvature of the stomach. It anastomoses with the left gastro-omental artery. A C

20 *Gastric branches.* Rami gastrici. Short branches
ascending to the stomach. A

21 *Omental branches.* Rami omentales. Long
branches for the supply of the greater omentum. A

22 Anterior superior pancreaticoduodenal
artery. A. pancreaticoduodenalis superior anteri-
or. Terminal branch passing inferiorly on the pancreas with anastomoses to the inferior pancreaticoduodenal artery. A C

23 *Pancreatic branches.* Rami pancreatici. A C

24 *Duodenal branches.* Rami duodenales. A C

25 **Splenic (lienal) artery.** A. splenica (lienalis).
Third branch of the celiac trunk. It runs along the
upper margin of the pancreas then through the
phrenicosplenic ligament to the spleen. C

26 Pancreatic branches. Rami pancreatici. Numerous small and several large branches to the
pancreas. A C

27 *Dorsal pancreatic artery.* A. pancreatica dorsalis.
Arising just at the beginning of the splenic artery,
it passes downward behind the neck of the pancreas partially embedded in pancreatic tissue. C

28 *Inferior pancreatic artery.* A. pancreatica inferior.
Branch of the dorsal pancreatic artery passing toward the left to the lower posterior surface of the
body of the pancreas. C

28 a *Prepancreatic artery.* A. praepancreatica. Anastomosis between the main branch of the dorsal
pancreatic artery and the anterior superior pancreaticoduodenal artery. C

29 *A. pancreatica magna.* It passes from near the
middle of the splenic artery downward onto the
posterior surface of the pancreas where it becomes
distributed and anastomoses with the inferior pan-
ceatic artery. C

30 **Artery to tail of pancreas.** A. caudae pancreatis.
It originates from the distal end of the splenic artery or from one of its terminal branches and
anastomoses with the inferior pancreatic artery in
the tail of the pancreas. C

31 **Left gastro-omental (gastro-epiploic) artery.** A.
gastro-omentalis (epiploica) sinistra. It lies at first
in the gastrosplenic ligament and then passes in the
greater omentum to anastomose with the right
gastro-omental artery. A C

32 Gastric branches. Rami gastrici. Long
branches to the stomach.

33 Omental branches. Rami omentales. Long
branches in the greater omentum. A

34 **Short gastric arteries.** Aa. gastrici breves. Small
vessels from the splenic or its branches passing
mainly to the fundus of the stomach. A

35 **Splenic branches.** Rami splenici. Five to six
~ branches of the splenic artery arising by division in front of the entrance into the spleen. A

35 a **Posterior gastric artery.** A. gastrica posterior.
Branch to the posterior wall of the stomach. A

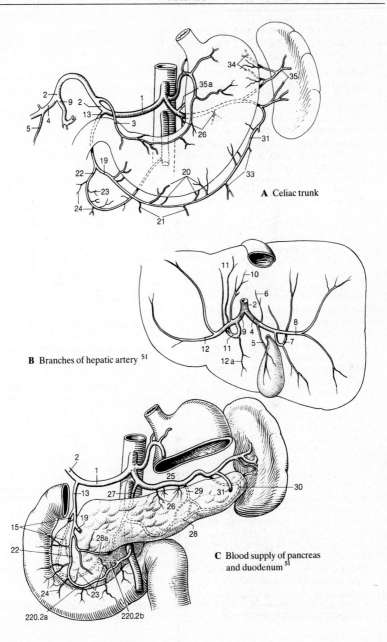

A Celiac trunk

B Branches of hepatic artery [51]

C Blood supply of pancreas and duodenum [51]

1 **Superior mesenteric artery.** A. mesenterica superior. Unpaired branch of the aorta arising about 1 cm below the celiac trunk. At first it lies behind the pancreas, then on the uncinate process and passes with its branches into the mesentery and mesocolon. A B

2 **Inferior pancreaticoduodenal artery.** A. pancreaticoduodenalis inferior. It arises behind the pancreas and passes between the duodenum and pancreas to anastomose with the superior pancreaticoduodenal artery. A

2a **Anterior branch.** Ramus anterior. It anastomoses with the anterior superior pancreaticoduodenal artery. See 219 C

2b **Posterior branch.** Ramus posterior. It anastomoses with the posterior superior pancreaticoduodenal artery. See 219 C

3 **Jejunal branches.** Aa. jejunales. Branches coursing in the mesentery to supply the jejunum. A

4 **Ileal branches.** Aa. ileales. Branches coursing
~ in the mesentery to supply the ileum. A

5 **Ileocolic artery.** A. ileocolica. It passes in the root of the mesentery downward and to the right toward the ileocecal junction. A

6 **Colic branch.** Ramus colicus. Ascending branch to the ascending colon. It anastomoses with the right colic artery. A

7 **Anterior cecal artery.** A. caecalis (cecalis)
~ anterior. It passes in the vascular cecal fold to the anterior surface of the cecum. A

8 A. caecalis (cecalis) posterior. It
~ courses behind the ileocecal junction to the posterior surface of the cecum. A

9 **Appendicular artery.** A. appendicularis. It courses at first behind the ileum, then in the free margin of the meso-appendix. It varies greatly in its origin; it is often doubled. A

9a **Ileal branch.** Ramus ilealis. Descending branch to the ileum. It anastomoses with the lowermost ileal artery. A

10 **Right colic artery.** A. colica dextra. It passes retroperitoneally to the ascending colon. Anastomoses: Ascending branch of ileocolic artery, middle colic artery. A

10a **Artery to right colic flexure.** A. flexura dextra. A

11 **Middle colic artery.** A. colica media. It passes in the mesocolon to the transverse colon. A

11a **Marginal colic artery [[of Drummond]].** A. marginalis coli. Anastomosis between the left colic artery and the sigmoid arteries. B

12 **Inferior mesenteric artery.** A. mesenterica inferior. Arising at the level of L3–4, it passes to the left to supply the descending colon, sigmoid colon and rectum. B

12a **Ascending [intermesenteric] artery.** A. ascendens [A. intermesenterica]. Anastomosis between the left colic artery and the middle colic artery. A B

13 **Left colic artery.** A. colica sinistra. It passes retroperitoneally to the descending colon. B

14 **Sigmoid arteries.** Aa. sigmoidea. They pass obliquely downward to the sigmoid colon. B

15 **Superior rectal artery.** A. rectalis superior. It passes behind the rectum into the lesser pelvis and divides into a right and left branch which, after penetrating the musculature, supply mainly the mucosa up to the anal valves. B

16 **Middle suprarenal artery.** A. suprarenalis (adrenalis) media. It originates directly from the aorta and supplies the suprarenal gland. C

17 **Renal artery.** A. renalis. It arises from the aorta in front of L1 and divides into several branches which enter the kidney. C D

17a **Capsular arteries.** Aa. capsulares (perirenales). C

18 **Inferior suprarenal artery.** A. suprarenalis inferior. Artery to the suprarenal gland. C

19 **Anterior branch.** Ramus anterior. It supplies the upper, anterior and lower segments of the kidney. C D

20 Superior segmental artery. A. segmenti superioris. It supplies the upper segment of the kidney as far as the posterior surface. C

21 Superior anterior segmental artery. A. segmenti anterioris superioris. It supplies the superior anterior segment of the kidney. C

22 Inferior anterior segmental artery. A. segmenti anterioris inferioris. It supplies the inferior anterior segment of the kidney. C

23 Inferior segmental artery. A. segmenti inferioris. It supplies the lower segment of the kidney extending up to the posterior surface. C

24 **Posterior branch.** Ramus posterior. It supplies the larger posterior segment of the kidney. C D

25 Posterior segmental artery. A. segmenti posterioris. It supplies the posterior segment of the kidney. D

26 **Ureteric branches.** Rami ureterici. Small branches for the ureter. C

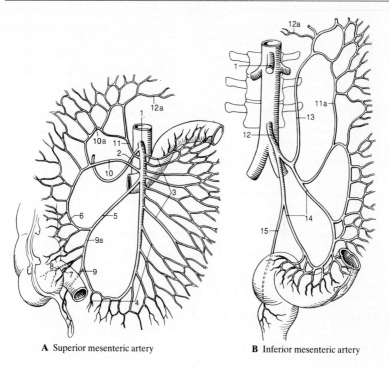

A Superior mesenteric artery

B Inferior mesenteric artery

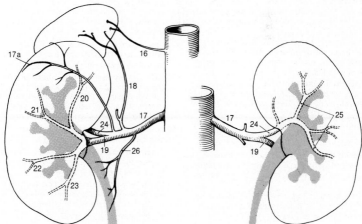

C Segmental arteries of the [37] kidney from front

D Segmental arteries of the [37] kidney from behind

1 **Testicular artery.** A. testicularis. It arises from the aorta at the level of L2, crosses over the ureter and, with the ductus deferens, passes through the inguinal canal into the testis. C

2 **Ureteric branches.** Rami ureterici. Small branches to the ureter. C

2a **Epididymal branches.** Rami epididymales. Branches to the epididymis.

3 **Ovarian artery.** A. ovarica. It arises from the aorta at the level of L2 and passes to the ovary within its suspensory ligament. It anastomoses with the uterine artery. C

4 **Ureteric branches.** Rami ureterici. Small branches to the ureter. C

4a **Tubal branches.** Rami tubarii (tubales). Branches to the infundibulum of the uterine tube. It anastomoses with the uterine artery. See 225 C

5 **Bifurcation of aorta.** Bifurcatio aortae. It occurs in front of L4, thus directly below the umbilicus. C

6 **Common iliac artery.** A. iliaca communis. It extends from the bifurcation of the descending aorta at L4 to its division into the internal and external iliac arteries in front of the sacro-iliac joint. It gives off only insignificant branches. C

7 **Internal iliac artery.** A. iliaca interna. It begins at the division of the common iliac artery, passes into the lesser pelvis and reaches as far as the upper margin of the greater sciatic foramen. Its branches vary greatly. C

8 **Iliolumbar artery.** A. iliolumbalis. It passes beneath the psoas muscle and the internal iliac artery into the iliac fossa. C

9 **Lumbar branch.** Ramus lumbalis. Branch leading into the psoas and quadratus lumborum muscles. C

10 Spinal branch. Ramus spinalis. Branch passing between the sacrum and L5 to enter the vertebral canal. C

11 **Iliac branch.** Ramus iliacus. Branch passing to the iliacus muscle in the ilac fossa; it lies parallel to the pelvis and anastomoses with the deep circumflex iliac artery. C

12 **Lateral sacral arteries.** Aa. sacrales laterales. Arteries passing downward lateral to the medial sacral artery. They can also arise from the superior gluteal artery. C

13 **Spinal branches.** Rami spinales. Arteries traversing the pelvic sacral foramina into the sacral canal. C

14 **Obturator artery.** A. obturatoria. It courses in the lateral wall of the pelvis and passes through the obturator foramen to supply the adductor muscles. B C

15 **Pubic branch.** Ramus pubicus. It anastomoses with the obturator branch of the inferior epigastric artery [[Corona mortis]]. C

16 **Acetabular branch.** Ramus acetabularis. It passes through the acetabular notch to the ligament for the head of the femur. B

17 **Anterior branch.** Ramus anterior. Located on the adductor brevis, it anastomoses with the medial circumflex femoral artery. B

18 **Posterior branch.** Ramus posterior. It is located beneath the adductor brevis. B

19 **Superior gluteal artery.** A. glutealis superior. It traverses the greater sciatic foramen above the piriformis [[suprapiriform foramen]] to enter the gluteal region. A C

20 **Superficial branch.** Ramus superficialis. It lies between the gluteus maximus and medius and anastomoses with the inferior gluteal artery. A

21 **Deep branch.** Ramus profundus. It lies between the gluteus medius and minimus. A

22 Superior branch. Ramus superior. It runs along the upper margin of the gluteus minimus as far as the tensor fasciae latae. A

23 Inferior branch. Ramus inferior. It courses in the gluteus medius as far as the greater trochanter. A

24 **Inferior gluteal artery.** A. glutealis inferior. Arriving through the greater sciatic foramen below the piriformis muscle [[infrapiriform foramen]], its branches are distributed beneath the gluteus maximus. They anastomose with the superior gluteal, obturator and circumflex femoral arteries. A C

25 **Accompanying artery of sciatic nerve (sciatic artery).** A. comitans n. ischiadici (sciatici). Phylogenetically, the major artery of the leg. It accompanies and supplies the sciatic nerve and anastomoses with the medial circumflex femoral artery and perforating branches. A C

26 **Umbilical artery.** A. umbilicalis. First inferior branch of the internal iliac artery. Postnatally, it becomes obliterated beyond the exit of the superior vesical arteries. C

26a **Patent part.** Pars patens. Portion of the fetal umbilical artery which does not become obliterated postnatally. It gives off the following vessels:

27 **Artery of ductus deferens.** A. ductus deferentis. It descends in the pelvis up to the base of the bladder and from there downward it accompanies the ductus deferens to eventually anastomose with the testicular artery. C

28 Ureteric branches. Rami ureterici. Three branches to the ureter. C

29 Superior vesical arteries. Aa. vesicales superiores. Arteries to the upper and middle segments of the urinary bladder. C

29a **Occluded part.** Pars occlusa. Portion of the fetal umbilical artery which becomes obliterated postnatally and forms the medial umbilical ligament.

30 **Medial umbilical ligament.** Ligamentum umbilicale mediale [[laterale]]. Fibrous cord remnant of the umbilical artery occupying the medial umbilical fold. C

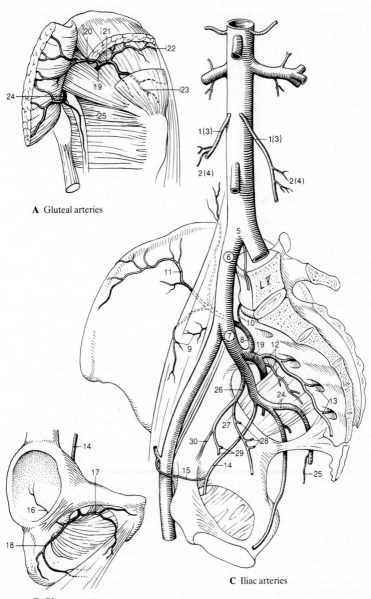

A Gluteal arteries

B Obturator artery

C Iliac arteries

1 **Inferior vesical artery.** A. vesicalis inferior. It supplies the inferior part of the urinary bladder and, in males, the prostate and seminal vesicle. A

1 a **Prostatic branches.** Rami prostatici. Branches to prostate and seminal vesicle.

2 **Uterine artery.** A. uterina. It corresponds to the artery of the ductus deferens. It passes to the cervix within the base of the broad ligament and very tortuously ascends lateral to the uterus. A C

2 a **Helicine branches.** Rami helicini. Corkscrew-like, coiled terminal branchings of the uterine artery. C

3 **Vaginal branches (azygos arteries of vagina).** Rami vaginales (aa. azygoi vaginae). Branches to the cervix with anastomoses to the opposite side for the supply of the upper part of the vagina. A C

4 **Ovarian branch.** Ramus ovaricus. It runs along the ovarian ligament proper and through the mesovarium to the ovary. It anastomoses with the ovarian artery and the tubal branch of the uterine artery. C

5 **Tubal branch.** Ramus tubarius (tubalis). It runs in the mesosalpinx of the tube as far as its anastomosis with the ovarian artery. C

6 **Vaginal artery.** A. vaginalis. It arises directly from the internal iliac artery. A

7 **Middle rectal artery.** A. rectalis media. It crosses the floor of the pelvis to the rectum and supplies its musculature. A E

7 a **Vaginal branches.** [Rami vaginales]. Branches to the lower part of the vagina. A

8 **Internal pudendal artery.** A. pudenda interna. It passes through the greater sciatic foramen [[*infrapiriform*]] from the pelvis and through the lesser sciatic foramen to the lateral wall of the ischio-anal fossa. A D E

9 **Inferior rectal artery.** A. rectalis inferior. It passes transversely through the ischio-anal fossa and supplies both sphincters, as well as the skin below the anal valves. D E

10 **Perineal artery.** A. perinealis. It arises at the posterior margin of the urogenital diaphragm and supplies the bulbospongiosus and ischiocavernosus muscles. D E

11 **Posterior scrotal branches.** Rami scrotales posteriores. Branches passing to the scrotum. E

12 **Posterior labial branches.** Rami labiales posteriores. Branches passing to the labium majus. D

13 **Urethral artery.** A. urethralis. It penetrates the corpus spongiosum at the junction of the crura of the penis and travels as far as the glans. It anastomoses with the dorsal and deep arteries of the penis. E

14 **Artery of bulb of penis.** A. bulbi penis. It also supplies the deep transversus perinei muscle and the bulbo-urethral gland. E

15 **Artery of bulb of vestibule.** A. bulbi vestibuli (vaginae). D

16 **Deep artery of penis.** A. profunda penis. It passes distally in the corpus cavernosum. E

17 **Dorsal artery of penis.** A. dorsalis penis. It passes beneath the fascia as far as the glans. E See 165 B

18 **Deep artery of clitoris.** A. profunda clitoridis. See 16

19 **Dorsal artery of clitoris.** A. dorsalis clitoridis. See 17

ARTERIES OF LOWER LIMB. ARTERIAE MEMBRI INFERIORIS.

20 **External iliac artery.** A. iliaca externa. Second branch of the common iliac artery; it continues as the femoral artery. A

21 **Inferior epigastric artery.** A. epigastrica inferior. It arises dorsal to the inguinal ligament and passes upward on the inner surface of the rectus abdominis. It produces the lateral umbilical fold and anastomoses with the superior epigastric artery. A B

22 **Pubic branch.** Ramus pubicus. Branch passing to the pubis. A

23 **Obturator branch.** Ramus obturatorius. Branch anastomosing with the pubic branch of the obturator artery [[*Corona mortis*]]. A

24 **Accessory obturator artery.** [A. obturatoria accessoria]. Obturator artery occasionally arising from the inferior epigastric artery.

25 **Cremasteric artery.** A. cremasterica. Branch for the cremaster muscle in the spermatic cord. It corresponds to the artery of the round ligament of the uterus.

26 **Artery of round ligament of uterus.** A. ligamenti teretis uteri. It supplies the connective tissue and smooth muscle of the round ligament. A C

27 **Deep circumflex iliac artery.** A. circumflexa iliaca profunda. Branch taking a curved course posterolaterally along the iliac crest beneath the transversalis fascia. A

28 **Ascending branch.** Ramus ascendens. It ascends between the transversus abdominis and internal abdominal oblique muscles to McBurney's point. It anastomoses with the iliolumbar artery. A

29 **Femoral artery.** A. femoralis. It extends from the inguinal ligament to the popliteal artery with which it is continuous. B

30 **Superficial epigastric artery.** A. epigastrica superficialis. It arises distal to the inguinal ligament and courses on the abdominal musculature toward the umbilicus. B

31 **Superficial circumflex iliac artery.** A. circumflexa iliaca superficialis. It proceeds parallel to the inguinal ligament in the direction of the anterior superior iliac spine. B

32 **External pudendal arteries.** Aa. pudendae externae. Usually two arteries for the lower abdominal wall and the external genitalia. B

33 **Anterior scrotal branches.** Rami scrotales anteriores. Branches for the scrotum. B

34 **Anterior labial branches.** Rami labiales anteriores. They supply the labia. B

35 **Inguinal branches.** Rami inguinales. Branches in the inguinal region. B

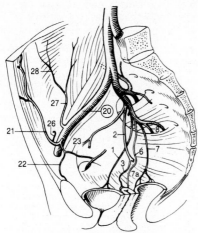

A Internal and external iliac arteries

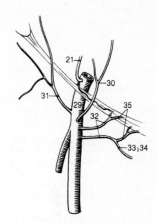

B Femoral artery

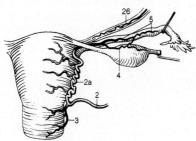

C Uterine artery

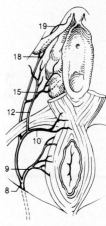

D Internal pudendal artery

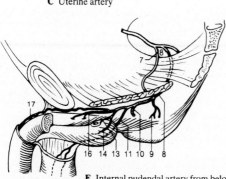

E Internal pudendal artery from below

1a Descending genicular artery. A. descendens ge-
nicularis. It arises in the adductor canal and penetrates the vasto-adductor membrane. A B

1b Saphenous branch. Ramus saphenus. It accompanies the saphenous nerve to the leg. A B

1c Articular branch. Ramus articularis. Forms
anastomoses between branches running in the
vastus medialis, then ends in the articular network of the knee. A

2 **A. profunda femoris.** Larger, deeper and
above all more lateral branch of the femoral artery.
It crosses under it and gives off the following
branches: A

3 **Medial circumflex femoral artery.** A. circumflexa femoris medialis. It passes medially and
posteriorly between the iliopsoas and pectineus
muscles. A

3a Superficial branch. Ramus superficialis. It
passes between the pectineus and adductor longus
muscles. A

4 Deep branch. Ramus profundus. It runs below
the lesser trochanter to the quadratus femoris, adductor magnus and ischiocrural muscles. It
anastomoses with the gluteal arteries. A

5 Ascending branch. Ramus ascendens. It
courses in the adductor brevis, adductor magnus
and obturator externus muscles and anastomoses
with the obturator artery. A

6 Descending branch. Ramus descendens. It
travels between the quadratus femoris and adductor magnus muscles to the ischiocrural musculature. A

7 Acetabular branch. Ramus acetabularis. It
goes through the acetabular notch into the ligament of the head of the femur and anastomoses
with the obturator artery. A

8 **Lateral circumflex femoral artery.** A. circumflexa femoris lateralis. It passes laterally beneath
the rectus femoris muscle. A

9 Ascending branch. Ramus ascendens. It ascends under the sartorius and rectus femoris and
terminates underneath the tensor fasciae latae. It
anastomoses with the medial circumflex femoral
and gluteal arteries. A

10 Descending branch. Ramus descendens. It
passes under the rectus femoris to the knee joint. A

11 Transverse branch. Ramus transversus. It
penetrates the vastus lateralis and has numerous
anastomoses. A

12 **Perforating branches.** Aa. perforantes. As terminal branches of the profunda femoris artery, they
pass posteriorly close to the femur via slits in the
adductor muscles and supply the long knee
flexors. A

12a **Nutrient arteries of femur.** Aa. nutrientes (nutriciae) femoris. They arise from the first and third
perforating arteries.

13 **Popliteal artery.** A. poplitea. It extends from
the end of the adductor canal to its division at the
lower margin of the popliteus muscle. B

14 **Lateral superior genicular artery.** A. superior
lateralis genus. It passes anteriorly above the
lateral femoral condyle and below the biceps tendon to join the articular network of the knee. A B

15 **Medial superior genicular artery.** A. superior
medialis genus. It runs anteriorly below the tendon
of the adductor magnus to join the articular network of the knee. B

16 **Middle genicular artery.** A. media genus. It runs
directly forward to enter the knee joint posteriorly
and supplies the cruciate ligaments and synovial
folds. B

17 **Sural arteries.** Aa. surales. Branches for the calf
musculature and the biceps tendon. B

18 **Lateral inferior genicular artery.** A. inferior
lateralis genus. It passes under the lateral head of
the gastrocnemius and under the lateral collateral
ligament to join the articular network of the knee.
A B

19 **Medial inferior genicular artery.** A. inferior medialis genus. It passes under the medial head of
the gastrocnemius and the medial collateral ligament
to join the articular network of the knee. A B

20 **Articular network of the knee.** Rete articulare genus. Arterial plexus primarily on the anterior side
of the knee joint. A

21 **Patellar network.** Rete patellare. Specific arteri-
~ al plexus on the patella. A

22 **Anterior tibial artery.** A. tibialis anterior. It
extends from its origin at the lower margin of the
popliteus muscle to the lower margin of the inferi-
or extensor retinaculum. After penetrating the interosseous membrane, it lies between the tibialis
anterior and the extensor digitorum longus, then
between the tibialis anterior and the extensor hallucis longus. A B C

23 **Posterior tibial recurrent artery.** [A. recurrens
tibialis posterior]. An inconstant branch which
passes under the popliteus to the knee joint. A B

24 **Anterior tibial recurrent artery.** A. recurrens tibialis anterior. It passes through the tibialis anteri-
or to join the articular network of the knee. A B

25 **Lateral anterior malleolar artery.** A. malleolaris anterior lateralis. It passes under the tendons of
the extensor digitorum to join the lateral malleolar
network. C

26 **Medial anterior malleolar artery.** A. malleolaris
anterior medialis. It passes under the tendon of the
tibialis anterior to join the medial malleolar network. C

27 **Lateral malleolar network.** Rete malleolare laterale. Arterial plexus over the lateral malleolus. C

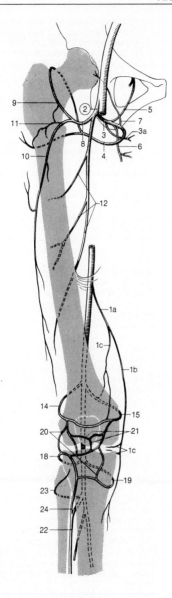

A Arteries of lower limb anterior view

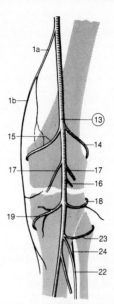

B Popliteal artery

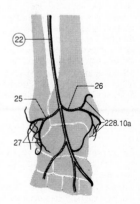

C Ankle joint with
arteries anterior view

1 **A. dorsalis pedis.** Continuation of anterior tibial artery on dorsum of foot. After crossing under the tendon of the extensor hallucis longus and passing the extensor retinaculum, it lies lateral to this tendon where it is palpable. B

2 **Lateral tarsal artery.** A. tarsalis lateralis. Arising at the level of the head of the talus, it passes under the short extensors of the toes in the direction of the cuboid bone. It anastomoses with the arcuate artery of the foot. B

3 **Medial tarsal arteries.** Aa. tarsales mediales. Several free branches to the inner margin of the foot. B

4 **Arcuate artery of foot.** [A. arcuata]. It takes a curved course laterally over the base of the metatarsals below the extensor digitorum brevis. B

5 Dorsal tarsal arteries. Aa. tarsales dorsales. Four branches which pass distally over the intermetatarsal areas, each dividing into two dorsal digital arteries. B

6 Dorsal digital arteries. Aa. digitales dorsales. Interdigital arteries arising from dorsal tarsal arteries. B

7 Deep plantar artery. A. plantaris profunda. Especially large perforating branch of a dorsal tarsal artery for anastomosis with the plantar arch. B

8 **Posterior tibial artery.** A. tibialis posterior. It arrives beneath the tendinous arch of the soleus muscle below the superficial flexor group and passes to the medial malleolus from behind. A C

9 **Fibular circumflex branch.** Ramus circumflexus fibularis ⟦Ramus fibularis⟧. Arising from the posterior tibial artery near its origin, it passes anteriorly around the fibula to join the articular network of the knee. A

10 **Medial malleolar branches.** Rami malleolares mediales. They pass behind the medial malleolus and join the medial malleolar network. A

10 a **Medial malleolar network.** Rete melleolare mediale. Arterial plexus over medial malleolus. A

11 **Calcanean branches.** Rami calcanei. Branches passing to medial surface of calcaneus. A

11 a **Nutrient artery of tibia.** A. nutriens (nutricia) tibialis. It courses below the soleil line of the tibia and enters the nutrient foramen. A

12 **Peroneal (fibular) artery.** A. fibularis. Passes to the calcaneus covered for the most part by the flexor hallucis longus. A

13 **Perforating branch.** Ramus perforans. Perforating the interosseous membrane shortly above the malleolus, it passes to the lateral malleolar network and dorsum of the foot. A

14 **Communicating branch.** Ramus communicans. Transversely coursing anastomotic branch to the posterior tibial artery. A

15 **Lateral malleolar branches.** Rami malleolares laterales. Branches to the lateral malleolus, frequently from the communicating branch. A

16 Calcanean branches. Rami calcanei. They pass mainly to the lateral side of the calcaneus. A

17 **Calcanean network.** Rete calcaneum. Arterial network on posterior aspect of calcaneus. A

17 a **Nutrient artery of fibula.** A. nutriens (nutricia) fibulae. A

18 **Medial plantar artery.** A. plantaris medialis. Generally the weaker medial terminal branch of the posterior tibial artery, it supplies the abductor hallucis and flexor digitorum brevis muscles. C

19 **Deep branch.** Ramus profundus. It usually joins the plantar arch. C

20 **Superficial branch.** Ramus superficialis. It takes a superficial course on the abductor hallucis as far as the big toe. C

21 **Lateral plantar artery.** A. plantaris lateralis. Larger lateral terminal branch of the posterior tibial artery. It takes a curved course anterolaterally as it passes between the flexor digitorum brevis and quadratus plantae. C

22 **Deep plantar arch.** Arcus plantaris profundus. Distal convex continuation of the lateral plantar artery between the interossei and the oblique head of the adductor hallucis. C

23 Plantar metatarsal arteries. Aa. metatarsales plantares. Four arterial trunks emanating from the plantar arch below the intervals between the metatarsal bones. C

24 Perforating branches. Rami perforantes. Usually two such branches arise from each plantar metatarsal artery and pass between the metatarsal bones to the dorsum of the foot. C

25 *Common plantar digital arteries.* Aa. digitales plantares communes. Arterial stems extending from the distal perforating branch to the division into the proper plantar digital arteries. C

26 *Proper plantar digital arteries.* Aa. digitales plantares propriae. Arteries coursing along the medial and lateral sides of the toes on the plantar aspect. C

26 a **Superficial plantar arch.** [Arcus plantaris superficialis]. Occasional superficial connection between the medial and lateral plantar arteries.

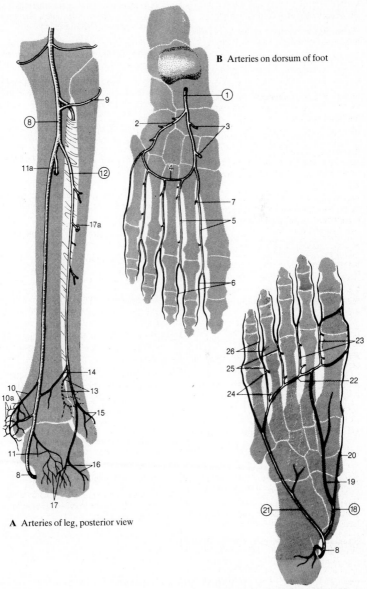

A Arteries of leg, posterior view

B Arteries on dorsum of foot

C Arteries on plantar surface of foot

1 VEINS. VENAE. Thin-walled blood vessels which return blood to the heart (atrium).

2 **Pulmonary veins.** Venae pulmonales. Veins leading from the lungs to the heart.

3 **The two superior right pulmonary veins.** [[Venae pulmonales dextrae]]. Occasionally they are united into a single trunk. A B

4 **Superior right pulmonary vein.** V. pulmonalis dextra superior. It comes from the upper and middle lobes. A B

5 Apical branch. Ramus apicalis. It comes from the apical segment of the upper lobe. A

6 *Intrasegmental part.* Pars intrasegmentalis. Twig coming out of the apical segment of upper lobe. A

7 *Intersegmental part.* Pars intersegmentalis. Twig situated between the apical and posterior segments of the upper lobe. A

8 Anterior branch. Ramus anterior. Branch from the anterior segment of the upper lobe.

9 *Intrasegmental part.* Pars intrasegmentalis. Twig coming from the anterior segment.

10 *Intersegmental part.* Pars intersegmentalis. Twig lying between the anterior and lateral segments. A

11 Posterior branch. Ramus posterior. Branch from the posterior segment of upper lobe. A

12 *Infralobar part.* Pars infralobaris. Twig coming from the posterior segment. A

13 *Intralobar part.* Pars intralobaris *[interseg-mentalis].* Twig lying between the posterior segment of the upper lobe and the apical (superior) segment of the lower lobe. A

14 Middle lobe branch. Ramus lobi medii. A

15 *Lateral part.* Pars lateralis. Twig coming from the lateral segment of the middle lobe. A

16 *Medial part.* Pars medialis. Twig coming from the medial segment of the middle lobe. A

17 **Inferior right pulmonary vein.** V. pulmonalis dextra inferior. It comes from the right lower lobe. A B

18 Superior branch. Ramus superior. Branch from the apical (superior) segment of the lower lobe. A

19 *Intrasegmental part.* Pars intrasegmentalis. Twig from the apical segment of the lower lobe.

20 *Intersegmental part.* Pars intersegmentalis. Twig lying between the apical and posterior basal segments of the lower lobe. A

21 Common basal vein. V. basalis communis. Common vein from the basal pulmonary segments. A

22 *Superior basal vein.* V. basalis superior. Vein for the drainage of blood from the lateral and anterior basal segments. A

23 *Anterior basal root.* Radix basalis anterior. Vein from the anterior and partly from the lateral basal segments. A

24 *Intrasegmental part.* Pars intrasegmentalis. Twig coming from the anterior basal segment. A

25 *Intersegmental part.* Pars intersegmentalis. Twig between the anterior and lateral basal segments. A

26 *Inferior basal segment.* V. basalis inferior. Vein from the posterior basal segment. A

27 **Left superior pulmonary veins.** Vv. pulmonalis sinistra superior. Both left pulmonary veins. They occasionally unite into a trunk. B

28 **Left superior pulmonary vein.** V. pulmonalis sinistra superior. It comes from the left upper lobe. B C

29 Apicoposterior branch. Ramus apicoposterior. It comes from the apicoposterior segment. C

30 *Intrasegmental part.* Pars intrasegmentalis. Twig from the apicoposterior segment. C

31 *Intersegmental part.* Pars intersegmentalis. Twig lying between the apicoposterior and anterior segments. C

32 Anterior branch. Ramus anterior. Branch from the anterior segment. C

33 *Intrasegmental part.* Pars intrasegmentalis. Twig from the anterior segment. C

34 *Intersegmental part.* Pars intersegmentalis. Twig between the anterior and superior lingular segments. C

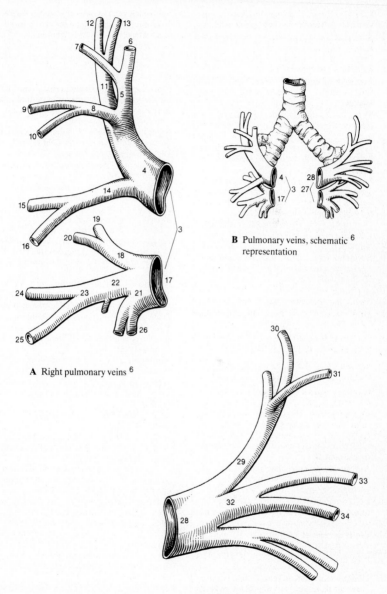

A Right pulmonary veins [6]

B Pulmonary veins, schematic [6] representation

C Superior left pulmonary vein [6]

1 Lingular branch. Ramus lingularis. Common branch from the two lingular segments. A

2 Superior part. Pars superior. Twig from the superior lingular segment. A

3 Inferior part. Pars inferior. Twig from the inferior lingular segment. A

4 **Left inferior pulmonary vein.** V. pulmonalis sinistra inferior. It comes from the left lower lobe. A

5 Superior branch. Ramus superior. Branch from the superior (apical) segment of the lower lobe. A

6 *Intrasegmental part.* Pars intrasegmentalis. Twig from the superior (apical) segment of the left lower lobe. A

7 *Intersegmental part.* Pars intersegmentalis. Twig lying laterally between the superior and anterior basal segments and medially between the superior and posterior basal segments. A

8 Common basal vein. V. basalis communis. Common trunk of superior and inferior basal veins. A

9 Superior basal vein. V. basalis superior. It lies between the anterior basal branch and the common basal vein. A

10 *Anterior basal branch.* Ramus basalis anterior. Branch from the anterior basal segment. A

11 *Intrasegmental part.* Pars intrasegmentalis. Twig from the anterior basal segment. A

12 *Intersegmental part.* Pars intersegmentalis. Twig between the medial and lateral basal segments. A

13 Inferior basal vein. V. basalis inferior. It comes from the posterior basal segment. A

14 **Cardiac veins.** Venae cordis. Veins from the heart wall. B

15 **Coronary sinus.** Sinus coronarius. Collecting vein situated on the posterior wall of the heart. It begins at the opening of the oblique vein of the left atrium and ends by opening into the right atrium. B

16 **Anterior interventricular vein.** V. interventricularis anterior. It runs in the anterior interventricular groove.

16 a **Left coronary vein.** V. coronaria sinistra. Continuation of the anterior interventricular vein in the left coronary (atrioventricular) groove.

17 **Posterior vein of left ventricle.** V. ventriculi sinistri posterior. It passes upwards from the left margin of the heart to empty into the great cardiac vein or the coronary sinus. B

18 **Oblique vein of left atrium.** V. obliqua atrii sinistri. Small, rudimentary vein at the posterior wall of the left atrium (remains of the left duct of Cuvier). B

19 **Fold of left vena cava.** Plica v. cavae sinistrae. Fold of serous pericardium thrown up by a fibrous strand between the brachiocephalic vein and the oblique vein (vestige of embryonic left superior vena cava). It lies in front of the left pulmonary vessels and can unite them together. B

20 **Posterior interventricular vein.** V. interventricularis posterior. It runs in the posterior interventricular groove and opens into the coronary sinus. B

20 a **Right marginal vein.** V. marginalis dextra. It lies at the outer margin of the right ventricle. B

20 b **Right coronary vein.** V. coronaria dextra. Accessory vein (32% of the cases) in the right coronary groove.

21 **Small cardiac vein.** V. cardiaca parva. It comes from the right margin of the heart and the right coronary groove in order to empty into the coronary sinus. B

22 Anterior vein of right ventricle. V. ventriculi dextri anterior. One to three small veins at the right anterior wall. It opens either into the small cardiac vein or directly into the right atrium. B

23 Smallest cardiac [[thebesian]] veins. Vv. cardiacae minimae [[Thebesii]]. Small veins opening directly into the cavities of the heart, especially that of the right atrium.

24 Right and left atrial veins. Vv. atriales dextrae and sinistrae. Small branches from the atrial walls. B

25 Ventricular veins. Vv. ventriculares. Small branches from the walls of the ventricles. B

26 Atrioventricular veins. Vv. atrioventriculares. Small veins from the atrioventricular borders. B

27 SUPERIOR VENA CAVA. VENA CAVA SUPERIOR. C

28 RIGHT AND LEFT BRACHIOCEPHALIC VEINS. VV. BRACHIOCEPHALICAE [DEXTRA ET SINISTRA]. Formed by the union of the internal jugular and subclavian veins on each side, they, in turn, unite to form the superior vena cava. C

29 **Inferior thyroid veins.** Vv. thyroideae inferiores. Veins passing into the left brachiocephalic vein, sometimes also the right, from the thyroideus impar plexus located below the thyroid gland. C

30 **Plexus thyroideus impar.** Venous plexus in front of the trachea below the caudal margin of the thyroid gland. C

31 Inferior laryngeal vein. V. laryngea inferior. It passes from the larynx into the thyroideus impar plexus. C

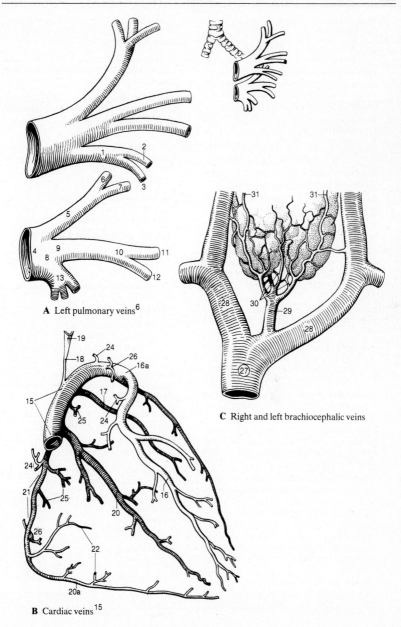

A Left pulmonary veins[6]

B Cardiac veins[15]

C Right and left brachiocephalic veins

1 **Thymic veins.** Vv. thymicae. Small branches from the thymus. A

2 **Pericardiac veins.** Vv. pericardiacae. Small branches from the pericardium. A

3 **Pericardiacophrenic veins.** Vv. pericardiaco-phrenicae. Veins accompanying the pericardiacophrenic arteries from the surface of the diaphragm and from the pericardium. A

4 **Mediastinal veins.** Vv. mediastinales. Small branches from the mediastinum. A

5 **Bronchial veins.** Vv. bronchiales. Small branches from the bronchi. A

6 **Tracheal veins.** Vv. tracheales. Small branches from the trachea. A

7 **Esophageal veins.** Vv. oesophageales. Small
~ branches from the esophagus. A

8 **Vertebral vein.** V. vertebralis. Companion vein of vertebral artery, usually as a plexus. A

9 Occipital vein. V. occipitalis. Arising in the venous network of the scalp, it frequently opens into the vertebral vein, but also into the internal or external jugular veins. A

10 Anterior vertebral vein. V. vertebralis anterior. Companion vein of ascending cervical artery. It opens inferiorly into the vertebral vein. A

11 **Accessory vertebral vein.** [V. vertebralis accessoria]. It is a continuation of the venous plexus of the vertebral artery and often appears by the foramen transversarium of C7. A

12 **Suboccipital venous plexus.** Plexus venosus suboccipitalis. Venous plexus between the occipital bone and atlas. A

13 **Deep cervical vein.** V. cervicalis profunda. Companion vein of same-named artery beneath the semispinalis capitis and cervicis muscles. A

14 **Internal thoracic veins.** Vv. thoracicae internae. Companion veins of internal thoracic artery, often doubled up to the third costal cartilage, then single and medial to the artery. A

15 Superior epigastric veins. Vv. epigastricae superiores. Companion vein of same-named artery. It empties parasternally into the internal thoracic veins behind the costal cartilages. A

16 Subcutaneous abdominal veins. Vv. subcutaneae abdominis. Cutaneous veins which empty into the superior epigastric veins. A

17 Musculophrenic veins. Vv. musculophrenicae. Companion veins of same-named arteries. A

18 Anterior intercostal veins. Vv. intercostales anteriores. Branches in the intercostal spaces. A

19 **Supreme intercostal vein.** V. intercostalis suprema. Carries blood from the first intercostal space to the brachiocephalic or vertebral vein. A

20 **Left superior intercostal vein.** V. intercostalis superior sinistra. Drains intercostal spaces 2–3(4) on the left side. It opens posteriorly into the left brachiocephalic vein. A

21 **Internal jugular vein.** V. jugularis interna. Main vein of the neck extending from the jugular foramen to the venous angle. A

22 **Superior bulb of jugular vein.** Bulbus superior venae jugularis. Dilatation of the internal jugular vein at its origin in the jugular foramen. A

23 **Vein of cochlear aqueduct.** V. aquaeductus cochleae. Minute companion vein of the perilymphatic duct. A

24 **Inferior bulb of jugular vein.** Bulbus inferior venae jugularis. Dilatation at the end of the internal jugular vein. It is closed cranially by a valve. A

25 **Pharyngeal plexus.** Plexus pharyngeus (pharyngealis). Venous plexus on the pharyngeal musculature. A

26 **Pharyngeal veins.** Vv. pharyngeales. Veins coming from the pharyngeal plexus. A

27 **Meningeal veins.** Vv. meningeae. Small venous branches from the dura. A

28 **Lingual vein.** V. lingualis. It is generally located by the lingual artery. A

29 Dorsal lingual veins. Vv. dorsales linguae. Numerous veins coming from the dorsum of the tongue. A

30 Companion vein of hypoglossal nerve. V. comitans n. hypoglossi. A

31 *Sublingual vein.* V. sublingualis. Larger vein situated lateral to the hypoglossal nerve. A

32 Deep lingual vein. V. profunda linguae. Companion vein of deep lingual artery lateral to the genioglossus. A

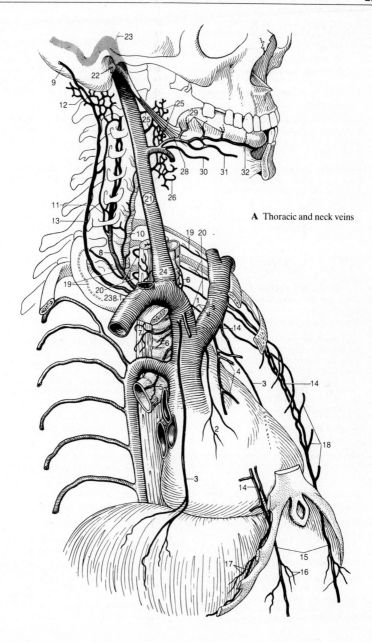

A Thoracic and neck veins

1 **Superior thyroid vein.** V. thyroidea superior. Companion vein of superior thyroid artery. It drains into the facial or internal jugular vein. A B

2 **Middle thyroid veins.** Vv. thyroideae mediae. One or more thyroid veins without corresponding arteries emptying into the internal jugular vein. A

3 **Sternocleidomastoid vein.** V. sternocleidomastoidea. It passes from the same-named muscle into the internal jugular or superior thyroid vein. A

4 **Superior laryngeal vein.** V. laryngea superior. Companion vein of superior laryngeal artery. It drains into the superior thyroid vein. A

5 **Facial vein.** V. facialis. It begins at the medial angle of the eye, lies behind the facial artery, then beneath the submandibular gland. A B

6 **Angular vein.** V. angularis. Formed by the union of the supratrochlear and supra-orbital veins, it becomes continuous with the facial vein at the medial angle of the eye and anastomoses with the ophthalmic vein. Via nasofrontal vein it is united with the superior ophthalmic vein and like the latter is devoid of valves. A B

7 **Supratrochlear veins.** Vv. supratrochleares [[V. frontalis]]. Beginning at the coronal suture, it drains the medial half of the forehead and joins the angular vein. A B

8 **Supra-orbital vein.** V. supraorbitalis. It comes from the lateral part of the forehead and joins the supratrochlear veins. A

9 **Superior palpebral veins.** Vv. palpebrales superiores. Veins of upper eyelid. A

10 **External nasal veins.** Vv. nasales externae. They come from the external parts of the nose. A

11 **Inferior palpebral veins.** Vv. palpebrales inferiores. They drain the lower eyelid. A

12 **Superior labial vein.** V. labialis superior. Vein of upper lip. A

13 **Inferior labial veins.** Vv. labiales inferiores. Usually several veins from the lower lip. A

14 **Deep facial vein.** V. profunda faciei (facialis). Arising from the pterygoid plexus, it passes anteriorly on the maxilla. A B

15 **Parotid branches.** Rami parotidei. A

16 **External palatine vein.** V. palatina externa.
~ Carries blood to the facial vein from the lateral tonsillar region of the palate and the pharyngeal wall. A B

17 **Submental vein.** V. submentalis. Accompanying vein of submental artery. It anastomoses with the sublingual and anterior jugular veins. A

18 **Retromandibular vein.** V. retromandibularis. It drains into the facial vein after receiving the confluence of many branches in front of the ear. A B

19 **Superficial temporal veins.** Vv. temporales superficiales. They accompany the superficial temporal artery. A

20 **Middle temporal vein.** V. temporalis media. Arising from the temporalis muscle, it opens into the superficial temporal veins. A

21 **Transverse facial vein.** V. transversa faciei (facialis). Companion vein of the transverse facial artery caudal to the zygomatic arch. A

22 **Maxillary veins.** Vv. maxillares. They unite the pterygoid plexus with the retromandibular vein. B

23 **Pterygoid plexus.** Plexus pterygoideus. Ve-
~ nous plexus between the temporalis and pterygoid (medial and lateral) muscles, predominantly around the lateral pterygoid muscle with the following tributaries. B

24 Middle meningeal veins. Vv. meningeae mediae. Companion veins of middle meningeal artery. B

25 Deep temporal veins. Vv. temporales profundae. Companion veins of deep temporal artery. B

26 Vein of pterygoid canal. V. canalis pterygoidei. Companion vein of artery of pterygoid canal. B

27 Anterior auricular veins. Vv. auriculares anteriores. Veins coming from the external acoustic meatus and pinna. A B

28 Parotid veins. Vv. parotideae. B

29 Articular veins. Vv. articulares. Branches from the temporomandibular joint. B

30 Tympanic veins. Vv. tympanicae. Branches from the tympanic cavity.

31 Stylomastoid vein. V. stylomastoidea. Companion vein of facial nerve from the tympanic cavity. B

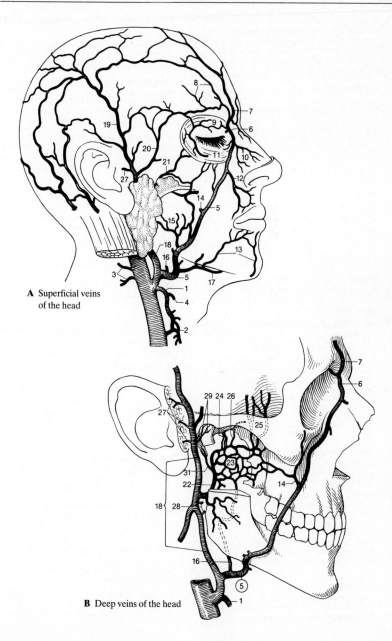

A Superficial veins of the head

B Deep veins of the head

1 **External jugular vein.** V. jugularis externa. Arising from the union of the occipital and posterior auricular veins, it courses between the platysma and superficial layer of the cervical fascia before emptying usually into the subclavian vein. A

2 **Occipital vein.** [[V. occipitalis]]. Companion vein of the occipital artery. A

3 **Posterior auricular vein.** V. auricularis posterior. Vein located superficially behind the ear. A

4 **Anterior jugular vein.** V. jugularis anterior. Beginning at the level of the hyoid bone, it crosses beneath the sternocleidomastoid and often opens into the external jugular vein. A

5 **Jugular venous arch.** Arcus venosus jugularis. Union of right and left anterior jugular veins in the suprasternal space. A

6 **Suprascapular vein.** V. suprascapularis. Generally two veins accompanying the same-named artery. A

7 **Transverse cervical veins.** Vv. transversae cervicis. Companion veins of the transverse cervical artery. A

8 *Dural sinuses.* Sinus durae matris. Incompressible venous conduits lying within the dura. They receive blood from the brain and meninges and drain into the internal jugular vein. B C

9 **Transverse sinus.** Sinus transversus. Dural sinus beginning at the confluence of the sinuses and continuous laterally with the sigmoid sinus. B C

10 **Confluence of sinuses.** Confluens sinum. Site of union of superior sagittal, straight, occipital and transverse sinuses at the internal occipital protuberance. B C

10a **Marginal sinus.** Sinus marginalis. It lies at the entrance of the foramen magnum and unites the venous plexus of the interior of the skull with that of the vertebral canal. B

11 **Occipital sinus.** Sinus occipitalis. Dural sinus beginning with a venous plexus at the foramen magnum and passing within the root of the falx cerebelli to the confluence of the sinuses. B C

12 **Basilar plexus.** Plexus basilaris. Venous plexus on the clivus with connections to the cavernous and petrosal sinuses as well as to the venous plexuses of the vertebral canal. B

13 **Sigmoid sinus.** Sinus sigmoideus. Continuous with the transverse sinus anteriorly, it takes an S-shaped turn medially to enter the jugular foramen. B C

14 **Superior sagittal sinus.** Sinus sagittalis superior. It lies within the root of the falx cerebri and extends from the crista galli to the confluence of the sinuses. B C

15 **Lateral lacunae.** Lacunae laterales. Lateral protrusions of the superior sagittal sinus. C

16 **Inferior sagittal sinus.** Sinus sagittalis inferior. Small dural sinus at the free margin of the falx cerebri. It terminates in the straight sinus. C

17 **Straight sinus.** Sinus rectus. It begins at the confluence of the great cerebral vein and the inferior sagittal sinus and passes to the confluence of the sinuses via the root of the falx cerebri at its junction with the tentorium cerebelli. C

18 **Inferior petrosal sinus.** Sinus petrosus inferior. It runs from the cavernous sinus to the jugular foramen along the posterior, lower margin of the petrous temporal. B

19 **Labyrinthine veins.** Vv. labyrinthales. Branches emanating from the internal acoustic meatus and entering the inferior petrosal sinus. C

20 **Superior petrosal sinus.** Sinus petrosus superior. It passes from the cavernous sinus to the sigmoid sinus along the upper margin of the petrous temporal. B

21 **Cavernous sinus.** Sinus cavernosum. Spongy venous space on both sides of the sella turcica into which the ophthalmic veins and others open. Within it lies the carotid artery and cranial nerve VI, its lateral walls housing cranial nerves III, IV and the ophthalmic and maxillary divisions of V. B

22 **Intercavernous sinus.** Sinus intercavernosi. Connections between the right and left cavernous sinus in front of and behind the hypophysis. B

23 **Sphenoparietal sinus.** Sinus sphenoparietalis. Blood channel passing beneath the lesser wing of the sphenoid to enter the cavernous sinus. B

24 **Diploic veins.** Vv. deploicae. Veins situated in the diploë of the calvaria. They take up the blood from the dura and roof of the skull and have connection both to the dural sinuses as well as the superficial cranial veins. A

25 **Frontal diploic vein.** V. diploica frontalis. Diploic vein running near the midline and opening into the supra-orbital vein and the superior sagittal sinus. A

26 **Anterior temporal diploic vein.** V. diploica temporalis anterior. Anteriorly situated diploic vein opening into the deep temporal vein and the sphenoparietal sinus. A

27 **Posterior temporal diploic vein.** V. diploica temporalis posterior. Posteriorly situated diploic vein opening into the posterior auricular vein and the transverse sinus. A

28 **Occipital diploic vein.** V. diploica occipitalis. Most posterior-lying diploic vein opening into the occipital vein and the transverse sinus. A

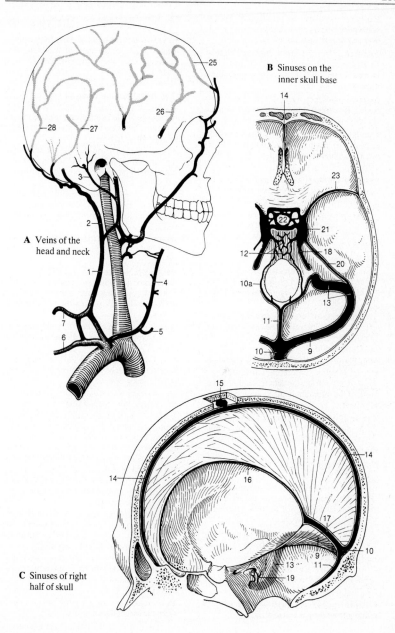

A Veins of the head and neck

B Sinuses on the inner skull base

C Sinuses of right half of skull

1   **Emissary veins.** Vv. emissariae. Venous connections between a venous sinus, diploic veins and superficial cranial veins.

2   **Parietal emissary vein.** V. emissaria parietalis. It connects the superior sagittal sinus with a superficial temporal vein via the parietal foramen. A

3   **Mastoid emissary vein.** V. emissaria mastoidea. It connects the sigmoid sinus with the occipital vein via the mastoid foramen. A

4   **Condylar emissary vein.** V. emissaria condylaris. It connects the sigmoid sinus with the external vertebral venous plexus via the condylar canal. A

5   **Occipital emissary vein.** V. emissaria occipitalis. Connection between the confluence of the sinuses and the occipital vein. A

6   **Venous plexus of hypoglossal canal.** Plexus venosus canalis hypoglossi. Occupying the hypoglossal canal, it lies between the venous plexus around the foramen magnum and the internal jugular vein. A

7   **Venous plexus of foramen ovale.** Plexus venosus foraminis ovalis. It lies in the foramen ovale between the cavernous sinus and the pterygoid plexus. D

8   **Venous plexus of internal carotid.** Plexus venosus caroticus internus. It occupies the carotid canal between the cavernous sinus and the pterygoid plexus. D

8 a **Hypophysial portal veins.** Vv. portales hypophysialis. Veins transporting blood to the cavernous sinus from the arterial capillary network of the infundibulum and the adenohypophysis. E

9   **Cerebral veins.** Vv. cerebri. Situated primarily in the subarachnoid space and without valves, they carry blood primarily into the dural sinuses.

10 **Superficial cerebral veins.** Vv. superficiales cerebri.

11 **Superior cerebral veins.** Vv. superiores cerebri. Arising from the lateral, medial and anterior aspects of the inferior surface of the brain, they drain into the superior sagittal sinus.

12 Prefrontal veins. Vv. praefrontales. They come from the frontal pole and its basal surface. B

13 Frontal veins. Vv. frontales. Veins from the upper third of the frontal lobe extending up to the central sulcus. B

14 Parietal veins. Vv. parietales. Sinus veins coming from the parietal lobe. B

15 Occipital veins. Vv. occipitales. Sinus veins coming from the occipital lobe. B

16 **Inferior cerebral veins.** Vv. inferiores cerebri. Veins located at the base of the brain with openings into the cavernous, petrosal and transverse sinuses.

17 Vein of the uncus. V. unci. C

18 **Superficial middle cerebral vein.** V. media superficialis cerebri. Coming from the lower two-thirds of the hemisphere, it passes to the cavernous sinus via the lateral sulcus of the cerebrum. B

19 Superior anastomotic vein. V. anastomotica superior [[Trolard]]. Well-developed vein occasionally present anastomosing with the superior sagittal sinus. B

20 Inferior anastomotic vein. V. anastomotica inferior [[Labbe]]. Well-developed anastomosis occasionally present with the transverse sinus. B

21 **Deep cerebral veins.** Vv. profundae cerebri. Cerebral veins lying predominantly concealed.

22 **Basal vein.** V. basalis [[*Rosenthal*]]. It begins at the anterior perforated substance, then courses along the optic tract and passes around the brainstem dorsally to join the great cerebral vein. C

23 Anterior cerebral veins. Vv. anteriores cerebri. Companion veins of the anterior cerebral artery. C
~

24 Deep middle cerebral vein. V. media profunda cerebri. It begins at the insula and opens into the basal vein. C

25 *Insular veins.* Vv. insulares. Origin branches of the deep middle cerebral vein. C

26 Inferior thalamostriate veins. Vv. thalamostriatae inferiores. Arising from the caudate and lentiform nucleus, as well as the thalamus, they penetrate the anterior perforated substance and open into the basal or deep middle cerebral vein. C
~

27 Vein of olfactory gyrus. V. gyri olfactorii. It comes from the region of the olfactory trigone and in front of it. C

28 Inferior ventricular vein. V. ventricularis inferior. Arising from the white matter of the temporal lobe, it passes through the choroid fissure at the level of the crus cerebri. C

29 Inferior choroid vein. V. choroidea inferior. It brings blood from the hippocampus, dentate gyrus and choroid plexus into the basal vein. C

30 Peduncular veins. Vv. pedunculares. Veins from the cerebral peduncle. C

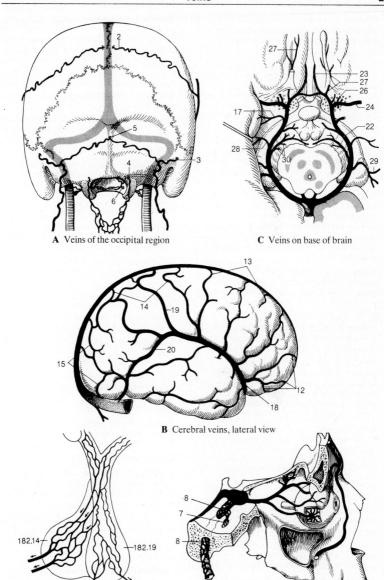

A Veins of the occipital region

C Veins on base of brain

B Cerebral veins, lateral view

E Portal vessel of the hypophysis

D Veins of orbit and middle cranial fossa

1 Great cerebral vein [[vein of Galen]]. V. magna cerebri [[Galeni]]. Short vein between the union of both internal cerebral veins and the beginning of the straight sinus. A C

2 Internal cerebral veins [[right and left]]. Vv. internae cerebri. Each runs in the transverse fissure, thus between the fornix and thalamus or the roof of the third ventricle. Both begin at the interventricular foramen and end at the union with that of the opposite side to form the great cerebral vein. A C

3 Superior choroid vein. V. choroidea superior. It lies in the entire length of the choroid plexus up to the interventricular foramen and receives branches from the hippocampus, fornix and corpus callosum. A

4 Superior thalamostriate vein. V. thalamo-
~ striata superior (V. terminalis). It runs in the angle between the thalamus and caudate nucleus (thus its name). It has no branches from the thalamus itself, but some from its vicinity. It ends by opening into the superior choroid vein in the interventricular foramen. A

5 Anterior vein of septum pellucidum. V. an-
~ terior septi pellucidi. From its drainage area, the medulla of the frontal lobe and the genu of the corpus callosum, it passes in the septum pellucidum to join the thalamostriate vein. A C

6 Posterior vein of septum pellucidum. V.
~ posterior septi pellucidi. It comes from the roof of the lateral ventricle and often opens into the internal cerebral vein. C

7 Medial atrial vein of lateral ventricle. V. medialis atrii ventriculi lateralis. Arising from the medulla of the parietal and occipital lobes, it passes in the medial wall of the lateral ventricle in front of the junction of the posterior horn. A

8 Lateral atrial vein of lateral ventricle. V. lateralis atrii ventriculi lateralis. Arising from the medulla of the parietal and occipital lobes, it courses in the lateral wall of the lateral ventricle in front of the exit of the posterior horn. A

9 *Veins of caudate nucleus.* Vv. nuclei caudati. Several veins. A

10 Lateral direct veins. Vv. directae laterales. Branches from the wall of the lateral ventricle opening directly into the internal cerebral vein. A

11 Posterior vein of corpus callosum. V. posterior corporis callosi. Branch coming from the end of the corpus callosum from below. A C

12 Dorsal vein of corpus callosum. V. dorsalis corporis callosi. Dorsal branch passing around the splenium. C

13 **Veins of brain stem.** Vv. trunci encephali.

14 **Anterior pontomesencephalic vein.** V. pontomesencephalica anterior. As a continuation of the vein of the medulla oblongata it extends as far as the interpeduncular fossa, often draining into the petrosal vein, and also into the basal vein. C

15 **Pontine veins.** Vv. pontis. Numerous branches from the pons which drain into the petrosal or pontomesencephalic veins, with an anastomosis between them. C

16 **Veins of medulla oblongata.** Vv. medullae oblongatae. Lower continuation of the pontomesencephalic vein with its branches from the medulla oblongata. C

17 **Vein of lateral recess of fourth ventricle.** V. recessus lateralis ventriculi quarti. It comes from the lateral recess and opens into the inferior petrosal sinus. C

18 **Cerebellar veins.** Vv. cerebelli.

19 **Superior vein of vermis.** V. superior vermis. Coming from the superior portion of the vermis, it empties into the great or internal cerebral vein. C

20 **Inferior vein of vermis.** V. inferior vermis. Arising from the lower half of the vermis, it opens into the straight sinus. C

21 **Superior veins of cerebellum.** Vv. superiores ce-
~ rebelli. They come mostly from the lateral hemispheres and usually open into the transverse sinus. A

22 **Inferior veins of cerebellum.** Vv. inferiores cere-
~ belli. They usually come from the inferior, lateral hemispheres and empty into the adjacent sinuses. C

23 **Precentral cerebellar vein.** V. praecentralis cerebelli. It begins between the lingula and central lobule and drains into the great cerebral vein. C

24 **Petrosal vein.** V. petrosa. It comes from the region of the flocculus, can be quite large and empties into the inferior or superior petrosal sinus. C

24 a **Orbital veins.** Vv. orbitae.

25 **Superior ophthalmic vein.** V. ophthalmica superior. Beginning medially above the eyeball with the nasofrontal vein, it passes through the superior orbital fissure to the cavernous sinus. B

26 **Nasofrontal vein.** V. nasofrontalis. Connects superior ophthalmic vein and the union of the supratrochlear with the angular vein. B

27 **Ethmoidal veins.** Vv. ethmoidales. B

28 **Lacrimal vein.** V. lacrimalis. B

29 **Vorticose veins (choroidal veins of eye).** Vv. vorticosae (Vv. choroideae oculi). Four or five branches from the choroid tunic of the eye. They penetrate the sclera laterally. B

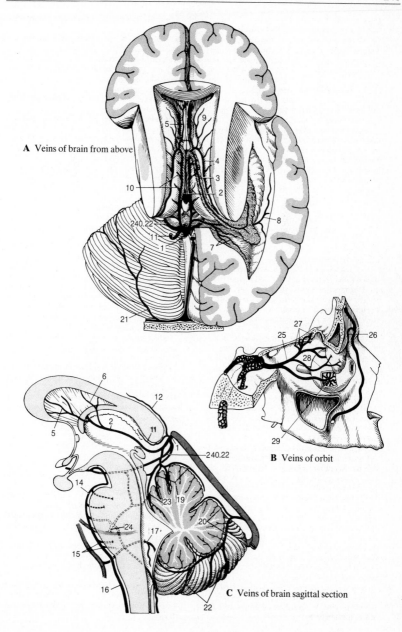

A Veins of brain from above

B Veins of orbit

C Veins of brain sagittal section

1 **Ciliary veins.** Vv. ciliares. Veins from the ciliary body which drain either into the veins of the ocular muscles or into the choroidal veins. A

2 **Anterior ciliary veins.** Vv. ciliares anteriores. Companion veins of the same-named arteries. They bring blood from the ciliary body to the veins of the ocular muscles at their attachments. A

2 a [Sinus venosus sclerae]. A See 354.30

3 Scleral veins. *Vv. sclerales.* Thin veins coursing mainly in the anterior sclera.

4 **Central vein of retina.** V. centralis retinae. Companion vein of central artery of retina. It drains either into the superior ophthalmic vein or directly into the cavernous sinus. A

5 **Episcleral veins.** Vv. episclerales. Branches located on the sclera and opening into the superior ophthalmic veins. A

6 **Palpebral veins.** Vv. palpebrales. Branches coming from the upper eyelids. A

7 Conjunctival veins. Vv. conjunctivales. A

8 **Inferior ophthalmic vein.** V. ophthalmica inferior. Arising from the lower eyelid and the lacrimal gland, it unites with the superior ophthalmic vein or passes directly into the cavernous sinus and the pterygoid plexus. A

9 **SUBCLAVIAN VEIN.** V. subclavia. It lies between the scalenus anterior and sternocleidomastoid muscles and extends from the internal jugular vein to the lateral margin of the first rib. B

10 **Pectoral veins.** Vv. pectorales. Veins passing from the area of the pectoral muscles directly into the subclavian vein. B

11 **Dorsal scapular vein.** V. scapularis dorsalis. Accompanying vein of the dorsal scapular artery. It frequently opens into the external jugular vein. B

12 **Thoracoacromial vein.** [V. thoracoacromialis]. Companion vein of the thoracoacromial artery with an occasional opening into the subclavian vein. B

13 **Axillary vein.** V. axillaris. Continuation of the subclavian vein extending from the lateral margin of the first rib to the lower margin of the tendon of the teres major. B D

13 a **Subscapular, circumflex scapular, thoracodorsal, posterior circumflex scapular, anterior circumflex scapular veins.** Vv. subscapularis, circumflexa scapulae, thoracodorsalis, circumflexa posterior humerais, circumflexa anterior humeralis. Newly named companion veins of the same-named arteries.

14 **Lateral thoracic vein.** V. thoracica lateralis. Companion vein of lateral thoracic artery located on the serratus anterior muscle. B

15 **Thoracoepigastric veins.** Vv. thoracoepigastricae. Subcutaneous veins from the lateral trunk wall. They represent collaterals between the superior and inferior venae cavae. B

16 **Areolar venous plexus.** Plexus venosus areolaris. Venous plexus around the nipple (areola). B

17 **Brachial veins.** Vv. brachiales. Companion veins of brachial artery. B

18 **Ulnar veins.** Vv. ulnares. Companion veins of ulnar artery. B

19 **Radial veins.** Vv. radiales. Companion veins of radial artery. B

19 a **Anterior interosseous veins.** Vv. interosseae anteriores. Two companion veins for each anterior interosseous artery.

19 b **Posterior interosseous veins.** Vv. interosseae posteriores. Two companion veins for each posterior interosseous artery.

20 **Cephalic vein.** V. cephalica. Epifascial vein beginning at the root of the thumb. It runs in the lateral bicipital groove and passes between the deltoid and pectoralis major muscle [[deltoideopectoral trigone]] to enter the axillary vein. C D

21 Thoracoacromial vein. V. thoracoacromialis. Accompanying vein of the thoraco-acromial artery. It drains into the axillary vein. B D

22 Accessory cephalic vein. [V. cephalica accessoria]. It runs from the extensor side of the forearm to the cephalic vein.

23 **Basilic vein.** V. basilica. Epifascial vein beginning above the distal ulna. It penetrates the brachial fascia in the middle of the medial bicipital groove and opens into the brachial vein. B D

24 **Median cubital vein.** V. mediana cubiti. Anasto-
~ motic branch between cephalic and basilic veins. It takes an oblique course in the vicinity of the elbow from inferolateral to superomedial. D

25 **Median antebrachial vein.** V. mediana antebra-
~ chii. Epifascial vein occasionally present between the cephalic and basilic veins. D

26 **Median cephalic vein.** V. mediana cephalica.
~ Branch or trunk of the median antebrachial vein to the cephalic vein. D

27 **Median basilic vein.** V. mediana basilica. Branch
~ or trunk of median antebrachial vein to the basilic vein. D

28 **Dorsal venous plexus of hand.** Rete venosum dorsale manus. Subcutaneous venous network on dorsum of hand. C

29 Intercapitular veins. Vv. intercapitulares. Located between the heads of the metatarsal bones, they connect the dorsal and palmar veins of the hand. C D

30 **Superficial palmar venous arch.** Arcus venosus palmaris superficialis. Companion vein of the arterial superficial palmar arch. D

31 **Palmar digital veins.** Vv. digitales palmares. Veins on the flexor side of the fingers. D

32 **Deep palmar venous arch.** Arcus venosus palmaris profundus. Companion veins of the arterial deep palmar arch. B D

33 Dorsal metacarpal veins. Vv. metacarpales dorsales. Three veins coming from the four ulnar fingers; they open into the dorsal venous plexus of the hand. C

34 Palmar metacarpal veins. Vv. metacarpales palmares. Companion veins of the metacarpal arteries; they open into the deep palmar venous arch. B D

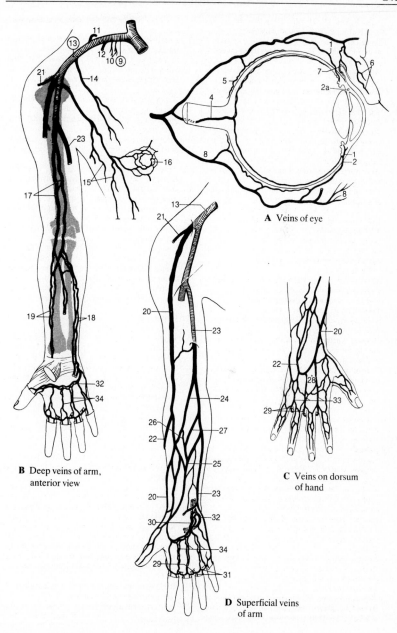

A Veins of eye

B Deep veins of arm,
anterior view

C Veins on dorsum
of hand

D Superficial veins
of arm

1 AZYGOS VEIN. VENA AZYGOS. Lying on the vertebral column, it begins with the ascending lumbar vein and opens into the superior vena cava at the level of T4–5 shortly before its entrance into the percardium. A

1 a **Arch of azygos vein.** Arcus venae azygos. Venous arch before entering the superior vena cava.

2 **Right superior intercostal vein.** V. intercostalis superior dextra. Formed by the union of 2nd and 3rd (4th) right superior intercostal veins, it opens into the azygos vein. A

3 **Hemiazygos vein.** V. hemiazygos. Frequently beginning at the left ascending lumbar vein, it receives intercostal veins 9–11 and drains into the azygos vein usually at the level of T9–10. A

4 **Accessory hemiazygos vein.** V. hemiazygos accessoria. After receiving intercostal veins 4–8, it opens into the azygos vein either alone or together with the hemiazygos vein. However, it can also take up the first three intercostal veins and then anastomose with the left brachiocephalic vein. A

5 **Esophageal veins.** Vv. oesophageales. Veins from
~ the esophagus draining into the azygos vein. A

6 **Bronchial veins.** Vv. bronchiales. Branches from the bronchi emptying into the azygos or hemiazygos veins. A

7 **Pericardial veins.** Vv. pericardiales. Branches from the pericardium destined for the azygos vein, superior vena cava or brachiocephalic vein. A

8 **Mediastinal veins.** Vv. mediastinales. Small branches from the mediastinum draining partially into the superior vena cava. A

9 **Superior phrenic veins.** Vv. phrenicae superiores. Small veins from the surface of the diaphragm. A

10 **Ascending lumbar vein.** V. lumbalis ascendens. Abdominal segments of the azygos on the right and the hemiazygos on the left. Collateral vein to the inferior vena cava via the common iliac vein. A B

11 Lumbar veins. Vv. lumbales. Segmental veins 1 and 2 opening into the ascending lumbar vein. A

12 **Subcostal vein.** V. subcostalis. Venous segment located below the 12th rib. From this tributary onward, the right and left longitudinal venous conduits are designated as the azygos and the hemiazygos veins, respectively. A B

13 **Posterior intercostal veins.** Vv. intercostales posteriores. Those from 4 to 11 drain into either the azygos or hemiazygos veins. A

14 Dorsal branch. Ramus dorsalis. Branch coming from the muscles and skin of the back. A B

15 Intervertebral vein. V. intervertebralis. Branch coming from the intervertebral foramen. B

16 Spinal branch. Ramus spinalis. Branch from the spinal cord and its meninges. B

16 a **Veins of the vertebral column.** Venae columnae vertebralis.

17 **Anterior/posterior external vertebral venous plexus.** Plexus venosus vertebralis externus anterior/posterior. Venous plexus in front of the verte-

bral body and behind the vertebral arch, respectively. B

18 **Anterior/posterior internal vertebral venous plexus.** Plexus venosus vertebralis internus anterior/posterior. Venous plexus situated at the anterior and posterior wall, respectively of the vertebral canal between the dura and periosteum or ligaments. B

19 Basivertebral veins. Vv. basivertebrales. Veins lying in the vertebral bodies and converging posteriorly to drain into the anterior internal vertebral venous plexus. B

20 Spinal cord veins. Vv. medullae spinalis. Venous plexus in the subarachnoid space for the drainage of the spinal cord.

20 a **Anterior spinal veins.** Vv. spinales anteriores. Cranially they are united with the network of the pons and pass caudally as the terminal vein.

20 b **Posterior spinal veins.** Vv. spinales posteriores. They terminate cranially at the rhomboid fossa, caudally at the conus medullaris.

21 INFERIOR VENA CAVA. VENA CAVA INFERIOR. Beginning at the union of the right and left common iliac veins, it lies to the right of the aorta and opens into the right atrium of the heart. A C

22 **Inferior phrenic veins.** Vv. phrenicae inferiores. Companion veins of inferior phrenic artery. C

23 **Lumbar veins.** Vv. lumbales. Segmental lumbar veins 3 and 4 open directly into the inferior vena cava. A C

24 **Hepatic veins.** Vv. hepaticae. Short intrahepatic veins. C

25 Right hepatic veins. Vv. hepaticae dextrae. Veins from right lobe of liver. C

26 Intermediate hepatic veins. Vv. hepaticae intermediae. Veins from caudate lobe of liver. C

27 Left hepatic veins. Vv. hepaticae sinistrae. Veins from left lobe of liver. C

28 **Renal veins.** Vv. renales. Right and left veins from kidney. C

28 a Capsular veins. Vv. capsulares. Venous network of the fatty capsule. Veins anastomose with veins of the region and the stellate veins. They can form a collateral circulation. C

29 Left suprarenal vein. V. suprarenalis (adrenalis) sinistra. Vein coming from the left suprarenal gland. C

30 Left testicular vein. V. testicularis sinistra. Vein from left testis. C

31 Left ovarian vein. V. ovarica sinistra. Vein from left ovary. C

32 **Right suprarenal vein.** V. suprarenalis (adrenalis) dextra. Vein from right suprarenal gland usually opening directly into the inferior vena cava. C

33 **Right testicular vein.** V. testicularis (adrenalis) dextra. It opens directly into the inferior vena cava. C

34 **Right ovarian vein.** V. ovarica dextra. It opens directly into the inferior vena cava. C

35 **Pampiniform plexus.** Plexus pampiniformis. Venous plexus around the spermatic cord. C

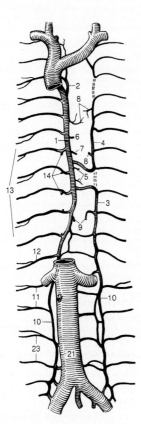

A Veins of posterior thoracic
and abdominal walls

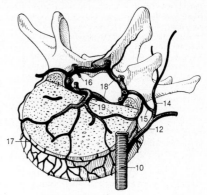

B Veins of vertebrae

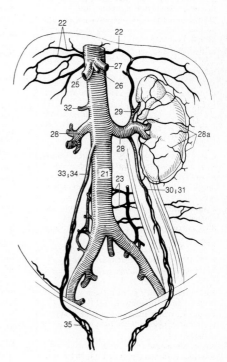

C Inferior vena cava

1 **Portal vein of liver.** Vena portae hepatis. It brings
~ blood from the intestinal tract to the liver. There are important anastomoses to esophageal veins, rectal venous plexus and the superficial veins of the abdominal skin. A

2 **Right branch.** Ramus dexter. Well developed, shorter right branch of portal vein. It splits up in the right lobe of the liver as far as the interlobular veins. A

3 Anterior branch. Ramus anterior. It supplies the anterior part of the right lobe. A

4 Posterior branch. Ramus posterior. It supplies the posterior part of the right lobe. A

5 **Left branch.** Ramus sinister. Longer and somewhat more slender branch supplying the left lobe as well as the caudate and quadrate lobes. A

6 Transverse part. Pars transversa. Initial segment of left branch coursing transversely into liver hilum. A

7 *Caudate branches.* Rami caudati. Twigs to caudate lobe. A

8 Umbilical part. Pars umbilicus. Sagittal continuation of left branch into the left lobe. A

9 *[Ductus venosus].* Embryonic vein uniting umbilical vein and inferior vena cava. Bypass of the liver. B

10 *Ligamentum venosum.* Lig. venosum. Connective tissue vestige of ductus venosus in groove for the ligamentum venosum. B

11 *Lateral branches.* Rami laterales. Branches leading to quadrate lobe and part of the caudate lobe.

12 Left umbilical vein. V. umbilicalis sinistra. Embryonic vein joining the portal vein in the liver. It carries umbilical cord blood to the right atrium partly via the ductus venosus and inferior vena cava. B

13 *Round ligament of liver.* Lig. teres hepatis. Connective tissue remains of left umbilical vein. A

14 *Medial branches.* Rr. mediales. Branches of umbilical part to anterior portion of left lobe of liver. A

15 **Cystic vein.** V. cystica. Vein from gallbladder emptying into right branch of portal vein. A

16 **Paraumbilical veins.** Vv. paraumbilicales. Small veins around the round ligament. They form anastomoses between the left branch of the portal vein and subcutaneous abdominal veins. A

17 **Left gastric vein.** V. gastrica sinistra. Companion vein of left gastric artery. A

18 **Right gastric vein.** V. gastrica dextra. Companion vein of right gastric artery. A

19 **Prepyloric vein.** V. praepylorica. Branch from anterior part of pylorus to the right gastric vein or portal vein. A

20 **Superior mesenteric vein.** V. mesenterica superior. Its drainage area extends from the distal half of the duodenum to the left colic flexure. It joins the splenic vein to form the portal vein. A

21 **Jejunal veins.** Vv. jejunales. Branches from the
~ jejunum and ileum. A

21 a **Ileal branches.** Vv. ileales. A

22 **Right gastro-omental (gastro-epiploic) vein.** V. gastro-omentalis (epiploica) dextra. Companion vein of right gastro-omental artery. A

23 **Pancreatic veins.** Vv. pancreaticae. Direct branches from the pancreas. A

24 **Pancreaticoduodenal veins.** Vv. pancreaticoduodenales. Companion veins of pancreaticoduodenal arteries. A

25 **Ileocolic vein.** V. ileocolica. Branch coming from the ileocecal region. A

26 Appendicular vein. V. appendicularis. Vein coming from the vermiform appendix. A

27 Right colic vein. V. colica dextra. Vein coming from the ascending colon. A

28 Middle colic vein. V. colica media (intermedia). Vein of transverse colon. It can also drain into the superior and inferior mesenteric veins. A

29 **Splenic vein.** V. splenica. It is found in the phreni-
~ colic ligament and then behind the pancreas. It joins the superior mesenteric vein to form the portal vein. A

30 Pancreatic veins. Vv. pancreaticae. They open directly into the splenic vein. A

31 Short gastric veins. Vv. gastricae breves. They course in the gastrosplenic ligament. A

32 **Left gastro-omental (gastro-epiploic) vein.** V. gastro-omentalis (epiploica) sinistra. Companion vein of left gastro-omental vein. A

33 **Inferior mesenteric vein.** V. mesenterica inferior. Extending from the left third of the colon to the upper rectum, it opens into the splenic vein. A

34 Left colic vein. V. colica sinistra. It comes from the descending colon. A

35 Sigmoid veins. Vv. sigmoideae. They drain the sigmoid colon. A

36 Superior rectal vein. V. rectalis superior. Branch from the upper rectum. A

37 COMMON ILIAC VEIN. V. ILIACA COMMUNIS. Venous trunk reaching from L4 to the sacroiliac joint. It unites with the contralateral vein to form the inferior vena cava. A

38 **Median sacral vein.** V. sacralis mediana. Unpaired branch to the left common iliac vein. A

39 **Iliolumbar vein.** V. iliolumbalis. Accompanying vein of the iliolumbar artery. It opens into the internal or common iliac vein. A

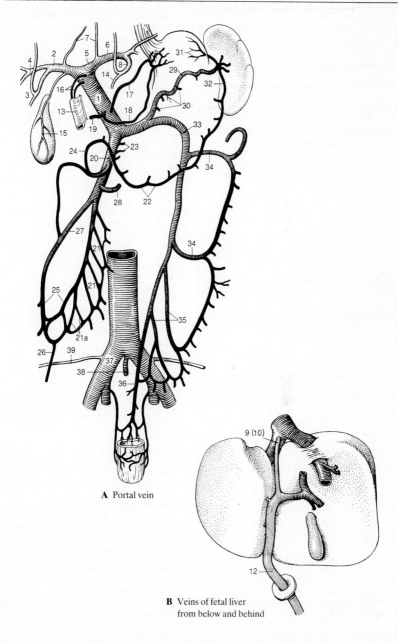

A Portal vein

B Veins of fetal liver
from below and behind

1 **Internal iliac [[hypogastric]] vein.** V. iliaca interna [[V. hypogastrica]]. Short trunk receiving veins from the pelvic viscera and perineum. A C

2 **Superior gluteal veins.** Vv. glutaeales[5] superiores. Companion veins of superior gluteal artery passing through the upper division of the greater sciatic foramen [[suprapiriform foramen]] to the pelvis. They converge into a trunk which opens into the internal iliac vein. A

3 **Inferior gluteal veins.** Vv. glutaeales[5] inferiores. Companion veins of inferior gluteal artery passing through the lower division of the greater sciatic foramen [[infrapiriform foramen]] into the pelvis. Uniting into a trunk, they open into the internal iliac vein. A C

4 **Obturator veins.** Vv. obturatoriae. Entering the pelvis via the obturator foramen, they usually open into both the internal iliac and common iliac veins. A

5 **Lateral sacral veins.** Vv. sacrales laterales. Lateral branches coming from the sacral venous plexus. A

6 **Sacral venous plexus.** Plexus venosus sacralis. Venous network lying in front of the sacrum. A

7 **Rectal venous (hemorrhoidal) plexus.** Plexus venosus rectalis [[Plexus haemorrhoidalis]]. It surrounds the rectum. A

8 **Vesical veins.** Vv. vesicales. Veins coming from the vesical venous plexus. A

9 **Vesical venous plexus.** Plexus venosus vesicalis. Occupying the base of the bladder, it communicates with the prostatic or vaginal venous plexus. A C

10 **Prostatic venous plexus.** Plexus venosus prostaticus. It surrounds the prostate and is united with the neighboring vesical venous plexus. C

11 **Deep dorsal vein of penis.** V. dorsalis profunda penis. Subfascial vein of dorsum of penis passing below the symphysis between the arcuate ligament of the pubis and the transverse perineal ligament to enter the prostatic venous plexus. It lies between the deep fascia of the penis and the tunica albuginea and is usually not paired. C 165 B

12 **Deep dorsal vein of clitoris.** V. dorsalis profunda clitoridis. Subfascial vein of dorsum of clitoris opening into vesical venous plexus. B

13 **Uterine veins.** Vv. uterinae. Anastomatic veins between uterine venous plexus and internal iliac vein. A

14 **Uterine venous plexus.** Plexus venosus uterinus. Network of veins primarily at the root of the broad ligament. It communicates with the vaginal venous plexus. A

15 **Vaginal venous plexus.** Plexus venosus vaginalis. Venous network around the vagina with numerous connections to the surrounding venous plexus. A

16 **Internal pudendal vein.** V. pudenda interna. It runs in the lateral wall of the ischio-anal fossa and enters the pelvis via the lower division of the greater sciatic foramen [[infrapiriform foramen]]. A B C

17 **Deep veins of penis.** Vv. profundae penis. They come from the roots of the corpus cavernosum and corpus spongiosum and drain into the prostatic venous plexus via the deep dorsal vein of the penis. C

18 **Deep veins of clitoris.** Vv. profundae clitoridis. They correspond to the deep veins of the penis. B

19 **Middle rectal veins.** Vv. rectales mediae. Branches from the rectal venous plexus. Located in the lesser pelvis, they anastomose with the superior rectal vein and the inferior rectal veins. A C

20 **Inferior rectal veins.** Vv. rectales inferiores. Arising from the anal region, they join the internal pudendal vein and form anastomoses to the middle rectal veins and the superior rectal vein. B C

21 **Posterior scrotal/labial veins.** Vv. scrotales/labiales posteriores. Coming from the scrotum or labia, they join the internal pudendal vein. B C

22 **Vein of bulb of penis/vestibule.** V. bulbi penis/vestibuli. Arising from the bulb of the corpus spongiosum, they convey their blood either to the deep dorsal vein of the penis (clitoris) or into the internal pudendal vein. B C

23 **External iliac vein.** V. iliaca externa. It begins at the upper end of the femoral vein below the inguinal ligament and ends when it joins the internal iliac vein to form the common iliac vein. A

24 **Inferior epigastric vein.** V. epigastrica inferior. Coming from the posterior side of the anterior abdominal wall, it forms the companion vein of the inferior epigastric artery. A

24a **Pubic branch (accessory obturator vein).** R. pubicus (V. obturatoria accessoria). It anastomoses with the branch of the obturator vein at the inner surface of the pubis. A

25 **Deep circumflex iliac vein.** V. circumflexa iliaca profunda. Companion vein of the deep circumflex iliac artery. A

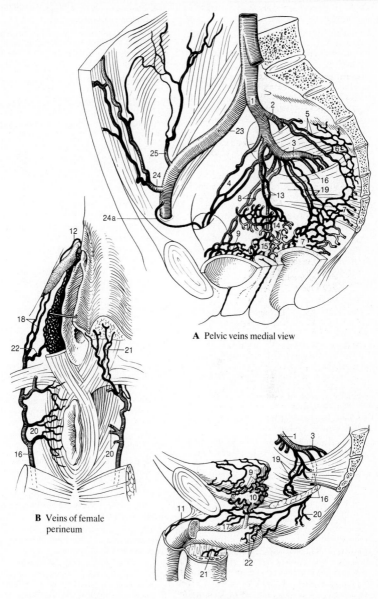

A Pelvic veins medial view

B Veins of female
perineum

C Veins of male urogenital organs

VEINS OF LOWER LIMB. VENAE MEMBRI INFERIORIS.

1 **Femoral vein.** V. femoralis. As the companion vein of the femoral artery, it extends from the hiatus tendineus of the adductor canal to the inguinal ligament. A

2 **External pudendal veins.** Vv. pudendae externae. Individual branches from the external genitalia. A

3 **Superficial circumflex iliac vein.** V. circumflexa iliaca superficialis. Subcutaneous companion vein of the superficial circumflex iliac artery. A

4 **Superficial epigastric vein.** V. epigastrica superficialis. Subcutaneous companion vein of the superficial epigastric artery. A

5 **Superficial dorsal veins of penis/clitoris.** Vv. dorsales superficiales penis/clitoridis. Paired epifascial veins of the penis (clitoris) with drainage into the femoral vein or external pudendal veins. They run between the superficial and deep fasciae of the penis. A. See also 165 B

6 **Anterior scrotal/labial veins.** Vv. scrotales/labiales anteriores. Arising from the scrotum or labia majora, they open into the femoral vein or the external pudendal veins. A

7 **Great saphenous vein.** V. saphena magna. Beginning at the medial side of the foot and ascending medially, this vein is provided with valves and receives most of the medial superficial cutaneous veins. It drains into the femoral vein via the saphenous opening. A B C D

8 **Accessory saphenous vein.** V. saphena accessoria. Anastomotic branch occasionally present from the small saphenous vein to great saphenous vein. Among its variants it receives blood from the thigh except for the deep and lateral regions. It runs parallel at times to the great saphenous vein before entering the latter. A

9 **Accompanying vein of the profunda femoris artery.** V. profunda femoris. A

10 Medial circumflex femoral veins. Vv. circumflexae mediales femorales. Companion veins of the same-named artery. A

11 Lateral circumflex femoral veins. Vv. circumflexae laterales femorales. Companion veins of the same-named artery. A

12 Perforating veins. Vv. perforantes. Arising from the ischiocrural musculature, they penetrate the adductors and open into the profunda femoris vein. A

13 **Popliteal vein.** V. poplitea. Lying between the popliteal artery and tibial nerve, it extends from the union of the anterior and posterior tibial veins to the hiatus tendineus of the adductor canal. C

13a **Sural veins.** Venae surales. Companion veins of the same-named artery.

14 **Genicular veins.** Vv. geniculares. Usually five veins coming from the knee. A

15 **Small saphenous vein.** V. saphena parva. It comes from the lateral margin of the foot, passes along the posterior side of the lower leg and drains into the popliteal vein. A B C D

16 **Anterior tibial veins.** Vv. tibiales anteriores. Companion veins of anterior tibial artery. A B C

17 Dorsal venous network of foot. Rete venosum dorsale pedis. Venous plexus on dorsum of foot with drainage into the great and small saphenous veins and into the anterior tibial veins. B

18 Dorsal venous arch of foot. Arcus venosus dorsalis pedis. Venous arch on dorsum of foot receiving the dorsal metatarsal veins of the foot. It also represents the main outlet for blood from the sole of the foot. B C D

19 Dorsal digital veins of foot. Vv. digitales dorsales pedis. Veins on the dorsum of the toes. B

20 Dorsal metatarsal veins. Vv. metatarsales dorsales. Companion veins of same-named arteries. They arise from the dorsal digital veins of the foot. B D

21 **Posterior tibial veins.** Vv. tibiales posteriores. Veins accompanying the posterior tibial artery. C

22 Peroneal (fibular) veins. Vv. fibulares. Companion veins of the peroneal artery found partly beneath the flexor hallucis longus. C

23 Plantar venous network. Rete venosum plantare. Dense subcutaneous network of veins at the sole of the foot. C

24 Plantar venous arch. Arcus venosus plantaris. Venous arch accompanying the arterial plantar arch. C

25 Plantar metatarsal veins. Vv. metatarsales plantares. Veins accompanying the same named arteries. C

26 Plantar digital veins. Vv. digitales plantares. Veins on the flexor side of the toes. C

26a Intercapitular veins. Vv. intercapitulares. Anastomotic branches between the plantar and dorsal venous arches. D

26b Lateral marginal vein. V. marginalis lateralis. Anastomotic vein as in 26a. It drains into the small saphenous vein. D

26c Medial marginal vein. V. marginalis medialis. Anastomotic vein as in 26a. It drains into the great saphenous vein. D

27 Perforating veins. Vv. perforantes. Anastomoses between cutaneous and subfascial veins especially at the lower leg. Their valves prevent the flow of blood from the deep veins to the epifascial veins

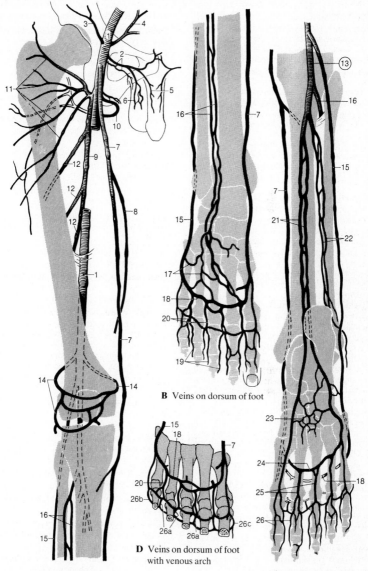

A Veins of lower limb,
anterior view

B Veins on dorsum of foot

D Veins on dorsum of foot
with venous arch

C Veins of leg and sole of foot

1 LYMPHATIC SYSTEM. SYSTEMA LYM-PHATICUM.

2 **Lymphatic vessels.** Vasa lymphatica.

3 **Lymphatic capillary.** Vas lymphocapillare. It ends blindly and its wall is quite permeable. C

4 **Lymphatic capillary network.** Rete lymphocapillare. Network of lymphatic capillaries near its beginning. C

5 **Lymphatic vessel.** Vas lymphaticum. It is continuous with the lymphatic capillaries and is provided with numerous valves. Its wall is quite thin and contains sparse smooth muscle. C

6 Lymphatic plexus. Plexus lymphaticus. Network of lymphatic vessels. It lies deeper than the lymphatic capillaries, e.g., in the skin it resides in the dermis and directly beneath it. C

7 **Superficial lymphatic vessel.** Vas lymphaticum superficiale. It is situated superficially on the fascia of the limbs.

8 **Deep lymphatic vessel.** Vas lymphaticum profundum. It lies beneath the fascia of the limbs and often, but not always, accompanies blood vessels.

9 **Lymphatic trunks.** Trunci lymphatici. Five main lymphatic branches of the lymphatic vascular system.

10 **Right/left lumbar trunk.** Truncus lumbaris dexter/sinister. Main branch which brings lymph to the cisterna chyli from the lower limb, pelvic viscera, urogenital system and from parts of the abdominal wall, as well as the abdominal viscera. B

11 **Intestinal trunks.** Trunci intestinales. Main conduits which transport lymph to the cisterna chyli from the supply region of the superior and inferior mesenteric arteries. B

12 **Right/left bronchomediastinal trunk.** Truncus bronchomediastinalis dexter/sinistra. It collects lymph from the heart, lungs and mediastinum. On the left side it opens into the thoracic duct, on the right side, the right lymphatic duct. Often, however, both may open directly into the subclavian veins. B

13 **Right/left subclavian trunk.** Truncus subclavius dexter/sinister. Exiting from the arm, it runs in company with the subclavian vein and usually opens on the right side into the right lymphatic duct, and on the left side into the angle between the left subclavian vein and internal jugular vein. B

14 **Right/left jugular trunk.** Truncus jugularis dexter/sinister. In company with the internal jugular vein, it passes to the angle between the internal jugular and subclavian veins (venous angle). B

15 **Lymphatic ducts.** Ductus lymphatici. The main excretory ducts of the lymphatic system.

16 **Right lymphatic duct (right thoracic duct).** Ductus lymphaticus dexter (Ductus thoracicus dexter). It is formed by the union of the right jugular, subclavian and bronchomediastinal trunks. It can be absent. B

17 **Thoracic duct.** Ductus thoracicus. Arising from the cisterna chyli a short distance below the diaphragm, it courses upward behind the aorta and opens into the venous angle, i.e., the angle between the left internal jugular and subclavian veins. B

18 Arch of thoracic duct. Arcus ductus thoracici. Arch formed by the thoracic duct before entering the venous angle. B

19 Cervical part. Pars cervicalis. Short cervical segment in front of C7. B

20 Thoracic part. Pars thoracica. It begins at the aortic hiatus and ends at the upper margin of T1. B

21 Abdominal part. Pars abdominalis. Very short segment in front of L1. B

22 **Cisterna chyli.** Not quite constant dilatation at the origin of the thoracic duct. It receives the lumbar and intestinal trunks. B

23 **Lymph node.** Nodus lymphaticus (Lymphonodus). Lymphoreticular filtering organ, 1–25 mm in diameter, inserted into the lymphatic vessels. Since lymph must usually traverse two lymph nodes before arriving in the blood stream at the venous angle, a double security exists against an invasion of pathogens or tumor cells into the blood stream. A

24 **Afferent lymphatic vessel.** Vas lymphaticum afferens. It enters the lymph node along its convex surface. A

25 **Efferent lymphatic vessel.** Vas lymphaticum efferens. It leaves the lymph node at the hilum. A

26 **Cortex.** Part of the lymphoreticular tissue beneath the capsule. A

27 **Medulla.** Lymphoreticular tissue between cortex and hilum. A

28 **Hilum.** Somewhat retracted area where blood
~ vessels enter and exit and lymphatic vessels leave. A

29 **Lymphatic nodule.** Nodulus lymphaticus
~ (lymphonodulus). Spherical condensation of lymphoreticular tissue predominantly occupying the cortex. It exhibits a lighter central area ("reaction center"). C

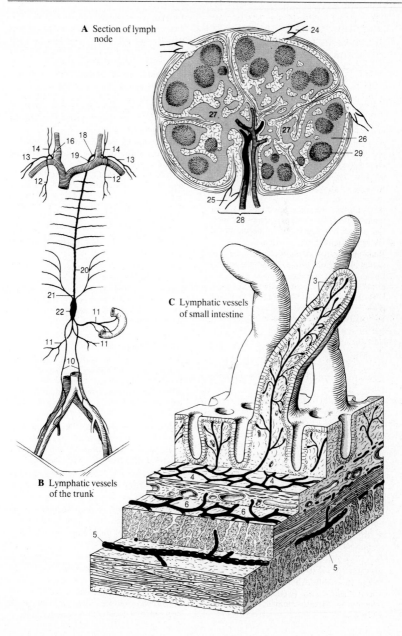

A Section of lymph node

B Lymphatic vessels of the trunk

C Lymphatic vessels of small intestine

1   REGIONAL LYMPH NODES. NODI LYM-
PHATICI REGIONALES.

2   HEAD AND NECK. CAPUT ET COLLUM.

3   **Occipital lymph nodes.** Nodi lymphatici occipitales. One to three lymph nodes lying close
to the margin of the trapezius. Afferent region:
scalp of occipital area. Efferents: deep cervical
lymph nodes. A

4   **Mastoid [retro-auricular] lymph nodes.**
Nodi lymphatici mastoidei [[retro-auricu-
lares]]. Usually 2 nodes on the mastoid process.
Afferent regions: posterior surface of pinna,
posterior wall of external acoustic meatus and
corresponding parts of scalp. Efferents: deep
cervical lymph nodes. A

5   **Superficial parotid lymph nodes.** Nodi lymphatici parotidei superficiales. They lie on the
parotid fascia in front of the tragus. Afferent
regions: junction of temporal region and anterior surface of pinna. Efferents: deep cervical
lymph nodes. A

6   **Deep parotid lymph nodes.** Nodi lymphatici
parotidei profundi. Group beneath the parotid
fascia. Afferent regions: tympanic cavity, external acoustic meatus, frontotemporal region,
eyelids, root of nose, eventually also the
posterior floor of the nose and nasopharyngeal
cavity. Efferents: deep cervical lymph nodes. A

7   Preauricular lymph nodes. Nodi lymphatici prae-auriculares. Group located in front of
the pinna. A

8   Infra-auricular lymph nodes. Nodi lymphatici infra-auriculares. Group beneath the
pinna. A

9   Intraglandular lymph nodes. Nodi lymphatici intraglandulares. Group situated directly within the parotid. A

10 **Facial lymph nodes.** Nody lymphatici faciales. Individually inconstant, they receive their
lymph from the eyelids, nose and the rest of the
face and buccal mucosa. Efferents: submandibular lymph nodes. The vessels accompany
the facial artery.

11 Buccinator node. [Nodus buccinatorius].
~   Lymph node situated deeply on the buccinator
muscle. A

12 Nasolabial node. [Nodus nasolabialis].
Lymph node located below the nasolabial fold.
A

13 Malar node. [Nodus malaris]. Lymph node
lying superficially on the cheek.

14 Mandibular node. [Nodus mandibularis].
Lymph node located externally on the mandible. A

14a **Lingual lymph nodes.** Nodi lymphatici linguales. They lie externally on the hyoglossus
muscle. Afferent regions: lower surface and
lateral margin of tongue as well as the medial
anterior two-thirds of its dorsal surface.

15 **Submental lymph nodes.** Nodi lymphatici
submentales. They lie between the anterior bellies of the digastric muscles. Afferent regions:
middle of lower lip, floor of mouth and tip of
tongue. Efferents: deep cervical and submental
lymph nodes. B

16 **Submandibular lymph nodes.** Nodi lymphatici submandibulares. They lie between the
mandible and submandibular gland and are
both first and second filter stations. Direct afferent area: inner canthus of eye, cheek, side of
nose, upper lip, lateral lower lip, gingiva and
anterior lateral margin of tongue. Indirect
afferents: facial and submental lymph nodes.
Efferents: deep cervical lymph nodes. B

17 **Anterior cervical lymph nodes.** Nodi lymphatici cervicales anteriores.

18 Superficial (anterior jugular) lymph
nodes. Nodi lymphatici superficiales (jug-
ulares anteriores). They lie on the internal
jugular vein. Afferent region: skin of anterior
side of neck. Efferents: bilateral deep cervical
lymph nodes. A

19 Deep lymph nodes. Nodi lymphatici profundi. Anterior group.

19a *Infrahyoid lymph nodes.* Nodi lymphatici infrahyoidei. They lie in the midline below the
body of the hyoid bone. Afferent areas: laryngeal vestibule, piriform recess and adjacent hy-
popharynx. Efferents: deep cervical lymph
nodes. B

20 *Prelaryngeal lymph nodes.* Nodi lymphatici
praelaryngeales[3]. They lie on the cricothyroid
ligament. Afferent area: lower half of larynx.
Efferents: deep cervical lymph nodes. B

21 *Thyroid lymph nodes.* Nodi lymphatici thyro-
idei. They lie on the thyroid gland. Efferents: as
in 20. B

22 *Pretracheal lymph nodes.* Nodi lymphatici
pretracheales. They lie in front of the trachea.
Afferent regions: trachea and larynx. Efferents: deep cervical lymph nodes. B

23 *Paratracheal lymph nodes.* Nodi lymphatici
paratracheales. They lie beside the trachea. Details as in 22. B

23a *Retropharyngeal lymph nodes.* Nodi lymphatici retropharyngeales. Deep cervical lymph
nodes in front of the arch of the atlas. 258.13

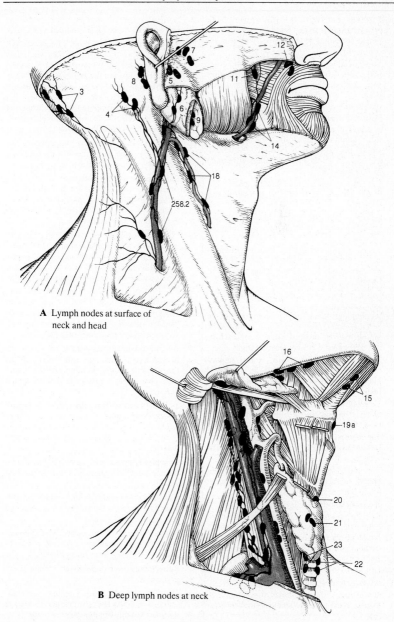

A Lymph nodes at surface of
neck and head

B Deep lymph nodes at neck

1 **Lateral cervical lymph nodes.** Nodi lymphatici cervicales laterales. Groups of lymph nodes lateral to the neck with the following divisions:

2 **Superficial lymph nodes.** Nodi lymphatici superficiales. They lie on the external jugular vein. Afferent regions: lower pinna and area below the parotid. Efferents: deep cervical lymph nodes. 257 A

3 **Superior deep lymph nodes.** Nodi lymphatici profundi superiores. They form the second filter station for almost all of the head lymph nodes but also receive direct peripheral tributaries from their surroundings. Efferents: jugular trunk. A

4 Lateral lymph nodes. Nodi lymphatici laterales. They lie lateral to the internal jugular vein. A

5 Anterior lymph nodes. Nodi lymphatici anteriores. Group in front of the internal jugular vein. A

6 Jugulodigastric node. Nodus jugulodigastricus. It is the most cranial of the deep cervical nodes and is palpable when the tonsil, tongue or pharynx is inflamed. A

7 **Inferior deep cervical lymph nodes.** Nodi lymphatici profundi inferiores. They form the second filter station for the lymph nodes of the cervical viscera and the last filter station for the lymph nodes of the head. They also receive direct tributaries. Efferents: jugular trunk.

8 Jugulo-omohyoid node. Nodus jugulo-omohyoideus. It lies between the omohyoid muscle and internal jugular vein. Afferent area: tongue. A

9 *Lateral lymphatic nodes.* Nodi lymphatici laterales. They lie lateral to the internal jugular vein. A

10 **Anterior lymph nodes.** Nodi lymphatici anteriores. Group in front of the internal jugular vein. A

11 Supraclavicular lymph nodes. Nodi lymphatici supraclaviculares. Nodes of the same group lying above the clavicle. A

12 **Accessory nodes.** Nodi accessorii.

13 Retropharyngeal lymph nodes. Nodi lymphatici retropharyngeales. Deep cervical lymph nodes at the level of the lateral mass of the atlas and at the lateral margin of the longus capitis muscle. A B

14 UPPER LIMB. MEMBRUM SUPERIUS.

15 **Axillary lymphatic plexus.** Plexus lymphaticus axillaris. Netlike connections of 20–30 axillary lymph nodes via their lymphatic vessels. C

16 **Axillary lymph nodes.** Nodi lymphatici axillares. They occupy the axilla. C

17 **Apical lymph nodes.** Nodi lymphatici apicales. Lying medial to the axillary vein, they extend from the upper margin of the pectoralis minor to the apex of the axilla. Afferent areas: upper lateral part of the breast and all remaining axillary lymph nodes. Efferents: on the left as the subclavian trunk to the thoracic duct or subclavian vein. On the right into the vein directly or after joining the jugular trunk. C

18 **Brachial lymph nodes.** Nodi lymphatici brachiales. They lie along the axillary artery for lymph drainage from the arm. C

19 **Subscapular lymph nodes.** Nodi lymphatici subscapulares. They are found alongside the subscapular artery for lymph drainage from the posterior thorax and shoulder, as well as from the lower nuchal region. C

20 **Pectoral lymph nodes.** Nodi lymphatici pectorales. Located at the lower margin of the pectoralis minor, they drain lymph from the anterior and lateral wall of the trunk as far as the navel, as well as the central and lateral part of the breast. C

21 **Central lymph nodes.** Nodi lymphatici centrales. Occupying the fat of the axilla, they are the filter stations for lymph from the brachial, subscapular and pectoral lymph nodes. C

22 **Interpectoral lymph nodes.** Nodi lymphatici interpectorales. Small group situated between the pectoralis major and minor. Afferent area: mammary gland. Efferents: apical lymph nodes. C

23 **Deltopectoral (infraclavicular) lymph nodes.** Nodi lymphatici deltopectorales (infraclaviculares). Located on the cephalic vein in the deltopectoral groove, receiving lymph from the arm. C

24 **Brachial lymph nodes.** Nodi lymphatici brachiales. Single lymph nodes along the brachial vessels.

25 **Cubital lymph nodes.** Nodi lymphatici cubitales. One to two lymph nodes on the brachial artery in the cubital fossa. C

26 **Supratrochlear lymph nodes.** Nodi lymphatici supratrochlearis. They lie medial to the basilic vein and above the elbow joint. C

27 **Superficial lymph nodes.** Nodi lymphatici superficiales.

28 **Deep lymph nodes.** Nodi lymphatici profundi. Individual lymph nodes which are inserted in the course of the deep lymphatic vessels.

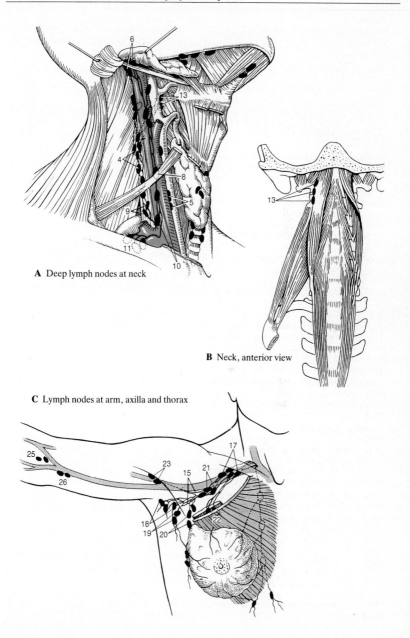

A Deep lymph nodes at neck

B Neck, anterior view

C Lymph nodes at arm, axilla and thorax

1 **THORAX.**

2 **PARAMAMMARY LYMPH NODES.** Nodi lymphatici paramammarii. Lymph nodes at the lateral margin of the mammary gland. A

3 **Parasternal lymph nodes.** Nodi lymphatici parasternales. They lie in the thorax along the internal thoracic vessels. Afferent regions: mammary gland, intercostal spaces, part of the liver and diaphragm. Efferents: either directly into the respective subclavian vein or internal jugular vein or into the thoracic duct or subclavian trunk. A

4 **Intercostal lymph nodes.** Nodi lymphatici intercostales. They lie in the paravertebral portion of the intercostal spaces. Afferent area: pleura and intercostal spaces. D

5 **Paravertebral lymph nodes.** Nodi lymphatici praevertebrales.[3] They lie between the esophagus and vertebral column. Afferent regions: surroundings, if not drained by others. C D

6 **Superior phrenic lymph nodes.** Nodi lymphatici phrenici superiores. They lie behind the cartilage-bone boundary of the 7th rib at the aortic opening in the diaphragm and at the inferior vena cava. Afferent areas: liver and diaphragm. D

7 **Prepericardial lymph nodes.** Nodi lymphatici prepericardiales. They are located between the sternum and pericardium. Afferent regions: sternum and anterior pericardium. Efferents: parasternal lymph nodes. B

8 **Lateral pericardial lymph nodes.** Nodi lymphatici pericardiales laterales. They are found between the pericardium and mediastinal pleura. B

9 **Anterior mediastinal lymph nodes.** Nodi lymphatici mediastinales anteriores. They lie at the brachiocephalic veins in front of the arch of the aorta and its branches. Afferent regions: thymus, pericardium and parasternal lymph nodes. Efferents: bronchomediastinal trunk. B

10 **Ligamentum arteriosum node.** [Nodus ligamenti arteriosi]. Inconstant. B

11 **Posterior mediastinal lymph nodes.** Nodi lymphatici mediastinales posteriores. Situated in the superior and posterior mediastinum, they receive lymph from the following organs: lungs, bronchi, trachea, esophagus, pericardium, diaphragm and diaphragmatic surface of the liver. Efferents: partly into the thoracic duct, partly into the bronchomediastinal duct. The following individual groups can be distinguished:

12 **Pulmonary juxtaesophageal lymph nodes.** Nodi lymphatici juxtaoesophageales pulmonales. Although situated beside the esophagus, they pertain to the lungs. C

13 **Tracheobronchial lymph nodes.** Nodi lymphatici tracheobronchiales. They are located on the bronchi near their entry into the lungs. C

14 **Superior tracheobronchial lymph nodes.** Nodi lymphatici tracheobronchiales superiores. Lymph nodes situated cranially on the stem bronchi and the trachea. C

15 **Inferior tracheobronchial lymph nodes.** Nodi lymphatici tracheobronchiales inferiores. Nodes located caudal to the tracheal bifurcation. C

16 **Paratracheal lymph nodes.** Nodi lymphatici paratracheales. They lie along the trachea. C

17 **Node of arch of azygos vein.** [Nodus arcus venae azygos]. Lymph node occasionally present at the arch which the azygos vein forms around the hilum of the right lung before its entry into the superior vena cava. B

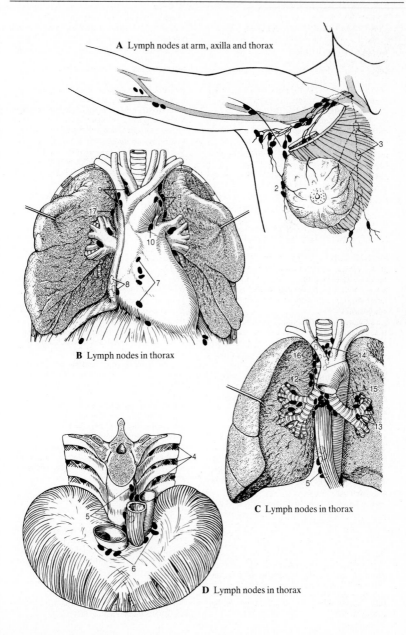

A Lymph nodes at arm, axilla and thorax

B Lymph nodes in thorax

C Lymph nodes in thorax

D Lymph nodes in thorax

1   **ABDOMEN. PARIETAL LYMPH NODES. NODI LYMPHATICI PARIETALES.** Lymph nodes in the abdominal wall.

2   **Left lumbar lymph nodes.** Nodi lymphatici lumbales (lumbares) sinistri. They lie at the abdominal aorta and are primarily second filter stations for lymph nodes located further below, and secondarily, first filter stations for the suprarenal gland, kidney, ureter, testis, ovary, uterine tubes, fundus of uterus and abdominal wall. Efferents: primarily into the lumbar trunk. Individually, the following three groups can be distinguished:

3   **Lateral aortic lymph nodes.** Nodi lymphatici aortici laterales. They lie on the left side of the aorta. A

4   **Pre-aortic lymph nodes.** Nodi lymphatici pre-aortici. They lie in front of the aorta. A

5   **Postaortic lymph nodes.** Nodi lymphatici postaortici. This group lies between the aorta and vertebral column. A

6   **Intermediate lumbar lymph nodes.** Nodi lymphatici lumbales (lumbares) intermedii. They lie between the aorta and inferior vena cava. They function as in 2A

7   **Right lumbar lymph nodes.** Nodi lymphatici lumbales (lumbares) dextri. They lie around the inferior vena cava and have the same function on their side as 2. Individually, the following groups can be identified:

8   Lateral caval lymph nodes. Nodi lymphatici cavales laterales. They lie on the right side of the inferior vena cava. A

9   Precaval lymph nodes. Nodi lymphatici precavales. They lie in front of the vena cava. A

10 Postcaval lymph nodes. Nodi lymphatici postcavales. They lie behind the vena cava. A

11 **Inferior phrenic lymph nodes.** Nodi lymphatici phrenici inferiores. They are situated at the inferior surface of the diaphragm near the aortic opening. A C

12 **Inferior epigastric lymph nodes.** Nodi lympha-
~   tici epigastrici inferiores. Three or four nodes at the inferior epigastric artery for its supply area. B

13 VISCERAL NODES. ABDOMEN – NODI LYMPHATICI VISCERALES. Lymph nodes of the abdominal viscera.

14 **Celiac lymph nodes.** Nodi lymphatici coeliaci. Lying around the celiac trunk, they form the second filter station for the stomach, duodenum, liver, gallbladder, pancreas and spleen. Efferents: some form the intestinal trunk, some pass directly into the cisterna chyli. A C

15 **Gastric lymph nodes [right and left].** Nodi lymphatici gastrici [dextri/sinistri]. Residing at the lesser curvature of the stomach, they follow the course of the right and left gastric arteries. Afferent region: stomach. Efferents: celiac lymph nodes. C

16 **[Anulus lymphaticus cardiae].** Lymphatic ring occasionally present around the cardia of the stomach. C

17 **Gastro-omental lymph nodes [right and left].**
~   Nodi lymphatici gastro-omentales [dextri/sinistri]. Located along the course of the right and left gastro-omental arteries at the greater curvature of the stomach, their afferents receive lymph from the stomach and the greater omentum and their efferents convey it, on the right side to the lymph nodes of the liver, and on the left side to the lymph nodes of the spleen and pancreas. C

18 **Pyloric lymph nodes.** Nodi lymphatici pylorici. Situated around the pylorus, their efferents drain into the hepatic or celiac lymph nodes.

19 Suprapyloric node. [Nodus suprapyloricus]. It lies above the pylorus. C

20 Subpyloric nodes. [Nodi subpylorici]. They lie caudal to the pylorus. C

21 Retropyloric nodes. [Nodi retropylorici]. Group located dorsal to the pylorus. C

22 **Pancreatic lymph nodes.** Nodi lymphatici pancreatici. Situated at the upper and lower margins of the pancreas, their efferents are conveyed partly into the splenic lymph nodes, partly into the mesenteric lymph nodes and partly into the pancreaticoduodenal lymph nodes.

23 **Superior pancreatic lymph nodes.** Nodi lymphatici pancreatici superiores. Group located at the upper margin of the pancreas. A C

24 **Inferior pancreatic lymph nodes.** Nodi lymphatici pancreatici inferiores. Group located at the lower margin of the pancreas. A C

25 **Splenic (lienal) lymph nodes.** Nodi lymphatici splenici (lienales). These lie at the hilum of the spleen and convey their lymph to celiac lymph nodes. A C

26 **Pancreaticoduodenal lymph nodes.** Nodi lymphatici pancreaticoduodenales. Small nodes between the pancreas and duodenum. Afferent regions: duodenum and pancreas.

27 Superior pancreaticoduodenal lymph nodes. Nodi lymphatici pancreaticoduodenales superiores. Cranially situated group. Efferents: hepatic nodes. C

28 Inferior pancreaticoduodenal lymph nodes. Nodi lymphatici pancreaticoduodenales inferiores. Caudal group. Efferents: mesenteric lymph nodes. C

29 **Hepatic lymph nodes.** Nodi lymphatici hepatici. They lie at the hilum of the liver, partly in the hepatoduodenal ligament. Their lymph is taken partly from the liver, partly from adjacent lymph nodes and transported to the celiac lymph nodes.

30 Cystic node. Nodus cysticus. Larger lymph node at the neck of the gallbladder. C

31 Foraminal node. Nodus foraminalis. Larger lymph node at the epiploic foramen. C

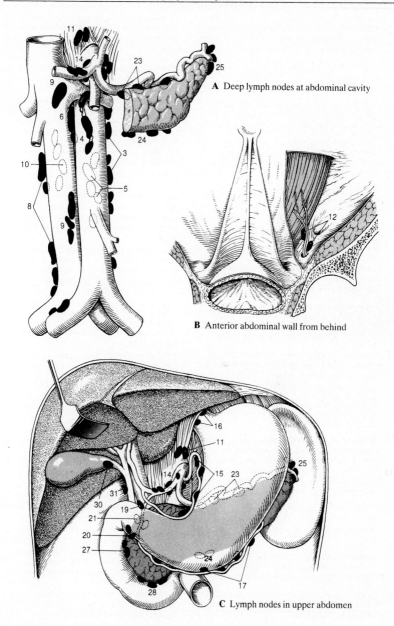

A Deep lymph nodes at abdominal cavity

B Anterior abdominal wall from behind

C Lymph nodes in upper abdomen

1 **Mesenteric lymph nodes.** Nodi lymphatici mesenterici. Numerous (100–150) lymph nodes important for the prevention of lipidemia, among other functions. Efferents: via celiac lymph nodes.

2 Juxtaintestinal lymph nodes. Nodi lymphatici juxtaintestinales. Portion of this group located close to the small intestine.

3 Superior [central] lymph nodes. Nodi lym-
~ phatici superiores [centrales]. Portion of this group lying at the stem of the superior mesenteric artery. A

4 **Ileocolic lymph nodes.** Nodi lymphatici ileocolici. Group of nodes situated along the ileocolic artery. Efferents: celiac lymph nodes. A

5 **Prececal lymph nodes.** Nodi lymphatici precaecales. Nodes lying along the anterior cecal artery. A

6 **Retrocecal lymph nodes.** Nodi lymphatici retrocaecales. They reside along the posterior cecal artery. A

7 **Appendicular lymph nodes.** Nodi lymphatici appendiculares. They lie at the appendicular artery. They may be absent (33–50%). A

8 **Mesocolic lymph nodes.** Nodi lymphatici mesocolici. Nodes for the greatest part of the colon. Predominantly located in the mesocolon, their efferents convey lymph to the celiac lymph nodes.

9 Paracolic lymph nodes. Nodi lymphatici paracolici. Portion of this group located at the colon. A

10 Right/middle/left colic lymph nodes. Nodi lymphatici colici [dextri/medii/sinistri]. Portion of this group situated at the stems of the right, middle and left colic arteries. A

11 **Inferior mesenteric lymph nodes.** Nodi lymphatici mesenterici inferiores. They are located at the inferior mesenteric artery. Afferent areas: part of descending colon, sigmoid and part of rectum. Efferents: pre-aortic lymph nodes at the level of the inferior mesenteric artery. A

12 Sigmoid lymph nodes. Nodi lymphatici sigmoidei. Located along the sigmoid artery, they drain the sigmoid and the adjoining segment of colon. A

13 Superior rectal lymph nodes. Nodi lymphatici rectales superiores. Nodes located at the superior rectal artery for drainage of the rectum. A

14 PARIETAL NODES OF PELVIS. PELVIS – NODI LYMPHATICI PARIETALES. Lymph nodes along wall of pelvis.

15 **Common iliac lymph nodes.** Nodi lymphatici iliaci communes. Group situated at the internal iliac vein. They serve as the second station for the lymph nodes of the pelvic organs, (= pelvic), interior pelvic wall, abdominal wall up to the navel, hip muscles, and gluteal muscles. Efferents: lumbar lymph nodes and lumbar trunk. Individually, the following subgroups are distinguished:

16 Medial common iliac lymph nodes. Nodi lymphatici iliaci communes mediales. Group situated medial to the vascular cord. B

17 Intermediate common iliac lymph nodes. Nodi lymphatici iliaci communes intermedii. Lymph nodes situated between the medial and lateral groups behind the vascular cord. B

18 Lateral common iliac lymph nodes. Nodi lymphatici iliaci communes laterales. Group located lateral to the vascular cord. B

19 Subaortic common iliac lymph nodes. Nodi lymphatici iliaci communes subaortici. They are located caudal to the aortic bifurcation in front of L4. B

20 Promontory common iliac lymph nodes. Nodi lymphatici iliaci communes promontorii. Group situated in front of the promontory. B

21 **External iliac lymph nodes.** Nodi lymphatici iliaci externi. Located on the external iliac vessels, they are the first lymph station for a part of the urinary bladder and vagina, and second lymph station for the inguinal lymph nodes. Efferents: common iliac lymph nodes. The following portions are distinguished:

22 Medial external iliac lymph nodes. Nodi lymphatici iliaci externi mediales. They are located medial to the vascular cord. B

23 Intermediate external iliac lymph nodes. Nodi lymphatici iliaci externi intermedii. Portion located between the lateral and medial groups and behind the artery. B

24 Lateral external iliac lymph nodes. Nodi lymphatici iliaci externi laterales. Portion lying lateral to the vascular bundle. B

25 Medial lacunar node. [Nodus lacunaris medialis]. It lies in the vascular lacuna medial to the vascular cord. B

26 Intermediate lacunar node. [Nodus lacunaris intermedius]. When present, it lies in the middle of the vascular lacuna. B

27 Lateral lacunar node. [Nodus lacunaris lateralis]. It lies laterally in the vascular lacuna. B

28 Interiliac external iliac lymph nodes. Nodi lymphatici iliaci externi interiliaci. Lymph nodes in the bifurcation between the internal and external iliac arteries. B

29 Obturator external iliac lymph nodes. Nodi lymphatici iliaci externi obturatorii. Portion located at the obturator artery. B

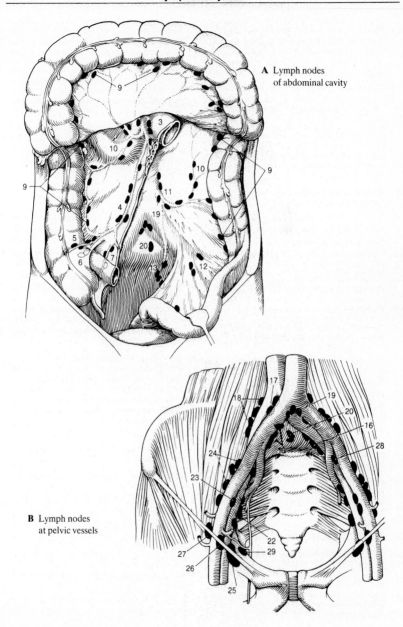

A Lymph nodes of abdominal cavity

B Lymph nodes at pelvic vessels

1 **Internal iliac lymph nodes.** Nodi lymphatici iliaci interni. Located at the internal iliac artery, they drain the pelvic organs, the deep perineal region and both the external and internal walls of the pelvis. Their efferents communicate with the common iliac lymph nodes.

2 Superior gluteal lymph nodes. Nodi lymphatici gluteales superiores. Nodes for the pelvic wall located at the superior gluteal artery. A

3 Inferior gluteal lymph nodes. Nodi lymphatici gluteales inferiores. Nodes for the prostate and proximal urethra are situated at the inferior gluteal artery. A

4 Sacral lymph nodes. Nodi lymphatici sacrales. Nodes for the prostate and cervix found at the sacrum. A

5 VISCERAL NODES OF PELVIS. PELVIS – NODI LYMPHATICI VISCERALES.

6 **Perivesicular lymph nodes.** Nodi lymphatici paravesiculares. Nodes for the urinary bladder and partly also for the prostate located at the bladder. A

7 Prevesicular lymph nodes. Nodi lymphatici prevesiculares. Subgroup located between the urinary bladder and symphysis. A

8 Postvesicular lymph nodes. Nodi lymphatici postvesiculares. Subgroup behind the urinary bladder. A

9 Lateral vesicular lymph nodes. Nodi lymphatici vesiculares laterales. Nodes situated at the lower end of the medial – formerly lateral – umbilical ligament. A

10 **Parauterine lymph nodes.** Nodi lymphatici parauterini. Nodes for the cervix uteri situated beside the uterus. A

11 **Paravaginal lymph nodes.** Nodi lymphatici paravaginales. Located beside the vagina, they drain part of this organ. A

12 **Pararectal (anorectal) lymph nodes.** Nodi lymphatici pararectales (anorectales). Located laterally directly on the musculature of the rectum, they drain this organ and a part of the vagina. A

13 LOWER LIMB. MEMBRUM INFERIUS.

14 **Superficial inguinal lymph nodes.** Nodi lymphatici inguinales superficiales. Group of nodes located in the subcutaneous adipose tissue, thus on the fascia lata and draining the anus, perineum, external genitalia, abdominal wall and surface of the leg. Efferents: external iliac lymph node.

15 Superomedial superficial inguinal lymph nodes. Nodi lymphatici inguinales superficiales superomediales. Medial portion of group located along the inguinal ligament. B

16 Superolateral superficial inguinal lymph nodes. Nodi lymphatici inguinales superficiales superolaterales. Lateral portion of group located below the inguinal ligament. B

17 Inferior superficial inguinal lymph nodes. Nodi lymphatici inguinales superficiales inferiores. Group arranged along a vertical line at the proximal end of the great saphenous vein. They drain the superficial lymphatic vessels of the leg. B

18 **Deep inguinal lymph nodes.** Nodi lymphatici inguinales profundi. Positioned below the fascia lata at the level of the saphenous hiatus, the uppermost can be especially large and occupy the femoral canal (Rosenmüller's node). Afferent region: deep lymphatic vessels of the leg. Efferents: external iliac lymph nodes. B

19 **Superficial popliteal lymph nodes.** Nodi
~ lymphatici popliteales superficiales. They lie at the proximal end of the small saphenous vein and receive lymph from the lateral margin of the foot and calf. Their efferents pass anteriorly through the hiatus tendineus into the deep inguinal lymph nodes. C

20 **Deep popliteal lymph nodes.** Nodi lymphatici popliteales profundi. Situated between the knee joint capsule and the popliteal artery, they receive lymph from the posterior side of the lower leg and their efferents convey it anteriorly through the hiatus tendineus to the deep inguinal lymph nodes. C

21 **Anterior tibial node.** [Nodus tibialis anterior]. Lymph node occasionally present at the anterior tibial artery.

22 **Posterior tibial node.** [Nodus tibialis posterior]. Lymph node occasionally present at the posterior tibial artery.

23 **Fibular node.** [Nodus fibularis]. Lymph node occasionally present at the peroneal (fibular) artery.

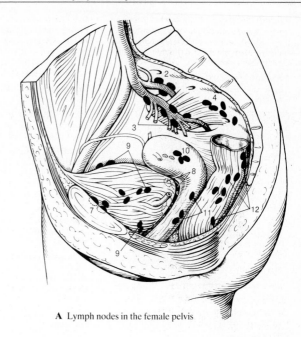

A Lymph nodes in the female pelvis

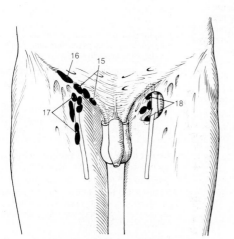

B Lymph nodes in the inguinal region

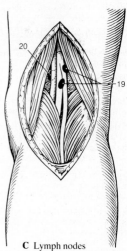

C Lymph nodes
in the popliteal fossa

1 SPLEEN. Splen (lien). Lymphoreticular organ inserted into the circulatory system. Functions: phagocytosis and destruction of red blood cells, lymphopoiesis, blood filtration and synthesis of antibodies. A B

2 **Accessory spleen.** [Splen accessorius]. Small islands of splenic tissue mostly in the greater omentum or gastrosplenic ligament.

3 **Diaphragmatic surface.** Facies diaphragmatica. Convex surface facing the diaphragm.

4 **Visceral surface.** Facies visceralis. Concave surface facing the viscera. A

5 Renal surface. Facies renalis. Lower surface in contact with the kidney. A

6 Gastric surface. Facies gastrica. Upper surface in contact with the stomach. A

7 Colic surface. Facies colica. Surface in contact with the colon. A

8 **Posterior end.** Extremitas posterior. A

9 **Anterior end.** Extremitas anterior. A

10 **Upper margin.** Margo superior. Border between gastric and diaphragmatic surfaces. A

11 **Lower margin.** Margo inferior. Border between diaphragmatic and renal surfaces. A

12 **Hilum of spleen.** Hilum splenicum. Entry and exit site of vessels between the gastric and renal surfaces. A

13 **Peritoneal covering.** Tunica serosa. B

14 **Connective tissue capsule of spleen.** Tunica fibrosa. B

15 **Trabeculae of spleen.** Trabeculae splenicae [lienales]. Connective tissue partitions penetrating into the spleen from the hilum and capsule and containing blood vessels. B

16 **Splenic pulp.** Pulpa splenica [lienalis]. It comprises white pulp (lymphoreticular tissue in form of arterial sheaths) and red pulp (venous sinuses with erythrocytes, reticular tissue). B

17 **Splenic sinus.** Sinus splenica [lienalis]. Thin-walled, strongly anastomosing venous spaces situated in the red pulp. B

18 **Splenic [lienal] branches.** Rami splenica [lienales]. Branches formed by the splenic artery before entering the spleen.

19 **Penicilli.** Brush-like arterial branches between the nodular arteries (in white pulp) and capillaries (or "sheathed capillaries"). B

20 **Lymphatic nodules (follicles) of spleen.** Folliculi lymphatici splenici [lienales] (Lymphonoduli splenici). Spherical or cylindrical aggregations of lymphoreticular tissue around an artery (Malpighian corpuscle). They are visible to the naked eye. B

21 NERVOUS SYSTEM. SYSTEMA NERVOSUM.

22 MENINGES. Connective tissue sheaths surrounding the central nervous system: dura mater, arachnoid and pia mater.

23 **Cranial dura mater [[pachymeninx]].** Dura mater cranialis (encephali). Tough fibrous sheet forming a supporting capsule for the brain and at the same time forming the periosteum for the inner aspect of the skull. E

24 **Falx cerebri.** Sickle-shaped part of the dura projecting downward into the longitudinal cerebral fissure. C

25 **Tentorium cerebelli.** Dural sheet spreading out between the ridge of the petrous temporal and the transverse sinus. It supports the occipital lobes. C

26 Tentorial notch. Incisura tentorii. Opening in the tentorium cerebelli for passage of the brainstem. C

27 **Falx cerebelli.** Small, sickle-shaped dural sheet between the right and left cerebellar hemispheres. C

28 **Diaphragma sellae.** Small horizontal sheet of dura spreading out between the clinoid processes above the hypophysis. C

29 **Cavitas trigeminalis (Cavum trigeminale).** Outpocketing of the dura enclosing the trigeminal ganglion. C

30 **Subdural space.** Spatium subdurale. Capillary space between the dura and arachnoid. It can be distended, for example, by a hemorrhage. E

31 Spinal dura mater. Dura mater spinalis. It is separated from the wall of the vertebral canal by an epidural space. D

32 **External filum terminale.** Filum terminale externum (durale). Filamentous end of the dura mater fused with the filum terminale. It extends from S2–3 to Co 2.

33 **Epidural space.** Spatium epidurale (peridurale). Space between the spinal dura mater and the wall of the vertebral canal. It is filled with fat and venous plexuses. D

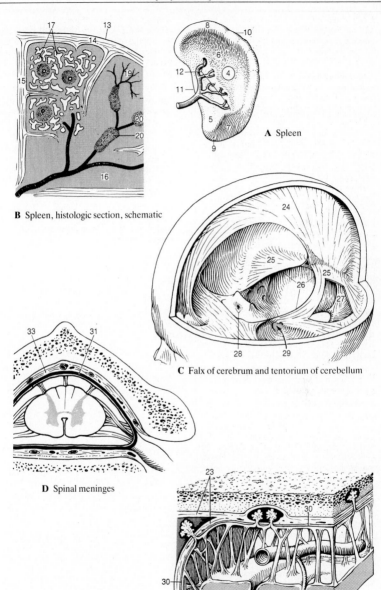

B Spleen, histologic section, schematic

A Spleen

C Falx of cerebrum and tentorium of cerebellum

D Spinal meninges

E Cranial meninges

1   **Cranial arachnoid.** Arachnoidea mater crani-
    alis (encephali). Thin, avascular membrane
    attaching to the cranial dura only by surface ad-
    hesion and communicating with the pia mater
    by connective tissue fibers. D

2   **Subarachnoid space.** Spatium subarachnoi-
    deum. Space between flat portion of arachnoid
    and pia mater. It is filled with arachnoidal
    connective tissue fibers and cerebrospinal
    fluid. D

3   Cerebrospinal fluid. Liquor cerebrospina-
    lis. Protein-poor fluid secreted by the choroid
    plexus with a cell content of 2–6 per mm. It
    flows into the subarachnoid space through
    openings in the fourth ventricle.

4   **Subarachnoid cisterns.** Cisternae sub-
    arachnoideae. Expansions of the subarachnoid
    space containing cerebrospinal fluid.

5   **Cerebellomedullary cistern (cisterna
    magna).** Cisterna cerebellomedullaris
    (magna). Space between the cerebellum and
    medulla oblongata filled with cerebrospinal
    fluid. It communicates with the fourth ventricle
    by a median aperture. It is accessible through
    the foramen magnum. B

6   **Cistern of lateral fossa of cerebrum.** Cister-
    na fossae lateralis cerebri. Space between the
    insula, temporal, frontal and parietal lobes. It is
    filled with cerebrospinal fluid and is accessible
    through the lateral sulcus. It contains branches
    of the middle cerebral and insular arteries. C

7   **Chiasmatic cistern.** Cisterna chiasmatica. En-
    larged space around the optic chiasma filled
    with cerebrospinal fluid. B

8   **Interpeduncular cistern.** Cisterna interpe-
    duncularis. Space situated behind the chias-
    matic cistern and bordered laterally by the tem-
    poral lobe and the cerebral crura. It is filled
    with cerebrospinal fluid and contains the
    oculomotor nerve, branches of the basilar
    artery, the origin of the superior cerebellar
    artery and the posterior cerebral artery. B

9   **Ambient cistern.** Cisterna ambiens. Enlarged
    cerebrospinal fluid-filled space lateral to the
    cerebral crus. It contains the posterior cerebral
    artery, superior cerebellar artery, basal vein
    (Rosenthal's) and the trochlear nerve. F

10 **Cisterna pericallosa.** Space filled with cere-
    brospinal fluid along the corpus callosum. F

11 **Pontocerebellar cistern.** Cisterna pontocere-
    bellaris. Expanded space in the cerebellopon-
    tine angle filled with cerebrospinal fluid. It
    communicates with the 4th ventricle by a
    lateral aperture. E

12 **Arachnoid granulations.** Granulationes
    arachnoideae. Avascular, villous-like evagina-
    tions of the subarachnoid space into the sagit-
    tal sinus and diploic veins. They develop more
    strongly somewhat after the tenth year of life
    and are concerned in the excretion of cerebro-
    spinal fluid. D

13 **Spinal arachnoid.** Arachnoidea mater
    spinalis. Thin avascular membrane attaching
    to the dura mater by surface adhesion and to the
    pia mater by its connective tissue fibers. A

14 **Subarachnoid space.** Spatium subarachnoi-
    deum. Space between the flat part of the arach-
    noid and the pia mater. It is filled with arach-
    noidal connective tissue fibers and cerebrospi-
    nal fluid. A

15 Cerebrospinal fluid. Liquor cerebrospina-
    lis. Fluid secreted predominantly by the cho-
    roid plexus. It is protein-poor with a cell con-
    tent of 2–6 per mm.

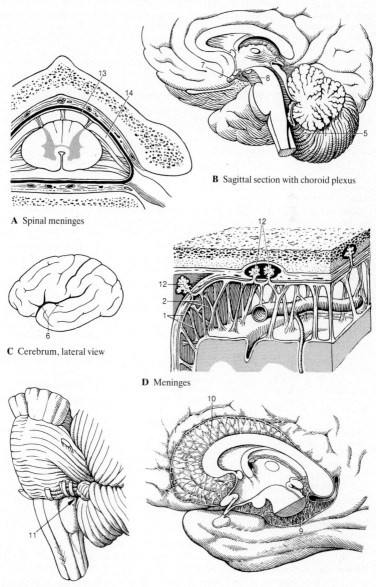

A Spinal meninges

B Sagittal section with choroid plexus

C Cerebrum, lateral view

D Meninges

E Pontocerebellar cistern

F System of cisterns in sagittal plane 7

1 **Cranial pia mater.** Pia mater cranialis (encephali). Delicate meninx bearing blood vessels and intimately covering the surface of the brain as well as extending into its sulci.

2 **Tela choroidea of fourth ventricle.** Tela choroidea ventriculi quarti. Thin membrane of pia mater and ependyma in lower part of roof of fourth ventricle. It is attached laterally to the tenia and exhibits lateral and median apertures. B

3 **Choroid plexus of fourth ventricle.** Plexus choroideus ventriculi quarti. Paired garland-like, ependymal-covered villous projections which extend into both lateral apertures. B

4 Tela choroidea of third ventricle. Tela choroidea ventriculi tertii. Thin, ependymal-covered membrane of pia mater between right and left teniae of thalamus. C

5 **Choroid plexus of third ventricle.** Plexus choroideus ventricul tertii. Paired, heavily vascularized villous formations projecting from the thin roof into the third ventricle and continuing anteriorly through the interventricular foramina into the choroid plexuses of the lateral ventricles. C

6 **Choroid plexus of lateral ventricle.** Plexus choroideus ventriculi lateralis. Villous, strongly vascularized garland invaginated into the lateral ventricle through the choroid fissure. It extends from the interventricular foramen to the inferior horn. C

7 **Choroid glomus.** Glomus choroideum. Enlargement of the choroid plexus in the region of the collateral trigone at the root of the inferior horn. C

8 **Spinal pia mater.** Pia mater spinalis. Vascularized connective tissue membrane firmly united to the surface of the spinal cord. A

9 **Denticulate ligament.** Lig. denticulatum. Frontally-placed connective tissue membrane connecting the spinal cord with the spinal dura mater. It has bow-shaped recesses at the level of the spinal nerve roots. A

10 **Intermediate cervical septum.** Septum cervicale intermedium. Connective tissue partition in the cervical segment of the spinal cord between the gracilis and cuneatus fasciculi extending from the pia mater to the depths of the posterior funiculus. A F

11 **Internal filum terminale.** Filum terminale internum (piale). Filamentous, caudal extension of the spinal cord and pia mater. It is contained in the filum of the spinal dura mater. D E

12 CENTRAL NERVOUS SYSTEM. SYSTEMA NERVOSUM CENTRALE. It comprises the brain and spinal cord.

13 SPINAL CORD. MEDULLA SPINALIS. Consisting of the myelin-rich white matter and the myelin-poor gray matter, it extends from the caudal end of the medulla oblongata, at the exit of the first spinal nerves, to the beginning of the filum terminale at L1–2. A D

14 **Cervical enlargement.** Intumescentia cervicalis. Enlargement of the spinal cord from C3 to T2 owing to the larger supply region for the arms. D

15 **Lumbosacral enlargement.** Intumescentia lumbosacralis. Expansion of the spinal cord from T9–10 to L1–2 caused by the greater supply region for the lower limbs. D

16 **Conus medullaris.** Tapered termination of the spinal cord at the level of L1–2 where it becomes continuous with the filum terminale. D

17 **Filum terminale (spinale):** Thin terminal prolongation of spinal cord attached inferiorly to the posterior surface of the coccyx. D E

18 **Terminal ventricle.** Ventriculus terminalis. Enlargement of the central canal at the end of the conus medullaris. E

19 Anterior median fissure. Fissura mediana anterior. Deep longitudinal fissure along the anterior aspect of the spinal cord. F

20 **Posterior median sulcus.** Sulcus medianus posterior. Median longitudinal groove between the right and left posterior funiculi. F

21 Posterior median septum. Septum medianum posterius. Thickening of the subarachnoid connective tissue within the posterior median sulcus, less in the cervical region, more in the thoracic segment. F

22 **Anterolateral sulcus.** Sulcus anterolateralis. Shallow furrow occasionally present at the exit of the ventral root fibers. F

23 **Posterolateral sulcus.** Sulcus posterolateralis. Longitudinal groove external to the boundary between the lateral and posterior funiculi. It marks the site of entry of the dorsal spinal nerve roots. F

24 **Posterior intermediate sulcus.** Sulcus intermedius posterior. Shallow longitudinal fissure on both sides of the median sulcus. Externally it marks the boundary between the funiculi gracilis and cuneatus. F

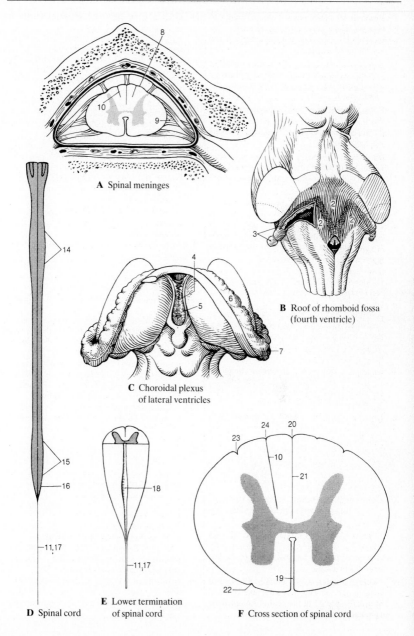

A Spinal meninges

B Roof of rhomboid fossa
(fourth ventricle)

C Choroidal plexus
of lateral ventricles

D Spinal cord

E Lower termination
of spinal cord

F Cross section of spinal cord

1 **Funiculi of spinal cord.** Funiculi medullae spinalis. Three columns of white matter segmented off by the posterior and anterior horns and their root fibers.

2 Anterior funiculus. Funiculus anterior.
~ Conduction bundle located between the anterior median fissure and the anterior horn with its root fibers. A

3 Lateral funiculus. Funiculus lateralis. Conduction bundle located lateral to the gray matter and between the posterior and anterior spinal nerve roots. A

4 Posterior funiculus. Funiculus posterior.
~ Posterior column situated between the posterior horn with its root fibers and the posterior median septum. A

5 **Segments of spinal cord.** Segmenta medullae spinalis. Spinal cord segments are considered here as regions where root fibers pass through a specific intervertebral foramen. The boundaries are not determinable in the isolated spinal cord.

6 Cervical segment. Segmenta cervicalia [1–8] = Pars cervicalis. Eight cervical segments represent the seven cervical vertebrae because the root fibers of segments 1–7 exit above the vertebra of the same number. Root fibers of the 8th cervical segment, on the other hand, exit below C7. The cervical portion of the spinal cord extends from the atlas to the middle of C7. C

7 Thoracic segment. Segmenta thoracica [1–12] = Pars thoracica. The 12 segments comprising this group extend from the middle of C7 to the middle of T11. C

8 Lumbar segment. Segmenta lumbaria [1–5] = Pars lumbaris. Comprised of five segments, it extends from the middle of the body of T11 to the upper border of the body of L1. C

9 Sacral segment. Segmenta sacralia [1–5] = Pars sacralis. These five sacral segments lie posterior to the body of L1. C

10 Coccygeal segment. Segmenta coccygea [1–3] = Pars coccygea. Three quite small segments. C

11 SPINAL CORD SECTIONS. SECTIONES MEDULLAE SPINALIS. These serve mostly as a foundation for the description of the following details.

12 **Central canal.** Canalis centralis. Obliterated remains of the embryonic neural tube lumen. It is usually located in the central intermediate substance (gray matter). A D

13 **Gray matter.** Substantia grisea. Spatially, it forms an H-shaped column (Columna grisea = gray column) consisting primarily of multipolar ganglion cells and enclosed by white matter. Sections of the spinal cord reveal that the "horns" (cornua) which correspond to the gray column S are characteristically different in the individual segments. A

14 **White matter.** Substantia alba. Consisting of myelinated nerves, it is organized into three cords (funiculi) which contain the nerve pathways. A

15 **Substantia gelatinosa centralis,** A narrow zone around the central canal with processes from ependymal cells.

16 GRAY COLUMNS. COLUMNAE GRI-
~ SEAE. Three columns of gray matter projecting ridge-like. B

17 **Anterior column.** Columna anterior. It is formed predominantly of motor neurons (anterior horn cells). B

18 **Anterior horn.** Cornu anterius. Anterior column as exhibited in cross section. D

19 Anterolateral nucleus. Nucleus anterolateralis. Lying anterolaterally in the anterior horn, it is localized in segments C4–8 and L2–S1 and innervates the muscles of the limbs. D

20 Anteromedial nucleus. Nucleus anteromedialis. Lying anteromedially in the anterior horn, it extends the entire length of the spinal cord. D

21 Posterolateral nucleus. Nucleus posterolateralis. It lies posterior to the anterolateral nucleus in segments C5–T1 and L2–S2 and innervates the musculature of the limbs. D

22 Retroposterolateral nucleus. Nucleus retroposterolateralis. It lies posterior to the posterolateral nucleus in segments C8–T1 and S1–3. D

23 Posteromedial nucleus. Nucleus posteromedialis. Located in the vicinity of the white matter, it extends over segments T1–L3 and probably innervates the trunk musculature. D

24 Central nucleus. Nucleus centralis. A less pronounced group in several cervical and lumbar segments. D

25 Nucleus of accessory nerve. Nucleus nervi accessorii (Nuc. accessorius). It lies in segments C1–6 in the area of the anterolateral nucleus and provides the root fibers of the spinal portion of the accessory nerve. D

26 Nucleus of phrenic nerve. Nucleus nervi phrenici (nuc. phrenicus). It lies in the middle of the anterior horn and extends from segments C4–C7. D

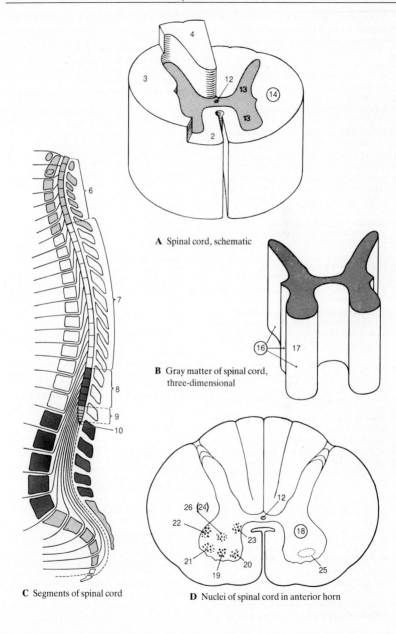

A Spinal cord, schematic

B Gray matter of spinal cord, three-dimensional

C Segments of spinal cord

D Nuclei of spinal cord in anterior horn

1 **Posterior column.** Columna posterior. It is
~ composed primarily of sensory neurons. B

2 **Posterior horn.** Cornu posterius. Posterior col-
~ umn as seen in transverse section. A

3 *Apex.* Apical cap of posterior horn consisting of
~ large nerve cells ventral to the substantia gelatinosa. A C

4 Head. Caput. Thickened middle part of posterior
~ horn in the lower cervical and thoracic spinal cord.
A

5 *Cervix.* Thinner segment of posterior horn between the head and base. A

6 Base. Basis. Broadened attachment of the posterior horn to the middle part of the gray matter. A

7 **Substantia gelatinosa.** Non-fixed, slightly glassy
substance above the apex of the posterior horn. It
consists primarily of glia and small ganglion cells.
A C

8 **Secondary visceral substance.** Substantia visceralis secundaria. Small field of autonomic ganglion cells anterior to the central intermediate
substance. A

9 **Lateral column.** Columna lateralis. Gray matter between the anterior and posterior horns. B

10 **Lateral horn.** Cornu laterale. Lateral prominence
of gray matter. A

11 **Interomediolateral (autonomic) column.** Co-
~ lumna intermediolateralis (autonomica). Lateral
horn visualized spatially. It contains cells of the
sympathetic nervous system and extends from
T1–L2. A B

12 **Central intermediate gray matter.** Substantia
[grisea] intermedia centralis. Ganglion cells at the
central canal. A C

13 **Lateral intermediate gray matter.** Substantia
[grisea] intermedia lateralis. Part of the sympathetic nervous system in the lateral horn. It extends from T1–L2. A C

14 Thoracic column. Columna thoracica (Nuc.
~ thoracicus) [[Stilling-Clarke]]. It lies at the base of
the posterior horn and extends usually from
C8–L2. It belongs partly to the posterior spinocerebellar tract. A C

15 **Sacral parasympathetic nuclei.** Nuclei pa-
rasympathici sacrales. Cells of the sacral para-
symphathetic nervous system in segments S2–4.
They lie between the anterior and posterior horns.

16 **Reticular formation.** Formatio reticularis. Netlike mixture of gray and white matter in the angle
between the lateral and posterior horns. A C

16a **Anterior/posterior gray commissure.** Commissura grisea anterior/posterior. Gray matter in front
of and behind the central canal. C

17 WHITE MATTER. SUBSTANTIA ALBA. It
~ consists primarily of myelinated nerve fibers.

18 **Anterior white commissure.** Commissura alba
anterior. White matter with decussating fibers between the central intermediate gray matter and the
anterior median commissure. C

18a **Posterior white commissure.** Commissura alba
posterior. Individual fibers decussating into the
posterior gray commissure.

19 **Anterior funiculus.** Funiculus anterior. Field
~ of white matter between anterior root fibers, anterior horn and anterior median fissure. A C

20 **Anterior fasciculi proprii.** Fasciculi proprii ante-
~ riores. Lying directly on the gray matter, these
bundles comprise longer and shorter fibers involved in connecting individual segments of the
spinal cord with one another. Reflex apparatus. C

21 **Sulcomarginal fasciculus.** Fasciculus sulcomar-
ginalis. Fibers of the reflex apparatus located at the
anterior median fissure.

22 **Anterior corticospinal (pyramidal) tract.** Trac-
~ tus corticospinalis (pyramidalis) anterior. Uncrossed portion of pyramidal tract lateral to the
anterior median fissure. C

23 **Vestibulospinal tract.** Tractus vestibulospinalis.
Fibers in the anterior funiculus for impulses from
the vestibular organ. C

24 **Reticulospinal tract.** Tractus reticulospinalis.
Arising from the reticular formation of the brain
stem, it forms a nondefinable tract in the middle of
the anterior funiculus and ends in the anterior horn.
C

25 **Anterior spinothalamic tract.** Tractus spinotha-
~ lamicus anterior. Fibers ascending to the thalamus
for pressure and tactile sensation. C

26 **Lateral funiculus.** Funiculus lateralis. It lies
between the anterior and posterior horns together
with their root fibers. A C

27 **Lateral fasciculi proprii.** Fasciculi proprii laterales. Shorter fibers at the gray matter for connection
to individual spinal cord segments. C

28 **Lateral corticospinal (pyramidal) tract.** Tractus
corticospinalis [pyramidalis] lateralis. Situated in
front of the posterior horn, it transmits conscious
motor impulses. C

29 **Rubrospinal tract.** Tractus rubrospinalis [[Mona-
kow]]. It passes from the red nucleus to the anteri-
or horn cells and lies in front of the lateral corticospinal tract. C

30 **Bulboreticulospinal tract.** Tractus bulboreticu-
lospinalis. A controversial tract in man.

31 **Pontoreticulospinal tract.** Tractus pontoreticu-
lospinalis. Likewise, a controversial tract in man.

32 **Tectospinal tract.** Tractus tectospinalis. Fibers in
the anterolateral region of the anterior funiculus
from the tectal lamina. They cross into the brain
stem and terminate in the anterior horns. C

33 **Olivospinal tract.** Tractus olivospinalis. Present
only in the cervical cord, its fibers pass from the
olive region to the anterior root fibers. C

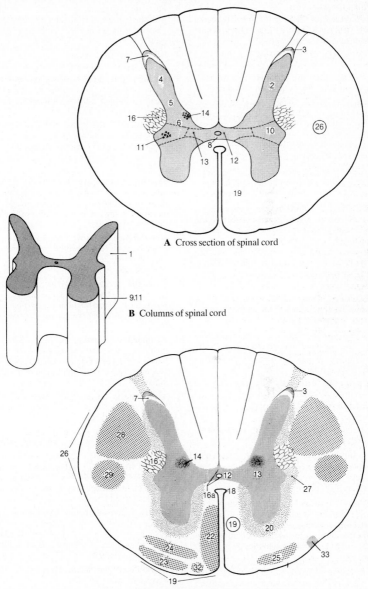

A Cross section of spinal cord

B Columns of spinal cord

C Cross section of spinal cord with tracts

1 **Spinotectal tract.** Tractus spinotectalis. Its fibers come from the posterior horn of the opposite side, run in the lateral spinothalamic tract and end in the tectal lamina. A

2 **Spinothalamic tract.** Tractus spinothalamicus. Lying in the lateral funiculus and coming primarily from the opposite side, its fibers transmit pain and temperature sensations. A

3 **Anterior spinocerebellar tract.** Tractus spi-
~ nocerebellaris anterior [[Gowers]]. It comes partly from the opposite side and transmits to the cerebellum information necessary for the coordination of movements concerning muscle extension and limb position. A

4 **Posterior spinocerebellar tract.** Tractus spi-
~ nocerebellaris posterior [[Flechsig]]. It courses uncrossed and is functionally like the anterior spinocerebellar tract. A

5 **Dorsolateral tract.** Tractus dorsolateralis [[Lissauer]]. Bundle of fine myelinated and nonmyelinated fibers between the apex of the posterior horn and the surface. The fibers are short and are partly lateral branches of posterior root fibers. A

6 **Spino-olivary tract.** Tractus spino-olivaris [[Hellweg]]. Predominantly crossed fibers to the olive. They lie by the anterior root fibers together with the olivospinal tract. A

7 **Spinoreticular tract.** Tractus spinoreticularis. Its fibers lie beside the spino-olivary tract and end in the reticular substance of the medulla oblongata. A

8 **Posterior funiculus.** Funiculus posterior.
~ White matter between the posterior horns. A

9 **Posterior fasciculi proprii.** Fasciculi proprii
~ posteriores. They lie directly on the gray matter and unite individual spinal cord segments for coordinated activity.

10 Septomarginal fasciculus. Fasciculus septomarginalis. Bundle of mostly descending fibers at the posterior median septum in the lower half of the thoracic cord. A

11 Interfascicular fasciculus. Fasciculus interfascicularis. Bundle of mostly descending fibers [comma tract of Schultze] located chiefly in the upper half of the thoracic cord between the fasciculi gracilis and cuneatus. A

12 **Fasciculus gracilis** [[Goll]]. It lies medially and contains fibers from the lower half of the spinal cord which function in the transmission of tactile and proprioceptive sensory information. A

13 **Fasciculus cuneatus** [[Burdach]]. It begins with the upper half of the thoracic cord and likewise contains fibers for tactile and proprioceptive transmission. A

14 BRAIN. ENCEPHALON.

15 BRAINSTEM. TRUNCUS ENCEPHALI. It extends from the medulla oblongata to the midbrain, inclusively. According to some, the diencephalon and insula likewise belong to the brainstem.

16 HINDBRAIN. RHOMBENCEPHALON. It includes the brain substance around the rhomboid fossa, thus the cerebellum, pons with substance attached dorsally and medulla oblongata. B

17 **Medulla oblongata (BULBUS).** Beginning at the lower margin of the pons, it extends up to the root fibers of C1. In the rhomboid fossa the beginning lies at the medullary striae of the 4th ventricle. B

18 **Anterior median fissure.** Fissura mediana anterior. Anterior groove continuous with that of the spinal cord. It is crossed over by the pyramidal decussation. C

19 **Pyramid.** Pyramis [medullae oblongatae]. Longitudinal elevation of pyramidal tract fibers to the right and left of the anterior median fissure. It ends with the pyramidal decussation. C

20 **Pyramidal decussation.** Decussatio pyrami-
~ dum (Dec. pyramidalis anterior motoria). 3–5 bundles of lateral pyramidal tract fibers crossing to the opposite side at the end of the medulla. C

21 **Anterolateral sulcus.** Sulcus anterolateralis.
~ Furrow lateral to the pyramid for the exit of the hypoglossal nerve. C

22 **Lateral funiculus.** Funiculus lateralis. Continuation of the lateral funiculus of the spinal cord up to the olive. C

23 **Olive.** Oliva. Bean-shaped prominence about 1.5 cm long between the roots of cranial nerves X and XII. It is produced by the nuclei lying beneath it. C

24 **Anterior external arcuate fibers.** Fibrae ar-
~ cuatae externae anteriores. Fibers from the arcuate nucleus coursing over the caudal end of the olive to the caudal cerebellar peduncle. Part of the pontocerebellar tract. C

25 **Retro-olivary sulcus.** Sulcus retro-olivaris. Furrow behind the olive. C

26 **Retro-olivary area.** Area retro-olivaris. Field behind the olive. C

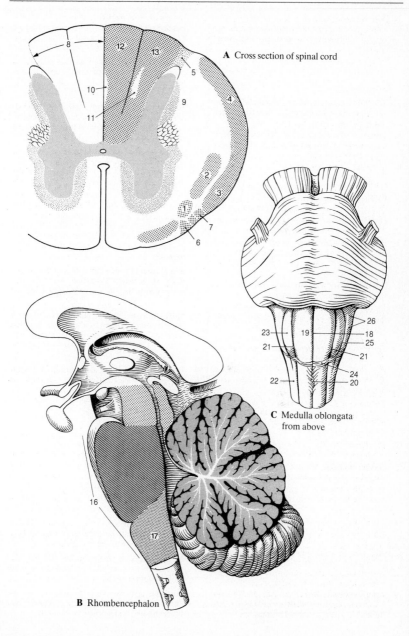

A Cross section of spinal cord

C Medulla oblongata from above

B Rhombencephalon

1 **Posterolateral sulcus.** Sulcus posterolateralis.
~ Furrow reaching up to the lateral recess of the 4th
ventricle. Site of exit of cranial nerves IX, X and
XI. A

2 **Inferior cerebellar peduncle.** Pedunculus cerebellaris inferior. Inferior connection to the cerebellum with fibers of the posterior spinocerebellar
tract and olive. A

3 **Trigeminal tubercle (tuber cinereum).** Tuberculum trigeminale. Low lateral elevation above the
spinal tract of the trigeminal nerve. B

4 **Cuneate fasciculus.** Fasciculus cuneatus. Lateral
part of posterior funiculus coming from the upper
half of the body. A

5 **Cuneate tubercle.** Tuberculum cuneatum.
~ Oblong prominence at the end of the cuneate fasciculus produced by the nucleus cuneatus. A

6 **Fasciculus gracilis.** Medial part of posterior funiculus coming from the lower half of the body. A

7 **Gracile tubercle (clava).** Tuberculum gracile.
Oblong bulge over the nucleus gracilis. A

8 **Posterior median sulcus.** Sulcus medianus posterior. Posterior furrow continued from the spinal
cord and closed above by a medullary lamella
(Obex). A

9 **Sections through the medulla oblongata.** Sectiones medullae oblongatae.

10 **Pyramidal fasciculus (tract).** Fasciculus pyramidalis. Nerve tract for the transmission of impulses
concerned with conscious movements. C D

11 Corticospinal fibers. Fibrae corticospinales.
Fibers from the precentral gyrus of the cortex to
the anterior horn cells of the spinal cord.

12 Corticonuclear fibers. Fibrae corticonucleares. Fibers from the precentral gyrus of the cortex
to the motor nuclei of cranial nerves.

13 **Decussation of the pyramids.** Decussatio pyra-
~ midum (Dec. motoria). Fibers of the lateral pyramidal tract crossing with 3–5 bundles at the end of
the medulla oblongata. B

14 **Fasciculus gracilis.** Medial part of posterior funiculus coming from the lower half of the body.

15 **Nucleus gracilis.** Nucleus of fasciculus gracilis
medial to cuneate nucleus. D

16 **Cuneate fasciculus.** Fasciculus cuneatus. Lateral
part of posterior funiculus coming from the upper
half of the body.

17 **Cuneate nucleus.** Nucleus cuneatus. Nucleus of
fasciculus cuneatus lateral to the nucleus gracilis.
D

18 **Accessory cuneate nucleus.** Nucleus cuneatus
accessorius. Gray matter lateral to upper part of
cuneate nucleus. Origin of external arcuate fibers
which pass to the cerebellum. D

19 **Internal arcuate fibers.** Fibrae arcuatae internae.
Fiber component of medial lemniscus arising from
the nucleus of the posterior funiculus. C

20 **Decussation of medial lemniscus.** Decussatio
~ lemniscorum medialium (Dec. sensoria). Formed
by fibers of nuclei gracilis and cuneatus, second
order neurons of posterior funiculus. C D

21 **Medial lemniscus.** Lemniscus medialis. Continuation of second order neuron of posterior funiculus after decussation of lemniscus [bulbothalamic
tract]. D

22 **Tectospinal tract.** Tractus tectospinalis. Decussa-
ted connection between the quadrigeminal
plate and the spinal cord. It lies between the facial
and trigeminal nuclei. D

23 **Medial longitudinal fasciculus.** Fasciculus longitudinalis medialis. Nerve fiber bundle for reciprocal connection to the motor nuclei of ocular
muscles, as well as vestibular, accessory and cervical muscle nuclei. C

24 **Posterior longitudinal fasciculus.** Fasciculus
longitudinalis posterior [[Schütz]]. Connection
between the hypothalamus, III, VII, XII cranial
nerve nuclei, nucleus ambiguus, tractus solitarius
and tractus salvatorius in the floor of the rhomboid
fossa. C

25 **Spinal tract of trigeminal nerve.** Tractus spinalis nervi trigeminalis. Descending fibers of the trigeminal nerve for pain and temperature stimuli. C
D

26 **Spinal nucleus of trigeminal nerve.** Nucleus
spinalis nervi trigeminalis. Continuous with the
substantia gelatinosa in the spinal cord, this nucleus receives the fibers of the spinal tract of the trigeminal nerve. C D

27 **Reticular formation (substance).** Formatio
(Substantia) reticularis. Cells lying scattered in the
tegmentum in the vicinity of the vagus, vestibular
and facial nuclei with regulating influence on the
muscles of the pharyngeal arch and other muscles
of the body. It extends cranially and caudally. C

28 **Inferior olivary nucleus.** Nucleus olivaris inferi-
~ or. Main olivary nucleus lying below the olive. It
has the form of a thick-walled pouch opened medially and is connected with the spinal cord and cerebellum. C

29 Amiculum of the olive. Amiculum olivare.
Fibrous sheath around the olive. It consists of afferent and efferent fibers of this nucleus. C

30 Hilum of inferior olivary nucleus. Hilum
~ nuclei olivaris inferioris. Opening of the medially
oriented pouch-like olivary nucleus. C

31 **Medial accessory olivary nucleus.** Nucleus olivaris accessorius medialis. It is located in front of
the hilum of the olivary nucleus. C

32 **Posterior accessory olivary nucleus.** Nucleus
olivaris accessorius posterior. It is situated between the olive and reticular formation. C

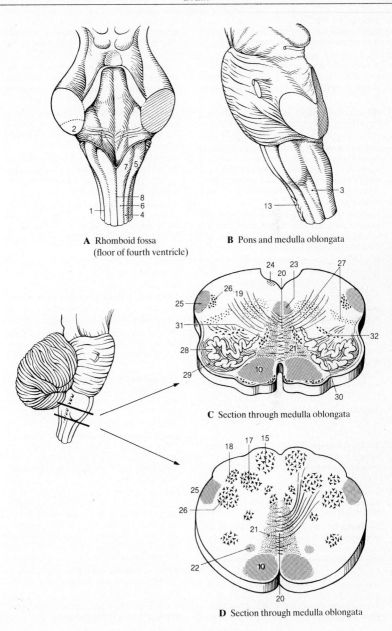

A Rhomboid fossa
(floor of fourth ventricle)

B Pons and medulla oblongata

C Section through medulla oblongata

D Section through medulla oblongata

1   **Olivospinal tract.** Tractus olivospinalis. Extrapyramidal tract limited to the cervical cord. It influences head and hand movements. D

2   **Spino-olivary tract.** Tractus spino-olivaris. Present in the entire spinal cord, it provides information for the olive, partly for its own needs, partly for forwarding to the cerebellum. D

3   **Olivocerebellar tract.** Tractus olivocerebellaris. It passes through the inferior cerebellar peduncle from the olive to the cerebellum. B

4   **Inferior cerebellar peduncle.** Pedunculus ce-
~   rebellaris inferior. Inferior connection to the cerebellum without a sharp boundary from the middle cerebellar peduncle. It contains fibers primarily from the spinocerebellar tract and olive. A B

5   **Nucleus of hypoglossal nerve (hypoglossal
~   nucleus).** Nucleus nerve hypoglossi (Nucleus hypoglossalis). It is located below the floor of the lower rhomboid fossa. C D

6   **Posterior paramedian nucleus.** Nucleus paramedianus posterior. Cell group in the vicinity of the hypoglossal nucleus with connection to the reticular formation.

7   **Dorsal nucleus of vagus nerve (dorsal vagal
~   nucleus).** Nucleus dorsalis nervi vagi (Nucleus vagalis dorsalis). Autonomic and sensory cell group located lateral and caudal to the hypoglossal nucleus. C D

8   **Nucleus intercalatus.** Nuclear group of unknown function between the nucleus of the hypoglossal nerve and the dorsal nucleus of the vagus. C

9   **Tractus solitarius.** Taste fibers of cranial nerves V, VII, IX and X for the nucleus of the tractus solitarius. C

10 **Nucleus solitarius.** Row of cells for the tractus
~   solitarius extending from the middle of the rhomboid fossa to the decussation of the pyramids. C

11 **Nucleus parasolitarius.** Dispersed cells ventrolateral to the nucleus solitarius with no known function.

12 **Vestibular nuclei.** Nuclei vestibulares. Four terminal nuclei of the vestibular division. They have connections to the spinal cord, cerebellum and medial longitudinal fasciculus. A

13 Inferior vestibular nucleus. Nucleus vestibularis inferior. Oblong nuclear group lying laterally beneath the medial nucleus with connection to the cerebellum and medial longitudinal fasciculus. A

14 Medial vestibular nucleus. Nucleus vestibularis medialis. Group of nuclei lateral to the limiting sulcus with fibers of origin for the medial longitudinal fasciculus of both sides. A

15 Lateral vestibular nucleus. Nucleus vestibularis lateralis. Smaller group of nuclei located toward the lateral recess with connection to the anterior horn of the spinal cord. A

16 **Cochlear nuclei.** Nuclei cochleares. Continuous nuclear mass below the lateral recess of the 4th ventricle where it can produce a slight elevation, the tuberculum acusticum. A

17 Anterior cochlear nucleus. Nucleus
~   cochlearis anterior. Its fibers pass to the opposite side primarily via the trapezoid body and joins the lateral lemniscus there. A

18 Posterior cochlear nucleus. Nucleus
~   cochlearis posterior. Its fibers pass mostly to the midline just beneath the floor of the rhomboid fossa where they go deeply in order to join the trapezoid body. A

19 **Commissural nucleus.** Nucleus commissuralis. Little-known nucleus in the medulla oblongata.

20 **Nucleus ambiguus.** Nucleus of origin for cranial nerves IX and X, as well as the cranial portion of XI. It is located behind the olive. C D

21 **Inferior salivary nucleus.** Nucleus salivarius
~   inferior. Autonomic nucleus for the parasympathetic fibers of the glossopharyngeal nerve. A C

22 **Arcuate nucleus.** Nucleus arcuati. Located in front of the pyramidal tract and medial to it, this group of nuclei gives origin to the external arcuate fibers. It corresponds to caudally displaced pontine nuclei. B

23 **Anterior external arcuate fibers.** Fibrae ar-
~   cuatae externae anteriores. Fibers from the arcuate nucleus which pass externally around and transversely across the olive into the cerebellar peduncles. C

24 **Posterior external arcuate fibers.** Fibrae ar-
~   cuatae externae posteriores. Fibers which pass uncrossed from the lateral part of the arcuate nucleus to the inferior cerebellar peduncle. They replace the posterior spinocerebellar tract for the region above C8. The thoracic nucleus is absent here. D

25 **Raphe of medulla oblongata.** Raphe medullae oblongatae. Suture-like midline in the decussation of the lemniscus. C

26 Nuclei raphae. Cells of the reticular formation located near the median plane.

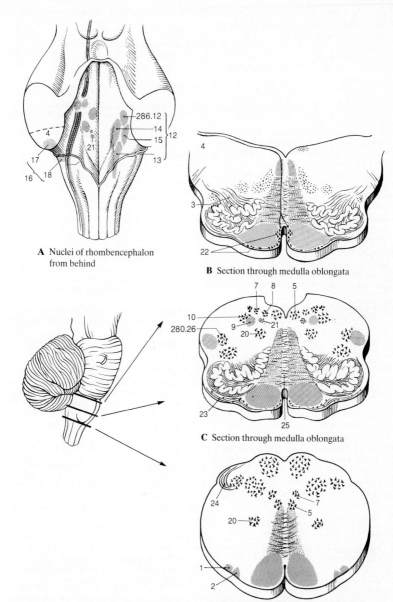

A Nuclei of rhombencephalon from behind

B Section through medulla oblongata

C Section through medulla oblongata

D Section through medulla oblongata

1　METENCEPHALON. Part of the rhombencephalon consisting of the pons, cerebellum and tegmentum.

2　PONS. Located between the interpeduncular fossa and pyramids, it consists mostly of crossing fibers and cells of the cerebral, pontine and cerebellar tracts. A B

3　**Bulbopontine (pontobulbar) sulcus.** Sulcus bulbopontines. Limiting furrow between the inferior margins of the medulla oblongata and pons. Site of exit of cranial nerves VI, VII and VIII. A

4　**Basilar sulcus of pons.** Sulcus basilaris. Median groove produced by pyramidal tract fibers situated to the right and left of the midline. It is occupied by the basilar artery. A C

5　**Middle (pontine) cerebellar peduncle.** Pedunculus cerebellaris medius (pontinus). Well developed middle peduncle containing the pontocerebellar tract. A

6　**Pontocerebellar trigone.** Trigonum pontocerebellare. Clinically important angle between the pons, medulla oblongata and cerebellum. A

7　SECTIONS OF PONS. SECTIONES PONTIS.

8　**Anterior (basilar) part of pons.** Pars anterior (basilaris) pontis. Portion of pons consisting mainly of fibers of the cerebropontocerebellar tract. C

9　**Longitudinal pontine fibers.** Fibrae pontis longitudinales. The following fiber tracts running longitudinally:

10　Corticospinal fibers. Fibrae corticospinales. Part of the pyramidal tract passing into the spinal cord. C

11　Corticonuclear (corticobulbar) fibers. Fibrae corticonucleares. Fibers of the pyramidal tract passing to the motor nuclei of cranial nerves. C

12　Corticoreticular fibers. Fibrae corticoreticulares. Fibers passing from the cerebral cortex to the reticular formation.

13　Corticopontine fibers. Fibrae corticopontinae. Fibers coming to the pontine nuclei from the frontal, occipital and temporal lobes. C

14　**Transverse pontine fibers.** Fibrae pontis transversae. Transversely-running fibers of the cerebropontocerebellar tract. C

15　**Pontocerebellar fibers.** Fibrae pontocerebellares. Fibers of the pontocerebellar tract passing from the pons to the cerebellum. C

16　**Pontine nuclei.** Nuclei pontis. Intercalary cells of the cerebropontocerebellar tract situated in the ventral part of the pons. C

17　**Posterior part of pons (tegmentum of pons).** Pars posterior pontis (Tegmentum pontis). Part of pons situated between the 4th ventricle and the transverse pontine fibers. C

18　**Pontine raphe.** Raphe pontis. Fibers from the trigeminal nucleus occupying the midline of the pons. C

19　**Medial longitudinal fasciculus.** Fasciculus longitudinalis medialis. Association tract between the nuclei of the ocular and neck muscles on one side and the vestibular organ on the other. C

20　**Posterior longitudinal fasciculus.** Fasciculus longitudinalis posterior [[Schütz]]. Reciprocal connections between the hypothalamus and the following nuclei: cranial nerves III, V, VII, X, XII, ambiguus, as well as the tractus solitarius and salivatorius in the mesencephalic central gray region. C

21　**Medial lemniscus.** Lemniscus medialis. Decussating connection between the nuclei of the posterior funiculus and the thalamus located, first of all medially, then laterally. C

22　**Tectospinal (spinotectal) tract.** Tractus tectospinalis. It begins in the superior colliculus, crosses to the opposite side and then lies ventral to the medial longitudinal fasciculus. It is concerned with optic reflexes. C

23　**Reticular formation.** Formatio reticularis. Located in the posterior part of the pons, this long group of cells is permeated by nerve fibers and is continued anterosuperiorly and caudally. It is concerned with the integration of visceral and muscular functions. C

24　**Spinal lemniscus.** Lemniscus spinalis. Cranial continuation of the lateral and anterior spinothalamic tracts. C

25　**Spinal tract of trigeminal nerve.** Tractus spinalis nervi trigeminalis. Trigeminal fibers descending as far as C4 to join the nucleus of the spinal tract of the trigeminal nerve. B

26　**Spinal (inferior) nucleus of trigeminal nerve.** Nucleus spinalis (inferior) nervi trigeminalis. Nucleus belonging to the spinal tract of the trigeminal nerve. B

27　**Pontine nucleus of trigeminal nerve.** Nucleus pontinus nervi trigeminalis. Main nucleus of trigeminal serving primarily for the sense of touch. B

28　**Trigeminal lemniscus (trigeminothalamic tract).** Lemniscus trigeminalis (Tractus trigeminothalamicus). Crossed fibers of the trigeminal nucleus on their way to the thalamus. C

29　**Mesencephalic tract of trigeminal nerve.** Tractus mesencephalicus nervi trigeminalis (Tractus mesencephalicus trigeminalis). Trigeminal fibers for the nucleus of the trigeminal nerve tract located lateral to the cerebral aqueduct and in the lateral part of the arch to the 4th ventricle. B C

30　**Mesencephalic nucleus of trigeminal nerve.** Nucleus mesencephalicus nervi trigeminalis [Nucleus mesencephalicus trigeminalis]. Upper sensory nucleus extending to below the tectal lamina. B

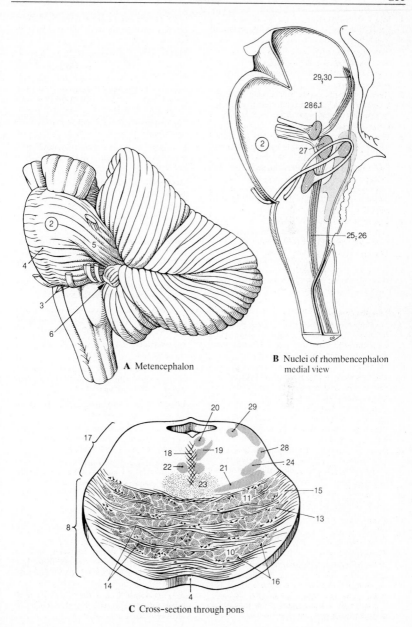

A Metencephalon

B Nuclei of rhombencephalon
medial view

C Cross-section through pons

1 ~ **Motor nucleus of trigeminal nerve.** Nucleus motorius nervi trigeminalis [nucleus motorius trigeminalis]. It is located at about the level of the exit of the trigeminal nerve. A B

2 ~ **Nucleus of abducens nerve.** Nucleus nervi abducentis [nucleus abducens]. It is found beneath the facial colliculus. A B

3 ~ **Nucleus of facial nerve.** Nucleus nervi facialis [nucleus facialis]. This motor nucleus lies laterally below the nucleus of the abducens. A B

4 **Genu of facial nerve.** Genu nervi facialis. Arch formed by fibers of facial nerve below the facial colliculus and above the nucleus of the abducens. B

5 **Superior salivary (salivatory) nucleus.** Nucleus salivarius superior. Autonomic nucleus for the parasympathetic fibers of the facial nerve. It supplies preganglionic fibers for the pterygopalatine and submandibular ganglia. A B

6 **Lacrimal nucleus.** Nucleus lacrimalis. Autonomic cells lying beside the superior salivary nucleus for the control of lacrimal secretion. A B

7 **Superior olivary nucleus.** Nucleus olivaris superioris. It lies lateral to the trapezoid body, contains fibers from the cochlear nuclei and integrates hearing via the olivocochlear tract. D

8 Olivocochlear tract. Tractus olivocochlearis. Tract from the superior olivary nucleus to the hair cells of the ear.

9 **Vestibular nuclei.** Nuclei vestibulares. Four terminal nuclei of the vestibular division with connections to the spinal cord, cerebellum and medial longitudinal fasciculus. A B

10 Medial vestibular nucleus. Nucleus vestibularis medialis. Nuclear group lateral to the sulcus limitans with fibers of origin for the medial longitudinal fasciculus of both sides. A D

11 Lateral vestibular nucleus. Nucleus vestibularis lateralis. Smaller group of nuclei situated toward the lateral recess with connection to the anterior horn of the spinal cord. A D

12 Superior vestibular nucleus. Nucleus vestibularis superior. Nucleus located above the lateral nucleus with connection to the medial longitudinal fasciculus and cerebellum. A D

13 **Cochlear nuclei.** Nuclei cochleares. Dorsal and ventral terminal nuclei of the cochlear division of the vestibulocochlear nerve. Both lie below the lateral recess. A

14 **Trapezoid body.** Corpus trapezoideum. Forming a part of the auditory pathway, its fibers arise from the cochlear nuclei. D

15 **Anterior nucleus of trapezoid body.** Nucleus corporis trapezoidei anterior. Smaller nucleus situated posterolaterally in the trapezoid body. D

16 **Posterior nucleus of trapezoid body.** Nucleus corporis trapezoidei posterior. It lies behind the anterior nucleus. D

17 **Lateral lemniscus.** Lemniscus lateralis. Ascending continuation of the trapezoid body. Part of the hearing pathway. D

18 **Nucleus of lateral lemniscus.** Nuclei lemnisci lateralis. Ganglion cells interspersed in the lateral lemniscus.

19 **Fourth ventricle.** Ventriculus quartus. Dilatation of the lumen of the embryonic neural tube in the rhombencephalon. D

20 **Rhomboid fossa.** Fossa rhomboidea. Floor of 4th ventricle. A C

21 **Lateral recess.** Recessus lateralis. Lateral corner of the 4th ventricle ending with the lateral aperture. C D

22 **Median sulcus.** Sulcus medianus. Median furrow passing through the rhomboid fossa. C

23 **Medial eminence.** Eminentia medialis. Oblong elevation located between the median sulcus and the sulcus limitans. C

24 **Facial colliculus.** Colliculus facialis. Prominence above the medullary striae produced by the genu of the facial nerve and the nucleus of the abducens nerve. C

25 **Limiting sulcus.** Sulcus limitans. Shallow furrow situated lateral to the medial eminence. C

26 **Vestibular area.** Area vestibularis. Field above the vestibular nuclei and lateral to the limiting sulcus at the beginning of the lateral recess. C

27 **Superior fovea.** Fovea superior. Pit situated lateral to the facial colliculus. C

28 **Locus ceruleus.** Locus caeruleus. Elongated bluish group of cells located in the lateral wall of the 4th ventricle and under it. C

29 **Inferior fovea.** Fovea inferior. Pit at the apex of the trigone of the vagus nerve. C

30 **Medullary striae.** Striae medullares. Strongly myelinated transverse nerve bundles from the arcuate nucleus to the cerebellum. C

31 ~ **Trigone of hypoglossal nerve.** Trigonum nervi hypoglossi (Trig. hypoglossale). Triangular bulge over the nucleus of the hypoglossal nerve located between the median sulcus and the sulcus limitans. C

32 **Funiculus separans.** Transparent stripe of ependyma between the trigone of the vagus nerve and the area postrema. C

33 ~ **Trigone of vagus nerve.** Trigonum nervi vagi (Trig. vagale). Triangle over the dorsal nucleus of the vagus nerve caudal to the trigone of hypoglossal nerve. C

34 **Area postrema.** A triangular field caudal to the trigone of the vagus with strongly vascularized, glia-rich tissue. C

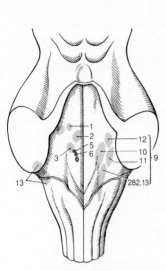

A Rhomboid fossa

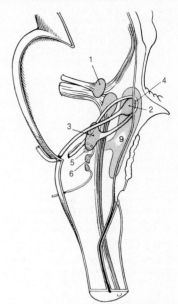

B Nuclei of rhombencephalon
medial view

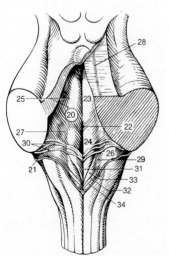

C Rhomboid fossa

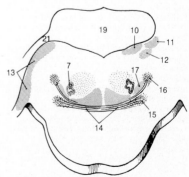

D Cross section through rhomboid fossa
at level of lateral recess

Brain

1 **Tegmen of fourth ventricle.** Tegmen ventriculi quarti. Roof of 4th ventricle. A

2 Superior medullary velum. Velum medulla-
~ re superius. Lamina of white matter spread out between the right and left superior cerebellar peduncles. It is fused with the lingula of the cerebellum. A

3 Frenulum of superior medullary velum.
~ Frenulum veli medullaris superioris. Band-like ridge from the superior medullary velum to the tectal lamina. A

4 Inferior medullary velum. Velum medullare
~ inferius. Plate of white matter in the upper part of the lower roof of the rhomboid fossa. It is fused with the peduncle of the flocculus and the nodulus of the cerebellum. A

5 **Tela choroidea of fourth ventricle [ventriculi quarti].** Clear pia mater carrying the choroid plexus and stretched between the inferior medullary velum and tenia of the fourth ventricle. A

6 **Choroid plexus of fourth ventricle.** Plexus choroideus [ventriculi quarti]. Paired, garland-like, ependymal-covered, highly vascularized tufted projection which extends into the two lateral apertures. A

7 **Tenia of fourth ventricle.** Taenia [ventriculi quarti]. Ridge on lower portion of roof of rhomboid fossa. A

8 **Obex.** Small bridge at lower end of roof of rhomboid fossa. A

9 **Median aperture of fourth ventricle [foramen of Magendie].** Apertura mediana [ventriculi quarti] [Magendie]. Unpaired opening directly above the obex for passage of cerebrospinal fluid. A

10 **Lateral aperture of fourth ventricle [foramen of Luschka].** Apertura lateralis [ventriculi quarti] [[Luschkae]]. Opening for passage of cerebrospinal fluid located at the end of the right and left lateral recess. A

11 **CEREBELLUM.** It is located above the rhomboid fossa.

12 **Folia of cerebellum.** Folia cerebelli. Delicate cerebellar convolutions (gyri) separated by fissures. B

13 **Cerebellar fissure.** Fissura cerebelli. Deeply branched furrow located between two cerebellar folia. B

14 **Vallecula.** Deep median groove inferiorly between right and left halves of the cerebellum. Into it fits the medulla oblongata. C

15 **Body of cerebellum.** Corpus cerebelli. Entire cerebellum except for the flocculonodular lobe.

16 **Vermis of cerebellum.** Vermis cerebelli. In part phylogenetically older, unpaired segment of the cerebellum. B

17 **Cerebellar hemisphere.** Hemisphaerium cerebelli. Each half of cerebellum. C

18 **Anterior lobe of cerebellum.** Lobus anterior cerebelli. Region cranial to primary fissure. B D

19 **Lingula.** Unpaired part of vermis fused with the superior medullary velum. It belongs to the archeocerebellum. C D

20 **Central lobule.** Lobulus centralis. It lies over the lingula and is continuous on both sides with the ala of the central lobule. C D

21 **Culmen.** Segment of vermis between the central lobule and primary fissure. B C D

22 **Ala of central lobule.** Ala lobuli centralis. Lateral extension of central lobule for connection with the cerebellar hemispheres. B C D

23 **Quadrangular lobule.** Lobulus quadrangularis
~ (pars anterior). Part attaching laterally to the declive. B C D

24 **Primary fissure.** Fissura prima. Indentation between the quadrangular and simplex lobules. B D

25 **Posterior lobe of cerebellum.** Lobus posterior cerebelli. Region located between the primary and dorsolateral fissures. D

26 **Declive.** Part of vermis declining posteriorly from the culmen. B D

27 **Folium of vermis.** Narrow midline connection between the left and right superior semilunar lobules. B D

28 **Tuber of vermis.** Median connection between right and left inferior semilunar lobules. B C D

29 **Pyramid of vermis.** Pyramis vermis. Segment situated between right and left biventral lobules. C D

30 Secondary (postpyramidal) fissure. Fissura secunda. Fissure between the pyramid and uvula of the vermis. C D

31 **Uvula vermis.** Part of vermis lying between the cerebellar tonsils. C D

32 **Lobulus simplex (Lobulus quadrangularis)**
~ **(Pars inferoposterior).** Portion located between the quandrangular and superior semilunar lobules. B C D

33 **Superior semilunar lobule.** Lobulus semilunaris
~ superior. Part situated between the inferior semilunar lobule and lobulus simplex. B C D

34 Horizontal fissure. Fissura horizontalis. Deep groove between the cranial and caudal semilunar lobules. B C D

35 **Inferior semilunar lobule.** Lobulus semilunaris
~ inferior. Part of cerebellum between the superior semilunar and biventral lobules. B C D

36 **Gracile (paramedian lobule).** Lobulus gracilis (Lob. paramedianus). It is located between the caudal semilunar and biventral lobules. D

37 **Biventral lobule.** Lobulus biventer. It lies between the paramedian lobule and cerebellar tonsil. C D

38 **Tonsil of cerebellum.** Tonsilla cerebelli. Small bean-shaped portion of the hemisphere lateral to the uvula. C D

39 **Posterolateral fissure.** Fissura posterolateralis.
~ Furrow separating the nodulus and flocculus on one side and the cerebellar tonsil with the biventral lobe on the other. C D

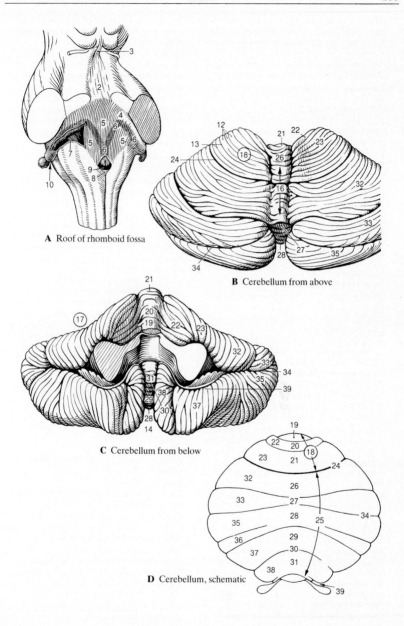

A Roof of rhomboid fossa

B Cerebellum from above

C Cerebellum from below

D Cerebellum, schematic

1 **Flocculonodular lobe.** Lobus flocculo-nodularis. Small archicerebellar portion of the cerebellum located caudal to the dorsolateral fissure.

2 **Nodulus.** Medial protuberance of the vermis united with the flocculus by the peduncles. E

3 **Flocculus.** Claw-like portion of the cerebellum between the inferior cerebellar peduncle and biventral lobule. E

4 Peduncle of flocculus. Pedunculus floccularis. Connecting band to the nodulus. It goes over partly into the inferior medullary velum. E

5 **Paraflocculus.** With respect to the human cerebellum, a small insignificant field of the caudal lobe where it contacts the flocculus.

6 **Archicerebellum.** Archaeocerebellum. Phylogenetically the oldest part of the cerebellum, it consists of the lingula and the flocculonodular lobe. A

7 **Paleocerebellum.** An old part of the cerebellum, it consists of the central lobule, culmen, pyramid, uvula, ala of central lobule and quadrangular lobule. A

8 **Neocerebellum.** Phylogenetically the young portion of the cerebellum, it comprises the declive, folium, tuber, lobulus simplex, cranial and caudal semilunar lobules, paramedian lobule and tonsil. A

9 CEREBELLAR SECTIONS. SECTIONES CEREBELLARES. Sections through the cerebellum.

10 **Arbor vitae [cerebelli].** Ramification pattern of the white matter in sectioned preparations suggestive of a living tree. C

11 **Medullary body.** Corpus medullare. White matter consisting of myelinated fibers. C

12 White laminae. Laminae albae. White matter extending into the folia from the medullary body. C

13 **Cerebellar cortex.** Cortex cerebellaris. About 1 mm thick, it consists primarily of nerve cells. B C

14 Molecular (plexiform) layer. Stratum moleculare (plexiforme). External cortical layer rich in dendrites and axons, poor in cell bodies. At its border with the granular layer are found the nuclei of the Purkinje cells. B

15 Purkinje cell layer. Stratum neurium piriformium. Perikarya of Purkinje cells located here. B

16 *Stratum granulosum.* Internal nuclear layer characterized by numerous closely packed small neurons. B

17 **Nuclei of cerebellum.** Nuclei cerebellaris.

18 Dentate nucleus. Nucleus dentatus. Located in the medullary body, it is a large nucleus resembling a folded pouch. C

19 Hilum of dentate nucleus. Hilum nuclei ~ dentati. Opening of dentate nucleus from which emerges most of the superior cerebellar peduncle. C

20 Emboliform nucleus. Nucleus emboliformis. It is found just in front of the hilum of the dentate nucleus. C

21 Globose nucleus. Nucleus globosus. It lies medial to the dentate nucleus. C

22 Fastigial nucleus. Nucleus fastigii. It lies ~ quite medially. C

23 **Cerebellar peduncles.** Pedunculi cerebellares. They provide connections from and to the cerebellum.

24 Inferior cerebellar peduncle (resti-~ form body). Pedunculus cerebellaris inferior. Inferior connection to the cerebellum with fibers of the posterior spinocerebellar tract and olive. E F

25 Middle cerebellar peduncle (brachium ~ pontis). Pedunculus cerebellaris medius (pontinus). Well developed peduncle containing fibers of the pontocerebellar tract. E F

26 Superior cerebellar peduncle (brachi-~ um conjunctivum). Pedunculus cerebellaris superior. Superior, paired (right and left) connection from the cerebellum to the brain stem with the superior medullary velum extending between them. E F

27 MIDBRAIN. MESENCEPHALON. It con-~ sists of cerebral crura, tegmentum and quadrigeminal plate (tectal lamina).

28 **Cerebral peduncle.** Pedunculus cerebri ~ (cerebralis). It comprises the cerebral crura and the tegmentum extending up to cerebral aqueduct. D

29 **Anterior part (cerebral crus, basis pedunculi).** Pars anterior (crus cerebri). It consists of the previously mentioned cerebral crura. D

30 **Pars posterior.** Posterior part of cerebral peduncle or tegmentum. See 292.10 D

31 **Oculomotor sulcus.** Sulcus oculomotorius. ~ Furrow on the medial surface of the cerebral crus, exit site of the oculomotor nerve. D

32 **Interpeduncular fossa.** Fossa interpeduncularis. It lies between the cerebral crura. D

33 **Interpeduncular (posterior) perforated substance.** Substantia perforata interpeduncularis [posterior]. Perforated floor of interpeduncular fossa produced by numerous vessels passing through holes. D

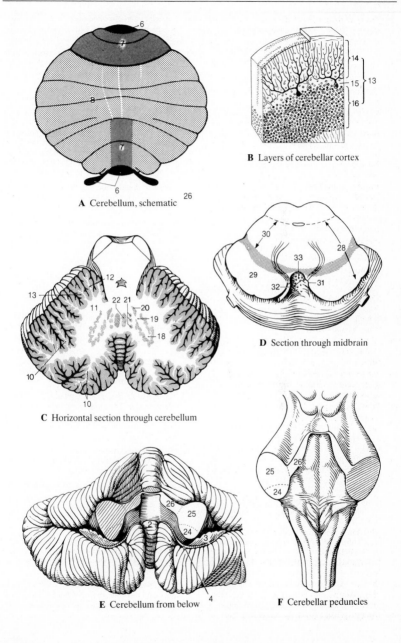

A Cerebellum, schematic

B Layers of cerebellar cortex

C Horizontal section through cerebellum

D Section through midbrain

E Cerebellum from below

F Cerebellar peduncles

1 **Basis pedunculi cerebri.** Synonymous with anterior part of cerebral peduncle, the cerebral crus. B

2 **Corticospinal fibers.** Fibrae corticospinales. Fibers of the pyramidal tract leading into the spinal cord. B C

3 **Corticonuclear (corticobulbar) fibers.** Fibrae corticonucleares. Pyramida tract fibers for the cranial nerve nuclei. B C

4 **Corticopontine fibers.** Fibrae corticopontinae.
~ Fibers of the cerebropontocerebellar tract.

5 **Parietotemporopontine fibers.** Fibrae parieto-
~ temporopontinae. Fibers of the cerebropontine tract which come from the parietal and temporal lobes. They lie in the lateral part of the cerebral crus. B C

6 **Frontopontine fibers.** Fibrae frontopontinae. Fi-
~ bers of the cerebropontine tract which arise from the frontal lobes and occupy the medial sixth of the cerebral crus. B C

7 **Substantia nigra.** Black nucleus lying on the cerebral crus. Its name is derived from its content of numerous pigmented ganglion cells rendering it visible with the naked eye. B C

8 **Compact part.** Pars compacta. Dense part of substantia nigra containing pigmented cells.

9 **Pars reticularis.** Reticular (fibrous) part of substantia nigra. It contains disaggregated pigmented fibers facing the cerebral crus. Its cells are irregularly dispersed between the fibers of the cerebral crus.

10 **Mesencephalic tegmentum.** Tegmentum mesencephalicum. It extends from the substantia nigra to an imaginary plane drawn through the cerebral aqueduct. B C

11 **Central gray matter.** Substantia grisea centralis. Gray matter around the cerebral aqueduct. B C

12 **Mesencephalic tectum.** Tectum mesencephalicum. Part of the mesencephalon located dorsal to the previous mentioned transverse plane through the cerebral aqueduct. B C

13 **Tectal lamina (quadrigeminal plate).** Lamina
~ tectalis [[quadrigemina]]. A

14 **Inferior colliculus.** Colliculus inferior. Inferior
~ hillock of quadrigeminal plate connected to the auditory pathway. A

15 **Superior colliculus.** Colliculus superior. Superi-
~ or hillock of quadrigeminal plate connected to the visual pathway. A

16 **Brachium of inferior colliculus.** Brachium colli-
~ culi inferioris. Connecting arm between the inferior colliculus and the medial geniculate body. A

17 **Brachium of superior colliculus.** Brachium col-
~ liculi superioris. Connecting arm between the superior colliculus and the lateral geniculate body. A

18 **Trigone of lemniscus.** Trigonum lemnisci. Triangular field laterally between the tectal lamina, superior cerebellar peduncle and cerebral crus. A

19 **Superior cerebellar peduncle.** Pedunculus cere-
~ bellaris superior. It carries fibers mainly from the dentate nucleus to the red nucleus and thalamus. A

20 **Mesencephalic (cerebral) aqueduct.** Aquaeductus mesencephali (cerebri). Narrow canal in the midbrain between the 3rd and 4th ventricle. B C D

21 **Sections through the mesencephalon.** Sectiones mesencephalici. B C D

22 **Reticular formation (substance).** Formatio (Substantia) reticularis. Mesencephalic portion of reticular formation extending up from the spinal cord. It lies around the cerebral aqueduct, its scattered ganglion cells functioning in the integration of muscular activities. B C D

23 **Corticoreticular fibers.** Fibrae corticoreticulares. Nerve fibers from the cerebral motor cortex to the ganglion cells of the reticular formation.

24 **Medial longitudinal fasciculus.** Fasciculus longitudinalis medialis. Fiber bundle with connections to the ocular muscles, neck muscles and vestibular nuclei for coordination of movements of the eyeball and head. B C D

25 **Posterior longitudinal fasciculus.** Fasciculus longitudinalis posterior [[Schütz]]. Descending and ascending fibers with connections between the hypothalamus and cranial nerve nuclei: III, V, VII, X, XII, as well as the nucleus ambiguus and the tractus solitarius and salivatorius. C

26 **Mesencephalic tract of trigeminal nerve.** Trac-
~ tus mesencephalicus nervi trigeminalis. Trigeminal fibers to the nucleus of the tract of the trigeminal nerve located lateral to the cerebral aqueduct and the 4th ventricle. D

27 Nucleus of mesencephalic tract of the trigeminal
~ nerve. Nucleus tractus mesencephalici nervi trigeminalis (Nucl. mes. trigeminalis). Upper sensory trigeminal nucleus extending to below the tectal lamina. D

28 **Nucleus of oculomotor nerve.** Nucleus nervi
~ oculomotorii (Nucleus oculomotorius). It is found in front of the cerebral aqueduct. B

29 Accessory nucleus of oculomotor nerve.
~ Nucleus oculomotorius accessorius (autonomicus). As parasympathetic portion of oculomotor nucleus, 96% supplies the ciliary muscle, the sphincter pupillae muscle receiving the rest.

30 **Nucleus of trochlear nerve.** Nucleus nervi
~ trochlearis (Nucleus trochlearis). It is located in the central gray matter caudal to the nucleus of the oculomotor nerve. C

31 **Interpeduncular nucleus.** Nucleus interpeduncularis. Located in the floor of the interpeduncular fossa, it is connected with the olfactory tract. C

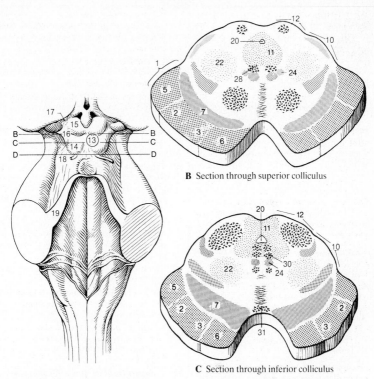

A Midbrain and rhomboid fossa

B Section through superior colliculus

C Section through inferior colliculus

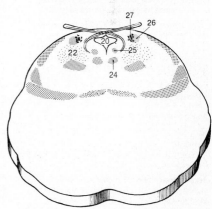

D Section through level of exit of trochlear nerve

1 **Interstitial nucleus of Cajal.** Nucleus interstitialis [[Cajal]]. Located lateral to the nucleus of the oculomotor nerve, this cell group is separated from it by the medial longitudinal fasciculus and contains fibers from the vestibular nuclei, globus pallidus and stratum griseum of the superior colliculus. B

2 **Tegmental nuclei.** Nuclei tegmenti (tegmentales). Nuclei in the reticular formation
~ dorsal to the trochlear nucleus and ventral to the medial longitudinal fasciculus. C

3 **Red nucleus.** Nucleus ruber. Iron-containing nucleus between the substantia nigra and central gray matter with tributaries from the cerebral cortex and thalamus. It is inserted in the tract from the cerebellum to the spinal cord. B

4 **Parvicellular part.** Pars parvocellularis. Characterized by small cells, this larger part of the red nucleus also partly forms the rubrospinal tract.

5 **Magnocellular part.** Pars magnocellularis. Characterized by large cells occupying the caudal part of the red nucleus, most of its fibers enter the rubrospinal tract.

6 **Endopeduncular nucleus.** Nucleus endopeduncularis. Cell group located medially in the cerebral crus directly after its entrance into the base of the brain. It is probably inserted in the tract between the globus pallidus and reticular formation.

7 **Decussations of tegmentum.** Decussationes tegmenti (tegmentales). Crossing of the rubrospinal, rubroreticular and tectospinal tracts. B

8 **Decussation of superior cerebellar peduncle.** Decussatio pedunculorum cerebellarium superiorum. Crossing of the superior cerebellar peduncle below the inferior colliculus and anterior to the medial longitudinal fasciculus. C

9 **Dentatorubral fibers.** Fibrae dentatorubrales. Component of the superior cerebellar peduncle which passes into the red nucleus.

10 **Rubrospinal tract.** Tractus rubrospinalis [[Monakow]]. Lying in front of the lateral pyramidal tract, this extrapyramidal tract passes from the red nucleus to the anterior horn cells.

11 **Tectobulbar tract.** Tractus tectobulbaris. It goes in the posterior tegmental decussation to the opposite side and then, lying anterior to the medial longitudinal fasciculus, it passes to the pontine nuclei, especially to the nuclei of the ocular muscles.

12 **Tectospinal tract.** Tractus tectospinalis. Initially behaving like the tectobulbar tract, it then descends in the anterior funiculus of the spinal cord.

13 **Lateral lemniscus.** Lemniscus lateralis. Partly crossing portion of auditory tract passing to the inferior colliculus. C D

14 **Lemniscus medialis.** Decussating connection between nuclei of posterior funiculus and thalamus. B C D

15 **Spinal lemniscus.** Lemniscus spinalis. Segment of spinothalamic tract residing in the midbrain adjacent to the medial lemniscus. D

16 **Trigeminal lemniscus.** Lemniscus trigeminalis. Crossing fiber tract between the sensory nuclei of the trigeminal and the thalamus. It also lies entirely in the vicinity of the medial lemniscus.

17 **Mesencephalic tectum.** Tectum mesencephalicum. Part of midbrain located dorsal to the aforementioned plane through the cerebral aqueduct. B C

18 **Tectal lamina.** Lamina tectalis [[quadrigemina]]. Quadrigeminal plate. A

19 **Nucleus of inferior colliculus.** Nucleus colli-
~ culi inferioris. It connects the auditory tract with the extrapyramidal system. C

20 **Brachium of inferior colliculus.** Brachium
~ colliculi inferioris. Connecting arm between the inferior colliculus and medial geniculate body. A

21 **Commissure of inferior colliculus.** Commissura colliculorum inferiorum. Connection between right and left inferior colliculi which also carries fibers from the lateral lemniscus of the opposite side. C

22 **Gray and white layers of superior colliculus.**
~ Strata [grisea et alba] colliculi superioris. Gray matter and the white matter surrounding it. B

23 **Brachium of superior colliculus.** Brachium
~ colliculi superioris. Connection between the superior colliculus and lateral geniculate body. A

24 **Commissure of superior colliculus.** Commissura colliculorum superiorum. Connection between the right and left superior colliculi. B

25 **Decussation of trochlear nerve.** Decussatio trochlearis (Decussatio nervorum trochlearium). Fibers of trochlear nerve crossing in the white matter. D

26 **Central tegmental tract.** Tractus tegmentalis centralis. Tract passing to the olive coming partially perhaps from the thalamus. B D

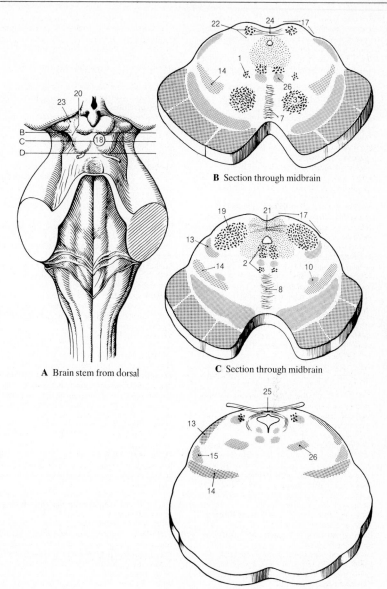

A Brain stem from dorsal

B Section through midbrain

C Section through midbrain

D Section through midbrain

1   FOREBRAIN. PROSENCEPHALON. Terminal portion of neural tube situated anterior to the anterior margin of the mesencephalon. It differentiates into the telencephalon and diencephalon.

2   DIENCEPHALON. It extends from the anterior margin of the anterior colliculus to the interventricular foramen.

3   **Epithalamus.** It consists essentially of the habenulae including their accessories and the epiphysis.

4   **Habenula.** Dorsal continuation of the stria medullaris of the thalamus. A B

5   **Habenular sulcus.** Sulcus habenuale (habenularis). Shallow furrow between the habenular trigone and the pulvinar. A

6   **Trigone of habenula.** Trigonum habenulae (T.
~   habenulare). Triangular field between the stria medullaris of the thalamus and the habenula. Beneath it lie the habenular nuclei. A

7   **Commissure of habenula.** Commissura habenu-
~   larum (habenularis). Fibers of the habenulae crossing over the midline. The decussation lies superior to the pineal recess. B

8   **Posterior (epithalamic) commissure.** Commis-
~   sura epithalamica (posterior). Lying between the pineal recess and entrance into the cerebral aqueduct, its fibers cross from a nearby area. B

9   **Pineal gland (body), epiphysis.** Corpus pineale (glandula pinealis). It lies topographically free on the quadrigeminal plate and is suspended from the habenula without functional connection. A B C

10   **Sections of epithalamus.** Sectiones epithalamici.

11   **Medial and lateral habenular nuclei.** Nuclei habenulares medialis et lateralis. Cell groups inserted in the reflex tract of the rhinencephalon. D

12   **Habenulointerpeduncular tract.** Tractus habenulointerpeduncularis. Connection between habenulae and interpeduncular nucleus. D

13   **Commissure of habenula.** Commissura habenu-
~   larum (habenularis). See 7. A B

14   **Pretectal area.** Area pretectalis. Region in front of upper margin of superior colliculus as far as the commissure of the epithalamus. C

15   **Pretectal nuclei.** Nuclei pretectales. Lying dorsolateral to the commissure of the epithalamus, they extend as far as the superior colliculus. They receive fibers from the occipital lobe and area in front of it, as well as the optic tract and send fibers to the accessory nucleus of the oculomotor nerve for the sphincter pupillae muscle.

16   **Posterior (epithalamic) commissure.** Commis-
~   sura epithalamica (posterior). See 8. B

17   **Pineal gland (body).** Corpus pineale (glandula pinealis). See 9. A B C

18   **Subfornical organ.** Organum subfornicale. Organ in the interventricular foramen between right and left fornix. It influences blood pressure and water excretion. B

19   **Subcommissural organ.** Organum subcommissurale. Group of specialized ependymal cells below the posterior commissure. They produce Reissner's fiber. B

20   **Dorsal thalamus.** Thalamus dorsalis. Portion of thalamus located cranial to the hypothalamic sulcus.

21   **Interthalamic adhesion (massa intermedia).** Adhesio interthalamica. Inconstant (70–85%) connection between right and left thalami. B

22   **Anterior tubercle of thalamus.** Tuberculum anterius thalamicum. Small protuberance dorsal to the anterior end of the thalamus above the anterior nucleus of the thalamus. A

23   **Internal/external medullary laminae.** Laminae medullares interna/externa. Layers of white matter located partly lateral to the thalamus and partly in it. They incompletely separate the individual thalamic nuclei. E

24   **Medullary stria of thalamus.** Stria medullaris thalamica. Bundle located at the medial side of the thalamus below the thalamic tenia. It continues dorsally into the habenula and receives fibers from the fornix of the stria terminalis and the precommissural septum. A B

25   **Pulvinar.** Posterior part of thalamus projecting freely. A

26   **Metathalamus.** Appendage of thalamus below the pulvinar. A C

27   **Medial geniculate body.** Corpus geniculatum mediale. United with the inferior colliculus, it is a part of the auditory pathway. A C

28   **Lateral geniculate body.** Corpus geniculatum laterale. Connected with the superior colliculus and visual cortex, it is the termination for most of the fibers of the optic tract. A C

29   **Ventral thalamus (subthalamus).** Thalamus ventralis (Subthalamus). Part of diencephalon situated basally from the hypothalamic sulcus.

30   **Hypothalamus.** Basal part of diencephalon. B

31   **Preoptic area.** Area preoptica. Area behind the lamina terminalis and in front of the paraventricular nucleus, partly also in front of the supra-optic nucleus. Its nuclei are probably inserted between the olfactory tract and tuber cinereum. B

32   **Optic chiasma.** Chiasma opticum. Decussation of medial optic nerve fibers between the optic tract and nerve. B C

33   **Optic tract.** Tractus opticus. Part of visual pathway between the optic chiasma and lateral geniculate body evident superficially at the base of the brain. C

34   Lateral root. Radix lateralis. Fibers of optic tract which end in the lateral geniculate body or superior colliculus. C

35   Medial root. Radix medialis. C

36   **Mamillary body.** Corpus mamillare. Paired, round elevation at the floor of the diencephalon connected with the thalamus and midbrain. B

37   **Tuber cinereum.** Gray matter in the posterior wall of the infundibulum. B

38   **Infundibulum.** Funnel-shaped passage to the posterior lobe of the hypophysis. B

39   **Neurohypophysis.** Posterior lobe of hypophysis suspended by the infundibulum. B

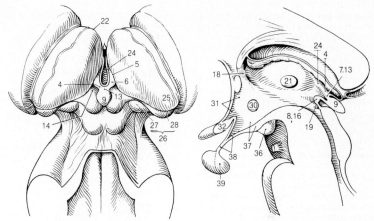

A Brain stem from dorsal

B Brain stem, sagittal section

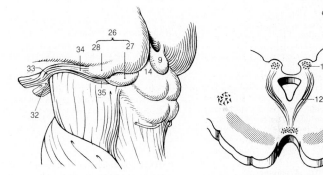

C Termination of optic tract

D Oblique section through midbrain

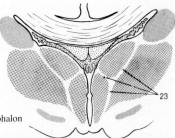

E Section through diencephalon

1 **Third ventricle.** Ventriculus tertius. Diencephalic portion of the cerebral ventricular system. It extends from the lamina terminalis to the beginning of the cerebral aqueduct. A C

2 **Hypothalamic sulcus.** Sulcus hypothalamicus. Furrow from the interventricular foramen to the entrance into the cerebral aqueduct. It separates the dorsal from the ventral thalamus. A

3 **Interventricular foramen.** Foramen interventriculare. Opening between the lateral ventricle and third ventricle behind the genu of the fornix. A

4 **Optic recess.** Recessus opticus. Recess of third ventricle above the optic chiasma. A

5 **Recess of infundibulum.** Recessus infundibu-
~ li (infundibularis). Recess of third ventricle into the infundibulum. A

6 **Pineal recess.** Recessus pinealis. Recess of third ventricle extending partially into the epiphysis. A

7 **Supraspinal recess.** Recessus suprapinalis. Recess between the roof of the third ventricle and the epiphysis. A

8 **Tela choroidea.** Thin, narrow roof of third ventricle with its choroid plexus. B C

9 **Tenia of thalamus.** Taenia thalami. Lateral attachment line of the upper wall of the third ventricle along the stria medullaris of the thalamus. B C

10 **Choroid plexus.** Plexus choroideus. Paired, heavily vascularized villous infolding which hangs down from the thin roof of the third ventricle and is continuous anteriorly via the interventricular foramen with the choroid plexus of the 4th ventricle. B C

11 **Sections of thalamus and metathala-**
~ **mus.** Sectiones thalamici et metathalamici. Annot. p. 409

12 **Reticular nucleus of thalamus.** Nucleus reticulatus [thalami]. Thin layer lying mainly laterally at the thalamus between the posterior limb of the internal capsule and external medullary lamina of the thalamus. It receives tributaries from the entire cerebral cortex, globus pallidus and reticular formation of the brainstem and gives off efferent fibers to the reticular formation of the midbrain and thalamus. B

13 **Anterior nuclei of thalamus.** Nuclei anteriores [thalami]. Cell group in the apex of the thalamus. They receive fibers from the mamillothalamic tract and have connection with the cingulate gyrus.

14 Anterodorsal nucleus. Nucleus anterodorsalis (anterosuperior). Narrow cell plate anterosuperiorly. B

15 Anteroventral nucleus. Nucleus anteroventralis (anteroinferior). Main nucleus of the anterior nuclei. B

16 Anteromedial nucleus. Nucleus anteromedialis. Degenerating nuclear remains medially and below the anteroventral nucleus. B

17 **Median nuclei of thalamus.** Nuclei mediani [thalami]. Collective term for the following three nuclei located quite medially and for the most part directly below the ependyma.

18 Anterior/posterior paraventricular
~ nuclei. Nuclei paraventriculares anteriores/ posteriores. Cell groups in the wall of the third ventricle with neuronal function (among others, vasopressin, angiotensin II, renin). C D E

19 Rhomboidal nucleus. Nucleus rhomboidalis. It often forms the interthalamic adhesion. D

20 Nucleus reuniens. It extends from the anterior end of the anterior tubercle to the middle of the interthalamic adhesion and can be concerned in its formation when it is present. It is absent in 28% of males, 14% of females. D

20a **Paratenial nucleus of thalamus.** Nucleus parataenialis [thalami]. Located between the stria medullaris, tenia, anterodorsal and paraventricular nuclei of the thalamus, it is probably involved in the processing of olfactory stimuli.

21 **Medial nuclei of thalamus.** Nuclei mediales [thalami]. Mass of nuclei medial to the internal medullary lamina with connections to other thalamic nuclei and to the frontal lobe.

22 Dorsal medial nucleus. Nucleus medialis
~ dorsalis. Principal nucleus of this group. C D

23 **Internal/external medullary lamina.** Lamina medullaris interna/externa. Layer of white matter which, provided it is located internally, has a Y-shape in sections and divides the thalamus into an anterior, a medial and a lateral region. B

24 **Reticular (intralaminar) nuclei of thalamus.** Nuclei reticulares (intralaminares thalami). Residing in the medullary lamina, they correspond functionally to the reticular formation and thus are integrative nuclei.

25 Centromedian nucleus. Nucleus centromedianus. It is the largest nucleus of this group and has connections, among others, with the corpus striatum and hypothalamus. E

26 Paracentral nucleus. Nucleus paracentralis. It lies in the internal medullary lamina lateral to the centromedian nucleus. C D

27 Parafascicular nucleus. Nucleus parafascicularis. It lies medial to the occipital region of the centromedian nucleus. E

28 Lateral central nucleus. Nucleus centralis lateralis. It lies first dorsolateral then medial to the centromedian nucleus. E

29 Medial central nucleus. Nucleus centralis medialis. It lies in the lower medial end of the internal medullary lamina.

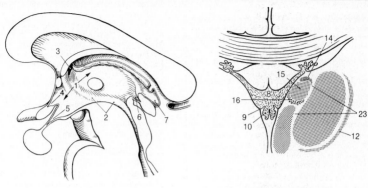

A Diencephalon, sagittal section

B Diencephalon, cross section

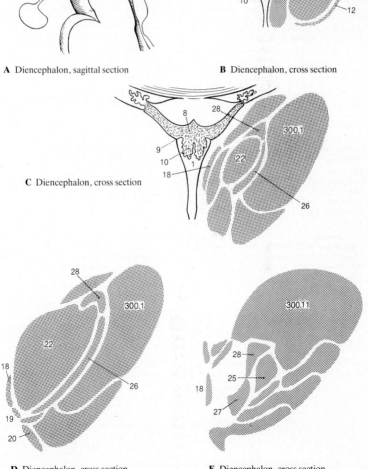

C Diencephalon, cross section

D Diencephalon, cross section

E Diencephalon, cross section

dullary lamina. B

2 Posterior lateral nucleus. Nucleus lateralis posterior. Area situated between the pulvinar and dorsal lateral nucleus with connections to the parietal lobe. A

3 Dorsal lateral nucleus. Nucleus lateralis dorsalis. Region of lateral group located anterosuperiorly with connections to the region of the posterior cingulum segment and the lower part of the parietal lobe. A

4 Anterior ventral nucleus. Nucleus ventralis
~ anterior. It lies anteriorly and has connections with the interlaminar nuclei, globus pallidus and dentate nucleus besides reciprocally with the precentral gyrus and the field anterior to it. It plays a role in Parkinson's disease. A

5 Intermediate ventral nucleus. Nucleus ven-
~ tralis intermedius. Lying behind the anterior ventral nucleus, it is a synaptic station between the cerebellum, red nucleus and motor cortex. A

6 Medial ventral nucleus. Nucleus ventralis medialis. Lying anterior to the posterior ventral nuclei and not sharply delimited, its function is unclear. A

7 Posterior ventral nuclei. Nuclei ventrales posteriores. Collective name for the following two nuclei.

8 *Posterolateral ventral nucleus.* Nucleus ventralis posterolateralis. As the lateral part of the posterior ventral nucleus, it receives the medial lemniscus and spinothalamic tract and relays their impulses to the postcentral gyrus via the thalamocortical tract. A

9 *Posteromedial ventral nucleus.* Nucleus ventralis posteromedialis. It lies between the centromedian and posterolateral nuclei and receives the trigeminal lemniscus. A

10 **Posterior nuclei of thalamus.** Nuclei posteriores [thalami]. Collective term for the following three parts of the thalamus:

11 Pulvinar nuclei. Nuclei pulvinares. Occupying
~ the posterior portion of the thalamus, they begin at the habenulae, receive tributaries from the auditory and visual pathways as well as from other thalamic nuclei and are connected with the visual cortex and the optic and acoustic control centers, among others. A

12 Lateral geniculate nucleus [dorsal part]. Nucleus [corporis geniculati] lateralis [Pars dorsalis]. Part of the visual pathway. A

13 Medial geniculate nucleus [dorsal part]. Nucleus [Corporis geniculati] medialis [Pars dorsalis]. Part of medial geniculate body containing small cells. A

14 **Sections of ventral thalamus.** Sectiones thalami ventralis.

15 **Lateral geniculate nucleus [ventral part].** Nucleus corporis geniculati lateralis [pars ventralis]. Small group of cells with fibers from the retina; part of a light reflex tract. C

16 **Medial geniculate nucleus [ventral part].** Nucleus corporis geniculati medialis [Pars ventralis]. Possibly the true acoustic part of the geniculate nucleus. C

17 **Subthalamic nucleus.** Nucleus subthalamicus [corpus Luysii]. It lies between the lower end of the internal capsule and the zona incerta. Of clinical importance is its reciprocal connection with the globus pallidus. B

18 **Reticular nuclei of thalamus.** Nuclei reticulares
~ [thalami]. Disaggregated cell layer at the external side of the thalamus between the external medullary lamina and internal capsule. B

19 **Zona incerta.** Basal continuation, among others, of the reticular nucleus of the thalamus. It is inserted in the path of the globus pallidus to the tegmentum of the diencephalon. B

20 Nuclear regions H, H1 and H2. Nuclei regionum H, H1 and H2. Dispersed neurons in the corresponding Forel's fields. Field H lies medial to the zona incerta and in front of the red nucleus, H1 between the thalamus and zona incerta, H2 between the zona incerta and subthalamic nucleus. B

21 **Thalamic tract and fasciculi.** Tractus et fasciculi thalamici.

22 **Lateral lemniscus.** Lemniscus lateralis. Auditory pathway passing into the medial geniculate body. A

23 **Medial lemniscus.** Lemniscus medialis. Continuation of the tract from the posterior funiculus radiating into the posterolateral ventral nucleus. A

24 **Spinal lemniscus.** Lemniscus spinalis. Pain pathway extending into the posterolateral ventral nucleus. A

25 **Trigeminal lemniscus.** Lemniscus trigeminalis. Fibers of the sensory trigeminal nucleus. They pass into the posteromedial ventral nucleus. A

26 **Brachium of inferior colliculus.** Brachium colli-
~ culi inferioris. Outwardly visible connection between the inferior colliculus and the medial geniculate body. C

27 **Acoustic radiation.** Radiatio acustica. Portion of auditory pathway from the medial geniculate body on its way to the transverse temporal gyri. It passes through the occipital part of the posterior limb of the internal capsule. A

28 **Brachium of superior colliculus.** Brachium colli-
~ culi superioris. Externally visible connection between the superior colliculus and the lateral geniculate body. Connection of the visual pathway with the extrapyramidal system. C

29 **Optic radiation.** Radiatio optica [[Gratiolet]]. Portion of visual pathway emanating from the lateral geniculate body. It passes through the occipital part of the posterior limb of the internal capsule and around the posterior horn of the lateral ventricle to the area striata. A

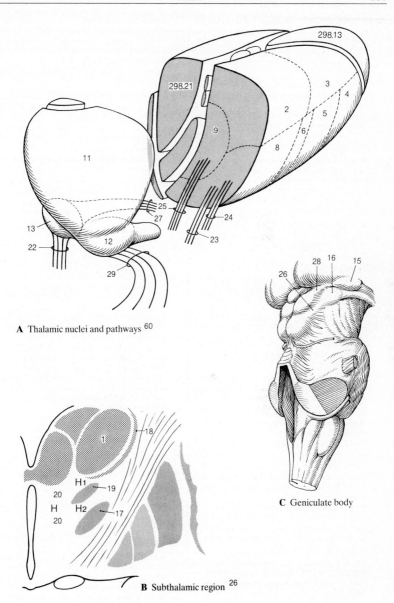

A Thalamic nuclei and pathways [60]

B Subthalamic region [26]

C Geniculate body

1　**Anterior thalamic radiations.** Radiationes thalamicae anteriores. Fibers of the anterior nucleus from and to the cingulate gyrus and likewise reciprocal connections between the lateral nucleus and frontal lobe. The fibers run in the anterior limb of the internal capsule. A

2　**Central thalamic radiations.** Radiationes thalamicae centrales. Reciprocal fibers passing fan-like through the posterior limb of the internal capsule from the posterior lateral, anterior ventral, lateral ventral and posterior ventral nuclei to the pre- and postcentral gyri in addition to the connecting fields of the cortex. A

3　**Posterior thalamic radiations.** Radiationes thalamicae posteriores. They lie in the occipital region of the posterior limb of the internal capsule and contain fibers from the lateral geniculate body (optic radiation) and the pulvinar for the occipital lobes and adjacent regions. A

4　**Dentatothalamic tract.** Tractus dentatothalamicus. It comes from the cerebellum and radiates in the thalamic fasciculus to the lateral ventral nucleus. C

5　**Thalamic fasciculus.** Fasciculus thalamicus. It lies below the thalamus, next to and above the zona incerta in field H1 and is composed of the ventricular fasciculus, ansa lenticularis and fibers from the cerebellum. Along with others, it is a conveyor for the anterior ventral and lateral ventral nuclei. C

6　**Subthalamic fasciculus.** Fasciculus subthalamicus. Fiber bundle from the globus pallidus to the subthalamic nucleus. C

7　**Mamillothalamic fasciculus.** Fasciculus mamillothalamicus. Fiber tract from the mamillary body to the anterior nucleus of the thalamus. D

8　**Inferior thalamic peduncle.** Pedunculus thalamicus inferior. Fibers between the hypothalamus and thalamus. According to other versions, it consists of fibers of the pulvinar from and to the occipital lobes and its vicinity, as well as fibers of the auditory tract.

9　**Ansa lenticularis and fasciculus lenticularis.**
~ 　Ansa et fasciculus lenticulares. Two fiber bundles from the lentiform nucleus to the ventral nuclei of the thalamus. One part passes around the anterior margin of the internal capsule (Ansa lenticularis); the other part passes through the internal capsule. Both tracts are united in the thalamic fasciculus. C

10　**Ansa peduncularis and fasciculus peduncula-**
~ 　**ris.** Ansa et fasciculus pedunculares. Fiber tract between the thalamus and claustrum coursing between the lentiform nucleus and the amygdaloid body. B C

11　**Intrathalamic fibers.** Fibrae intrathalamicae. Conncetions of individual thalamic nuclei.

12　**Periventricular fibers.** Fibrae periventriculares. Fibers coursing beneath the ependyma of the third ventricle between the medial nucleus and the hypothalamic nucleus to enter the posterior longitudinal fasciculus.

13　**Sections of the hypothalamus.** Sectiones hypothalami.

14　**Dorsal (posterior) hypothalamic region.** Regio (area) hypothalamica dorsalis. Area of the hypothalamus next to the apex.

15　**Nucleus of ansa lenticularis.** Nucleus ansae lenticularis. Groups of cells dispersed in the ansa lenticularis.

16　**Anterior (ventral) region of hypothalamus.** Regio hypothalamica anterior.

17　**Medial/lateral preoptic nucleus.** Nucleus preopticus medialis/lateralis. Group of nuclei located beneath the anterior commissure and at the lamina terminalis with connections to the stria terminalis, medial telencephalic fasciculus and medial thalamic nuclei. D

18　**Supraoptic nucleus.** Nucleus supraopticus. Nucleus lying above the optic chiasma with neurosecretory fibers (oxytocin and vasopressin) to the posterior pituitary. D

19　**Paraventricular nuclei.** Nuclei paraventriculares. Group of autonomic nuclei with neurosecretory fibers (oxytocin and vasopressin) to the posterior lobe of the hypophysis. They lie superiorly toward the base of the hypothalamic sulcus and behind the anterior hypothalamic nucleus. D

20　**Anterior hypothalamic nucleus.** Nucleus hypothalamicus anterior. Located behind the preoptic nucleus with connections to the hemispheres, stria terminalis and thalamus, its efferent fibers communicate with motor and autonomic nuclei. It influences heat regulation, glandular activity and circulation. D

21　**Intermediate hypothalamic region.** Regio hypothalamica intermedia. Area situated between the anterior and posterior hypothalamic regions.

22　**Arcuate nucleus.** [[Nucleus arcuatus]]. It lies in the wall of the entrance to the infundibulum and belongs to the tuberal nuclei, i.e., it regulates the release of hormones from the anterior lobe by delivering an active substance (neurohormone) into blood vessels of the hypophysial stalk where its processes (axons) are found. D

23　**Tuberal nuclei.** Nuclei tuberales. Groups of nuclei in the posterior wall of the infundibulum. Function as in 22. D

24　**Lateral hypothalamic region.** Regio hypothalamica lateralis. Area separated from the medial hypothalamus by the fornix, mamillothalamic fasciculus and medial telencephalic fasciculus. It is occupied, among others, by the lateral preoptic nucleus and the supraoptic nucleus with its lateral portion. D

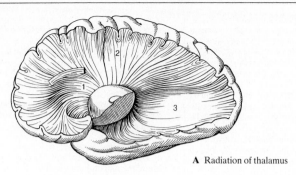

A Radiation of thalamus

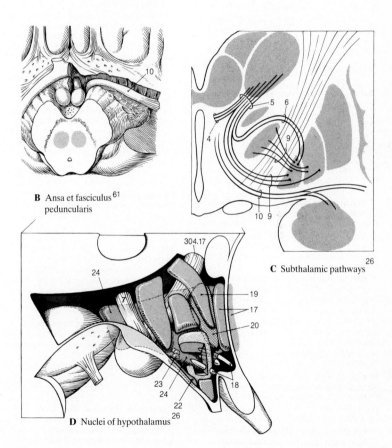

B Ansa et fasciculus [61] peduncularis

C Subthalamic pathways

D Nuclei of hypothalamus

1 **Ventromedial hypothalamic nucleus.** Nucle-
~ us hypothalamicus ventromedialis. Lying at
the entrance into the infundibulum and above
it, this nucleus belongs to the group of tuberal
nuclei and, like them, controls the release of
regulating hormones for the anterior lobe via
the hypophysial stalk. A

2 **Dorsomedial hypothalamic nucleus.** Nucleus hypothalamicus dorsomedialis. It lies toward the apex of the ventromedial hypothalamic nucleus and resembles it in its function. A

3 **Dorsal hypothalamic nucleus.** Nucleus hypothalamicus dorsalis. Group of cells located
below the dorsal hypothalamic area (302.14).
A

4 **Posterior periventricular nucleus.** Nucleus
periventricularis posterior. Cell group located
below the ependyma in the posterior segment
of the 3rd ventricle. A

5 **Infundibular (arcuate) nucleus.** Nucleus infundibularis (arcuatus). It lies somewhat at the
apex of the funnel of the infundibulum and is
compared functionally to the tuberal nuclei. A

6 **Posterior hypothalamic area.** Regio hypothalamica posterior. It contains, among others,
the lateral and medial nuclei of the mamillary
body.

7 **Medial and lateral nuclei of mamillary
body.** Nuclei corporis mamillaris mediales/
laterales. Medial nucleus forms the mamillary
body and is the origin of the mamillothalamic
fasciculus. Lateral nucleus lies ventrolateral
and receives the fornix. A B

8 **Posterior hypothalamic nucleus.** Nucleus
hypothalamicus posterior. It lies toward the occiput from the dorsomedial and ventromedial
nucleus, somewhat toward the apex of the mamillary body up to the hypothalamic sulcus and
influences circulation, peristalsis and the
blood-sugar level. A B

9 **Neurohypophysis.** In contrast to the two
other posterior lobes of the hypophysis, it is of
neurogenic origin as is the continuation of the
infundibulum. B

10 **Hypothalamic tract and fasciculi.** Tractus et
fasciculi hypothalamici. Tracts and fiber bundles of the hypothalamus.

11 **Periventricular fibers.** Fibrae periventriculares. Fiber tract directly under the ependyma of
the 3rd ventricle. Permeated by cells, it connects the thalamus with the hypothalamus and continues posteriorly into the posterior longitudinal fasciculus. B

12 **Dorsal supraoptic commissure.** Commissura
supraoptica dorsalis [[Meynert]]. Decussation
lying directly above the chiasma. Passing to the

other side, it connects perhaps the subthalamic
nucleus with the globus pallidus of the opposite
side.

13 **Ventral supraoptic commissure.** Commissura supraoptica ventralis [[Gudden]]. Crossing
fibers lying partially still in the chiasma
perhaps connect, among others, the medial geniculate bodies with one another.

14 **Posterior (dorsal) longitudinal fasciculus.**
Fasciculus longitudinalis dorsalis [[Schütz]].
Cranial continuation of a large portion of the
ventricular fibers. In the midbrain they lie close
to the cerebral aqueduct and connect the
hypothalamus with the rest of the brainstem. B

15 **Mamillotegmental fasciculus.** Fasciculus
mamillotegmentalis. Dissectible fiber bundle
between the mamillary body and the tegmental
nuclei of the midbrain. It arises in a common
trunk together with the mamillothalamic fasciculus and then branches off into the mesencephalic tegmentum. B

16 **Mamillothalamic fasciculus.** Fasciculus mamillothalamicus. After arising in common with
the mamillotegmental fasciculus, it passes to
the anterior thalamic nuclei. B

17 **Fornix.** It brings some fibers from the hippocampal formation into the medial thalamic
nuclei and the hypothalamus, and further fibers
into the lateral nuclei of the mamillary body. B

18 **Fibers of stria terminalis.** Fibrae striae terminalis. Fibers from the amygdaloid body which
communicate with the stria terminalis in the
hypothalamus. B

19 **Medial prosencephalic fasciculus.** Fasciculus prosencephalicus medialis. Fibers lying between the medial and lateral hypothalamus.
They connect individual hypothalamic nuclei
with one another and continue toward the occiput in the posterior longitudinal fasciculus. B

20 **Hypothalamohypophysial tract.** Tractus hy-
pothalamohypophysialis. Bundle with neurosecretory fibers after the union of the fiber
groups from the supra-optic and paraventricular nuclei. B

21 **Supraoptic fibers.** Fibrae supraopticae. Fibers coming from the supraoptic nucleus. B

22 **Paraventricular fibers.** Fibrae paraventriculares. Fibers coming from the paraventricular nucleus. B

23 **Supraopticohypophysial tract.** Tractus su-
praopticohypophysialis. Fibers of the supraoptic nucleus before forming a part of the hypothalamohypophysial tract.

24 **Paraventriculohypophysial tract.** Tractus
paraventriculohypophysialis. Fibers of the paraventricular nucleus before forming a part of
the hypothalamohypophysial tract.

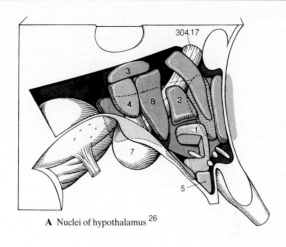

A Nuclei of hypothalamus [26]

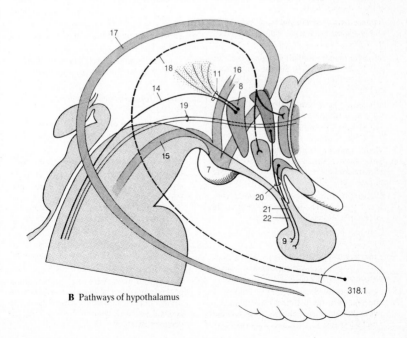

B Pathways of hypothalamus

1 ENDBRAIN. Telencephalon. Developed from the prosencephalon (forebrain), it consists of the cerebral cortex with the corpus callosum, corpus striatum and olfactory brain.

2 CEREBRUM. In the present context, the cerebral hemispheres with their contents.

3 **Cerebral cortex.** Cortex cerebralis (Pallium). Paired portion of the hemispheres covering most of the brainstem.

4 **Cerebral gyri.** Gyri cerebrales. Convolutions about 1 cm wide.

5 **Cerebral sulci.** Sulci cerebrales. Fissures between gyri.

6 **Cerebral lobes.** Lobi cerebrales. There are four lobes of the cerebrum: frontal, parietal, temporal and occipital.

7 **Longitudinal fissure of cerebrum.** Fissura longitudinalis cerebralis. Deep longitudinal groove between the right and left cerebral hemispheres. It is occupied by the falx cerebri. B

8 **Transverse fissure of cerebrum.** Fissura transversa cerebralis [[Fissura telodiencephalica]]. Fissure beneath the corpus callosum and fornix as well as above the thalamus and roof of the 3rd ventricle. B

9 **Lateral fossa of cerebrum.** Fossa lateralis cerebralis. Space in the depth of the lateral sulcus. B

10 **Superior (superomedial) margin.** Margo superior (superomedialis). Superior border of a hemisphere between the superolateral and medial surface. B

11 **Inferior (inferolateral) margin.** Margo inferior (inferolateralis). Inferolateral border of a hemisphere between the superolateral and inferior surfaces. B

12 **Medial (inferomedial) margin.** Maro medialis (inferomedialis). Inferomedial border of a hemisphere between the inferior and medial surfaces. B

13 **[[Fissura limitans]].** Fissure between the insula and opercula. The floor of this cleft, as the sulcus limitans, receives the insula.

14 **Cerebral hemisphere.** Hemispharium (cerebralis). Half of the telencephalon. B

15 **Superolateral surface of hemisphere.** Facies superolateralis hemispherii. Upper and lateral surface of the hemisphere. B

16 **Central sulcus.** Sulcus centralis. Furrow located between the pre- and postcentral gyri and at the same time between the frontal and parietal lobes. A

17 **Lateral sulcus.** Sulcus lateralis. Deep cleft between the temporal lobe below and the frontal and parietal lobes above.

18 Anterior ramus. Ramus anterior. Short anteriorly directed branch of the lateral sulcus. A

19 Ascending ramus. Ramus ascendens. Short branch of the lateral sulcus ascending into the frontal lobe. A

20 Posterior ramus. Ramus posterior. Long posterior branch of the lateral suclus terminating at the supramarginal gyrus. A

21 **Interlobar sulci.** Sulci interlobares. Furrows which separate the cerebral lobes from one another: central sulcus, parieto-occipital sulcus and the lateral sulcus with its posterior ramus.

22 **Frontal lobe.** Lobus frontalis. It extends from the frontal pole to the central sulcus. A

23 **Frontal pole.** Polus frontalis. Anterior end of frontal lobe. A

24 **Precentral sulcus.** Sulcus precentralis. Furrow in front of the precentral gyrus. A

25 **Precentral gyrus.** Gyrus precentralis. Motor convolution of the frontal lobe lying in front of the central sulcus. A

26 **Superior frontal gyrus.** Gyrus frontalis superior. A

27 **Superior frontal sulcus.** Sulcus frontalis superior. Furrow below the superior frontal gyrus. A

28 **Middle frontal gyrus.** Gyrus frontalis medius. A

29 **Inferior frontal sulcus.** Sulcus frontalis inferior. Furrow lying between the middle and inferior frontal gyrus. A

30 **Inferior frontal gyrus.** Gyrus frontalis inferior.

31 Opercular part (frontal operculum). Pars opercularis [Operculum frontale]. Part of inferior frontal gyrus lying behind the ascending ramus and at the same time covering the insula. A

32 Orbital part. Pars orbitalis. Part of the inferior frontal gyrus located below the anterior ramus of the lateral cerebral sulcus. A

33 Triangular part. Pars triangularis. Portion of the inferior frontal gyrus located between the anterior and descending rami of the lateral cerebral sulcus. Region of the motor speech center of Broca. A

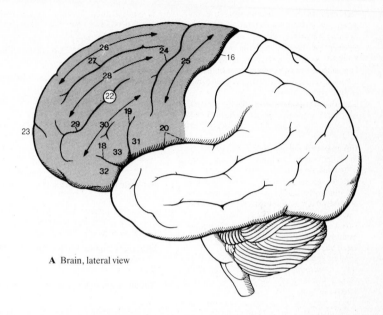

A Brain, lateral view

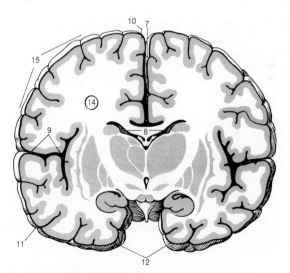

B Brain, frontal section

1 **Parietal lobe.** Lobus parietalis. It is bordered anteriorly by the central sulcus, posteriorly by the parieto-occipital sulcus. A

2 **Postcentral sulcus.** Sulcus postcentralis. Posterior boundary of the postcentral gyrus. A

3 **Postcentral gyrus.** Gyrus postcentralis. Predominantly sensory, it lies between the central and postcentral sulci. A

4 **Superior parietal lobule.** Lobulus parietalis superior. Upper half of parietal lobe behind the postcentral gyrus and above the intraparietal sulcus. A

5 **Intraparietal sulcus.** Sulcus intraparietalis. Inconstant sagittal furrow between the superior and inferior parietal lobules. A

6 **Inferior parietal lobule.** Lobulus parietalis inferior. Lower half of parietal lobe behind the postcentral gyrus and below the intraparietal sulcus. A

7 **Frontoparietal operculum.** Operculum frontoparietale. Part of the cerebral segment located above the posterior ramus of the lateral cerebral sulcus and covering the insula. It extends toward the occiput somewhat up to the place where the posterior ramus makes a bend upwards. A

8 **Supramarginal gyrus.** Gyrus supramarginalis. Convolution curving around the posterior end of the posterior ramus of the lateral sulcus. A

9 **Angular gyrus.** Gyrus angularis. Convolution curving around the posterior end of the superior temporal sulcus. A

10 **Occipital lobe.** Lobus occipitalis. It is incompletely bordered by the parietal and parieto-occipital sulci and the pre-occipital incisure. A

11 **Occipital pole.** Polus occipitalis. Posterior end of occipital lobe. A

12 **Transverse occipital sulcus.** Sulcus occipitalis transversus. Continuation of the intraparietalis sulcus on the occipital lobe. A

13 **Lunate sulcus.** Sulcus lunatus. Well developed arched furrow occasionally present as the anterior boundary of the visual cortex. It lies at the superolateral surface of the cerebrum near the occipital pole at the posterior end of the calcarine fissure. A

14 **Preoccipital incisure.** Incisura preoccipitalis. Notch at the inferolateral margin marking the boundary between the occipital and temporal lobes at the lower border of the brain. On the bony skull it corresponds to the site where the petrous ridge goes over into the lateral wall of the skull. A

15 **Temporal lobe.** Lobus temporalis. It is bordered superiorly by the posterior ramus of the lateral sulcus. A

16 **Temporal pole.** Polus temporalis. Anterior end of temporal lobe. A

17 **Transverse temporal sulci.** Sulci temporales transversi. Transverse furrows between the transverse temporal gyri in the floor of the posterior ramus of the lateral sulcus. C

18 **Transverse temporal gyri.** Gyri temporales transversi [Heschl's transverse convolutions]. 2–4 transverse convolutions located in the floor of the posterior ramus of the lateral sulcus. Acoustic center. C

19 **Superior temporal gyrus.** Gyrus temporalis superior. A C

20 **Temporal operculum.** Operculum temporale. Part of superior temporal gyrus which covers the insula. A

21 **Superior temporal sulcus.** Sulcus temporalis superior. Cleft between the superior and middle temporal gyri. A

22 **Middle temporal gyrus.** Gyrus temporalis medius. A C

23 **Inferior temporal sulcus.** Sulcus temporalis inferior. Cleft between the middle and inferior temporal gyri. A

24 **Inferior temporal gyrus.** Gyrus temporalis inferior. A

25 **Insula (insular lobe).** Lobus insularis (Insula). Originally exposed cerebral cortex overlapped during ontogenesis. It lies in the floor of the lateral cerebral fossa. B

26 **Insular gyri.** Gyri insulae.

27 **Short gyri of insula.** Gyri breves insulae. Short, anterior convolutions. B

28 **Long gyrus of insula.** Gyrus longus insulae. Long horizontal convolution located posteriorly. B

29 **Limen insulae.** Terminal portion of insular surface directed anteroinferiorly toward the anterior perforated substance. It is covered by the middle cerebral artery. B

30 **Central sulcus of insula.** Sulcus centralis insulae. Cleft between the long gyrus and short gyri of the insula. B

31 **Circular sulcus of insula.** Sulcus circularis insulae. Limiting furrow of the insula. It is interrupted at the limen. B

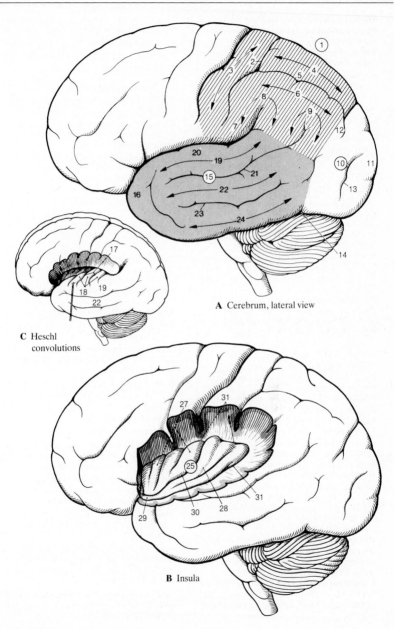

A Cerebrum, lateral view

C Heschl convolutions

B Insula

1 **Medial and inferior surface of cerebral hemisphere.** Facies medialis et inferior hemispherii.

2 **Sulcus of corpus callosum.** Sulcus corporis callosi. Cleft between the corpus callosum and the cingulate gyrus. A

3 **Cingulate gyrus.** Gyrus cinguli (cingulatum). Convolution between cingulate sulcus and sulcus of corpus callosum coursing parallel to the corpus callosum. It belongs to the limbic cortex. A

4 Isthmus of cingulate gyrus. Isthmus gyri cinguli (cingulatum). Constriction at the transition of the cingulate gyrus into the parahippocampal gyrus posterior and inferior to the splenium of the corpus callosum. A

5 Cingulate sulcus. Sulcus cinguli (cingulatus). Furrow bordering anterior portion of cingulate gyrus anteriorly and superiorly. A

6 **Subparietal sulcus.** Sulcus subparietalis. Furrow bordering the posterior portion of the cingulate gyrus superiorly and posteriorly. A

7 **Medial frontal gyrus.** Gyrus frontalis medialis. Convolution superior to the medial surface of the frontal lobe, bordered inferiorly by the cingulate sulcus. A

8 **Paracentral lobule.** Lobulus paracentralis. Hooklike connection between the pre- and postcentral gyri on the medial surface. A

9 **Precuneus.** Precuneus.[3] Field situated in front of the parieto-occipital sulcus and bordered anteriorly partly by the subparietal sulcus. A

10 **Parieto-occipital sulcus.** Sulcus parieto-occipitalis. Deep cleft in front of the cuneus separating the occipital and parietal lobes. A

11 **Cuneus.** Field between the calcarine and parieto-occipital sulci. A

12 **Calcarine sulcus.** Sulcus calcarinus. Deep furrow below the cuneus in the region of the primary visual area. Anteriorly, it meets the parieto-occipital sulcus at an acute angle. A

13 **Dentate gyrus.** Gyrus dentatus. Curved convolution of gray matter appearing serrated owing to numerous indentations. It forms the inferior continuation of the fasciolar gyrus, reaches up to the medial surface of the uncus and lies between the hippocampus and parahippocampal gyrus. A

14 **Hippocampal sulcus.** Sulcus hippocampi (hippocampalis). Furrow situated between the parahippocampal and dentate gyri. It meets the uncus anteriorly. A

15 **Parahippocampal gyrus.** Gyrus hippocampi (parahippocampalis). Well-developed convolution located below the hippocampal sulcus. A B

16 Uncus. Anterior hook-shaped termination of the parahippocampal gyrus. A B

17 **Lingual gyrus.** Gyrus lingualis. Continuation of the parahippocampal gyrus toward the occiput. A B

18 **Collateral sulcus.** Sulcus collateralis. Furrow between the parahippocampal and medial occipitotemporal gyri extending into the occipital lobe. A B

19 **Rhinal sulcus.** Sulcus rhinalis. Continuation of the collateral sulcus occasionally present lateral to the uncus. A B

20 **Medial occipitotemporal gyrus.** Gyrus occipitotemporalis medialis. Basal convolution between the collateral and occipitotemporal sulci. A B

21 **Occipitotemporal sulcus.** Sulcus occipitotemporalis. Cleft between the medial and lateral occipitotemporal gyri located on the inferior surface of the brain lateral to the collateral sulcus. A B

22 **Lateral occipitotemporal gyrus.** Gyrus occipitotemporalis lateralis. Convolution adjoining the occipitotemporal sulcus laterally. At the inferior margin of the temporal lobe it becomes continuous with the inferior temporal gyrus without interruption. A B

23 **Gyrus rectus.** Elongated convolution located above the orbit at its medial margin. B

24 **Olfactory sulcus.** Sulcus olfactorius. Groove for the olfactory tract on the inferior surface of the frontal lobe. B

25 **Orbital gyri.** Gyri orbitales. Frontal convolutions located lateral to the gyrus rectus.

26 **Orbital sulci.** Sulci orbitales. Furrows between the orbital gyri. B

26 a **Olfactory brain.** Rhinencephalon.

27 **Olfactory bulb.** Bulbus olfactorius. Knob-like enlargement containing dendrite-rich mitral cells at the beginning of the olfactory tract. B

28 **Olfactory tract.** Tractus olfactorius. Connection between the olfactory bulb and trigone on the inferior surface of the frontal lobe. B

29 **Olfactory trigone.** Trigonum olfactorium. Triangular widening at the end of the olfactory tract. B

30 **Medial and lateral olfactory striae.** Striae olfactoriae medialis et lateralis. Diverging fiber bundles of the olfactory tract radiating fanlike at the olfactory trigone. B

31 **Medial and lateral olfactory gyri.** Gyri olfactorii medialis et lateralis. Cellular continuations of same named striae.

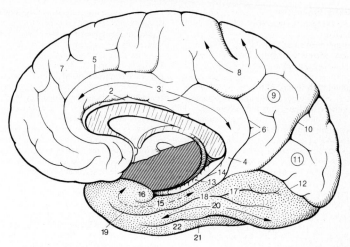

A Cerebrum, medial view

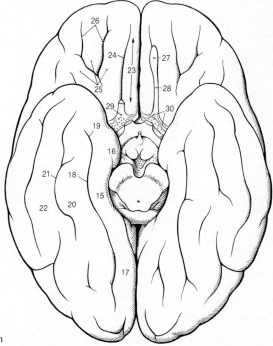

B Base of brain

1 **Olfactory brain.** Rhinencephalon. In the present context, it consists of the following four parts:

2 **Anterior perforated substance.** Substantia perforata anterior. Perforated field posterior to the olfactory trigone caused by the passage of cerebral vessels. A

3 **Diagonal stria (band) of Broca.** Stria diagonalis [Broca]. Bundle of myelinated fibers often coursing obliquely over the anterior perforated substance. It connects the precommissural septum with the uncus. A

4 **Subcallosal area.** Area subcallosa. Field at the medial surface of the frontal lobe below the genu and rostrum of the corpus callosum. A

5 Paraterminal gyrus. Gyrus paraterminalis. Convolution located at the medial surface below the rostrum and in front of the laminal terminalis. A

6 **Corpus callosum.** A massive transverse fiber connection between the right and left hemispheres at the base of the longitudinal fissure of the cerebrum. A B C

7 **Splenium.** Posterior, thicker, free end of the corpus callosum. B

8 **Trunk.** Truncus. Portion of corpus callosum between the splenium and genu. B

9 **Genu.** Bend of the corpus callosum located anteriorly above the rostrum. B

10 **Rostrum.** Anterior end of corpus callosum tapering to a point inferiorly where it joins the lamina terminalis. B

11 **Radiation of corpus callosum.** Radiatio corporis callosi. Fibers radiating out from the corpus callosum to the cerebral cortex. A D

12 Forceps minor. Forceps frontalis (minor). U-shaped fibers passing through the genu of the corpus callosum and connecting the frontal lobes with one another. D

13 Forceps major. Forceps occipitalis (major). U-shaped fibers passing through the splenium of the corpus callosum and connecting the posterior parts of the occipital lobes with one another. D

14 Tapetum. Continuous layer of fibers from the corpus callosum passing bow-like laterally and inferiorly and forming the lateral wall of the inferior and posterior horns of the lateral ventricle as well as the roof of the posterior horn. C

15 **Indusium griseum.** Thin layer of gray matter on the superior surface of the corpus callosum. B C

16 Medial longitudinal stria. Stria longitudinalis medialis. Medial longitudinal white stripe embedded in the indusium griseum bilaterally. It is part of the so-called olfactory brain. B C

17 Lateral longitudinal stria. Stria longitudinalis lateralis. Paired longitudinal stripe embedded in the indusium griseum and covered laterally by the cingulate gyrus. It is part of the so-called olfactory brain. B C

18 **Gyrus fasciolaris.** Passing around the splenium of the corpus callosum, it forms a connection between the longitudinal striae, including the indusium griseum and dentate gyrus. B

19 **Lamina terminalis.** Thin walled, anterior border of the 3rd ventricle. A B

20 **Anterior commissure.** Commissura anterior. Anterior, transverse connection between
~ the right and left halves of the cerebrum. It lies behind the lamina terminalis and is visible in the most anterior segment of the 3rd ventricle. A

21 **Fornix.** Curved fiber bundle with fibers, among others, passing in both directions between the mamillary body and hippocampus. B

22 **Posterior limb of fornix.** Crus. It arises from the hippocampus as hippocampal fimbria, circles around the pulvinar and joins up with the contralateral limb to form the body of the fornix. B

23 **Body of fornix.** Corpus. Unpaired middle part of fornix situated below the corpus callosum and formed by the union of both crura. B

24 **Tenia.** Taenia. Thin, lateral margin of fornix giving attachment to the choroid plexus of the lateral ventricle. B

25 **Column.** Columna. Anterior part of fornix located partly in the lateral wall of the 3rd ventricle. It extends as far as the mamillary body. B

26 **Commissure.** Commissura. Triangular connecting plate between the crura of the fornix below the posterior part of the corpus callosum. It contains fibers crossing from the hippocampal fimbriae of both sides. B

27 **Septum pellucidum (lucidum).** Bilayered, thin plate stretched out between the corpus callosum and fornix. It separates the anterior horns of the lateral ventricles from one another. B

28 **Lamina of septum pellucidum.** Lamina septi pellucidi. Paired sheet forming the septum pellucidum and the lateral wall of its cavity. B

29 **Cavity of septum pellucidum.** Cavum septi pellucidi. Enclosed cavity of variable size between the two laminae of the septum pellucidum. B

30 **Precommissural septum.** Septum precommissurale. Area at the free medial surface of the frontal lobe in front of the lamina terminalis.

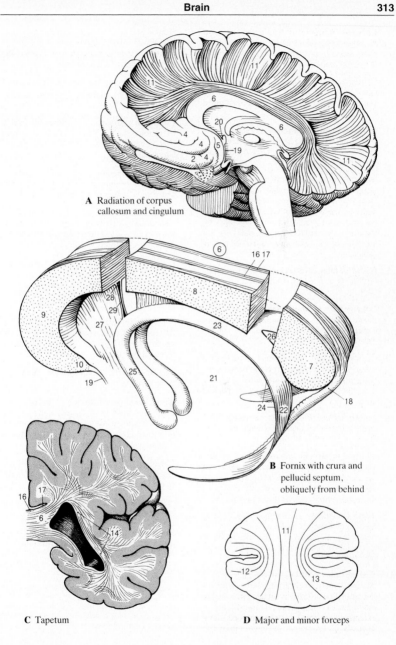

A Radiation of corpus callosum and cingulum

B Fornix with crura and pellucid septum, obliquely from behind

C Tapetum

D Major and minor forceps

1 **Lateral ventricle.** Ventriculus lateralis. Paired ventricle which communicates with the third ventricle via the interventricular foramen. It consists of the following three parts: A

2 **Central part.** Pars centralis. Middle portion of lateral ventricle located above the thalamus and below the corpus callosum. It contains a part of the choroid plexus. A

3 **Interventricular foramen.** Foramen interventriculare. Opening between the lateral ventricle and 3rd ventricle behind and below the genu of the fornix. D

4 **Anterior horn of lateral ventricle.** Cornu frontale (anterius). Extending anteriorly from the interventricular foramen, it is bordered medially by the septum pellucidum, laterally by the head of the caudate nucleus, superiorly by the trunk of the corpus callosum, anteriorly and inferiorly by the genu or rostrum of the corpus callosum. A

5 **Posterior horn of lateral ventricle.** Cornu occipitale (posterius). It extends into the occipital lobe. A

6 **Inferior horn of lateral ventricle.** Cornu temporale (inferius). It accompanies the hippocampus laterally and contains a part of the choroid plexus. A

7 **Stria terminalis.** Longitudinal stripe formed by myelinated fibers in the angle between the thalamus and caudate nucleus above the thalamostriate vein. It comes from the amygdaloid body. B

8 **Lamina affixa.** Floor of lateral ventricle between the stria terminalis and tenia choroidea. B

9 **Choroid fissure.** Fissura choroidea. Cleft between the thalamus and fornix for passage of the choroid plexus into the lateral ventricle. In the inferior horn it lies between the fimbria of the hippocampus and the stria terminalis. B

10 **Tenia choroidea.** Taenia choroidea. Attachment line of the choroid plexus of the lateral ventricle to the thalamus. It becomes visible as a detachment line after removal of the choroid plexus. B

11 **Choroid plexus of lateral ventricle.** Plexus choroideus ventriculi lateralis. Strongly vascularized, villous fringe invaginated into the lateral ventricle through the choroid fissure. It extends anteriorly to the interventricular foramen and posteriorly into the inferior horn. B

12 **Bulb of posterior horn.** Bulbus cornus occipitalis (posterioris). Enlargement at the medial side of the posterior horn caused by fibers of the splenium of the corpus callosum. C

13 **Calcar avis.** Enlargement at the medial side of the posterior horn produced by the calcarine fissure. C

14 **Collateral eminence.** Eminentia collateralis. Elevation in the lateral floor of the inferior horn near the hippocampus. It is caused by the collateral sulcus. C

15 **Collateral trigone.** Trigonum collaterale. Broadened beginning of the collateral eminence at the border to the posterior horn. C

16 **Hippocampus.** Elongated elevation in the inferior horn caused by the hippocampal sulcus. It is a specifically structured part of the rhinencephalon. C

17 **Pes.** Paw-like anterior end of the hippocampus. C

18 **Alveus.** Thin layer of white matter on the hippocampus. C

19 **Fimbria.** Bundle of white fibers emanating from the alveus and passsing medially and upward on the hippocampus to continue into the fornix as its crus. C

19a **Sections of the telencephalon.** Sectiones telencephalici.

20 **Archicortex** (archipallium). Archaecortex. Phylogenetically the older part of the cerebral cortex, it is not six-layered as the neocortex, but only three-layered and is formed by the hippocampus and dentate gyrus.

21 **Paleocortex.** Palaeocortex. Oldest part of cortex. It corresponds to the region which is derived from the piriform lobe.

22 **Neocortex.** It constitutes the largest part of the cerebral cortex and is six-layered.

22a **Mesocortex.** Incompletely differentiated zone in the region of the insular cortex. It has visceral functions.

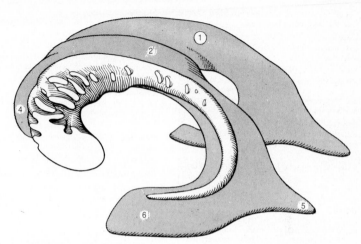

A Right and left lateral ventricles with left caudate nucleus

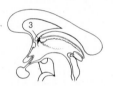

D Interventricular foramen

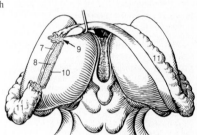

B Thalamus with fornix

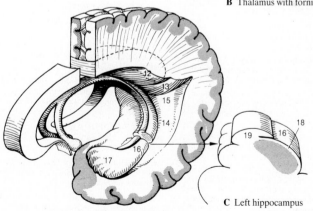

C Left hippocampus

1 **Sections through telencephalon.** Sectiones telencephali.

2 **Cerebral cortex.** Cortex cerebralis (pallium). Gray matter, 1.5–4.5 mm thick, consisting mostly of 6 cellular layers: A

3 **Molecular (plexiform) layer.** Layer 1. Lamina molecularis (plexiformis). It contains a few horizontal cells and a thick, tangential network of fibers from dendrites of pyramidal cells and axons of other cells without having its own processes extend beyond its cortical field. A

4 **External granular layer.** Layer 2. Lamina granularis externa. A layer of small cells in a fine fiber network. A

5 **External pyramidal layer (pyramidal cell layer).** Layer 3. Lamina pyramidalis externa. It contains, among others, medium-sized pyramidal cells which, however do not form long tracts. A

6 **Internal granular layer.** Layer 4. Lamina granularis interna. It consists predominantly of closely packed stellate cells and receives impulses primarily from thalamocortical fibers. Densely stratified tangential fibers form its stria. A

7 **Internal pyramidal (ganglionic) layer. Layer 5.** Lamina pyramidalis interna (ganglionaris). It contains larger pyramidal cells and is in the corresponding field of areas 4 and 6, exit of the corticonuclear and corticospinal tract. A

8 **Multiform (fusiform) layer. Layer 6.** Lamina multiformis. It is made up of many, mostly small, fusiform cells and extends into the white matter without sharp boundaries. A

9 **Tangential neurofibers.** Neurofibrae tangentiales. It is made up of the following four fiber layers running parallel to the surface:

10 Stria of molecular layer. Stria laminae molecularis (plexiformis). Tangential fibers in layer 1. A

11 Stria of external granular layer. Stria laminae granularis externa. Less pronounced tangential fiber stripes in layer 2 . A

12 Stria of internal granular layer. Stria laminae granularis interna. Stripe of tangential fibers in layer 4 [[external band of Baillarger]]. A

13 Stria of internal pyramidal layer. Stria laminae pyramidalis interna (ganglionaris). Tangential fiber band in layer 5 [[internal band of Baillarger]]. A

14 **Arcuate fibers of cerebrum.** Fibrae arcuatae cerebri. Arcuate connecting fibers between adjacent cerebral gyri. F

15 **Cingulum.** Fiber bundle lying in the medulla of the cingulate gyrus. Arising from the area subcallosa, it arches around the corpus callosum, passes the splenium and then turns anteriorly up to the uncus. C

16 **Superior longitudinal fasciculus.** Fasciculus longitudinalis superior. Largest association bundle extending from the frontal lobe to the temporal lobe via the occipital lobe. E

17 **Inferior longitudinal fasciculus.** Fasciculus longitudinalis inferior. Association fibers between the temporal and occipital lobes. E

18 **Uncinate fasciculus.** Fasciculus uncinatus. Association fibers between the inferior surface of the frontal lobe and the anterior part of the temporal lobe. E

19 **Radiation of corpus callosum.** Radiatio corporis callosi. Connecting fibers between the right and left cerebral cortex. See also 312.11–14. C

20 **Basal nuclei.** Nuclei basales. Basal ganglion.

21 **Corpus striatum.** Basal ganglia (caudate nucleus and putamen) united by bundles of gray matter. Central synaptic station of the extrapyramidal system. D

22 **Caudate nucleus.** Nucleus caudatus. Elongated nucleus curving around the thalamus. It is formed from the ganglionic mass of the telencephalon.

23 Head of caudate nucleus. Caput [[nuclei caudati]]. Situated anteriorly, it forms the lateral wall of the anterior horn of the lateral ventricle. B D

24 Body of caudate nucleus. Corpus [[nuclei caudati]]. Middle part of caudate nucleus lying on the thalamus. B D

25 Tail of caudate nucleus. Cauda [[nuclei caudati]]. It accompanies the inferior horn and forms the tapering posterior and inferior segment of the caudate nucleus. D

26 **Lentiform nucleus.** Nucleus lentiformis (lenticularis). It arises partly from the telencephalon, partly from the diencephalon. D

27 **Putamen.** Lateral, telencephalic portion of the lentiform nucleus. B

28 Lateral medullary lamina. Lamina medullaris lateralis. Medullary layer between the globus pallidus and putamen. B

29 Lateral globus pallidus. Globus pallidus lateralis. Part of the diencephalic globus pallidus located between the lateral and medial medullary lamina. B

30 Medial medullary lamina. Lamina medullaris medialis. Medullary layer between the medial and lateral globus pallidus. B

31 Medial globus pallidus. Globus pallidus medialis. Part of the globus pallidus located medial to the medial medullary lamina. B

32 **Claustrum.** Layer of gray matter between the lentiform nucleus and the insular cortex. B

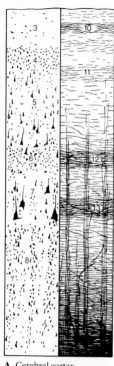

A Cerebral cortex
Cells at left
Medullary sheaths at right

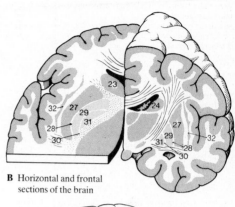

B Horizontal and frontal
sections of the brain

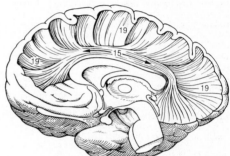

C Radiation of corpus callosum and cingulum

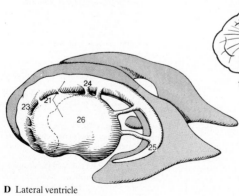

D Lateral ventricle
with left striate body

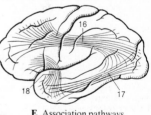

E Association pathways

F Arcuate fibers

1   **Amygdaloid body (amygdala).** Corpus amygdaloideum. Nuclear group in front of the inferior horn of the lateral ventricle. Connecting with the medial cerebral cortex, it belongs partly to the rhinencephalon and has some autonomic functions, influencing emotional behavior. D

2   **Anterior amygdaloid area.** Area amygdaloidea anterior. Anterior group of cells directed toward the anterior perforated substance. It receives fibers from the lateral olfactory tract and the diagonal band of Broca begins from this area. D

3   **Basolateral part.** Pars basolateralis. In humans, this part contains the largest group of nuclei of the amygdala complex. It receives no olfactory fibers but is connected with the hypothalamus, hippocampus and other parts of the brain, as well as with the stria terminalis. D

4   **Corticomedial part.** Pars corticomedialis [olfactoria]. Smaller nuclear group located superomedially. It receives fibers from the olfactory tract and is likewise involved in the formation of the stria terminalis. D

5   **Extreme capsule.** Capsula extrema. White matter between the cortex of the insula and the claustrum. A B

6   **External capsule.** Capsula externa. White matter between the claustrum and lentiform nucleus. A B

7   **Internal capsule.** Capsula interna. Very important conduction band lying on the one hand medial to the lentiform nucleus, on the other hand lateral to the thalamus and caudate nucleus. A

8   **Anterior limb of internal capsule.** Crus anterius capsulae internae. It lies between the lentiform nucleus and the head of the caudate nucleus. A

9   Anterior thalamic radiations. Radiationes thalamicae anteriores. It contains connecting fibers between the frontal lobe and the medial nucleus of the thalamus, as well as between the anterior nucleus of the thalamus and the anterior region of the cingulate gyrus. B

10 Frontopontine tract. Tractus frontopontinus. Fibers from the frontal lobe to the nuclei of the pons. B

11 **Genu of internal capsule.** Genu capsulae internae. It lies between the anterior and posterior limbs of the internal capsule and forms part of the lateral wall of the ventricular system. A B

12 Corticonuclear tract. Tractus corticonuclearis. Part of the pyramidal tract passing into the motor nuclei of the cranial nerves. B

13 **Posterior limb of internal capsule.** Crus posterius capsulae internae. It lies between the lentiform nucleus on the one hand and the thalamus and body of caudate nucleus on the other hand. A

14 Thalamolentiform part. Pars thalamolentiformis. Portion of posterior limb of internal capsule reaching up to the posterior margin of the lentiform nucleus. B

15 *Corticospinal fibers.* Fibrae corticospinales. Spinal cord portion of pyramidal tract. It is organized somatotopically in such a way that the fibers for the most caudal region of the body lie farthest toward the occiput. B

16 *Corticorubral fibers.* Fibrae corticorubrales. Fibers from the frontal lobe to the red nucleus. B

17 *Corticoreticular fibers.* Fibrae corticoreticulares. Fibers passing from the region in front of and behind the central sulcus to the reticular formation. B

18 *Corticothalamic fibers.* Fibrae corticothalamicae. Part of the thalamic radiation in the thalamus. B

19 *Thalamoparietal fibers.* Fibrae thalamoparietales. Part of the thalamic radiation passing into the cerebral cortex. B

20 *Central thalamic radiations.* Radiationes thalamicae centrales. Superior thalamic radiation. B See also 302.2.

21 Sublentiform part. Pars sublentiformis. Portion of internal capsule lying below the posterior part of the lentiform nucleus. A B

22 *Optic radiation [[Gratioleti]].* Radiatio optica. Fiber tract on its way from the lateral geniculate body to the area striata in the occipital lobe. A B

23 *Acoustic radiation.* Radiatio acustica. Auditory tract on its way from the medial geniculate body to the transverse temporal gyrus [[Heschl]]. A B

24 *Corticotectal fibers.* Fibrae corticotectales. Connecting fibers between the cerebral cortex and the tectum. B

25 *Temporopontine fibers.* Fibrae temporopontinae. Fibers of the cerebropontocerebellar tract coming from the temporal lobe. B

26 Retrolentiform part. Pars retrolentiformis. Portion of internal capsule situated occipital to the lentiform nucleus. A B

27 *Posterior thalamic radiations.* Radiationes thalamicae posteriores. B

28 *Parieto-occipitopontine fasciculus.* Fasciculus parieto-occipitopontinus. Portion of cerebropontocerebellar tract coming from the parietal and occipital lobes. B

29 **Corona radiata.** Fibers of the internal capsule radiating out fanlike in all directions toward the cerebral cortex. A

30 **Anterior commissure.** Commissura anterior. It lies in front of the column of the fornix and is freely visible in the anterior wall of the third ventricle. A C

31 *Anterior part.* Pars anterior. It radiates into the area subcallosa and belongs to the phylogenetic rhinencephalon. C

32 *Posterior part.* Pars posterior. Larger portion of anterior commissure. It connects the two temporal lobes. C

33 **Association neurofibers.** Neurofibrae associationes. Association fibers connecting adjacent or farther removed cerebral parts of the same side with one another. They form named tracts, e.g., cingulum, superior longitudinal fasciculus, etc.

34 **Commissural neurofibers.** Neurofibrae commissurales. They connect the same cerebral fields of both hemispheres.

35 **Projecting neurofibers.** Neurofibrae projectiones. They form the longer tracts, e.g., pyramidal tract, optic and acoustic radiations, thalamic radiation.

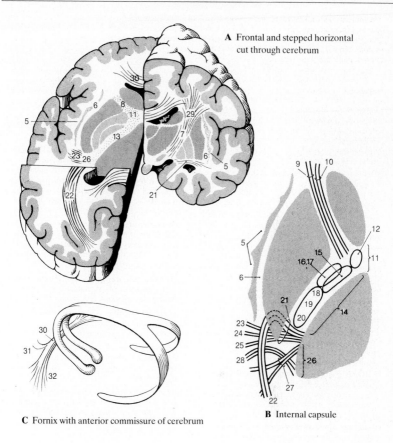

A Frontal and stepped horizontal cut through cerebrum

B Internal capsule

C Fornix with anterior commissure of cerebrum

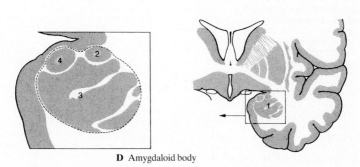

D Amygdaloid body

1 **Peripheral nervous system.** Pars peripherica (systema nervosum periphericum). It includes all peripheral conducting tracts (nerves). Its separation from the central nervous system lies at the surface of the brain and spinal cord.

2 CRANIAL NERVES. NERVI CRANIALES (ENCEPHALICI). There are 12 pairs of cranial nerves all of which, with the exception of the trochlear (IV), pass out of the base of the brain and leave the skull through its base (in contrast to the spinal nerves). Area of distribution: head, neck, as well as the thorax and abdomen (via vagus nerve).

3 OLFACTORY NERVE (I). NN. OLFACTORII (I). First cranial nerve. Formed by about 20 small fiber bundles of nonmyelinated axons of olfactory cells, it passes through the cribriform plate of the ethmoid into the olfactory bulb (synaptic site). A

4 OPTIC NERVE (II). N. OPTICUS [II]. Second cranial nerve. Leaving the eyeball medial to the posterior optic pole, it extends up to the optic chiasma. B C

5 OCULOMOTOR NERVE (III). N. OCULOMO-TORIUS [III]. Third cranial nerve. Exiting from the sulcus on the medial side of the cerebral peduncle, this motor nerve (somatic and visceral) passes into the orbit through the superior orbital fissure. B C

6 **Superior ramus (division).** Ramus superior. Superior branch for the superior rectus and levator palpebrae superioris muscles. B

7 **Inferior ramus (division).** Ramus inferior. Inferior branch for the medial and inferior recti and inferior oblique muscles. B

8 **Ciliary ganglion.** Ganglion ciliare. Located about 2 cm behind the eyeball and lateral to the optic nerve, this parasympathetic ganglion serves as a relay station for fibers innervating the ciliary and sphincter pupillae muscles. B

9 **Parasympathetic (motor) root.** Radix parasympathetica (oculomotoria). Branch from the oculomotor nerve with preganglionic, parasympathetic fibers for the ciliary ganglion. B

10 **Short ciliary nerves.** Nn. ciliares breves. Short nerves (up to 20) penetrating the sclera above and below the optic nerve and carrying postganglionic, parasympathetic and sympathetic fibers. B

11 **Sympathetic root.** Radix sympathetica. Fine, postganglionic fiber tract from the internal carotid plexus without synapsing in the ciliary ganglion. B

12 **Sensory root.** Radix sensoria (nasociliaris). Fine, long connection with afferent fibers to the nasociliary nerve. B

13 TROCHLEAR NERVE (IV). N. TROCHLEA-RIS [IV]. Fourth cranial nerve. Thin nerve exiting dorsal and caudal to the tectal lamina and supplying the superior oblique muscle. B

14 **Decussation of trochlear nerve.** Decussatio nervorum trochlearium. It takes place in the superior medullary velum. B

15 TRIGEMINAL NERVE (V). N. TRIGEMINUS [V]. Fifth cranial nerve (nerve of the 1st pharyngeal arch). Exiting laterally from the pons with two groups of fibers, it supplies the masticatory muscles and provides sensory innervation to the face. B C

16 **Sensory root.** Radix sensoria [Portio major]. Sensory part which exits from the pons caudally and enters the trigeminal ganglion. C

17 **Trigeminal (semilunar, gasserian) ganglion.** Ganglion trigeminale [[semilunare; Gasseri]]. Semilunar in shape and equivalent to a spinal ganglion, it is located in an outpocketing of the subarachnoid space (cavum trigeminale) above the foramen lacerum at the medial, anterior border of the petrous temporal bone. C

18 **Motor root.** Radix motoria [Portio minor]. Motor portion of trigeminal nerve for innervation of the masticatory muscles. It is situated cranially at the exit of the trigeminal nerve and then below the trigeminal ganglion. C

19 **Ophthalmic nerve.** N. ophthalmicus. First division (branch) of trigeminal nerve. It passes through the superior orbital fissure. C

20 **Tentorial (meningeal) branch.** Ramus tentorii (meningeus). Recurrent nerve for the tentorium cerebelli and falx cerebri. C

21 **Lacrimal nerve.** N. lacrimalis. Passing laterally through the superior orbital fissure, it supplies the lacrimal gland, conjunctiva and lateral portion of upper eyelid. C

22 Communicating ramus with zygomatic nerve. Ramus communicans [cum n. zygomatico]. Connection to the zygomatic nerve with autonomic fibers from the pterygopalatine ganglion to the lacrimal gland. C

23 **Frontal nerve.** N. frontalis. Passing through the superior orbital fissure, it lies on the levator palpebrae superioris and continues toward the forehead. C See also 323 A

24 Supraorbital nerve. N. supraorbitalis. Thickest branch of frontal nerve. It supplies the conjunctiva, upper eyelid, frontal sinus and the skin of the forehead. C

25 *Lateral branch.* Ramus lateralis. It passes through the supra-orbital notch. C

26 *Medial branch.* Ramus medialis. It passes medially through the frontal notch. C

27 Supratrochlear nerve. N. supratrochlearis. Thin, medial branch of frontal nerve. It divides at the medial angle of the eye into an ascending and descending branch. C

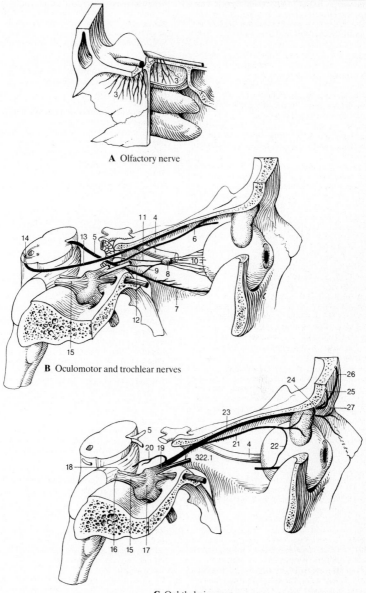

A Olfactory nerve

B Oculomotor and trochlear nerves

C Ophthalmic nerve

1 **Nasociliary nerve.** N. nasociliaris. Branch of the ophthalmic nerve situated most medially. At first it lies below the superior rectus, then between the superior oblique and medial rectus. A

2 Communicating branch with the ciliary ganglion. Ramus communicans [cum ganglio ciliari]. Sensory fibers from the eye passing through the ciliary ganglion. A

3 Long ciliary nerves. Nn. ciliares longi. Two long, fine twigs with sympathetic fibers for the dilatator pupillae muscle and afferent fibers from the iris, ciliary body and cornea. A

4 Posterior ethmoidal nerve. N. ethmoidalis posterior. Thin nerve at the posterior end of the orbit for the sphenoidal sinus and posterior ethmoidal cells. A

5 Anterior ethmoidal nerve. N. ethmoidalis anterior. Passing through the anterior ethmoidal foramen into the cranial cavity where it is extradural, it then courses through the cribriform plate of the ethmoid into the nasal cavity. A B C

6 Nasal branches of anterior ethmoidal nerve. Rami nasales [n. ethmoidalis ant.]. Collective term for the following four branches of the anterior ethmoidal nerve:

7 *Internal nasal branches*. Rami nasales interni. Rami for the nasal mucosa in front of the conchae and for the anterior nasal septum. B

8 *Lateral nasal branches.* Rami nasales laterales. Rami for the anterior part of lateral nasal wall. B

9 *Medial nasal branches.* Rami nasales mediales. Rami for the anterior part of the nasal septum. C

10 *External nasal branch.* Ramus nasalis externus. Ramus for the skin of the tip of the nose and the nasal ala; it passes through the ethmoidal sulcus of the nasal bone. A

11 Infratrochlear nerve. N. infratrochlearis. It passes below the trochlea of the superior oblique at the inner angle of the eye and supplies the lacrimal sac, lacrimal caruncle a. surrounding skin. A

12 *Palpebral branches*. Rami palpebrales. Rami for a part of the upper and lower eyelids. A

13 **Maxillary nerve.** N. maxillaris. Second division (branch) of trigeminal nerve. It passes through the foramen rotundum to the pterygopalatine fossa and subsequently through the inferior orbital fissure into the orbit. A C

14 **Meningeal nerve.** Ramus meningeus [medius]. Given off in front of the foramen rotundum, it supplies the dura in the region of the frontal branch of the middle meningeal artery. A

15 **Ganglionic branches.** Rami ganglionici (ganglionares). Usually two rami from the pterygopalatine ganglion. They contain autonomic fibers for the lacrimal gland and sensory fibers, among others, from the periosteum of the orbit. A

16 **Pterygopalatine ganglion.** Ganglion pterygopalatinum. Parasympathetic ganglion located in the same named fossa close to the sphenopalatine foramen. Their postganglionic fibers innervate the lacrimal and nasal glands. A B C

16a **Parasympathetic root.** Radix parasympathetica. It arrives via the greater petrosal nerve and nerve of the pterygoid canal.

16b **Sympathetic root.** Radix sympathetica. It arrives via the deep petrosal nerve and nerve of the pterygoid canal.

16c **Sensory root.** Radix sensoria. Fibers of maxillary nerve.

17 **Orbital branches.** Rami orbitales. Two to three fine rami which pass into the orbit through the inferior orbital fissure, then through the bone to the posterior ethmoidal cells and to the sphenoidal sinus. B C

18 **Lateral posterior superior nasal branches.** Rami nasales posteriores superiores laterales. Up to 10 fine rami which pass through the sphenopalatine foramen to the superior and middle nasal conchae and to the posterior ethmoidal cells. B

19 **Medial posterior superior nasal branches.** Rami nasales posteriores superiores mediales. Two to three branches which pass through the sphenopalatine foramen to the upper part of the nasal septum. C

20 Nasopalatine nerve. N. nasopalatinus [[incisivus]]. It passes between the periosteum and mucosa of the nasal septum, then through the incisive canal to the anterior part of the palatine mucosa and the gingiva of the upper incisor teeth. C

20a Long nasopalatine nerve. Nervus nasopalatinus longus. Annot. p. 409

20b Branches to nasal septum. Rami septales nasales. Annot. p. 409

20c Short nasopalatine nerves. Nervi nasopalatini breves. Annot. p. 409

20d Lateral nasal branches. Rami nasales laterales. Annot. p. 409

20e Branches to maxillary sinus. Rami sinus maxillaris. Annot. p. 409

21 **Pharyngeal nerve.** Nervus pharyngeus. Fine nerve for the pharyngeal mucosa. B

22 **Greater palatine nerve.** N. palatinus major. After passing through the greater palatine canal, it courses through the same-named foramen and supplies the mucosa of the hard palate and its glands. B

23 Posterior inferior nasal branches. Rami nasales posteriores inferiores. Rami for the middle and inferior nasal meatuses as well as the inferior nasal concha. B

24 **Lesser palatine nerves.** Nn. palatini minores. They travel in the same named, slender canals, exit through the lesser palatine foramina and supply the soft palate. B

24a **Tonsillar branches.** Rami tonsillares. Branches to the palatine tonsil.

25 **Zygomatic nerve.** N. zygomaticus. Branching off in the pterygopalatine fossa, it passes through the inferior orbital fissure to the lateral wall of the orbit and provides an anastomotic branch to the lacrimal gland. A

26 Zygomaticotemporal branch. Ramus zygomaticotemporalis. It passes through the same-named foramen to the lateral wall of the orbit. A

27 Zygomaticofacial branch. Ramus zygomaticofacialis. It passes through the same-named foramen to the skin over the zygomatic bone. A

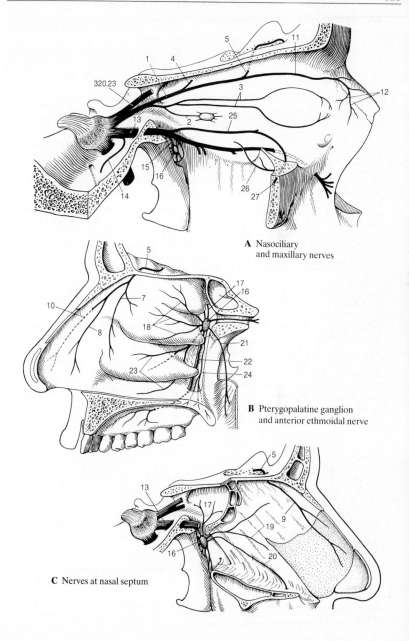

A Nasociliary
and maxillary nerves

B Pterygopalatine ganglion
and anterior ethmoidal nerve

C Nerves at nasal septum

1 **Infraorbital nerve.** N. infraorbitalis. Terminal branch of maxillary nerve. It passes through the inferior orbital fissure and the same-named sulcus and foramen to the skin of the upper eyelid, nose, upper lip and cheek. C

2 Superior alveolar nerve. Nn. alveolares superiores. Branches to the maxillary teeth.

3 *Posterior superior alveolar branches*. Rami alveolares superiores posteriores. Two to three branches passing through the alveolar foramina to the inner surface of the maxilla. They supply the maxillary sinus and the molars with their buccal gingiva. C

4 *Middle superior alveolar branch*. R. alveolaris superior medius. It runs in the infraorbital sulcus to the maxilla and passes along the lateral wall of the maxillary sinus up to the superior dental plexus. C

5 *Anterior superior alveolar branches*. Rami alveolares superiores anteriores. They run in their own canal and via the superior dental plexus to the incisors, canines, premolars and first molar tooth. C

6 *Superior dental plexus*. Plexus dentalis superior. Nerve plexus situated in the bone above the roots of the teeth and formed by the superior alveolar rami. C

7 *Superior dental branches*. Rami dentales superiores. Branches for the individual roots of the teeth. C

8 *Superior gingival branches*. Rami gingivales superiores. Rami for the gingiva. C

9 Inferior palpebral branches. Rami palpebrales inferiores. Rami given off to the lower eyelid outside of the infraorbital foramen. C

10 External nasal branches. Rami nasales externi. Branches to the outside of the nasal ala. C

11 Internal nasal branches. Rami nasales interni. Branches to the skin of the nasal vestibule. C

12 Superior labial branches. Rami labiales superiores. Rami to the skin and mucosa of the upper lip. C

13 **Mandibular nerve.** N. mandibularis. Third division (branch) of the trigeminal nerve. It passes through the foramen ovale and into the infratemporal fossa. Besides sensory fibers, it contains motor fibers for the masticatory muscles. A

14 **Meningeal branch (nervus spinosus).** Ramus meningeus (n. spinosus). It passes through the foramen spinosum accompanied by both branches of the middle meningeal artery and supplies the dura, a part of the sphenoidal sinus and the mastoid air cells. A

15 **Masseteric nerve.** N. massetericus. Motor nerve for the masseter muscle passing above the lateral pterygoid muscle and through the mandibular notch. A

16 **Deep temporal nerves.** Nn. temporales profundi. Motor nerves passing to the temporalis muscle from below. A

17 **Nerve to lateral pterygoid.** N. pterygoideus lateralis. Motor nerve for the same named muscle. It frequently arises in common with the buccal nerve. A

18 **Nerve to medial pterygoid.** N. pterygoideus medialis. Motor nerve for the same named muscle. It also sends small twigs to the tensor veli palatini and tensor tympani muscles. A

19 **Otic ganglion.** Ganglion oticum. Parasympathetic ganglion located medial to the mandibular nerve below the foramen ovale. It receives its tributaries from the glossopharyngeal nerve via the lesser petrosal nerve and sends secretory fibers to the parotid gland. B

20 Ramus communicans [cum nervo pterygoideo mediali]. Branch which communicates with the nerve to the medial pterygoid muscle. B

21 Nerve to tensor veli palatini muscle. N. musculi tensoris veli palatini. It sometimes comes from the nerve to the medial pterygoid muscle. B

22 Nerve to tensor tympani muscle. N. musculi tensoris tympani. It also sometimes comes from the nerve to the medial pterygoid muscle. B

23 **Buccal nerve**. N. buccalis. Sensory nerve for the skin and mucosa of the cheek and the buccal gingiva in the region of the first molar. A

24 **Auriculotemporal nerve.** N. auriculotemporalis. It usually encircles the middle meningeal artery, sends a small branch to the temporomandibular joint and then passes upward between the ear and superficial temporal artery to the skin of the temporal region. A

25 Nerve to external acoustic meatus. N. meatus acustici externi. Usually two small branches for the skin of the external acoustic meatus. A

26 Fine branches to the tympanic membrane. *Rami membranae tympani*. A

27 Parotid branches. Rami parotidei. Small branches for the parotid gland. A

28 Branches communicating with the facial nerve. Rami communicantes [cum n. faciali]. They carry parasympathetic fibers from the otic ganglion to the parotid gland via the facial nerve. A

29 Anterior auricular nerves. Nn. auriculares anteriores. They supply the anterior surface of the pinna. A

30 Superficial temporal rami. Rami temporales superficialis. Branches for the skin of the temporal region in front of and above the ear. A

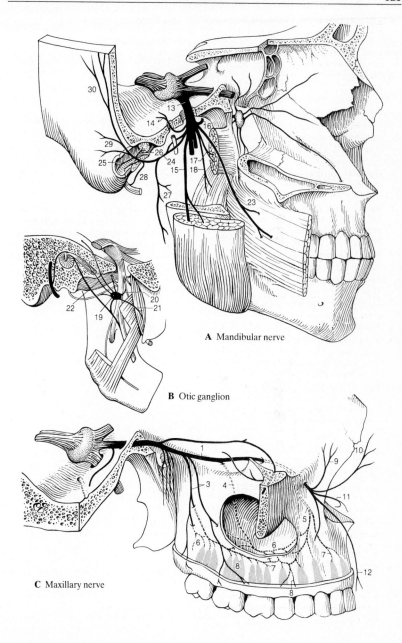

A Mandibular nerve

B Otic ganglion

C Maxillary nerve

1 **Lingual nerve.** N. lingualis. As a branch of the mandibular nerve, it passes between the lateral and medial pterygoid muscles in an arch anteriorly to the floor of the mouth where it lies near the wisdom tooth directly below the mucosa. A B C

2 Branches to isthmus of the fauces. Rami isthmi faucium (rami fauciales). It also provides branches to the tonsils. A

3 Communicating rami to the hypoglossal nerve Rami communicantes [cum n. hypoglosso]. It lies on the hyoglossus muscle. A

4 Communicating ramus to the chorda tympani nerve. Ramus communicans [cum chorda tympani]. A

5 Sublingual nerve. N. sublingualis. It passes lateral to the sublingual gland into the mucosa of the floor of the mouth and into the gingiva of the anterior mandibular teeth. A

6 Lingual branches. Rami linguales. Numerous rami containing sensory and taste fibers from the anterior two-thirds of the lingual mucosa. A

7 Ganglionic branches. Rami ganglionares. Rami communicating with the submandibular ganglion. A

8 Submandibular ganglion. Ganglion submandibulare. Parasympathetic ganglion above or in front of the submandibular gland. Synaptic station for preganglionic fibers of the chorda tympani with postganglionic fibers for the sublingual and submandibular glands. A

9 **Inferior alveolar nerve.** N. alveolaris inferior. Largest branch of mandibular nerve with sensory and motor components. It passes 1 cm behind the lingual nerve and through the mandibular foramen into the mandibular canal. A B C

10 Mylohyoid nerve. N. mylohyoideus. Coursing in the mylohyoid groove and then below the mylohyoid muscle, this motor nerve supplies the same-named muscle and the anterior belly of the digastric. A B C

11 Inferior dental plexus. Plexus dentalis inferior. Plexus of nerves within the mandibular canal. B

12 *Inferior dental branches.* Rami dentales inferiores. Rami for the mandibular teeth. B

13 *Inferior gingival branches.* Rami gingivales inferiores. Rami for the buccal gingiva of the mandibular teeth (except for the first molar). B

14 **Mental nerve.** N. mentalis. Sensory nerve exiting from the mental foramen below the 2nd premolar tooth. B

15 Mental branches. Rami mentales. From the chin. B

16 Labial branches. Rami labiales. From the lower lip. B

16a Gingival branches. Rami gingivales. B

17 **Otic ganglion.** Ganglion oticum. Parasympathetic ganglion located medial to the mandibular nerve below the foramen ovale. It communicates with the glossopharyngeal nerve via the lesser petrosal nerve and sends secretory fibers into the parotid gland. C

18 ABDUCENT NERVE (VI). N. ABDUCENS [VI]. Sixth cranial nerve. It exits the brain in the angle between the pons and pyramid, penetrates the dura at the level of the middle of the clivus, passes laterally into the cavernous sinus and then through the inferior orbital fissure into the orbit where it supplies the lateral rectus muscle. D

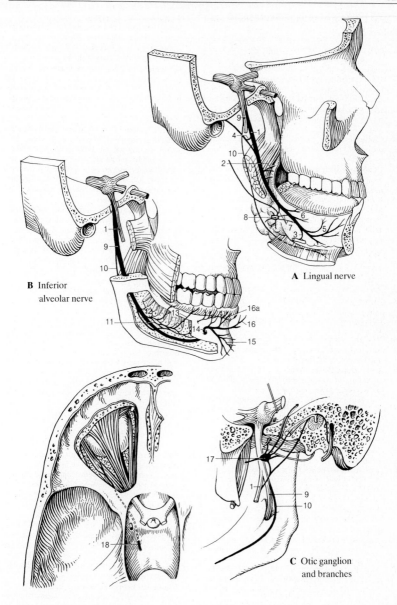

A Lingual nerve

B Inferior
alveolar nerve

C Otic ganglion
and branches

D Abducent nerve

1 FACIAL NERVE (VII). N. FACIALIS (N. IN-TERMEDIOFACIALIS) [VII]. Seventh cranial nerve (nerve of the 2nd pharyngeal arch). It exits between the pons and olive, passes with the vestibulocochlear nerve into the petrous temporal bone and leaves it through the stylomastoid foramen. It supplies the muscles of facial expression. A B C D

2 **Genu of facial nerve.** Geniculum [n. facialis]. Bend in the facial nerve just below the anterior wall of the petrous temporal. A

3 **Nerve to the stapedius.** N. stapedius. Slender branch for the stapedius muscle. A

4 **Communicating ramus with the tympanic plexus.** Ramus communicans [cum plexus tympanico]. A

5 **Communicating ramus with the vagus nerve.** Ramus communicans [cum nervo vago]. Directly below the stylomastoid foramen.

6 **Posterior auricular nerve.** N. auricularis posterior. Branches off beneath the stylomastoid foramen, passes upward between the mastoid process and the external acoustic meatus and supplies the posterior ear muscles and the occipital belly of the occipitofrontalis muscle. B

7 **Occipital branch.** Ramus occipitalis. Ramus for the occipital belly of the occipitofrontalis muscle. B

8 **Auricular branch.** Ramus auricularis. It passes to the muscles of the pinna. B

9 **Digastric branch.** Ramus digastricus. It supplies the posterior belly of the digastric muscle. A B

10 **Stylohyoid branch.** Ramus stylohyoideus. Often arising in common with the lingual branch, it supplies the stylohyoid muscle. A

11 **Communicating ramus with the glosso-pharyngeal nerve.** Ramus communicans [cum n. glossopharyngeo]. A

12 **Intraparotid plexus.** Plexus intraparotideus. Facial nerve plexus situated in the space accessible anteriorly between the two parotid lobes. B

13 **Temporal branches.** Rami temporales. Rami ascending over the zygomatic arch for the muscles of facial expression above the palpebral fissure and at the ear. B

14 **Zygomatic branches.** Rami zygomatici. Rami for the lateral part of the orbicularis oculi and the muscles of facial expression between the palpebral and oral fissures. B

15 **Buccal branches.** Rami buccales. Rami for the buccinator muscle and the muscles of facial expression around the mouth. B

16 **Lingual branch.** Ramus lingualis. Inconstant ramus to the tongue. It sometimes arises in common with the stylohyoid ramus.

17 **Marginal mandibular branch.** Ramus marginalis mandibularis. It passes to the chin and supplies the muscles of facial expression below the oral fissure. B

18 **Cervical branch.** Ramus colli (cervicalis). Motor branch for the platysma. It anastomoses with the transverse cervical nerve. B

19 **Sensory root of facial nerve.** N. intermedius. It arises from the brainstem independently between the facial and vestibular nerves and transports autonomic and taste fibers. After various anastomoses, it is finally united with the facial nerve in the petrous temporal. D

20 **Geniculate (facial) ganglion.** Ganglion geniculi (geniculatum). Equivalent to a spinal ganglion with pseudo-unipolar ganglion cells, it is located in the petrous temporal bone at the bend of the facial nerve. It receives taste fibers from the chorda tympani. A

21 **Chorda tympani.** Nerve bundle with parasympathetic fibers for the submandibular gland and sensory fibers from the taste buds occupying the anterior two-thirds of the tongue. It takes a recurrent course into the tympanic cavity where it passes between the malleus and incus, then goes through the petrotympanic fissure [[Glaser]] to subsequently join the lingual nerve. A

22 **Pterygopalatine ganglion.** Ganglion pterygopalatinum. Parasympathetic ganglion located in the same named fossa near the sphenopalatine foramen. It receives preganglionic fibers from the facial nerve via the greater petrosal nerve and sends postganglionic secretory fibers to the lacrimal and nasal glands. C

23 **Nerve of pterygoid canal.** N. canalis pterygoidei [Radix facialis]. Located in the same-named canal at the root of the pterygoid process, it contains parasympathetic (facial nerve), sympathetic and sensory fibers destined for the pterygopalatine ganglion. C

24 **Greater petrosal nerve.** N. petrosus major. Branch of facial nerve appearing at the anterior wall of the petrous temporal. Incorporating parasympathetic and sensory fibers, it penetrates the covering plate of the foramen lacerum lateral to the internal carotid artery where it is joined by the deep petrosal nerve. A C

25 **Deep petrosal nerve.** N. petrosus profundus. Carrying sympathetic fibers from the internal carotid plexus, it joins up with the greater petrosal nerve to form the nerve of the pterygoid canal. C

26 **Submandibular ganglion.** Ganglion submandibulare. Located above or in front of the submandibular gland, this parasympathetic ganglion is the synaptic site between preganglionic fibers from the chorda tympani and postganglionic fibers destined for the sublingual and submandibular glands. C

27 **Sympathetic branch (to the submandibular ganglion).** Ramus sympatheticus (ad ganglion submandibulare). From the internal carotid plexus. Its fibers arrive at the submandibular ganglion above the facial artery and pass through the ganglion without synapsing. C

28 **Glandular branches.** Rami glandulares. Small rami at the inferior margin of the submandibular ganglion destined for the submandibular gland. C

29 **Sublingual ganglion.** [Ganglion sublinguale]. Small group of cells occasionally present at the glandular rami. C

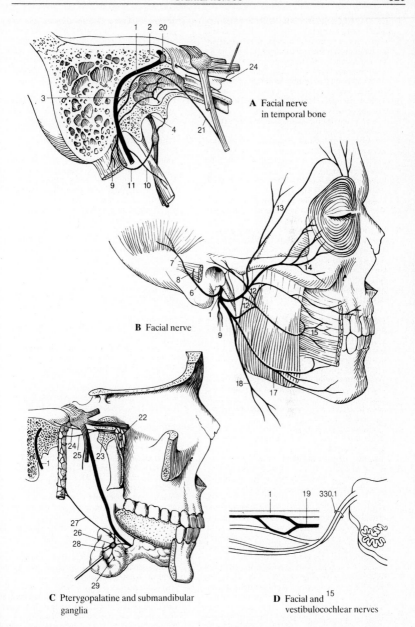

A Facial nerve in temporal bone

B Facial nerve

C Pterygopalatine and submandibular ganglia

D Facial and vestibulocochlear nerves

1   **VESTIBULOCOCHLEAR NERVE (VIII).** N. VESTIBULOCOCHLEARIS [VIII]. Eighth cranial nerve. Exiting at the lower margin of the pons, it passes through the internal acoustic meatus to the vestibular (equilibrium) and auditory organs. A

2   **Vestibular nerve.** N. vestibularis. Superior, ventral, ~   vestibular portion of vestibulocochlear nerve. A

3   **Cochlear nerve.** Nervus cochlearis. Inferior, dorsal, ~   cochlear part of vestibulocochlear nerve. A

4   **Vestibular nerve.** Nervus vestibularis. Portion of ~   VIII nerve passing from the vestibular nucleus to the maculae and ampullary crest. A

5   **Vestibular ganglion.** Ganglion vestibulare. Located in the floor of the internal acoustic meatus, it contains bipolar neurons associated with the vestibular nerve. A

6   **Communicating branch with cochlear nerve.** Ramus communicans cochlearis.

7   **Upper part of vestibular ganglion.** Pars superior. It supplies the anterior and lateral semicircular canals, utricle and anterior part of saccule. A

8   **Utriculoampullar nerve.** N. utriculoampullaris. Superior branch of vestibular nerve with fibers from the macula and ampullary crest of the superior (anterior) and lateral semicircular canals. A

9   **Utricular nerve.** N. utricularis. Branch from the macula utriculi. A

10   **Anterior ampullar nerve.** N. ampullaris anterior. Branch from the ampullary crest of the anterior semicircular canal. A

11   **Lateral ampullar nerve.** N. ampullaris lateralis. Branch from the ampullary crest of the lateral semicircular canal. A

12   **Inferior part of the vestibular ganglion.** Pars inferior. It supplies the posterior semicircular canal and a part of the sacculus. A

13   **Posterior ampullar nerve.** N. ampullaris posterior. Branch from the ampullary crest of the posterior semicircular canal. A

14   **Saccular nerve.** N. saccularis. Branch from the macula sacculi. A

15   **Cochlear nerve.** Nervus cochlearis. Part of the ve~   stibulocochlear nerve for the auditory organ located in the cochlea. A

16   **Cochlear (spiral) ganglion.** Ganglion cochleare (spiral cochleae). Helical-shaped band of ganglion cells oriented to the axis of the cochlea and situated along the base of the osseous spiral lamina. A

17   GLOSSOPHARYNGEAL NERVE (IX). N. GLOSSOPHARYNGEUS [IX]. Ninth cranial nerve (nerve of the 3rd pharyngeal arch). Exiting from the brain in the posterolateral sulcus behind the olive, it courses through the jugular foramen and passes obliquely downward posterior to the stylopharyngeus muscle. It contains motor fibers for the pharyngeal constrictors and the stylopharyngeus muscle, as well as sensory fibers for the pharyngeal mucosa, tonsils and posterior $1/3$ of the tongue (taste fibers) and parasympathetic fibers to the otic ganglion via the tympanic and lesser petrosal nerves. B

18   **Superior (jugular) ganglion.** Ganglion superius [[intracraniale]]. Smaller ganglion in the jugular foramen. It contains cell bodies of afferent fibers. B C

19   **Inferior (petrous) ganglion.** Ganglion inferius [[ex-

tracraniale]]. Larger ganglion directly below the jugular foramen. It contains cell bodies of afferent fibers. B C

20   Tympanic nerve. N. tympanicus. First branch of IX nerve. Branching off from the inferior ganglion, it passes between the jugular foramen and carotid canal and through the tympanic canaliculus to the tympanic cavity. C

21   Tympanic enlargement (ganglion). Intumescentia tympanica (ganglion tympanicum). Irregular~   ly scattered ganglion cells forming an enlargement in the course of the tympanic nerve. C

22   **Tympanic plexus.** Plexus tympanicus. N. plexus in the mucosa over the promontory. It is formed by the tympanic n. internal carotid plexus a. communicating ramus with the tympanic plexus of the facial n. C

23   Tubal branch of tympanic plexus. Ramus tubarius (tubalis). Ramus for the auditory tube. C

24   Caroticotympanic nerves. Nn. caroticotympanici. Sympathetic fibers of the tympanic plexus derived from the internal carotid plexus. C

25   Branch communicating with the auricular branch of the vagus nerve. Ramus communicans [cum ramo auriculari nervi vagi]. Fine branch from the inferior ganglion to the auricular ramus of the vagus. B

26   Pharyngeal branches of IX nerve. Rami pharyngeales (pharyngei). Three to four rami passing into the pharyngeal plexus. B

27   Ramus to stylopharyngeus muscle. Ramus m. stylopharyngei. B

28   Branch to carotid sinus. Ramus sinus carotici. It also passes to the carotid body and communicates with the sympathetic trunk and vagus nerve. B

29   Tonsillar branches. Rami tonsillares. It supplies the mucosa of the palatine tonsil and its surroundings. B

30   Lingual branches. Rami linguales. Taste fibers from the posterior $1/3$ of the tongue including the vallate papillae which are also supplied by the lingual nerve via the chorda tympani. B

31   **Otic ganglion.** Ganglion oticum. Parasympathetic ganglion located medial to the mandibular nerve below the foramen ovale. It receives preganglionic fibers from the glossopharyngeal nerve via the lesser petrosal nerve and sends postganglionic secretory fibers to the parotid gland. D

32   Lesser petrosal nerve. N. petrosus minor. Containing parasympathetic fibers from the glossopharyngeal nerve, it emerges from the tympanic plexus, penetrates the anterior wall of the petrous temporal and leaves the middle cranial fossa through the sphenopetrosal fissure. Its fibers synapse in the otic ganglion. C D

33   Communicating ramus with the meningeal branch of the mandibular nerve. Ramus communicans [cum ramo meningeo]. D

34   Communicating branch with the auriculotemporal nerve. Ramus communicans [cum n. auriculotemporali]. It includes postganglionic parasympathetic fibers for the parotid gland. D

35   Communicating ramus with chorda tympani. Ramus communicans [com chorda tympani]. It incorporates sensory nerve fibers. D

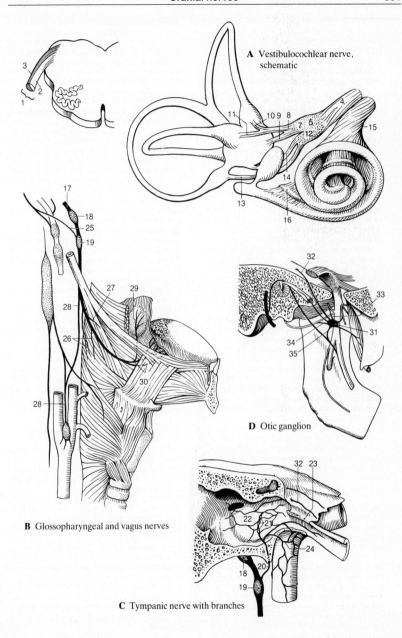

A Vestibulocochlear nerve, schematic

B Glossopharyngeal and vagus nerves

D Otic ganglion

C Tympanic nerve with branches

1 VAGUS NERVE (X). N. VAGUS [X]. Tenth cranial nerve (nerve of 4th and 5th pharyngeal arches). Together with the IX nerve, it exits the brain in the posterolateral sulcus and passes through the jugular foramen. Its supply region extends into the thoracic and abdominal cavities. A

2 **Superior (jugular) ganglion.** Ganglion superius. Smaller and superior sensory ganglion of vagus situated in the jugular foramen. A

3 **Inferior (nodose) ganglion.** Ganglion inferius. Larger and inferior, spindle-shaped ganglion of vagus. A

4 **Meningeal branch.** Ramus meningeus. Recurrent branch from the superior ganglion for the dura of the posterior cranial fossa in the region of the transverse and occipital sinuses. A

5 **Auricular branch.** Ramus auricularis. It arises from the superior ganglion of the vagus, passes through the mastoid canal, exits through the tympanomastoid fissure and supplies the posterior surface of the pinna and the postero-inferior wall of the external acoustic meatus. A

6 Communicating branch with IX nerve. Ramus communicans [cum n. glossopharyngeo]. Anastomotic branch from the auricular ramus to the glossopharyngeal nerve. A

7 **Pharyngeal branch.** Ramus pharyngealis (pharyngei). Branch radiating into the pharyngeal plexus. A

8 **Pharyngeal plexus.** Plexus pharyngealis. Nerve plexus below the middle pharyngeal constrictor and formed by the glossopharyngeal and vagus nerves and the cervical sympathetic trunk. A

9 **Superior cervical cardiac branches.** Rami cardiaci cervicales superiores. Given off at variable high cervical levels, they travel to the deep part of the cardiac plexus. A

10 **Superior laryngeal nerve.** N. laryngealis superior. It arises from the inferior ganglion and passes downward medial to the internal carotid artery to supply the larynx. A

11 External branch of superior laryngeal nerve (external laryngeal nerve). Ramus externus. It provides branches to the inferior pharyngeal constrictor and then, covered by the infrahyoid musculature, passes to the cricothyroid muscle. A

12 Internal branch (internal laryngeal nerve). *Ramus internus.* Together with the superior laryngeal artery, it penetrates the thyrohyoid membrane and arriving below the mucosa of the piriform recess, it supplies the mucosae of the epiglottic valleculae, the epiglottis and the larynx as far down as the level of the vocal folds. A

13 *Branch communicating with the recurrent laryngeal nerve. Ramus communicans [cum n. laryngeali recurrenti].* A

14 **Inferior cervical cardiac branches.** Rami cardiaci cervicales inferiores. They pass, on the right side, to the deep part of the cardiac plexus, on the left side to the superficial part of the cardiac plexus in company with the vagus nerve. A

15 **Recurrent laryngeal nerve.** N. laryngealis recurrens. On the right side it loops around the subclavian artery whereas on the left side it curves around the arch of the aorta. Then, ascending in the groove between the trachea and esophagus, its terminal branch penetrates the inferior pharyngeal constrictor and enters the larynx where it supplies the mucosa up to the vocal folds, as well as all intrinsic laryngeal muscles except the cricothyroid. It also provides a communicating branch to the internal laryngeal nerve. A

16 Tracheal branches. Rami tracheales. A

17 Esophageal branches. Rami oesophageales. A

17a Rami pharyngeales. Pharyngeal branches to the inferior pharyngeal constrictor.

18 **Inferior laryngeal nerve.** [[N. laryngeus inferior]]. Term sometimes employed for the terminal branch of the recurrent laryngeal nerve supplying the intrinsic muscles of the larynx except the cricothyoid and giving off a communicating branch to the internal laryngeal nerve. A

19 *[[R. communicans [cum ramo laryngeo interno]].* Communicating branch of the inferior (recurrent) laryngeal nerve to the internal laryngeal nerve. A

20 **Thoracic cardiac branches.** Rami cardiaci thoracici. Rami to the thoracic inlet. A

21 **Bronchial branches.** Rami bronchiales. Rami given off to the hilum of the lung below the recurrent laryngeal nerve. A

22 **Pulmonary plexus.** Plexus pulmonalis. Nerve plexus located anterior and posterior to the hilum of the lung for innervation of bronchi, vessels and visceral pleura. A

23 **Esophageal plexus.** Plexus oesophagealis. Nerve plexus around the esophagus formed directly by the two vagus nerves as well as superiorly also by the left recurrent laryngeal nerve. A

24 **Anterior vagal trunk.** Truncus vagalis anterior. Weak anterior plexus emerging from the esophageal plexus and containing fibers from the both vagi. A

25 **Posterior vagal trunk.** Truncus vagalis posterior. Better developed posterior nerve plexus arising from the esophageal plexus and containing fibers from both vagi. A

26 **Anterior gastric branches.** Rami gastrici anteriores. Rami from the anterior vagal trunk to the anterior surface of the stomach. A

27 **Posterior gastric branches.** Rami gastrici posteriores. Rami from the posterior vagal trunk to the posterior surface of the stomach. A

28 **Hepatic branches.** Rami hepatici. Rami to the hilum of the liver. A

29 **Celiac branches.** Rami coeliaci. Rami to the celiac plexus. A

30 **Renal branches.** Rami renales. Rami to the renal plexus. A

31 ACCESSORY NERVE (XI). N. ACCESSORIUS [XI]. Eleventh cranial nerve. Its two roots are united temporarily in the skull and pass through the jugular foramen together with the IX and X nerves. B

32 **Cranial roots (vagal part).** Radices craniales (pars vagalis). Fibers from the nucleus ambiguus which leave the accessory nerve in the jugular foramen and join the vagus nerve. B

33 **Spinal roots (spinal part).** Radices spinales (pars ~ spinalis). They arise from the base of the anterior horn of the cervical spinal cord (C1–6) and form a trunk which ascends into the subarachnoid space of the skull where it unites temporarily with fibers from the cranial roots. B

34 **Accessory nerve trunk.** Truncus nervi accessorii. It is formed by the union of both roots. B

35 Internal branch. Ramus internus. Fiber tract associated with the vagus nerve and formed by the united cranial roots of the accessory nerve. B

36 External branch. Ramus externus. United spinal root fibers of the accessory nerve. They supply the sternocleidomastoid and trapezius muscles. B

37 Muscular branches. Rami musculares. Branches supplying the sternocleidomastoid and trapezius muscles. B

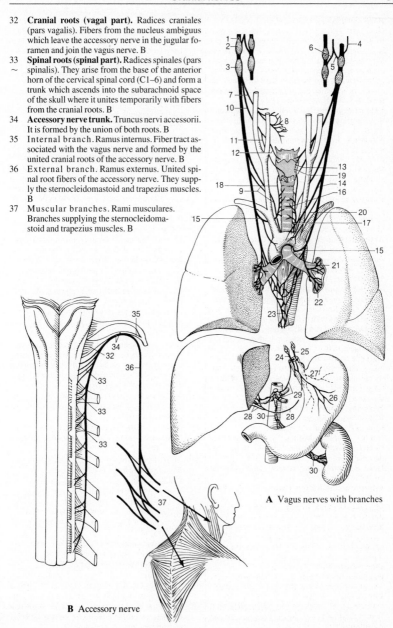

A Vagus nerves with branches

B Accessory nerve

1 HYPOGLOSSAL NERVE (XII). N. HYPO-GLOSSUS [XII]. Twelfth cranial nerve. Formed by numerous roots emerging from the brain between the pyramid and olive, it passes through the hypoglossal canal and descends between the internal jugular vein and internal carotid artery. At the level of the angle of the mandible it then proceeds anteriorly above the posterior margin of the floor of the mouth to enter the tongue. B

2 **Lingual branches.** Rami linguales. Rami beginning lateral to the hyoglossus muscle and supplying the styloglossus, hyoglossus and genioglossus muscles as well as the intrinic muscles of the tongue. B

3 SPINAL NERVES. NERVI SPINALES. They are formed by two roots and, in constrast to the cranial nerves, they exit through the intervertebral foramina. A C

4 **Root filaments.** Fila radicularia. Fine root fibers emerging from the spinal cord. They are packaged into the anterior and posterior roots of the individual spinal nerves. A

5 **Anterior (ventral) root.** Radix anterior (motoria). Motor root. A

6 **Posterior (dorsal) root.** Radix posterior (sensoria). Sensory root. A

7 Spinal (dorsal root) ganglion. Ganglion spinale (sensorium). Situated in the intervertebral foramen and possessing pseudo-unipolar cells, this sensory ganglion resides in the posterior root just before its union with the anterior root. A

8 **Spinal nerve trunk.** Truncus nervi spinalis. Segment between the union of both roots and the first branch. A C

9 **Anterior (ventral) branch.** Ramus anterior. A
~ Larger anterior branch of a spinal nerve. It communicates with adjacent anterior rami to form large plexuses. In the thoracic region it becomes an intercostal nerve. A

10 **Posterior (dorsal) branch.** Ramus posterior. A
~ Weaker branch for the skin of the back and autochthonous back musculature. A

11 **Rami communicantes.** Communicating branches between the spinal nerve and the sympathetic trunk. A

11a **Gray communicating ramus.** Ramus griseus. Postganglionic part. A

11b **White communicating ramus.** Ramus albus. Preganglionic part. A

12 **Meningeal branch.** Ramus meningeus. Delicate, recurrent ramus. It passes in front of the spinal nerve to re-enter the vertebral canal through the intervertebral foramen and supply the meninges of the spinal cord where it unites with other meningeal rami into a plexus. Its fibers are sensory and sympathetic. A

13 **Cauda equina.** Collection of all spinal nerve roots extending from L1–2 caudally in addition to the filum terminale. C

14 CERVICAL NERVES. NERVI CERVICALES. Eight spinal nerves emerging from the cervical spinal cord. B

15 **Posterior (dorsal) branches.** Rami posteriores. Branching off from the spinal nerve posteriorly, they supply the nuchal muscles and the skin lateral to the nuchal region and at the occiput. A

16 **Medial branch of posterior ramus.** Ramus medialis. Possessing motor and sensory fibers, it courses to the musculature and skin. A

17 **Lateral branch of posterior ramus.** Ramus lateralis. It passes obliquely laterad into the musculature and is purely motor. A

18 **Suboccipital nerve.** N. suboccipitalis. Posterior branch of the first cervical spinal nerve. It exits between the vertebral artery and posterior arch of the atlas and supplies the short muscles of the neck. D

19 **Greater occipital nerve.** N. occipitalis major. Posterior branch of the second cervical spinal nerve. It emerges between the axis and obliquus capitis inferior muscle, pierces the trapezius and supplies the nuchal muscles and skin of the occipital region. D

20 **Third occipital nerve.** N. occipitalis tertius. Posterior branch of the third cervical spinal nerve. It supplies the skin of the nuchal region close to the midline. D

21 **Anterior (ventral) branches.** Rami anteriores. Anterior rami of cervical spinal nerves. They form the cervical and brachial plexuses. A

22 CERVICAL PLEXUS. PLEXUS CERVICALIS. Nerve plexus formed by the anterior rami of spinal nerves C1–4. They supply the skin and musculature of the neck.

23 **Nerve loop from C1–3.** Ansa cervicalis (hypoglossi). Its fibers are partly attached to the hypoglossal nerve and partly come directly from spinal nerves. They supply the infrahyoid musculature except the thyrohyoid. B

24 Anterior (ventral) root. Radix anterior. Fibers from C1–3 attached temporarily to the hypoglossal nerve. B

25 Posterior (dorsal) root. Radix posterior. Fibers of the ansa cervicalis coming directly from C1–3. B

26 Thyrohyoid branch. Ramus thyrohyoideus. Ramus passing to the thyrohyoid muscle. B

27 **Lesser occipital nerve.** N. occipitalis minor. Uppermost cutaneous branch of the cervical plexus. It passes upward at the posterior margin of the sternocleidomastoid and at the occiput ramifies as a lateral communicating nerve of the greater occipital nerve. D

28 **Great auricular nerve.** N. auricularis magnus. In its course to the ear, it crosses the sternocleidomastoid vertically somewhat above its middle. D

29 Posterior (dorsal) branch. Ramus posterior. It supplies the skin of the posterior surface of the pinna and the adjacent area. D

30 Anterior (ventral) ramus. Ramus anterior. It supplies the skin of the anterior surface of the ear up to the angle of the mandible. D

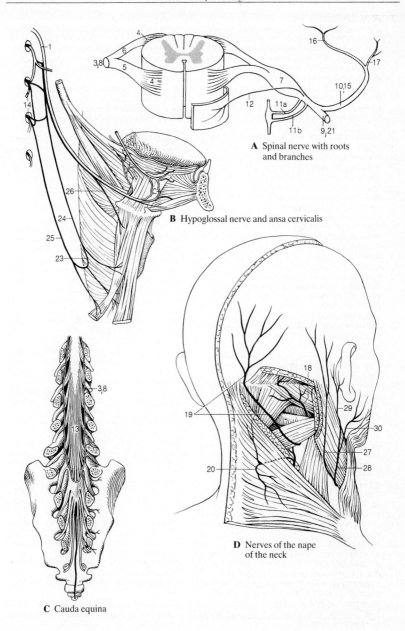

A Spinal nerve with roots and branches

B Hypoglossal nerve and ansa cervicalis

C Cauda equina

D Nerves of the nape of the neck

1 **Transverse cervical (colli) nerve.** N. transversus colli. Transverse cutaneous nerve of neck. Arising from C3, it is the third nerve occupying the "nerve point" at the posterior margin of the middle third of the sternocleidomastoid muscle where it turns anteriorly and passes beneath the platysma to supply the skin. It receives motor fibers for the platysma from the cervical branch of the facial nerve. B

2 Superior branches. Rami superiores. They ascend to the suprahyoid region. B

3 Inferior branches. Rami inferiores. They descend to the infrahyoid region. B

4 **Supraclavicular nerves.** Nn. supraclaviculares. Cutaneous branches from C3–4. They spread out fanlike to the shoulder and clavicular regions. B

5 Medial supraclavicular nerves. Nn. supraclaviculares mediales. They pass over the middle third of the clavicle and supply the skin of the neck in this region and the thorax as far as the sternal angle, as well as the sternoclavicular joint. B

6 Intermediate supraclavicular nerves. Nn. supraclaviculares intermedii. They descend beneath the platysma and over the middle third of the clavicle up to the skin up to the 4th rib. B

7 Lateral (posterior) supraclavicular nerves. Nn. supraclaviculares laterales (posteriores). Posterior group of nerves supplying the skin over the acromion, deltoid muscle and the acromioclavicular joint. B

8 **Phrenic nerve.** N. phrenicus. It arises from C4 with additional rami from C3 and C5, lies on the scalenus anterior muscle, then passes through the middle mediastinum to the diaphragm and, in part, further into the peritoneum. A C

9 Pericardial branch. Ramus pericardiacus. Slender branch to the anterior surface of the pericardium. A

10 Phrenicoabdominal branches. Rami phrenicoabdominales. Fibers destined for the peritoneum up to the gallbladder and pancreas. On the right side they pass through the foramen for the vena cava, on the left side further anteriorly through the diaphragm near the left margin of the heart. A

11 **Accessory phrenic nerves.** Nn. phrenici accessorii. Frequent additional roots of the phrenic nerve from C5 and C6 via the nerve to the subclavius. A C

12 BRACHIAL PLEXUS. PLEXUS BRACHIALIS. Nerve plexus formed by the anterior rami of spinal nerves C5–T1. Supplying the arm and part of the shoulder girdle, it passes between the scalenus anterior and medius extending as far as the head of the humerus. C

12 a **Nerve roots.** Radices.

13 **Trunks.** Trunci. Three primary trunks make up the brachial plexus and each is usually formed from one or two anterior rami of spinal nerves.

14 **Upper trunk.** Truncus superior. Formed by the union of C5 and C6 spinal nerves, it generally arises lateral to the scalenus gap. C

15 **Middle trunk.** Truncus medius. A continuation of C7 spinal nerve itself. C

16 **Lower trunk.** Truncus inferior. Formed by the union of C8 and T1 spinal nerves, it lies within the scalenus gap posterior to the subclavian artery. C

17 Anterior divisions. Divisiones anteriores. Portions of brachial plexus formed by the anterior branches of the three trunks. They supply the flexor muscles.

18 Posterior divisions. Divisiones posteriores. Portions of brachial plexus formed by the posterior branches of the three trunks. They unite to form the posterior cord and supply the extensor muscles.

18 a **Cords.** Fasciculi. Three nerve bundles formed by the union of branches (anterior and/or posterior) from the three trunks.

19 SUPRACLAVICULAR PART. PARS SUPRACLAVICULARIS. Part of brachial plexus extending up to the superior margin of the clavicle. C

20 **Dorsal scapular nerve.** N. dorsalis scapulae. Arising from C5 directly lateral to the intervertebral foramen, it penetrates the scalenus medius and then courses below the levator scapulae and the two rhomboid muscles which it innervates. C

21 **Long thoracic nerve.** N. thoracicus longus. Arising from C5–7, it penetrates the scalenus medius and then travels on the serratus anterior which it supplies. C

22 **Nerve to subclavius.** N. subclavius. Slender nerve from the upper trunk with fibers from C4–6 for the subclavius muscle. It frequently sends a branch (11) to the phrenic nerve. C

23 **Suprascapular nerve.** N. suprascapularis. Arising from C5–6, it passes over the brachial plexus to the scapular notch and then goes under the superior transverse ligament of the scapula to innervate the supra- and infraspinatus muscles. C

24 INFRACLAVICULAR PART. PARS INFRACLAVICULARES. Portion of brachial plexus below the clavicle. It extends from the upper margin of the clavicle to the level where the cords divide into the individual nerves. C

25 **Lateral cord.** Fasciculus lateralis. Located lateral to the axillary artery, it is formed by the union of the anterior divisions of the upper and middle trunks, thus from C5–7. C

26 **Medial cord.** Fasciculus medialis. Located medial to the axillary artery, it is formed solely by the anterior division of the lower trunk, thus from C8–T1. C

27 **Posterior cord.** Fasciculus posterior. Located posterior to the axillary artery, it is formed by the union of the posterior divisions of all three trunks, thus from C5–T1. C

28 **Medial pectoral nerve.** N. pectoralis medialis. It is formed by fibers from the medial cord, thus from C8–T1 and supplies the pectoralis major and minor muscles. C

29 **Lateral pectoral nerve.** N. pectoralis lateralis. It is made up of fibers from C5–7 for the two pectoral muscles. C

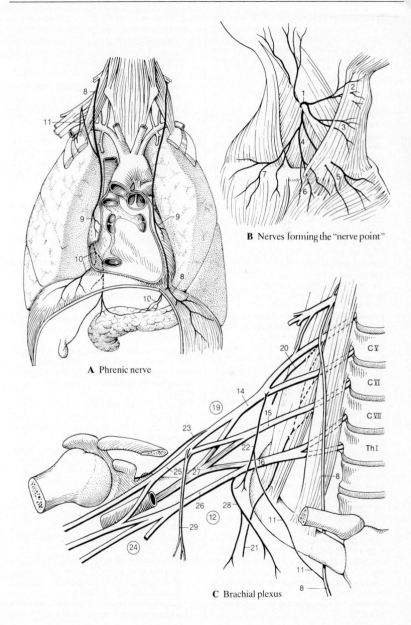

A Phrenic nerve

B Nerves forming the "nerve point"

C Brachial plexus

1 **Musculocutaneous nerve.** N. musculocutaneus. Arising from the lateral cord (C5–7), it penetrates the coracobrachialis and supplies it as well as the biceps and brachialis muscles. It ends as the lateral antebrachial cutaneous nerve. A

2 **Muscular branches.** Rami musculares. Branches to the coracobrachialis, biceps and brachialis muscles. A

3 **Lateral antebrachial cutaneous nerve.** N. cutaneus antebrachii lateralis. Terminal branch of musculocutaneous nerve. It penetrates the fascia at the bend of the elbow and supplies the skin of the lateral forearm. A

4 **Medial brachial cutaneous nerve.** N. cutaneus brachii medialis. Originating from the medial cord (C8, T1), it supplies the skin of the medial upper arm together with the intercostobrachial nerve. A

5 **Medial antebrachial cutaneous nerve.** N. cutaneus antebrachii medialis. Arising from the medial cord (C8, T1), it penetrates the fascia at about the middle of the upper arm and accompanies the basilic vein. It supplies the skin on the medial side of both the distal upper arm and the forearm. A

6 **Anterior branch.** Ramus anterior. It supplies the medial flexor side of the forearm. A

7 **Posterior (ulnar) branch.** Ramus posterior [ulnaris]. It supplies the medial upper ⅔ of the posterior aspect of the forearm. A B

8 **Median nerve.** N. medianus. It is formed by the union of medial and lateral roots from the medial and lateral cords, respectively (C6–T1). A

9 **Medial root.** Radix medialis. Contributor of the median nerve coming from the medial cord with fibers from C8 and T1. A

10 **Lateral root.** Radix lateralis. Contributor of the median nerve arising from the lateral cord with fibers from C6–7. A

11 **Anterior interosseous nerve of forearm.** N. interosseus (antebrachii) anterior. Arising at the bend of the elbow from the posterior side of the median nerve, it runs on the interosseous membrane and supplies the radiocarpal joint, intercarpal joints, flexor pollicis longus, flexor digitorum profundus (radial part) and pronator quadratus. A

12 **Muscular branches.** Rami musculares. They supply the pronator teres, flexor carpi radialis, palmaris longus and flexor digitorum superficialis muscles. A

13 **Palmar branch of median nerve.** Ramus palmaris n. mediani. It arises in the distal third of the forearm and supplies the skin of the lateral palm. A

14 **Communicating branch to the ulnar nerve.** Ramus communicans [cum nervo ulnari]. A

15 **Common digital nerves.** Nn. digitales communes. They run in the intervals between the first four fingers and then divide. A

16 **Proper palmar digital nerves.** Nn. digitales palmares proprii. Terminal branches of common palmar digital nerves. They supply the palmar aspect of the skin of the radial 3½ fingers and dorsal aspect of the skin of the radial 2½ distal phalanges. A

17 **Ulnar nerve.** N. ulnaris. Arising from the medial cord (C8, T1), it initially lies in the medial bicipital groove, breaks through the medial intermuscular septum and then, after passage in the groove for the ulnar nerve, penetrates the flexor carpi ulnaris. C

18 **Muscular branches.** Rami musculares. They supply the flexor carpi ulnaris and the ulnar part of the flexor digitorum profundus. C

19 **Dorsal branch of ulnar nerve.** Ramus dorsalis n. ulnaris. Cutaneous branch passing between the distal and middle third of the forearm beneath the flexor carpi ulnaris to innervate the dorsum of the hand. B C

20 **Dorsal digital nerves.** Nn. digitales dorsales. Individual branches to the little finger, ring finger and the ulnar side of the middle finger. This area of innervation can be displaced by the radial nerve. B

21 **Palmar branch of ulnar nerve.** Ramus palmaris nervi ulnaris. Arising in the distal third of the forearm, it penetrates the deep fascia and supplies the skin on the palmar surface of the hand. C

22 **Superficial branch.** Ramus superficialis. It lies beneath the palmar aponeurosis and divides into the common palmar digital nerves and a fine branch to the palmaris brevis. C

23 **Common palmar digital nerves.** Nn. digitales palmares communes. Usually only one branch which runs in the region between the ring and little fingers. C

25 *Proper palmar digital nerves.* Nn. digitales palmares proprii. Cutaneous nerves to the little finger and to the ulnar side of the ring finger. In addition, they supply the dorsal aspect of the middle and distal phalanges of the 1½ ulnar fingers. C

25 **Deep branch (of ulnar nerve).** Ramus profundus. Curving around the hamulus, it supplies the muscles of the hypothenar eminence, the interossei, the two ulnar lumbricals, the adductor pollicis and the deep head of the flexor pollicis brevis. C

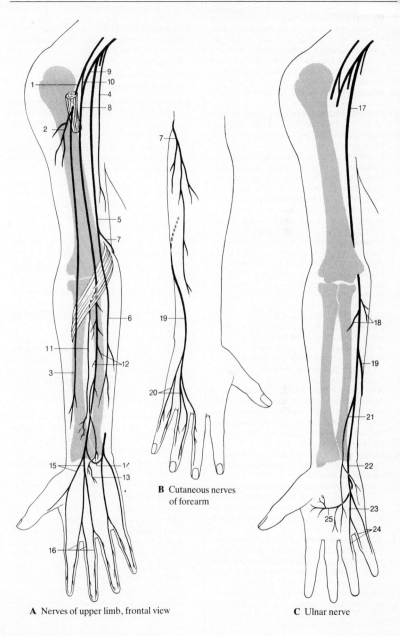

A Nerves of upper limb, frontal view

B Cutaneous nerves of forearm

C Ulnar nerve

...dial nerve. N. radialis. Originating from the posterior cord (usually with fibers from C5–T1), it takes a spiral course around the posterior aspect of the humerus as it occupies the groove for the radial nerve, then proceeds laterally between the brachialis and brachioradialis as well as both extensor carpi radialis muscles. At the elbow it divides into its deep and superficial ramus. A B D

2 **Posterior brachial cutaneous nerve.** N. cutaneus brachii posterior. Small cutaneous branch for the skin at the extensor side of the upper arm. A

3 **Lateral brachial cutaneous nerve.** N. cutaneus brachii lateralis inferior. Second cutaneous branch for the lateral and dorsal surfaces of the upper arm below the deltoid muscle. A

4 **Posterior antebrachial cutaneous nerve.** N. cutaneus antebrachii posterior. Cutaneous branch for the field between the lateral and medial antebrachial cutaneous nerves. B

5 **Muscular branches.** Rami musculares. Motor rami to the triceps, anconeus, brachioradialis and extensor carpi radialis longus muscles. A

6 **Deep branch.** Ramus profundus. It supplies the extensors of the forearm. It penetrates the supinator, supplying it and all extensors (except the extensor carpi radialis longus) and the abductor pollicis longus. A B

7 Posterior interosseous nerve of forearm. N. interosseus (antebrachii) posterior. Terminal branch of the deep ramus. It lies on the interosseous membrane in the distal third of the forearm beneath the extensors and extends to the wrist joint. A

8 **Superficial branch.** Ramus superficialis. It runs along the brachioradialis together with the radial artery, crosses under its accompanying muscle and then arrives at the dorsum of the hand and fingers as a cutaneous nerve. A B

9 Communicating branch to the ulnar nerve. Ramus communicans ulnaris. It joins the dorsal ramus of the ulnar nerve on the dorsum and the hand. A

10 Dorsal digital nerves. Nn. digitales dorsales. Terminal rami of the superficial branch passing on the radial and ulnar sides of the extensor aspect of the lateral 2$\frac{1}{2}$, sometimes also 3$\frac{1}{2}$ fingers. A

11 **Subscapular nerves.** Nervi subscapulares. Two to three branches from the brachial plexus (supraclavicular part or posterior cord) for the subscapularis and teres major muscles. D

12 **Thoracodorsal nerve.** N. thoracodorsalis. Longest subscapular nerve with fibers from C6–8. It courses along the lateral margin of the scapula and supplies the latissimus dorsi. D

13 **Axillary nerve.** N. axillaris. Arising from the posterior cord (C5–6), it passes, accompanied by the posterior circumflex humeral artery, through the axilla to the teres minor and deltoid muscles. D

14 **Muscular branches.** Rami musculares. Fibers to the teres minor and deltoid muscles. D

15 **Superior lateral brachial cutaneous nerve.** N. cutaneus brachii lateralis superior. It supplies the area of the skin located somewhat over the deltoid muscle. D

16 **Thoracic nerves.** Nn. thoracici. Twelve thoracic spinal nerves emerging below thoracic vertebrae 1–12, respectively. C

17 **Posterior branches.** Rami posteriores. Rami passing dorsally through the autochthonous musculature of the back. After supplying these muscles, they divide into a lateral and medial cutaneous branch. C

18 Lateral/medial muscular branches. Ramus muscularis lateralis/medialis. C

19 Posterior cutaneous branch. Ramus cutaneus posterior. C

20 **Anterior branches (intercostal nerves).** Rami anteriores (Nn. intercostales). Rami forming the intercostal nerves ventrally in the thoracic region. C

21 Lateral cutaneous branch (pectoral/abdominal). Ramus cutaneus lateralis (pectoralis/abdominalis). Arising from the intercostal nerve at about its middle, it passes obliquely ventrad and appears between the slips of the serratus anterior muscle and the latissimus dorsi. C

22 *Lateral mammary branches.* Rami mammarii laterales. Rami of lateral cutaneous branches coming from T4–6 and passing anteriorly to the mammary region. C

23 **Intercostobrachial nerves.** Nn. intercostobrachiales. Lateral cutaneous rami arising usually from T1, but also from T1–3 and passing to the upper arm. C

24 Anterior cutaneous branch (pectoral/abdominal). Ramus cutaneus anterior (pectoralis/abdominalis). Emerging medially and anteriorly, it divides again into medial and lateral branches. C

25 *Medial mammary branches.* Rami mammarii mediales. Medial branches from the anterior cutaneous rami of intercostal nerves 2–4. C

26 **Subcostal nerve.** N. subcostalis. Anterior branch of the 12th thoracic nerve located below the 12th rib.

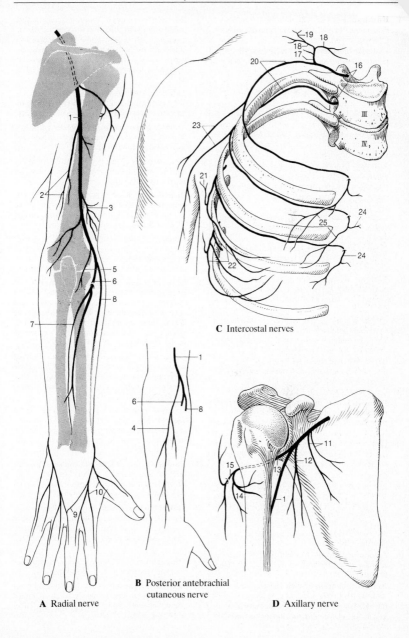

A Radial nerve

B Posterior antebrachial
cutaneous nerve

C Intercostal nerves

D Axillary nerve

1 ...ar nerves. Nn. lumbales (lumbares). Five lumbar spinal nerves each emerging below its respective lumbar vertebra.

2 **Posterior branches.** Rami posteriores. They supply the autochthonous back musculature and the skin overying it. C

3 Medial branch. Ramus medialis. Weak motor branch in the lumbar region. C

4 Lateral branch. Ramus lateralis. Predominantly sensory. C

5 *Superior clunial (gluteal) branches.* Rami clunium (gluteales) superiores. Lateral rami of L1–3 supplying the skin up to the greater trochanter (buttock region). B

6 **Anterior branches.** Rami anteriores. Ventral branches forming the lumbar plexus. C

7 **Sacral nerves and coccygeal nerve.** Nn. sacrales et n. coccygeus. Five sacral and one coccygeal nerves.

8 **Posterior branches.** Rami posteriores. Sensory and motor rami emerging from the posterior sacral foramina. A B

9 Medial branch. Ramus medialis. It supplies the multifidus and the skin over the sacrum and coccyx. A B

10 Lateral branch. Ramus lateralis. Sensory branch for the skin over the coccyx formed by the union of sensory fibers from the dorsal rami of S1–3. A B

11 *Medial clunial (gluteal) nerves.* Rami clunium (gluteales) mediales. Sensory nerves from S1–3. They penetrate the gluteus maximus and supply the skin of the medial, upper gluteal region. B

12 **Anterior branches.** Rami anteriores. They pass through the pelvic sacral foramina and form the sacral plexus. A C

13 LUMBOSACRAL PLEXUS. PLEXUS LUMBOSACRALIS. Collective term for the combined lumbar and sacral plexuses joined together by fibers from L4 and mutually supplying the lower limb. C

14 LUMBAR PLEXUS. PLEXUS LUMBALIS (LUMBARIS). Nerve network formed by spinal nerves L1–4 which lie at the anterior side of the leg.

15 **Iliohypogastric nerve.** N. iliohypogastricus. It contains sensory and motor fibers from T12 and L1 for the abdominal musculature. It traverses the psoas major, then comes to lie between the transversus abdominis and internal abdominal muscles and pierces the latter medial to the anterior superior iliac spine. C

16 **Lateral cutaneous branch.** Ramus cutaneus lateralis. It can reach as far as the lateral gluteal region. C

17 **Anterior cutaneous branch.** Ramus cutaneus anterior. It frequently penetrates the aponeurosis of the external oblique just above the superficial inguinal ring and supplies the skin in this area. C

18 **Ilioinguinal nerve.** N. ilioinguinalis. Formed from L1, possibly also T12, it appears at the lateral margin of the psoas and courses between the kidney and quadratus lumborum, then between the transversus abdominis and internal abdominal oblique (muscular branches) to enter the inguinal canal. C

19 **Anterior scrotal nerves.** Nn. scrotales anteriores. Sensory branches to the anterior skin of the scrotum, mons pubis and adjacent skin of the thigh. C

20 **Anterior labial nerves.** Nn. labiales anteriores. Sensory rami to the labium majus, mons pubis and adjacent skin of the thigh. C

21 **Genitofemoral nerve.** N. genitofemoralis. Formed from L1–2, it penetrates the psoas major and lies on it. C

22 **Genital branch.** Ramus genitalis. It courses through the inguinal canal and supplies the cremaster muscle, skin of scrotum (labium majus) and adjacent skin of the thigh. C

23 **Femoral branch.** Ramus femoralis. It passes through the vascular lacuna (between femoral artery and iliopectineal arch), then through the saphenous hiatus to supply the skin located there. C

24 **Lateral femoral cutaneous nerve.** N. cutaneus femoris lateralis. Formed from L2–3, it appears at the lateral margin of the psoas and courses beneath the iliac fascia and through the lateral part of the muscular lacuna into the thigh where it proceeds below or above the sartorius to the lateral skin of the thigh. C

25 **Obturator nerve.** N. obturatorius. Formed from L2–4, it passes beneath the psoas, behind the internal iliac artery and lateral to the ureter, then through the obturator canal to the adductor group and to the medial skin of the thigh. C

26 **Anterior branch.** Ramus anterior. It lies on the adductor brevis and obturator externus muscles and beneath the adductor longus and pectineus. It supplies these muscles in addition to the gracilis. C

27 Cutaneous branch. Ramus cutaneus. Variable terminal branch which appears between the adductor longus and gracilis muscles and supplies the distal 2/3 of the skin of the thigh. C

28 **Posterior branch.** Ramus posterior. It pierces the obturator externus and supplies it and the adductor magnus and brevis. With a sensory branch it extends as far as the posterior wall of the knee joint. C

29 **Muscular branches.** Rami musculares. Branches supplying the previously named muscles. C

30 **Accessory obturator nerve.** N. obturatorius accessorius. It frequently appears as an additional obturator nerve from L3–4 supplying the pectineus and hip joint.

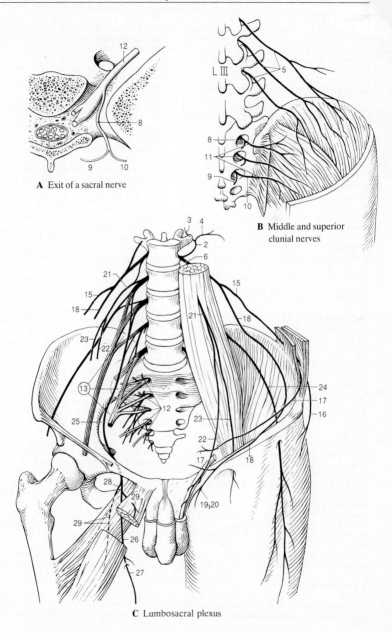

A Exit of a sacral nerve

B Middle and superior clunial nerves

C Lumbosacral plexus

nerve. N. femoralis. Derived from
..., it appears at the lateral margin of the psoas and
runs between the iliacus and psoas major muscles to
pass through the muscular lacuna. A

2 **Muscular branches.** Rami musculares. Branches to
the sartorius, pectineus and quadriceps femoris
muscles. A

3 **Anterior cutaneous branches.** Rami cutanei anteriores. Main branches for the distal ³/₄ of the anterior
surface of the thigh up to the patella. A

4 **Saphenous nerve.** N. saphenus. Longest, purely
sensory ramus of the femoral nerve. It begins in the
femoral triangle, passes beneath the "vasto-adductor
membrane", which it pierces, arrives beneath the
skin between the sartorius and gracilis muscles and,
in company with the great saphenous vein, proceeds
as far as the medial side of the foot. A

5 **Infrapatellar branch.** Ramus infrapatellaris. It
penetrates the sartorius and arrives at the skin below
the patella. A

6 **Medial cutaneous branches of the leg.** Rami
cutanei cruris mediales. Branches of saphenous
nerve to skin of the lower leg and foot. A

7 **Lumbosacral trunk.** Truncus lumbosacralis.
Connection to the lumbar plexus formed by L5 and a
part of L4. A

8 SACRAL PLEXUS. PLEXUS SACRALIS. Formed
by L5–S3 and a part of L4 and S4, it lies anterior to
the piriformis muscle beneath its fascia. Its nerves
pass to the posterior side of the lower limb. A

9 **Nerve to obturator internus muscle.** N. musculi
obturatorii interni. It arises from L5–S2 and passes
through the greater sciatic foramen into the ischio-
anal fossa from where it arrives at the obturator internus muscle.

10 **Nerve to piriformis muscle.** N. musculi piriformis.
Formed from S1–2, it proceeds to the anterior side of
the piriformis.

11 **Nerve to quadratus femoris.** N. musculi quadrati
femoris. Originating from L4–S1, it passes through
the greater sciatic foramen and proceeds further
deeply to the quadratus femoris and the hip joint.

12 **Superior gluteal nerve.** N. gluteus superior.
Formed from L4–S1, it passes through the greater
sciatic foramen cranial to the piriformis [["suprapiri-
form foramen"]] and then between the gluteus medius and minimus as far as the tensor fasciae latae. It
supplies all of the above-mentioned muscles except
for the piriformis. B

13 **Inferior gluteal nerve.** N. gluteus inferior.
Arising from L5–S2, it passes through the infrapiriform foramen and supplies the gluteus maximus. B

14 **Posterior femoral cutaneous nerve.** N.
cutaneus femoralis posterior. Arising from S1–3, it
passes through the greater sciatic foramen below the
piriformis [["infrapiriform foramen"]] and supplies
the skin at the posterior side of the thigh and proximal portion of lower leg. B

15 **Inferior clunial (gluteal) rami.** Rami clunium
(gluteales) inferiores. Cutaneous branches passing
upward around the lower margin of the gluteus maximus. B

16 **Perineal branches.** Rami perineales. They
branch off at the lower margin of the gluteus maximus, pass beneath the ischial tuberosity medially to
the scrotum (labia) and have one branch which ascends as far as the coccyx. B

16a **Perforating cutaneous nerve.** N. cutaneus perforans. Ramus of the posterior femoral cutaneous
nerve supplying the skin of the anus. B

17 **Sciatic nerve.** N. ischiaticus (sciaticus). Arising
from L4–S3, it is the thickest nerve of the body. It
leaves the pelvis through the greater sciatic foramen
below the piriformis [[infrapiriform foramen]] and
passes downward lateral to the ischial tuberosity,
beneath the gluteus maximus and the long head of
the biceps. B

18 **Common peroneal (fibular) nerve.** N. fibularis
communis. Arising from L4–S2, it branches off from
the sciatic nerve at a variable level, passes in company with the biceps tendon as far as the posterior
aspect of the head of the fibula and then crosses
obliquely forward between the skin and fibula. B

19 **Lateral sural cutaneous nerve.** N. cutaneus surae lateralis. It usually arises in the popliteal fossa
and supplies the skin on the lateral aspect of the proximal ²/₃ of the posterior side of the lower leg. A B

20 **Communicating branch of common peroneal (fibular) nerve.** Ramus communicans fibularis. It passes beneath the fascia over the lateral head
of the gastrocnemius and joins the medial sural cutaneous nerve to form the sural nerve. B

21 **Superficial peroneal (fibular) nerve.** N. fibularis
superficialis. One of the terminal branches of the
common peroneal nerve. It descends between the
peroneal muscles and extensor digitorum longus. A
B

22 **Muscular branches.** Rami musculares. Branches
to the peroneus longus and brevis.

23 **Medial dorsal cutaneous nerve.** N. cutaneus
dorsalis medialis. It runs over the extensor retinacula and supplies the skin of the dorsum of the foot, the
medial side of the big toe and the halves of the 2nd
and 3rd toes facing one another. A

24 **Intermediate dorsal cutaneous nerve.** N.
cutaneus dorsalis intermedius. Lateral cutaneous
branch of the superficial peroneal nerve to the middle and lateral aspect of the dorsum of the foot. A

25 *Dorsal digital nerves of foot.* Nn. digitales dorsales
pedis. Branches for the toes except for the distal phalanges. A

26 **Deep peroneal (fibular) nerve.** N. fibularis profundus. It proceeds beneath the peroneus longus, then
lateral to the tibialis anterior muscle to supply the
dorsum of the foot. A B

27 **Muscular branches.** Rami musculares. Rami
passing to the tibialis anterior, extensor hallucis longus and brevis, and extensor digitorum longus and
brevis muscles. A

28 **Dorsal digital nerves of lateral surface of
great toe and of medial surface of second
toe.** Nn. digitales dorsales, hallucis lateralis et digiti secundi medialis. Sensory branches. A

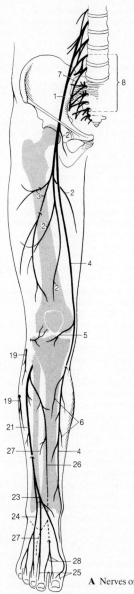

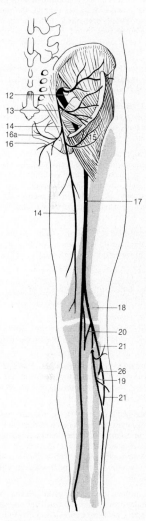

B Nerves of lower limb from behind

A Nerves of lower limb from front

...ve. N. tibialis. Formed from ...e second terminal branch of the ... nerve. It passes through the popliteal fossa, disappears beneath the tendinous arch of the soleus muscle and proceeds, accompanied by the posterior tibial artery, around the medial malleolus to the sole of the foot. A

2 **Muscular branches.** Rami musculares. Rami to the gastrocnemius, plantaris, soleus and the deep flexors at the lower leg. A

3 **Interosseous nerve of leg.** N. interosseus cruris. In company with the anterior tibial artery, it contains fibers for the bones and tibiofibular joint. A

4 **Medial sural cutaneous nerve.** N. cutaneus surae medialis. It arises from the tibial nerve in the popliteal fossa, then descends subfascially lateral to the small saphenous vein and joins the peroneal communicating branch of the common peroneal nerve to form the sural nerve. A B

5 **Sural nerve.** N. suralis. Continuation of the medial sural cutaneous nerve after its union with the peroneal communicating ramus. B

6 Lateral dorsal cutaneous nerve. N. cutaneus dorsalis lateralis. It passes to the lateral aspect of the dorsum of the foot and anastomoses with the intermediate dorsal cutaneous nerve. B

7 Lateral calcaneal branches. Rami calcanei laterales. Lateral branches to the calcaneus. B

8 **Medial calcaneal branches.** Rami calcanei mediales. Coming directly from the tibial nerve, they pass to the medial aspect of the calcaneus. B

9 **Medial plantar nerve.** N. plantaris medialis. The larger terminal branch of the tibial nerve. It proceeds beneath the flexor retinaculum and the abductor hallucis to the sole of the foot which it supplies, as well as the skin and the flexor hallucis brevis and flexor digitorum brevis. A

10 Common plantar digital nerves. Nn. digitales plantares communes. They course in the interval between toes 1–4 and divide into the proper plantar digital nerves. A

11 *Proper plantar digital nerves.* Nn. digitales plantares proprii. Cutaneous nerves passing on the tibial and fibular sides of the flexor aspect of the medial $3^1/_2$ toes. They supply the distal phalanges, including their dorsal aspect. A

12 **Lateral plantar nerve.** N. plantaris lateralis. Smaller terminal branch of the tibial nerve. It passes beneath the flexor digitorum brevis medial to the lateral plantar artery as far as the base of the 5th metatarsal bone. A

13 Superficial branch. Ramus superficialis. Predominantly sensory branch of lateral plantar nerve. A

14 *Common plantar digital nerves.* Nn. digitales plantares communes. Two branches, one passing to the little toe and giving off a branch to the flexor digiti minimi brevis, the other proceeding to the interval between the 4th and 5th toes. A

15 *Proper plantar digital nerves.* Nn. digitales plantares proprii. They pass to the fibular and tibial sides of the little toe as well as to the fibular side of the 4th toe. A

16 Deep branch. Ramus profundus. Muscular branch passing in company with the plantar arch to the interossei, adductor hallucis and the lateral three lumbrical muscles. A

17 **Pudendal nerve.** N. pudendus. Arising from S2–4, it passes through the greater sciatic foramen below the piriformis [["infrapiriform foramen"]] to the ischio-anal fossa. C

18 **Inferior rectal nerves.** Nn. rectales (anales) inferiores. Fibers from S3–4 for the external anal sphincter and the anal skin. C

19 **Perineal nerves.** Nn. perineales. Collective term for the nerves of the perineum.

20 Posterior scrotal (labial) nerves. Nn. scrotales/labiales posteriores. They reach the scrotum (labium majus) from behind. C

21 Muscular branches. Rami musculares. They supply the muscles of the perineum.

22 **Dorsal nerve of penis.** N. dorsalis penis. Paired nerves lying on the dorsum of the penis with branches also to the underside of the penis. C

23 **Dorsal nerve of clitoris.** N. dorsalis clitoridis. Smaller nerve corresponding to the dorsal nerve of the penis. C

24 **Coccygeal nerve.** N. coccygeus. Last spinal nerve. It emerges between the coccyx and sacrum and anastomoses with S4–5 nerves. C

25 **Coccygeal plexus.** Plexus coccygeus. Nerve plexus formed by fibers from a part of S4, all of S5 and the coccygeal nerve. It supplies the skin over the coccyx. C

26 **Anococcygeal nerves.** Nn. anococcygei. Several fine nerves from the coccygeal plexus. They pierce the anococcygeal ligament and supply the skin lying over it. C

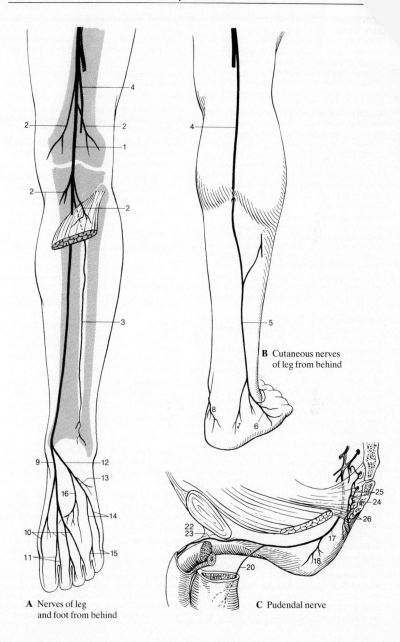

A Nerves of leg
and foot from behind

B Cutaneous nerves
of leg from behind

C Pudendal nerve

NERVOUS SYSTEM. PARS
SYSTEMA NERVORUM AU-
It regulates the functions of the
(viscera) by its influence on
....uscle, cardiac muscle and glands.

2 **Autonomic (visceral) plexus.** Plexus autonomici (viscerales). Autonomic nerve plexuses mainly in front of the vertebral column at the branches of the aorta.

3 **Ganglia of autonomic plexus.** Ganglia plexuum autonomicorum (visceralium). Groups of ganglion cells scattered in the autonomic plexuses for synaptic connections between pre- and postganglionic fibers.

4 **Thoracic aortic plexus.** Plexus aorticus thoracicus. Autonomic nerve plexus around the aorta with fibers from the first five thoracic ganglia and the splanchnic nerve. It also contains afferent vagal fibers. B

5 **Cardiac plexus.** Plexus cardiacus. Autonomic nerve plexus from sympathetic and vagal fibers at the base of the heart, especially around the arch of the aorta and at the root of the pulmonary trunk, as well as along the coronary vessels and between the aorta and tracheal bifurcation. B

6 **Cardiac ganglia.** Ganglia cardiaca. Small macroscopic accumulations of ganglion cells especially to the right of the ligamentum arteriosum. B

7 **Esophageal plexus.** Plexus oesophagealis. Network of autonomic nerve fibers around the esophagus.

8 **Pulmonary branches.** Rami pulmonales. Rami from the 3rd to 4th thoracic sympathetic ganglia, particularly to the posterior part of the pulmonary plexus. B

9 Pulmonary plexus. Plexus pulmonalis. Plexus in front of and behind the hilum of the lung formed by vagal and sympathetic fibers. It is connected across the midline with the pulmonary plexus of the opposite side and with the cardiac plexus. B

10 **Abdominal aortic plexus.** Plexus aorticus abdominalis. Nerve plexus in front of and on both sides of the aorta. It extends from the celiac plexus to the aortic bifurcation, receives fibers from both upper lumbar ganglia and continues caudally into the superior hypogastric plexus.

11 **Celiac plexus.** Plexus coeliacus. Nerve plexus around the celiac trunk. It communicates with adjacent plexuses and receives fibers from both splanchnic nerves and from the vagus. A C

12 **Celiac ganglia.** Ganglia coelica. Aggregations of ganglion cells communicating with the celiac plexus and lying to the right and left of the aorta by the celiac trunk. A

13 **Aorticorenal ganglia.** Ganglia aorticorenalia. Accumulations of ganglion cells at the exit of the renal artery. They receive the lesser splanchnic nerve and can be fused with the celiac ganglia. A

14 **Superior mesenteric ganglion.** Ganglion mesentericum superius. Group of ganglion cells at the right and left of the aorta near the superior mesenteric artery and its branches. It is often fused with adjacent ganglia. A

15 **Intermesenteric plexus.** Plexus intermesentericus. Nerve plexus between the superior and inferior mesenteric plexuses. A

16 **Inferior mesenteric ganglion.** Ganglion mesentericum inferius. Ganglion cells located entirely within the inferior mesenteric plexus. A

17 **Phrenic ganglia.** Ganglia phrenica. Small accumulation of ganglion cells in the nerve plexus accompanying the inferior phrenic artery. A

18 **Hepatic plexus.** Plexus hepaticus. Continuation of the celiac plexus at the liver with fibers from the vagus and phrenic nerves. A C

19 **Splenic (lienal) plexus.** Plexus splenicus (lienalis). Extensions of the celiac plexus along the splenic artery to the spleen. A C
~

20 **Gastric plexus.** Plexus gastrici. Autonomic nerve plexus for the stomach. The anterior and posterior part is formed by the vagus, the left part is a continuation of the celiac plexus along the left gastric artery. C

21 **Pancreatic plexus.** Plexus pancreaticus. Continuation of the celiac plexus along the pancreatic vessels. C

22 **Suprarenal plexus.** Plexus suprarenalis. Continuation of the celiac plexus along the suprarenal vessels with, among others, preganglionic fibers for the suprarenal medulla. A

23 **Renal plexus.** Plexus renalis. Nerve plexus continued onto the renal artery. It also comtains vagal fibers. A

24 **Renal ganglia.** Ganglia renalis. Microscopically small groups of ganglion cells dispersed within the renal plexus. A

25 **Ureteric plexus.** Plexus uretericus. Nerve plexus along the ureter with fibers from the renal and abdominal aortic plexuses and the aorticorenal ganglia. A

26 **Testicular plexus.** Plexus testicularis. Nerve plexus along the testicular artery. It extends as far as the testis and receives fibers from the renal and abdominal aortic plexuses. A

27 **Ovarian plexus.** Plexus ovaricus. Autonomic nerve plexus along the ovarian artery with fibers from the abdominal aortic and renal plexuses. A

28 **Superior mesenteric plexus.** Plexus mesentericus superior. Nerve plexus accompanying the superior mesenteric artery and its branches. It contains sympathetic fibers from the celiac plexus and parasympathetic fibers from the vagus nerve. A

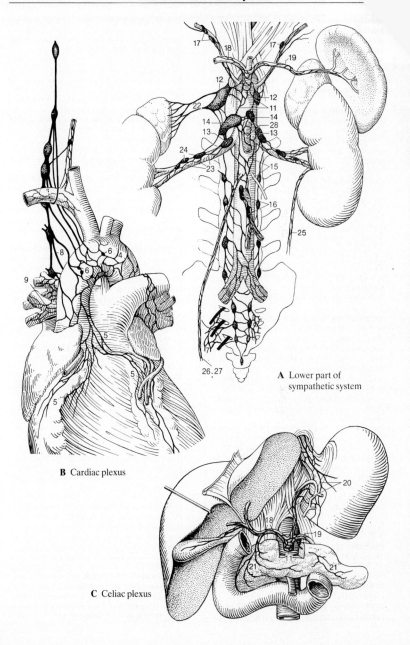

A Lower part of
sympathetic system

B Cardiac plexus

C Celiac plexus

Autonomic nervous system

349

eric plexus. Plexus mesentericus ...ation of the abdominal aortic : inferior mesenteric artery in- ...es. D

...perior rectal plexus. Plexus rectalis superior. Continuation of the inferior mesenteric plexus on the superior rectal artery and rectum. It also contains parasympathetic fibers from the pelvic plexus. D

3 **Enteric plexus.** Plexus entericus. Collective term for the autonomic plexuses in the wall of the intestinal tract.

4 Subserosal plexus. Plexus subserosus. Fine autonomic plexus located directly beneath the serosa. C

5 Myenteric (Auerbach's) plexus. Plexus myentericus [[Auerbach]]. Well developed plexus situated between the longitudinal and circular muscle layers. It contains ganglion cells and regulates the peristaltic action of the intestine. C

6 Submucosal (Meissner's) plexus. Plexus submucosus [[Meissner]]. Well developed plexus occupying the submucosa. It contains ganglion cells and regulates the activity of the muscularis mucosae and villi. C

7 **Iliac plexus.** Plexus iliaci. Continuation of the abdominal aortic plexus onto both iliac arteries. D E

8 **Femoral plexus.** Plexus femoralis. Continuation of the iliac plexus onto the femoral artery. E

9 **Superior hypogastric plexus (presacral nerve).** Plexus hypogastricus superior (N. praesacralis). Plexus-like connection between the abdominal aortic and pelvic plexuses located predominantly in front of the 5th lumbar vertebral body and receiving branches from the lumbar sympathetic ganglia. D E

10 **Right/left hypogastric nerve.** N. hypogastricus dexter/sinister. Right and left branch of the superior hypogastric plexus to the pelvic viscera. They communicate with the inferior hypogastric plexus. D E

11 **Inferior hypogastric plexus (pelvic plexus).** Plexus hypogastricus inferior (plexus pelvicus). Network of sympathetic and parasympathetic fibers located to the right and left of the rectum and in front of it. D

12 **Middle rectal plexus.** Plexus rectalis medius. Continuation of the inferior hypogastric plexus onto the wall of the rectum. E

13 **Inferior rectal plexus.** Plexus rectalis inferior. Autonomic nerve plexus located around the branches of the internal iliac artery and passing to both sides of the rectum. E

14 **Prostatic plexus.** Plexus prostaticus. Nerve plexus mainly at the posterior and inferior surfaces of the prostate and extending as far as the membranous part of the urethra. E

15 **Deferential plexus.** Plexus deferentialis. Nerve plexus around the ductus deferens. E

16 **Uterovaginal plexus.** Plexus uterovaginalis. Nerve plexus occupying the parametrium and infiltrated with many ganglia. It sends branches to the uterus, vagina, uterine tube and ovary. It communicates with the pelvic plexus in the recto-uterine fold. D

17 Vaginal nerves. Nervi vaginales. Branches of the uterovaginal plexus passing to the vagina. D

18 **Vesical plexus.** Plexus vesicalis. Plexus situated on both sides of the urinary bladder. It contains parasympathetic fibers and is involved in regulating the voiding mechanism of the urinary bladder. E

19 **Cavernous nerves of penis.** Nn. cavernosi penis. Rami from the prostatic plexus to the cavernous bodies of the penis. E

20 **Cavernous nerves of clitoris.** Nn. cavernosi clitoridis. Nerves corresponding to the cavernous nerves of the penis. E

21 SYMPATHETIC PART (SYSTEM). PARS SYMPATHETICA. Thoracolumbar part of the autonomic nervous system represented in the sympathetic trunk. Excitable by adrenalin (adrenergic), it has a stimulatory effect upon the circulation, an inhibiting action on the intestinal tract.

22 **Sympathetic trunk.** Truncus sympatheticus. Chain of ganglia connected by nerve fibers. It lies to the right and left of the vertebral column and extends from the base of the skull to the coccyx. B

23 **Ganglia of sympathetic trunk.** Ganglia trunci sympathetici. Groups of small, mostly multipolar ganglion cells producing macroscopic thickenings and forming synaptic sites between myelinated preganglionic and nonmyelinated postganglionic fibers. B

24 **Interganglionic branches.** Rami interganglionares. Bundles of white and gray fibers linking the sympathetic ganglia. B

25 **Rami communicates.** Communicating branches (afferent and efferent) between the spinal nerves and sympathetic trunk. B

26 **Intermediate ganglia.** Ganglia intermedia. Additional accumulations of sympathetic ganglion cells mainly in the rami communicantes of the cervical and lumbar regions. B

27 **Superior cervical ganglion.** Ganglion cervicale superius. Uppermost sympathetic trunk ganglion, about 2.5 cm long and lying 2 cm below the base of the skull between the longus capitis and posterior belly of the digastric. A

28 **Jugular nerve.** N. jugularis. Branch to the inferior ganglion of the glossopharyngeal nerve and to the superior ganglion of the vagus. A

29 **Internal carotid nerve.** N. caroticus internus. It contains postganglionic fibers and forms the internal carotid plexus in the carotid canal. A

30 **Internal carotid plexus.** Plexus caroticus internus. Nerve plexus in the carotid canal giving rise to the deep petrosal nerve and branches to the inner ear. It supplies the eye with sympathetic fibers. A

31 **External carotid nerves.** Nn. carotici externi. Nerves for the external carotid plexus descending along the external carotid artery. A

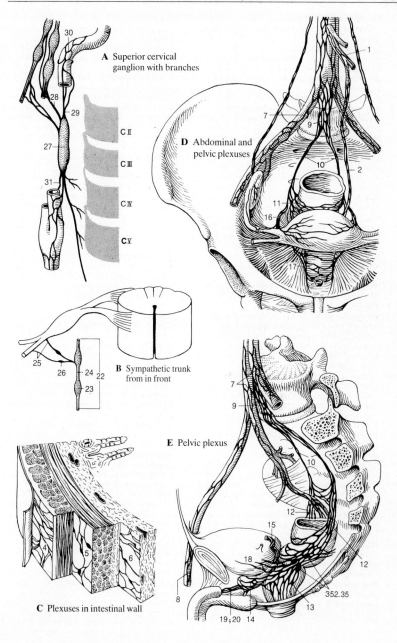

A Superior cervical
ganglion with branches

D Abdominal and
pelvic plexuses

B Sympathetic trunk
from in front

E Pelvic plexus

C Plexuses in intestinal wall

1 **External carotid plexus.** Plexus caroticus externus. Autonomic nerve plexus around the external carotid artery. A

2 **Common carotid plexus.** Plexus caroticus communis. It surrounds the common carotid artery. A

3 **Laryngopharyngeal branches.** Rami laryngopharyngeales. Postganglionic fibers to the pharyngeal plexus. A

4 **Superior cervical cardiac nerve.** N. cardiacus cervicalis superior. Fibers to the cardiac plexus. A

5 **Middle cervical ganglion.** Ganglion cervicale medium. Often very small, this ganglion of the sympathetic trunk lies at the level of C6 in front of or behind the inferior thyroid artery. A E

6 **Vertebral ganglion.** Ganglion vertebrale. Small accessory ganglion usually on the vertebral artery in front of its entrance into the foramen transversarium. A

7 **Middle cervical cardiac nerve.** N. cardiacus cervicalis medius. It passes from the middle cervical ganglion to the deep part of the cardiac plexus. A

8 **Cervicothoracic (stellate) ganglion.** Ganglion cervicothoracicum (stellatum). Fusion of the inferior cervical with the 1st, and often the 2nd thoracic ganglia (about 75%). A E

9 **Ansa subclavia.** Cord of nerve fibers forming a loop around the subclavian artery. A

10 **Inferior cervical cardiac nerve.** N. cardiacus cervicalis inferior. It passes to the deep part of the cardiac plexus. A

11 **Subclavian plexus.** Plexus subclavius. Autonomic nerve plexus around the subclavian artery. A

12 **Vertebral nerve.** N. vertebralis. Located behind the vertebral artery, it forms the vertebral plexus. A

13 **Vertebral plexus.** Plexus vertebralis. Network of nerves around the vertebral artery. A

14 **Thoracic ganglia.** Ganglia thoracica. 11–12 thickenings in the thoracic sympathetic trunk. A E

15 **Thoracic cardiac branches.** Rami cardiaci thoracici. Rami with efferent and afferent (pain) fibers passing from T2–4(5) thoracic ganglia to the cardiac plexus. A E

15a **Thoracic pulmonary branches.** Rami pulmonales thoracici. Efferent fibers from T2–4 ganglia to the pulmonary plexus at the lung hilum. E

15b **Esophageal branches.** Rami oesophageales. Efferent fibers from T2–5 ganglia.

16 **Greater splanchnic nerve.** N. splanchnicus major. It passes from sympathetic trunk ganglia 5–9(10) to the celiac ganglion and contains pre- and postganglionic fibers which conduct, among others, pain sensations from the upper abdominal organs. E

17 **Thoracic splanchnic ganglion.** Ganglion thoracicum splanchnicum. Accessory ganglion at the level of T9. It is incorporated into the greater splanchnic nerve. E

18 **Lesser splanchnic nerve.** N. splanchnicus minor. Arising from sympathetic trunk ganglia 9–11, it is similar to the greater splanchnic nerve. E

19 **Renal branch.** Ramus renalis. Occasional branch from the lesser splanchnic nerve to the renal plexus. E

20 **Lowest splanchnic nerve.** N. splanchnicus imus. It often arises independently from the T12 ganglion and passes to the renal plexus. E

21 **Lumbar ganglia.** Ganglia lumbalia (lumbaria). Often four sympathetic ganglia of the lumbar vertebral column. B

22 **Lumbar splanchnic nerves.** Nervi splanchnici lumbales (lumbares). Usually four nerves from the lumbar sympathetic trunk forming a plexus on L5. B

23 **Sacral ganglia.** Ganglia sacralia. Four smaller ganglia lying medial to the pelvic sacral foramina. B

24 **Sacral splanchnic nerves.** Nervi splanchnici sacrales. Two to three fine nerves from sacral ganglia 2–4. B

25 **Ganglion impar.** Last unpaired sympathetic trunk ganglion lying in front of the coccyx. B

26 PARASYMPATHETIC PART (SYSTEM). PARS PARASYMPATHETICA. Craniosacral component of the autonomic nervous system involving cranial nerves III, VII, IX, and X and sacral spinal nerves. 2–4. Antagonistic to the sympathetic division, it slows down the heart beat and stimulates intestinal and sexual functions.

26a **Cranial part.** Pars cranialis.

27 **Terminal nerve.** N. terminalis. A slender, partly interwoven nerve of unknown function, but probably autonomic. It unites the olfactory region with the anterior perforated substance. C

28 **Terminal ganglion.** Ganglion terminale. It comprises all of the ganglion cells dispersed in the terminal nerves.

29 **Ciliary ganglion.** Ganglion ciliare. Located lateral to the optic nerve, it receives preganglionic fibers from the oculomotor nerve and gives off postganglionic fibers which constrict the pupil and contract the ciliary musculature during accommodation. D

30 **Pterygopalatine ganglion.** Ganglion pterygopalatinum. Lying lateral to the pterygopalatine foramen, it receives motor fibers from the facial nerve via the nerve of the pterygoid canal and supplies the lacrimal and nasal glands. D

31 **Otic ganglion.** Ganglion oticum. Situated below the foramen ovale and medial to the mandibular nerve, it receives motor fibers from the glossopharyngeal nerve via the lesser petrosal nerve and innervates the parotid gland. D

32 **Submandibular ganglion.** Ganglion submandibulare. Located at the lingual nerve below the mandible, it receives motor fibers from the facial nerve via the chorda tympani and sends efferent fibers to the sublingual and submandibular glands. D

33 **Sublingual ganglion.** Ganglion sublinguale. Small accumulations of cells occasionally present on the glandular branches.

33a **Pelvic part** (Pars pelvica). Sacral part of parasympathetic division.

34 **Pelvic splanchnic nerves.** Nn. pelvici splanchnici (nn. erigentes). Parasympathetic fibers from S2–4 spinal nerves to the pelvic ganglia for the pelvic and genital organs. They also contain afferent fibers. B

35 **Pelvic ganglia.** Ganglia pelvica. Groups of autonomic cells in the inferior hypogastric plexus. They give rise to the postganglionic axons. See 351 E

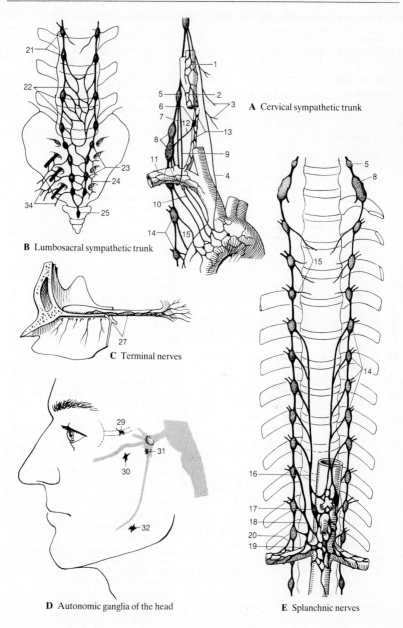

A Cervical sympathetic trunk

B Lumbosacral sympathetic trunk

C Terminal nerves

D Autonomic ganglia of the head

E Splanchnic nerves

1 SENSE ORGANS. ORGANA SENSORIA (SENSUUM). In the narrow sense: organs of vision, hearing, smell and taste.

2 ORGAN OF VISION. ORGANUM VISUS (VISUALE).

3 **Eye.** Oculus.

4 **Optic nerve.** N. opticus. Fiber bundle beginning in the retina and extending as far as the optic chiasma. It is histologically and embryologically a tract of the brain and accordingly is enclosed by meninges up to the posterior aspect of the eyeball. Its axons have no neurilemma (sheath of Schwann) but are myelinated, the myelin sheath being formed by the oligodendroglia. A C E

5 Intracranial part. Pars intracranialis. Segment of the optic nerve between the optic canal and the chiasma. E

6 Intracanalicular part. Pars intracanicularis. Segment of the optic nerve located in the optic canal. It is partially connected with the canal wall. E

7 Orbital part. Pars orbitalis. Slightly tortuous segment of the optic nerve measuring about 3 cm in length and occupying the orbit. E

8 Intraocular part. Pars intraocularis. Segment of optic nerve located in the wall of the eyeball.

9 *Postlaminar part.* Pars postlaminaris. Intraocular segment located behind the lamina cribrosa and thus at the site where the external sheath of the optic nerve (dura) blends into the sclera. A

10 *Intralaminar part.* Pars intralaminaris. Intraocular segment lying within the lamina cribrosa. A

11 *Prelaminar part.* Pars prelaminaris. Intra-ocular segment extending between the lamina cribrosa and the nerve fiber layer of the retina. A

12 **External sheath.** Vagina externa. Dural covering of the optic nerve extending up to the eyeball. A

13 **Internal sheath.** Vagina interna. Pia and arachnoid coverings accompanying the optic nerve to the eyeball. A

14 Intervaginal spaces. Spatia intervaginalia. Subarachnoid space accompanying the optic nerve and the capillary space between the arachnoid and dura. A

15 **Eyeball.** Bulbus oculi. Globe of the eye. It consists of the cornea and sclera together with all of the structures they enclose. D

16 **Anterior pole.** Polus anterior. It is determined by the corneal vertex and represents the central point of the anterior curvature of the eyeball. D

17 **Posterior pole.** Polus posterior. It lies lateral to the optic nerve exit and opposite to the anterior pole. D

18 **Equator.** Aequator. Greatest circumference of the eyeball located equidistant between the anterior and posterior poles. D

19 **Meridians.** Meridiani. Semicircles oriented at right angles to the equator between the anterior and posterior poles. D

20 **External axis of eyeball.** Axis bulbi externus. Line connecting anterior and posterior poles. C

21 **Internal axis of eyeball.** Axis bulbi internus. Distance from posterior surface of cornea to inner surface of retina measured along a line (external axis of eyeball) going through the anterior and posterior poles. C

22 **Optic axis.** Axis opticus. Line passing through the midline of the cornea and lens and bisecting the retina between the fovea centralis and optic disc. C

23 **Fibrous tunic of eyeball.** Tunica fibrosa bulbi. External wall of eyeball comprising the cornea and sclera. C

24 **Sclera.** Consisting of irregularly arranged collagenous fibers, it appears bluish-white through the conjunctiva. A B C

25 Scleral sulcus. Sulcus sclerae. Shallow groove between cornea and sclera caused by the greater curvature of the cornea. B C D

26 *Corneoscleral junction.* Limbus. The concave border of the sclera adjacent to the cornea. B

27 *Trabecular meshwork (pectinate ligament).* Reticulum trabeculare (lig. pectinatum) [[Spongium iridocorneale]]. Connective tissue framework at the iridocorneal (filtration) angle.

28 Corneoscleral part. Pars corneoscleralis. Part of the meshwork attached to the sclera. B

29 *Uveal part.* Pars uvealis. Part of the trabecular meshwork attached to the iris. B

30 **Canal of Schlemm.** Sinus venosus sclerae. Circular vessel occupying the interior aspect of the trabecular meshwork. It can be interrupted or doubled and is involved in the discharge of aqueous humor from the anterior chamber. B

31 **Episclera.** Lamina episcleralis. Delicate displaceable connective tissue between the outer surface of the sclera and [[Tenon's capsule]] (bulbar fascia).

32 **Substantia propria sclerae corneal stroma.** It consists of irregularly arranged collagenous fibers with sparse elastic fibers. A B

33 **Lamina fusca sclerae.** Layer of loose connective tissue between the sclera and the choroid lying deep to it. It appears yellowish owing to the pigment-containing cells dispersed within it. A

34 **Lamina cribrosa.** Fine, perforated plate in the sclera for the passage of the optic nerve fibers from the retina. A

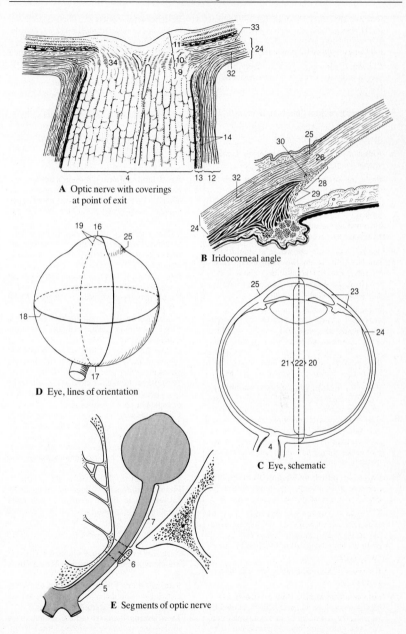

A Optic nerve with coverings at point of exit

B Iridocorneal angle

D Eye, lines of orientation

C Eye, schematic

E Segments of optic nerve

1 **Cornea.** It forms the transparent anterior part ($^1/_6$) of the eyeball with an anterior convex and a posterior concave curvature. It is 0.9 mm thick in its middle, 1.2 mm at its margins. B D

2 **Conjunctival ring.** Anulus conjunctivae. Junction between bulbar conjunctival epithelium and the anterior epithelium of the cornea. D

3 **Corneoscleral junction.** Limbus corneae. D

4 **Vertex corneae.** Widest projecting point of the anterior surface of the cornea.

5 **Anterior surface.** Facies anterior. Corneal surface facing the outside air. D

6 **Posterior surface.** Facies posterior. Corneal surface facing the anterior chamber. D

7 **Anterior epithelium.** Epithelium anterius. Stratified (about 5 layers) squamous epithelium covering the anterior surface of the cornea. Its surface is especially smooth. B D

8 **Anterior limiting (Bowman's) membrane.** Lamina limitans anterior [[Bowman]]. Basement membrane of the anterior epithelium. About 10–20 mm thick, it is continuous posteriorly with the substantia propria. B

9 **Substantia propria.** Predominant part of the avascular cornea consisting of highly organized lamellar connective tissue embedded within a mucopolysaccharide ground substance. State of turgescence of the fibers and the distribution of the colloidal matrix affect the transparency of the cornea. B

10 **Posterior limiting (Descemet's) membrane.** Lamina limitans posterior [[Descemet]]. Basement membrane of the corneal (posterior) endothelium. At its lateral margin it breaks up into fibers which radiate into the trabecular meshwork of the sclera and iris. Aqueous humor passas through its interstices to drain into the sinus venosus sclerae. B D

11 **Posterior epithelium (endothelium).** Epithe-
~ lium posterius. Simple squamous epithelium lining the posterior surface of the cornea. B D

12 **Vascular tunic of eyeball (uveal tract).** Tunica vasculosa bulbi (tractus uvealis). Representing the middle layer of the wall of the eyeball, it consists of the choroid, ciliary body and iris.

13 **Choroid.** Choroidea. It lies between the retina and sclera. A

14 **Suprachoroid lamina (lamina fusca).** Lamina suprachoroidea. Displaceable layer directly beneath the sclera. Poor in vessels and containing pigment, its fibers are partly covered by endothelium. A

15 **Perichoroidal space.** Spatium perichoroideale. Spatial system in the suprachoroid lamina. Belonging partly to the lymph pathways, it houses the ciliary nerves, long and short posterior ciliary arteries and the vorticose veins. A

16 **Vascular lamina.** Lamina vasculosa. It contains the branchings of the short posterior ciliary arteries. A

17 **Choriocapillaris.** Lamina choroidocapillaris. Pigment-free layer of connective tissue with a dense network of capillaries extending as far as the ora serrata. It is often delimited from the vascular lamina by a special connective tissue layer. A

18 **Basal lamina [[Bruch's membrane]].** Complexus (lamina) basalis. Homogeneous zone about 2–4 mm thick between the choriocapillaris and the pigment epithelium of the retina. A

19 **Ciliary body.** Corpus ciliare. Enlarged uveal segment situated between the ora serrata and root of the iris. It contains the ciliary musculature and ciliary processes. C

20 **Pars plicata** (Corona ciliaris). Circular zone occupied by ciliary processes. C

21 **Ciliary processes.** Processus ciliares. 70–80 radially positioned, capillary-rich folds, 0.1–0.2 mm wide, 1 mm high and 2–3 mm long. Its lining epithelium produces the aqueous humor. C

22 **Ciliary folds.** Plicae ciliares. Low folds in the region of the corona ciliaris, partly also between the ciliary processes. C

23 **Pars plana.** Orbiculus ciliaris. Circular zone lying between the corona and ora serrata. It is occupied by ciliary folds. C

24 **Ciliary muscle.** M. ciliaris. Smooth muscle occupying the ciliary body. It pulls the choroid forward and, in so doing, relaxes the zonule fibers so that the lens can assume a more strongly curved shape for accommodation to near objects. D

25 **Meridional (longitudinal) fibers.** Fibrae meridionales [fibrae longitudinales]. Larger muscle fibers oriented meridionally (longitudinally). Anteriorly they are attached to the posterior limiting lamina above the trabecular meshwork; posteriorly, they insert into the choroid. D

26 **Circular fibers.** Fibrae circulares. Circular muscle lying internal to the meridional fibers. D

27 **Radial fibers.** Fibrae radiales. Muscle fibers crossing perpendicular to the two other muscle systems and coursing from within outward. D

28 **Basal lamina.** Lamina basalis. Continuation of the basement membrane of the choroid. It supports the epithelium. D

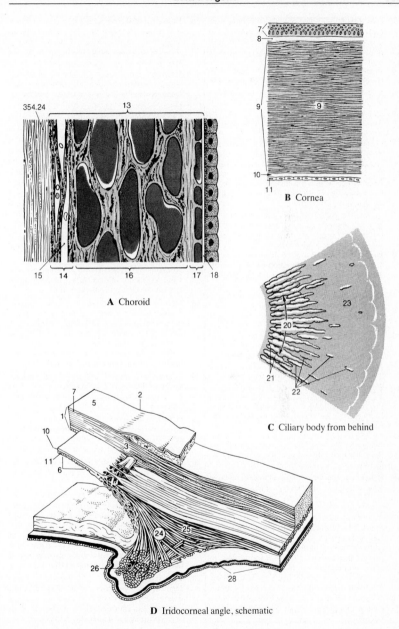

354.24

13

15 14 16 17 18

A Choroid

7
8

9 9

10
11

B Cornea

23

20

21

22

C Ciliary body from behind

7 2
5
1

10
11
6

3

24 25

26

28

D Iridocorneal angle, schematic

1 **Iris.** Frontally-located, round, variably colored diaphragm about 10–12 mm in diameter with a central aperture (pupil). It forms the posterior border of the anterior chamber and is continuous at its lateral margin with the ciliary body. A

2 **Pupillary margin.** Margo pupillaris. Medial (internal) margin of the iris bordering the pupil. A B

3 **Ciliary margin.** Margo ciliaris. Lateral (external) margin of iris attached to ciliary body at the iridocorneal angle. B

4 **Anterior surface.** Facies anterior. It faces the anterior chamber. B

5 **Posterior surface.** Facies posterior. It faces the posterior chamber. A B

6 **Greater ring (circle) of iris.** Anulus iridis major. Ciliary segment of iris. Outer circular zone on anterior surface of iris. It is distinguished from the lesser ring by its coarser structure and larger breadth. A

7 **Lesser ring (circle) of iris.** Anulus iridis minor. Pupillary segment of iris. Narrower inner, circular zone on anterior surface of iris. It possesses a finer structure than the greater ring. A

8 **Iridial folds.** Plicae iridis. Folds passing around the pupillary margin on the anterior side of the iris. They produce the slight serration of the pupillary margin. A

9 **Pupil.** Pupilla. Aperture in the iris surrounded by the pupillary margin of the iris. Its diameter varies depending upon the intensity of light and the focal distance of the object. A

10 **M. sphincter pupillae.** Network of spirally coursing muscle fibers the longitudinal axes of which run approximately parallel to the pupillary margin when the pupil is dilated. It is innervated by parasympathetic fibers from the oculomotor nerve. B

11 **M. dilator pupillae.** Thin layer of smooth muscle oriented primarily in a radial direction. It is innervated by sympathetic fibers from the carotid plexus.

12 **Stroma iridis.** Vascular framework of the iris infiltrated by pigmented connective tissue cells. It is thicker anteriorly and posteriorly with a fine fibrous network inbetween. A B

13 **Pigmented (posterior) epithelium.** Epithelium pigmentosum. Bilayered, pigment-bearing epithelium on the posterior surface of the iris. It is so heavily pigmented that no nuclei are visible on the surface facing the posterior chamber. A

14 **Spaces of iridocorneal angle [spaces of Fontana].** Spatia anguli iridocornealis. Interstices between the fibers of the trabecular meshwork. They provide passageways for the aqueous fluid to reach the sinus venosus sclerae. A

15 **Greater arterial circle of iris.** Circulus arteriosus iridis major. Ring-like vascular system with radiating branches. It is formed by anastomoses between the long and short posterior ciliary arteries. A

16 **Lesser arterial circle of iris.** Circulus arteriosus iridis minor. Ring-like vascular system in the vicinity of the pupillary margin formed by anastomoses between the radial branches of the greater arterial circle. A

17 **Pupillary membrane.** [Membrana pupillaris]. Anterior part of embryonically-present vascular membrane around the lens. Situated behind the pupil, it is fused to the pupillary margin and receives blood vessels from there.

18 **Internal (sensory) tunic of eyeball.** Tunica interna bulbi. It comprises the retina with its pigment epithelium.

19 **Retina.** Inner lining of eyeball developed from the two layers of the optic cup. Most of it is light-sensitive (**P**ars optica). B

20 **Pars optica retinae.** Retinal segment capable of transforming light stimuli into nerve impulses. It lines the posterior aspect of the eyeball and extends as far anteriorly as the ora serrata. B

21 **Pigmented part.** Pars pigmentosa. Pigment epithelium arising from the external layer of the optic cup. B

22 **Nervous part.** Pars nervosa. Retina proper consisting essentially of three nuclear layers lying internal to the pigment epithelium. B

23 *Neuroepithelial (photosensitive) layer.* Stratum
~ neuroepitheliale (photosensorium). Outer layer of the cerebral stratum. It consists of rods and cones the outer segments of which effect the transformation of light stimuli into nerve impulses. Cell bodies of rods and cones form the outermost layer of retinal nuclei (external nuclear layer). D

24 *Internal nuclear layer.* [[Stratum ganglionare retinae]]. Middle layer of cell nuclei consisting of the cell bodies of bipolar and amacrine cells, among others. D

25 *Ganglion cell layer.* [[Stratum ganglionare n. optici]]. Internal layer of nuclei consisting of multipolar cell bodies of ganglion cells the axons of which, initially nonmyelinated, form the optic nerve. D

26 **Ora serrata.** Serrated margin between the light-sensitive and light-insensitive parts of the neural retina. B C

27 **Pars ciliaris retinae.** Light-insensitive retinal segment consisting of a bilayered cuboidal epithelium (ciliary epithelium) forming the posterior surface of the ciliary body. Its outer layer of epithelium is continuous with the pigment epithelium of the retina and is pigmented whereas the innermost epithelium is continous with the pars nervosa of the retina and is devoid of pigment. B

28 **Pars iridica retinae.** Light-insensitive retinal segment on the posterior surface of the iris. Continuous with the pars ciliaris retinae, it forms the bilayered posterior epithelium of the iris, both layers being heavily pigmented, however. B

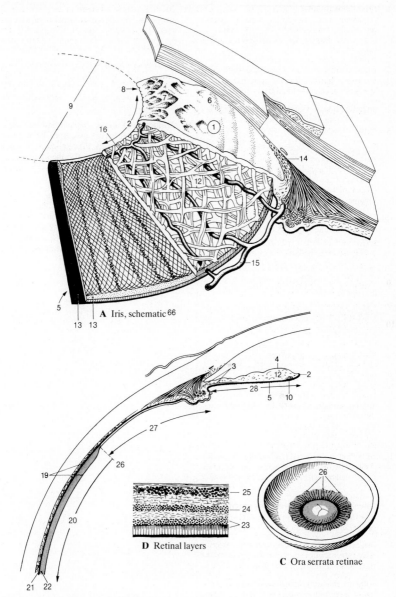

A Iris, schematic 66

D Retinal layers

C Ora serrata retinae

B Sections of retina

1 **Optic disc (papilla).** Discus nervi optici [papilla nervi optici]. Beginning of the optic nerve as visualized in the fundus about 3–4 mm medial to the macula. Its diameter is about 1.6 mm. C

2 Physiological cup. Excavatio disci. Depression in the middle of the optic disc with the stems of the central retinal artery and vein. C

3 **Macula** [[lutea]]. Transversely oval, yellowish area, 2–4 mm in diameter, at the posterior pole of the retina. C

4 Fovea centralis. Central depression in the macula produced by a localized spreading aside of the internal retinal layers. Its diameter measured from the beginning of the decrease in retinal thickness of one side to that of the other amounts to approximately 1–2 mm. B C

5 Foveola. Thinnest area of fovea centralis with a diameter of about 0.2–0.4 mm. Here, the retina is comprised entirely of cones, 2500 packed closely together. B

6 **Retinal blood vessels.** Vasa sanguinea retinae. Branches of the central retinal artery and vein lie on the internal aspect of the retina.

7 **Circle of arteries around the optic nerve.** Circulus vasculosus nervi optici. Small vascular ring penetrating the sclera around the optic nerve.

8 **Superior temporal arteriole/venule of retina.** Arteriola/venula temporalis retinae superior. Lateral upper branch of central retinal artery/vein. C

9 **Inferior temporal arteriole/venule of retina.** Arteriola/venula temporalis retinae inferior. Lateral lower branch of central retinal artery/vein. C

10 **Superior nasal arteriole/venule of retina.** Arteriola/venula nasalis retinae superior. Upper medial branch of central retinal artery/vein. C

11 **Inferior nasal arteriole/venule of retina.** Arteriola/venula nasalis retinae inferior. Lower medial branch of central retinal artery/vein. C

12 **Superior macular arteriole/venule.** Arteriola/venula macularis superior. It supplies/drains the upper part of the macula. C

13 **Inferior macular arteriole/venule.** Arteriola/venula macularis inferior. It supplies/drains the lower part of the macula. C

14 **Medial arteriole/venule of retina.** Arteriola/venula medialis retinae. Small branch for the medial part of retina close to the optic disc. C

14a **Chambers of the eye.** Camerae bulbi

15 **Anterior chamber.** Camera anterior. It extends from the anterior surface of the iris to the posterior surface of the cornea and communicates with the posterior chamber via the pupil. A

16 **Iridocorneal angle.** Angulus iridocornealis. Angle between the iris and cornea. It houses the trabecular meshwork the interstices of which serve as passageways for the drainage of aqueous humor into the sinus venosus sclerae. A

17 **Aqueous humor.** Humor aquosus. Fluid produced by the epithelium of the ciliary processes. Occupying the anterior and posterior chambers, its total quantity is 0.2–0.3 ml consisting of 98% water, 1.4% NaCl and traces of protein and sugar. It is clear, with a refractive index of 1.336.

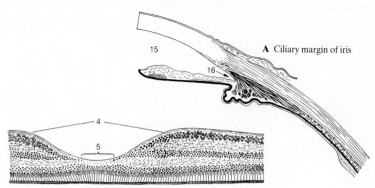

A Ciliary margin of iris

B Fovea centralis

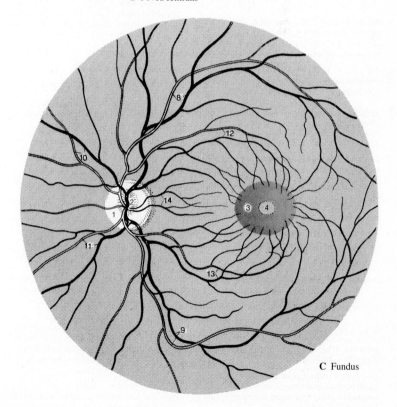

C Fundus

1 **Posterior chamber.** Camera posterior. It extends from the iris and ciliary body to the anterior surface of the vitreous. A

2 **Aqueous humor.** Humor aquosus. Produced by the ciliary processes, it flows between the interstices of the suspensory ligaments of the lens to the anterior surface of the lens and then between the iris and lens to the pupil by means of which it enters the anterior chamber.

3 **Vitreous chamber.** Camera vitrea. Space filled up by the vitreous body. B

4 **Vitreous body.** Corpus vitreum. It consists of about 98% water and contains, among others, traces of protein and NaCl, as well as a mixture of fine fibrils which are thicker toward the surface and form a limiting membrane. Its gelatinous consistency is caused by the high content of hyaluronic acid. A

5 **Hyaloid artery.** [A. hyaloidea]. Branch of ophthalmic artery to the vascular membrane of the lens. Present only during embryonic development, its proximal portion persists in the optic nerve as the central retinal artery. B

6 **Hyaloid canal.** Canalis hyaloideus. Canal within the vitreous body formerly occupied by the embryonic hyaloid artery which has degenerated in this region. Assuming a corkscrew shape sagging downward, it extends from the optic disc to the posterior surface of the lens. Its wall is formed by condensed fibers. A

7 **Hyaloid (lenticular, patellar) fossa.** Fossa hyaloidea. Fossa at the anterior surface of the vitreous body adjacent to the lens. A

8 **Vitreous (hyaloid) membrane.** Membrana vitrea. Condensation of fibers on the surface of the vitreous body. See 4. A

9 **Stroma of vitreous body.** Stroma vitreum. Fine network of fibers in the vitreous body. It is condensed at its surface to form the vitreous membrane.

9a **Vitreous humor.** Humor vitreus. Fluid part of vitreous body. Characterized by mucopolysaccharides, it lies between the fibers of the stroma.

10 **Lens.** Suspended between the pupil and vitreous body by the ciliary zonule (suspensory ligaments), it has a diameter of 9–10 mm and is about 4 mm thick. B C D

11 **Substantia lentis.** Lens substance situated beneath the lens epithelium and organized into a lens nucleus and lens cortex with a refractive index of 1.44–1.55. C

12 **Lens cortex.** Cortex lentis. External zone of the lens. It is softer owing to its high water content and blends into the lens nucleus without a sharp boundary. C

13 **Nucleus of lens.** Nucleus lentis. Hardend core of lens, especially in the elderly. It has a low water content. C

14 **Lens fibers.** Fibrae lentis. Corresponding to the lens epithelium from which they develop, they form the lens substance measuring 2.5–12 µm thick and up to 10 mm long. C

15 **Epithelium of lens.** Epithelium lentis. Confined to the anterior surface and extending as far as the equator, it is derived embryologically from the anterior epithelium of the lens vesicle. C

16 **Lens capsule.** Capsula lentis. Transparent membrane up to 15 µm thick covering the lens including its epithelium. It is thicker at the anterior pole than at the posterior pole. It serves for the attachment of the suspensory ligaments. C

17 **Anterior pole.** Polus anterior. D

18 **Posterior pole.** Polus posterior. D

19 **Anterior surface.** Facies anterior. More weakly curved lens surface with a radius of 8.3–10 mm. C

20 **Posterior surface.** Facies posterior. More strongly curved lens surface with a radius of about 6.5 mm. C

21 **Axis.** Line connecting anterior and posterior poles. D

22 **Equator.** Margin of lens. D

23 **Radii of lens.** Suture line of the individual lens fibers. In the young it resembles a triradiate suture. D

24 **Ciliary zonule.** Zonula ciliaris. Suspensory apparatus together with its interstices. Encircling the lens equator, it consists of a radially oriented system of fibers of variable length and the folds situated between them. C

25 **Zonular fibers (suspensory ligaments).** Fibrae zonulares. Suspensory fibers attached to the equator and the adjacent anterior and posterior surfaces of the lens. They arise distally at the basal lamina of the ciliary body and the pars ciliaris retinae. C

26 **Zonular spaces.** Spatia zonularia. Spaces between the zonule fibers filled with percolating aqueous humor. C

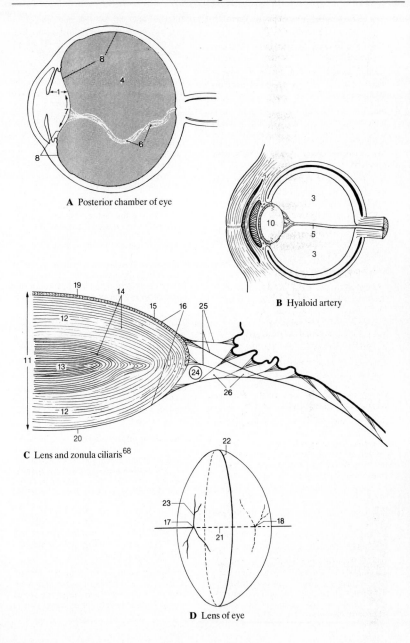

A Posterior chamber of eye

B Hyaloid artery

C Lens and zonula ciliaris [68]

D Lens of eye

1 ACCESSORY ORGANS OF EYE. ORGANA OCULI ACCESSORIA.

2 **Muscles of eye.** Musculi bulbi. Extrinsic ocular muscles.

3 **Orbital muscle.** M. orbitalis. Thin layer of smooth muscle which bridges the inferior orbital fissure. C

4 **Superior rectus.** M. rectus superior. o: Common tendinous ring. i: Along an oblique line in front of the equator, 7–8 mm posterior to the corneal margin. F: Elevation and medial rotation of superior pole of eyeball. I: Oculomotor nerve. B C D

5 **Inferior rectus.** M. rectus inferior. o: Common tendinous ring. i: Along an oblique line about 6 mm behind the corneal margin. F: Depression and lateral rotation of superior pole of eyeball. I: Oculomotor nerve. B C D

6 **Medial rectus.** M. rectus medialis. o: Common tendinous ring. i: About 5.5 mm from the corneal margin. F: Adduction of corneal pole. I: Oculomotor nerve. B C

7 **Lateral rectus.** M. rectus lateralis. o: Common tendinous ring and lesser wing. i: 5.5 mm behind corneal margin. F: Abduction of corneal pole. I: Abducent nerve. B C D

8 Tendon of origin of lateral rectus at greater wing. *Lacertus musculi recti lateralis.* C

9 **Common tendinous ring (common annular
~ tendon).** Anulus tendineus communis. Tendinous ring for the origin of the recti ocular muscles. It surrounds the optic canal and medial part of the superior orbital fissure. C

10 **Superior oblique.** M. obliquus superior. o: Body of sphenoid medial to common tendinous ring. i: Posterolateral aspect of sclera behind the equator after its tendon passes through the trochlea and approaches sclera obliquely from the medial margin of orbit. F: Abduction, medial rotation and depression. I. Trochlear nerve. B

11 *Trochlea.* Cartilaginous sling attached to the medial wall of the orbit [[trochlear spine]] and serving as a pulley for the tendon of the superior oblique. B

12 *Tendon sheath of superior oblique muscle (synovial bursa of trochlea).* Vagina tendinis m. obliqui superioris [[Bursa synovialis trochlearis]]. Synovial sheath (bursa) for the tendon of the superior oblique separating the tendon from the trochlea. B

13 **Inferior oblique.** M. obliquus inferior. o: Laterally, beside the nasolacrimal canal. i: Posterior to equator. F: Elevation, abduction and lateral rotation. I: Oculomotor nerve. D

14 **M. levator palpebrae superioris.** o: Bone above optic canal and dura of optic nerve. Its tendon of insertion broadens anteriorly and splits into an upper and lower layer. I: Oculomotor nerve. A C D.

15 Superificial lamina of levator tendon. Lamina superficialis. It passes between the tarsus and orbicularis oculi to insert into the subcutaneous connective tissue of the upper eyelid. It is so broad that it reaches the wall of the orbit mainly laterally. A

16 Deep lamina of levator tendon. Lamina profunda. It is inserted into the upper margin and the anterior surface of the tarsus. A

17 **Orbital fasciae.** Fasciae orbitales.

18 **Periosteum of orbit.** Periorbita. It is delicate and fused solidly to bone at the inlet and outlet of the orbit. Anteriorly, it is continuous with the adjacent periosteum, posteriorly with the dura. A

19 **Orbital septum.** Septum orbitale. Connective tissue septum partly reinforced by tendon. It passes from the orbital margin below the orbicularis oculi to the external margins of the tarsi and forms the anterior end of the orbit. A

20 **Muscular fasciae.** Fasciae musculares. Sheaths of Tenon's capsule enveloping the tendons and muscular bellies of the 6 extrinsic ocular muscles. A

21 **Tenon's capsule (fascia bulbi).** Vagina bulbi. Connective tissue gliding membrane between the eyeball and orbital fat. It is fused to the sclera posteriorly at the optic nerve. Anteriorly it ends beneath the conjunctiva. It is separated from the sclera primarily by the episcleral space. A

22 **Episcleral space.** Spatium episclerale [[intervaginale]]. Gliding space between the eyeball and Tenon's capsule. It is traversed by long, delicate connective tissue fibers. A

23 **Orbital fat body.** Corpus adiposum orbitae. Adipose tissue fills the spaces around the ocular muscles, the eyeball and the optic nerve and is bordered anteriorly by the orbital septum. A D

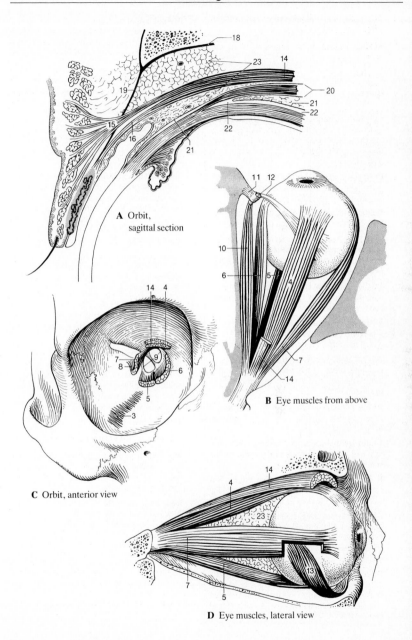

A Orbit, sagittal section

B Eye muscles from above

C Orbit, anterior view

D Eye muscles, lateral view

1 **Eyebrow.** Supercilium. It possesses somewhat thicker, bristle-like hairs. A

2 **Eyelids.** Palpebrae.

3 **Upper eyelid.** Palpebra superior. A

4 **Lower eyelid.** Palpebra inferior. A

5 **Anterior palpebral surface.** Facies anterior palpebralis. It is covered by external skin. E

6 **Epicanthus (mongolian fold).** [Plica palpebronasalis] [[Epicanthus]]. Vertical fold covering the medial angle of the eye. It is a continuation of the upper eyelid at the lateral nasal wall. C

7 **Posterior palpebral surface.** Facies posterior palpebralis. It is lined by conjunctival epithelium possessing dispersed goblet cells. E

8 **Palpebral fissure.** Rima palpebrarum. Space between the margins of the upper and lower eyelids. A E

9 **Lateral palpebral commissure.** Commissura palpebralis lateralis. Lateral junction of upper and lower eyelids. A

10 **Medial palpebral commissure.** Commissura palpebralis medialis. Medial junction of upper and lower eyelids. A

11 **Lateral angle (canthus) of eye.** Angulus oculi lateralis. Acutely angled, it is also the lateral end of the palpebral fissure. A

12 **Medial angle (canthus) of eye.** Angulus oculi medialis. More rounded medial end of palpebral fissure which delimits a triangular space, the lacrimal lake. A

13 **Limbi palpebrales anteriores.** Anterior edges of the free margins of the eyelids adjacent to the external skin. E

14 **Limbi palpebrales posteriores.** Posterior edges of the free margins of the eyelids adjacent to the conjunctiva. E

15 **Eyelashes.** Cilia. They are organized into 3–4 rows in the vicinity of the anterior edge of the free margin of the eyelids. E F

16 **Superior tarsal plate.** Tarsus superior. Curved plate about 10 mm high occupying the upper eyelid and consisting of compact, interwoven collagenous connective tissue with tarsal glands. B E

17 **Inferior tarsal plate.** Tarsus inferior. Plate about 5 mm high within the lower eyelid. It likewise consists of firm, interwoven collagenous connective tissue with tarsal glands. B E

18 **Medial palpebral ligament.** [[Lig. palpebrale mediale]]. Band of connective tissue between the medial palpebral commissure and the medial wall of the orbit. It lies in front of the lacrimal sac. B D

19 **Lateral palpebral raphe.** [[Raphe palpebralis lateralis]]. Delicate band on the lateral palpebral ligament. It is reinforced by the orbicularis oculi muscle. D

20 **Lateral palpebral ligament.** Lig. palpebrale laterale. Attachment of the lateral palpebral commissure to the lateral wall of the orbit in front of the orbital septum. B

21 **Tarsal [[Meibomian]] glands.** Glandulae tarsales. Elongated holocrine glands located in the superior and inferior tarsal plates with openings near the posterior edge of the free margin of the eyelids. They produce a sebaceous secretion for lubrication of the lid margins; it prevents tears from overflowing. E

22 **Superior tarsal muscle.** M. tarsalis superior. Smooth muscle fibers between the muscle-tendon border of the levator palpebrae muscle and the superior tarsal plate. E

23 **Inferior tarsal muscle.** M. tarsalis inferior. Smooth muscle fibers between the inferior fornix of the conjunctiva and the inferior tarsal plate. E

24 **Tunica conjunctiva.** It lines the inner surface of the eyelids as the palpebral conjunctiva where it consists of a bilayered or multilayered columnar epithelium with goblet cells and a loose, vascular-rich and cell-rich lamina propria. It then continues around the fornix of the conjunctiva to cover the eyeball up to the corneal margin as the bulbar conjunctiva containing stratified squamous epithelium. E

25 **Semilunar fold of conjunctiva.** Plica semilunaris conjunctivae. It lies in the medial angle of the eye between the fornix of the upper and lower eyelid. F

26 **Lacrimal caruncle.** Caruncula lacrimalis. Mucosal mass in the medial angle of the eye covered by stratified squamous or columnar epithelium. F

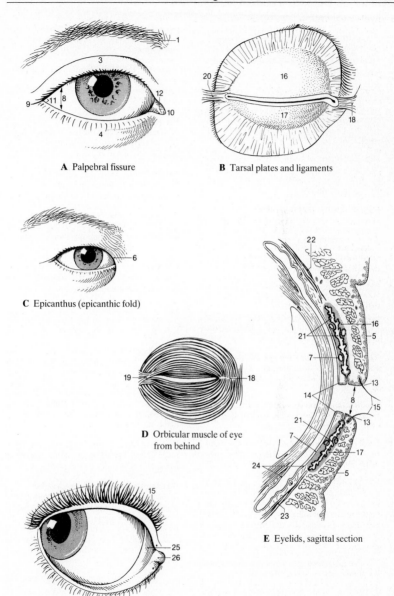

A Palpebral fissure

B Tarsal plates and ligaments

C Epicanthus (epicanthic fold)

D Orbicular muscle of eye from behind

E Eyelids, sagittal section

F Inner (nasal) canthus of eye

1 **Bulbar conjunctiva.** Tunica conjunctiva bulbaris. Part of conjunctiva covering the eyeball. It consists of stratified squamous, nonkeratinized epithelium with only a few goblet cells and a loose, cell-poor lamina propria permeated with elastic fibers. A

2 **Palpebral conjunctiva.** Tunica conjunctiva palpebralis. Conjunctiva lining the posterior surface of the eyelid. It consists of two to several layers of columnar epithelium with goblet cells and a loose, vascular-rich lamina propria. A

3 **Superior fornix of conjunctiva.** Fornix conjunctivae superior. Reflected fold of conjunctiva from the eyeball (bulbar) on to the upper eyelid (palpebral). A

4 **Inferior fornix of conjunctiva.** Fornix conjunctivae inferior. Reflected fold of conjunctiva from the eyeball (bulbar) on to the lower eyelid (palpebral). A

5 **Conjunctival sac.** Saccus conjunctivalis. Space between palpebral and bulbar conjunctivae. Its upper and lower ends form the superior and inferior fornices of the conjunctiva. A

6 **Ciliary glands (of Moll).** Glandulae ciliares [[Moll]]. Apocrine glands at the lid margin. They open either into the hair follicles of the eyelashes or at the lid margin. A

7 **Sebaceous glands (of Zeis).** Glandulae sebaceae [[Zeis]]. Small sebaceous glands with openings into the hair follicles of the eyelashes. A

8 **Conjunctival glands.** Glandulae conjunctivales. Follicle-like aggregations of lymphocytes at the medial angle of the eye.

9 **Lacrimal apparatus.** Apparatus lacrimalis. It serves for the lubrication of the cornea and conjunctiva. B

10 **Lacrimal gland.** Glandula lacrimalis. Located above the lateral angle of the eyelids, it is separated into an upper and lower portion by the tendon of levator palpebrae muscle. It excretory ducts open laterally into the superior fornix of the conjunctiva. B

11 **Orbital part.** Pars orbitalis. Larger portion of lacrimal gland located above the tendon of the levator palpebrae muscle. B

12 **Palpebral part.** Pars palpebralis. Smaller portion of lacrimal gland located below the tendon of the levator palpebrae muscle. B

13 Excretory ducts of lacrimal gland. Ductuli excretorii [[glandulae lacrimalis]]. 6–14 ducts opening into the superior fornix of the conjunctiva. B

14 **Accessory lacrimal glands.** [Gll. lacrimales accessoriae]. Additional smaller lacrimal glands found scattered especially in the vicinity of the superior conjunctival fornix. A

15 **Rivus lacrimalis.** Pathway taken by tears from the excretory ducts to the lacrimal lake. It lies within the conjunctival sac between the closed eyelids and the eyeball.

16 **Lacrimal lake.** Lacus lacrimalis. Space in the medial angle of the eye around the lacrimal caruncle. B C

17 **Papilla lacrimalis.** Small cone-shaped elevation medial to the inner edge of both the upper and lower eyelids. Each apex houses an opening or lacrimal punctum. C

18 **Lacrimal punctum.** Punctum lacrimale. Small opening marking the beginning of the lacrimal fluid drainage system. C

19 **Lacrimal canaliculus.** Canaliculus lacrimalis. Small canal, up to 1 cm long, from each lacrimal punctum to the lacrimal sac. C

20 **Ampulla of lacrimal canaliculus.** Ampulla canaliculi lacrimalis. Slight enlargement at the bend of the lacrimal canaliculus. C

21 **Lacrimal sac.** Saccus lacrimalis. It is located in the lacrimal fossa and is about 1.5 cm long and about 0.5 cm wide. It descends directly into the nasolacrimal duct. C

22 Fornix of lacrimal sac. Fornix sacci lacrimalis. Dome-shaped upper margin of lacrimal sac. C

23 **Nasolacrimal duct.** Ductus nasolacrimalis. Directly continuous with the lacrimal sac and measuring 1.2–2.4 cm in length, it passes through the nasolacrimal canal and opens into the inferior nasal meatus. Its flattened lumen is lined by a mucosa containing two or more layers of columnar epithelium bearing cilia at some sites. C

24 Lacrimal fold. Plica lacrimalis. Mucosal fold at the opening of the nasolacrimal duct into the inferior nasal meatus, 3–3.5 cm posterior to the external naris. C

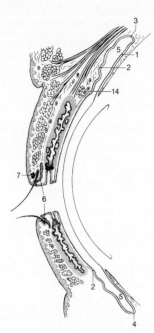

A Eyelids, sagittal section

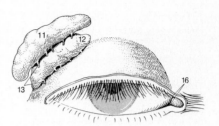

B Lacrimal gland

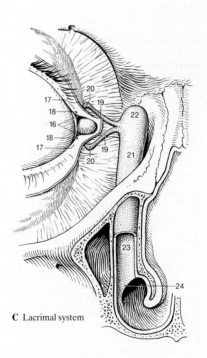

C Lacrimal system

1 VESTIBULOCOCHLEAR ORGAN. ORGA-
NUM VESTIBULOCOCHLEARE. Sensory
apparatus housed in the temporal bone for the
perception of sound, equilibrium and positional
changes.

2 INTERNAL EAR. AURIS INTERNA. Part of the
vestibulocochlear organ residing in the petrous
temporal bone.

3 **Membranous labyrinth.** Labyrinthus membranaceus. Complicated system of ducts and dilatations containing sensory epithelium and suspended within a bony labyrinth by connective
tissue. A

4 **Endolymph.** Fluid contained within the membranous labyrinth.

5 **Perilymph.** Fluid occupying the osseous labyrinth and surrounding the membranous labyrinth.

6 **Vestibular labyrinth.** Labyrinthus vestibularis. Portion of membranous labyrinth constitut-
ing the organ of equilibrium. It includes the semicircular ducts.

7 **Endolymphatic duct.** Ductus endolymphaticus
[[Aquaeductus vestibuli]]. Slender duct arising
from the utriculosaccular duct and passing
through the osseous aqueduct of the vestibule to
terminate as the endolymphatic sac. A

8 **Endolymphatic sac.** Saccus endolymphaticus.
Blind sac of endolymphatic duct. It is located between two dural layers at the posterior wall of the
petrous temporal. A

9 **Utriculosaccular duct.** Ductus utriculosaccula-
ris. Slender duct between the saccule and utricle.
It gives rise to the endolymphatic duct. A

10 **Utricle.** Utriculus. Sac, 2.5–3.5 mm in diameter,
serving as the base for the three semicircular ducts.
A

11 **Semicircular duct.** Ductus semicirculares. Three
in all, each membranous duct cooresponds somewhat to two-thirds of a circular arch and occupies
its own osseous semicircular canal oriented perpendicular to one another.

12 Anterior (superior) semicircular duct.
Ductus semicircularis anterior. It is oriented vertically and somewhat perpendicular to the petrous
temporal. A

13 Posterior semicircular duct. Ductus semicircularis posterior. It is oriented somewhat vertically in a plane which runs parallel to the longitudinal axis of the petrous temporal. A

14 Lateral semicircular duct. Ductus semicircularis lateralis. It is oriented horizontally, lies
broadest laterally and can bulge the medial wall of
the tympanic cavity. A

15 **Proper membrane of semicircular duct.** Membrana propria ductus semicircularis. Layer below
the basement membrane consisting, at first, of
somewhat densely packed fibers which then extends into the looser network of the perilymphatic
space. C

16 **Basal membrane of semicircular duct.** Membrana basalis ductus semicircularis. By light
microscopy a homogeneous appearing basement
membrane situated directly below the epithelium.
C

17 [[**Epithelium of semicircular duct**]]. [[Epitheli-
um ductus semicircularis]]. Simple epithelium lining the inner aspect of the membranous semicircular duct. The cells are flat and become cuboidal
on their concava side. C

18 **Membranous ampullae.** Ampullae mem-
branaceae. Dilatations of the semicircular ducts in
the vicinity of the utricle.

19 Anterior membranous ampulla. Ampulla
membranacea anterior. Ampulla of anterior (superior) semicircular duct located anteriorly near
the lateral membranous ampulla. A

20 Posterior membranous ampulla. Ampulla
membranacea posterior. Expansion of the posteri-
or semicircular duct located far from the two other
ampullae. A

21 Lateral membranous ampulla. Ampulla
membranacea lateralis. Ampulla of the lateral semicircular duct located close beside the anterior
membranous ampulla. A

22 **Sulcus ampullaris.** Indentation below the ampullary crest bearing branches from the ampullar
nerve for innervation of the ampullary crest. B

23 **Ampullary crest.** Crista ampullaris. Crescent-
shaped ridge projecting into the ampullary space.
It is covered by sensory epithelium and has a base
of nerve fibers and connective tissue. B

24 [[Neuroepithelium]]. Sensory epithelium of
ampullae consisting of supporting cells and sensory cells with hairs (microvilli) projecting from
the surface into an overlying cupula. B

25 Cupula. Gelatinous body suspended above the
ampullary crest as far as the roof of the ampulla
and penetrated by hairs from the sensory cells. B

26 **Membranous crura.** Crura membranacea. Limbs
of semicircular ducts opening into the utricle.

27 Simple membranous crus. Crus mem-
branaceum simplex. Posterior limb of lateral semicircular duct opening into the utricle by itself. A

28 Ampullary membranous crura. Crura membranacea ampullaria. Semicircular duct segments
situated between the ampullae and the utricle. A

29 Common membranous crus. Crus mem-
branaceum commune. Common limb formed by
the anterior and posterior semicircular ducts and
opening into the utricle. A

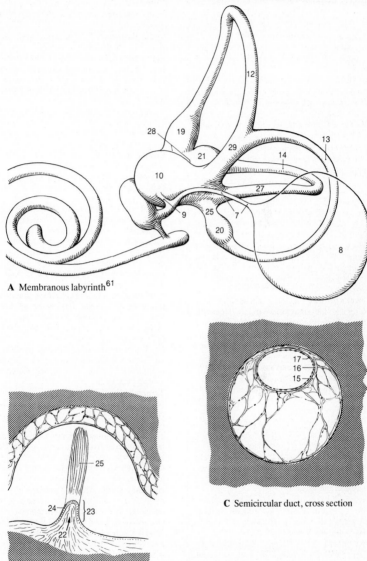

A Membranous labyrinth[61]

B Ampulla of semicircular duct

C Semicircular duct, cross section

1 **Ductus reuniens.** Fine tube connecting the saccule with the cochlear duct. B

2 **Saccule.** Sacculus. Round vesicle, 2–3 mm in size, equipped with a sensory field. B

3 **Maculae** [[staticae]]. Sensory field for the perception of the position of the head in space. A B

4 Utricular macula. Macula utriculi. Horizontally oriented sensory field, 2.3–3 mm in size, occupying the floor of the utricle. B

5 Saccular macula. Macula sacculi. Vertically oriented, arched sensory field, about 1.5 mm wide, at the medial wall of the saccule. B

6 Statoconia. Calcium concretions, up to 15 μm in size, embedded in a gelatinous substance together with the sensory hairs. A

7 Statoconial membrane. Membrana statoconiorum. Membrane covering the maculae and consisting of a gelatinous ground substance with statoconia lying on its surface. It is penetrated by bristle-like processes from underlying macular sensory cells. A

8 [[Neuroepithelium]]. Pseudostratified, prismatic, sensory epithelium of the macula consisting of supporting and sensory cells. The sensory cells bear 20–25 μm long bristle-like processes which project into the statoconial membrane. A

9 Cochlear labyrinth. Labyrinthus cochlearis. Complicated content of the osseous cochlea. C

10 **Perilymphatic space.** Spatium perilymphaticum. Space occupied by perilymph and partially permeated by connective tissue fibers. It includes the scala vestibuli and tympani. A B

11 Scala vestibuli. Perilymphatic canal located above the osseous spiral lamina and cochlear duct. It ascends as far as the apex of the cochlea (helicotrema). C

12 Scala tympani. Perilymphatic canal below the osseous spiral lamina and basilar membrane. C

13 Cochlear aqueduct (perilymphatic duct). Aquaeductus cochleae. Pathway connecting the perilymphatic space with the subarachoid space. B

14 External aperture of perilymphatic duct. Apertura externa aquaeductus cochleae. It opens in the vicinity of the canaliculus for the tympanic nerve. See 14.22

15 **Cochlear duct.** Ductus cochlearis. Endolymphatic tube, triangular in cross section, taking $2\frac{1}{2}$–$2\frac{3}{4}$ turns around a bony axis (modiolus) before ending blindly at the apex of the cochlea. It houses the sensory epithelium for the perception of sound. B C E

16 **Cupular cecum.** Caecum cupulare. Blind end
~ of cochlear duct located at the apex of the cochlea. B

17 **Vestibular cecum.** Caecum vestibulare. Blind
~ end of the cochlear duct facing the vestibule. B

18 **Tympanic wall of cochlear duct (spiral membrane).** Paries tympanicus ductus cochlearis (membrana spiralis). Inferior wall of cochlear duct situated above the scala tympani. E

19 **Spiral organ (of Corti).** Organum spirale [[Corti]]. Sensory field lying on the basilar membrane. It transforms sound waves into nerve impulses. D

20 **Basilar membrane.** Lamina basilaris. Plate of connective tissue between the cochlear duct and scala tympani. It is stretched out between the tympanic lip of the osseous spiral lamina and the spiral ligament. E

21 **Spiral crest (ligament).** Crista spiralis (lig. spirale). Fiber system, triangular in cross section, arising from the periosteum of the cochlear canal and radiating into the basilar lamina. E

22 **Nerve foramina.** Foramina nervosa. Holes in the basilar lamina for the passage of cochlear nerve fibers on their way from the hair cells to the spiral ganglion. D

23 **Limbus of osseous spiral lamina.** Limbus laminae spiralis osseae. Thickening and transformation of the endosteum on the upper layer of the osseous spiral lamina indented externally by the internal spiral sulcus. E

24 **Vestibular lip of limb of osseous spiral lamina.** Labium limbi vestibulare. Upper, shorter process of the limbus. Site of attachment for the tectorial membrane. E

25 **Tympanic lip of limb of osseous spiral lamina.** Labium limbi tympanicum. Lower, longer process of limbus. It lies on the basilar membrane. D E

26 **Tectorial membrane.** Membrana tectoria. Fibrous membrane lying above the organ of Corti. It is narrow at its attachment to the vestibular lip and ends freely beyond the row of outer hair cells. D E

27 **Auditory teeth.** Dentes acustici. Cell rows projecting ridge-like on the surface of the vestibular lip. The tectorial membrane is anchored in this area. D

28 **Internal spiral sulcus.** Sulcus spiralis internus. Groove between the vestibular and tympanic lips. D E

29 **External spiral sulcus.** Sulcus spiralis externus. Groove at the outer wall of the cochlear duct between the spiral prominence and the spiral organ. E

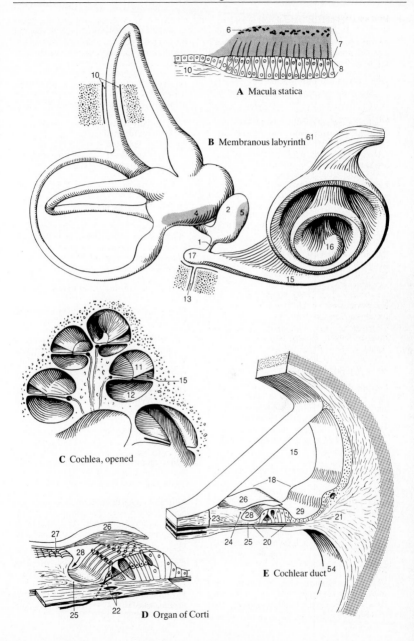

A Macula statica

B Membranous labyrinth

C Cochlea, opened

D Organ of Corti

E Cochlear duct

1 **Reticular membrane.** Membrana reticularis. Covering membrane of the organ of Corti with gaps penetrated by the microvilli of the hair cells. It is composed of the head plates of pillar and Deiter's cells. B

2 **Spiral vessel.** Vas spirale. Small blood vessel running in the tympanic covering layer of the basilar lamina beneath the tunnel. A

3 **Vestibular wall of cochlear duct (vestibular [[Reissner's]] membrane).** Paries vestibularis ductus cochlearis (membrana vestibularis) [[Reissner]]. Upper wall of cochlear duct. It is about 3 μm thick. A

4 **External wall of cochlear duct.** Paries externus ductus cochlearis. Lateral wall. A

5 **Basilar crest.** Crista basilaris. Pointed margin of spiral ligament going over into the basilar lamina. A

6 **Spiral prominence.** Prominentia spiralis. Marginal ridge projecting above the external spiral sulcus. It consists of connective tissue and a blood vessel. A

7 **Vas prominens.** The blood vessel coursing in the spiral prominence. A

8 **Stria vascularis.** Broad, specialized band of strongly vascularized stratified squamous epithelium above the spiral prominence. It is said to secrete endolymph. A

9 **Spiral ganglion of cochlea.** Ganglion spirale cochlearis. Accumulation of bipolar ganglion cells in the spiral canal of the modiolus. The afferent, peripheral fibers of these cells arise from the hair cells; the central, efferent fibers form the cochlear branch of the vestibulocochlear nerve. C

10 **Vessels of inner ear.** Vasa auris internae. C

11 **Labyrinthine artery.** A. labyrinthina. It arises from the basilar artery in front of the anterior inferior cerebellar artery, passes through the internal acoustic meatus with the vestibulocochlear nerve and enters the petrous temporal bone where it ramifies and supplies the inner ear. C

12 Vestibular branches. Rami vestibulares. Branches for the supply of the ampullae, maculae, semicircular ducts and the lower third of the basal turn of the cochlea. C

13 Cochlear branch. Ramus cochlearis. It passes into the modiolus where it supplies the spiral ganglion and the cochlear duct together with its contents except for the lower third of the basal turn. C

14 Arterial glomeruli of cochlea. Glomeruli arteriosi cochleae. Spirally oriented arterial network accompanying the spiral vein. C

15 **Labyrinthine veins.** Vv. labyrinthinae. Companion veins of labyrinthine artery. They pass through the internal acoustic meatus and open either into the inferior petrosal sinus or directly into the internal jugular vein. C

16 Spiral vein of modiolus. V. spiralis modioli. It takes a spiral course in the modiolus and empties into the labyrinthine vein. C

17 Vestibular veins. Vv. vestibulares. They arise from the semicircular ducts in the region of the utricle and saccule and drain partly into a labyrinthine vein, partly into the vein of the vestibular aqueduct. C

18 Vein of vestibular aqueduct. V. aqueductus vestibuli. Companion vein of endolymphatic duct. It opens into the inferior petrosal sinus. C

19 Vein of cochlear aqueduct. V. aqueductus cochleae. Companion vein of perilymphatic duct. It carries blood from the basal turn of the cochlea through the cochlear canaliculus. C

20 **Osseous labyrinth.** Labyrinthus osseus. Bony capsule enclosing the membranous labyrinth. D

21 **Vestibule.** Vestibulum. Part of osseous labyrinth enclosing the utricle and saccule. D

22 **Spherical recess of vestibule.** Recessus sphericus. Rounded recess in the medial wall of the vestibule. It is occupied by the saccule. D

23 **Elliptical recess of vestibule.** Recessus ellipticus. Oval depression in the medial wall of the vestibule. It is occupied by the portion of the utricle between the posterior ampulla and common crus. D

24 **Crest of vestibule.** Crista vestibuli. Ridge between the spherical and elliptical recesses. D

25 **Pyramid of vestibule.** Pyramis vestibuli. Upper broadened part of the crest of the vestibule. D

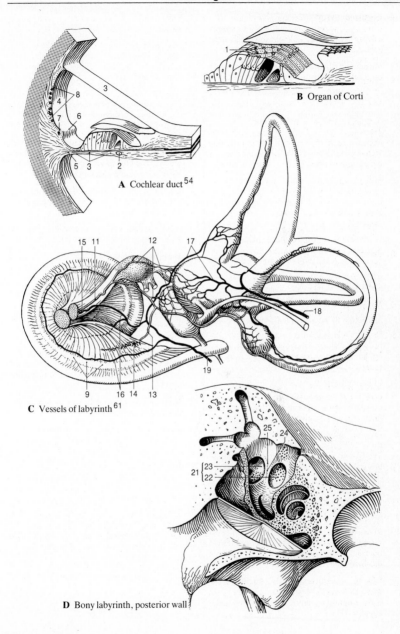

A Cochlear duct [54]

B Organ of Corti

C Vessels of labyrinth [61]

D Bony labyrinth, posterior wall

1 **Cochlear recess.** Recessus cochlearis. Depression lying below and in front of the spherical recess. It is occupied by the lower end of the cochlear duct. C

2 **Maculae cribrosae.** Perforated bony areas transmitting fibers of the vestibulocochlear nerve.

3 Macula cribrosa superior. Perforated bony area transmitting fibers of the utriculo-ampullar nerve. C

4 Macula cribrosa media. Perforated bony area in the vicinity of the base of the cochlea for the passage of fibers of the saccular nerve. C

5 Macula cribrosa inferior. Perforated bony area in the wall of the posterior osseous ampulla for the passage of fibers of the posterior ampullar nerve. C

6 **Osseous semicircular canals.** Canales semicirculares ossei. Bony canals containing perilymph and enclosing the membranous semicircular ducts (filled with endolymph). C

7 Anterior (superior) semicircular canal. Canalis semicircularis anterior. It shares a common crus with the posterior semicircular canal and is oriented vertically, somewhat perpendicular to the axis of the petrous temporal. B

8 Posterior semicircular canal. Canalis semicircularis posterior. Situated widest inferiorly, it lies somewhat parallel to the axis of the petrous temporal. B

9 Lateral semicircular canal. Canalis semicircularis lateralis. Oriented horizontally, it can bulge the medial wall of the tympanic cavity. B

10 **Osseous ampulla.** Ampullae osseae. Dilatations close to the base of the semicircular crura. They are occupied by the membranous ampullae. C

11 Anterior osseous ampulla. Ampulla ossea anterior. Ampulla of the anterior semicircular canal. It lies anteriorly close beside the ampulla of the lateral semicircular canal. B

12 Posterior osseous ampulla. Ampulla ossea posterior. Ampulla of posterior semicircular canal. It lies posteriorly below the plane of the lateral semicircular canal. B

13 Lateral osseous ampulla. Ampulla ossea lateralis. Ampulla of lateral semicircular canal. It lies anteriorly near the anterior semicircular ampulla. B

14 **Crura ossea.** Osseous crura of semicircular canals.

15 Common osseous crus. Crus osseum commune. Posteriorly situated common limb formed by the union of the crura from the superior and posterior semicircular canals. B

16 Simple osseous crus. Crus osseum simplex. Posteriorly situated crus of lateral semicircular canal opening by itself into the wall of the vestibule. B

17 Ampullary osseous crura. Crura ossea ampullaria. Crura of semicircular canals which are expanded for the occupation of the ampullae of the membranous labyrinth. B

18 **Cochlea.** It comprises 2½–2¾ turns, measures 8–9 mm at its base and is altogether 4–5 mm high. B

19 **Apex of cochlea.** Cupula cochlea. In the skull it points anteriorly, inferiorly and laterally. B

20 **Base of cochlea.** Basis cochlea. Its surface faces somewhat in the direction of the internal acoustic meatus. A

21 **Spiral canal of cochlea.** Canalis spiralis cochleae. It is partitioned into three canals by the osseous spiral lamina and the basilar lamina on one side and by the vestibular membrane on the other. A

22 **Modiolus.** Cone-shaped axis of cochlea. It is hollowed out for the occupation of the cochlear nerve and forms the medial wall of the spiral canal. A

23 Base of modiolus. Basis modioli. Beginning of the cochlear axis. A

24 Lamina of modiolus. Lamina modioli. Bony plate extended upward as the end of the osseous spiral lamina. A

25 Spiral canal of modiolus. Canalis spiralis modioli. Fine channel in the axial wall near the base of the osseous spiral lamina. It contains the spiral ganglion. A

26 Longitudinal canals of modiolus. Canales longitudinales modioli. Centrally located bony channels containing fibers of the cochlear nerve leaving the spiral ganglion. A

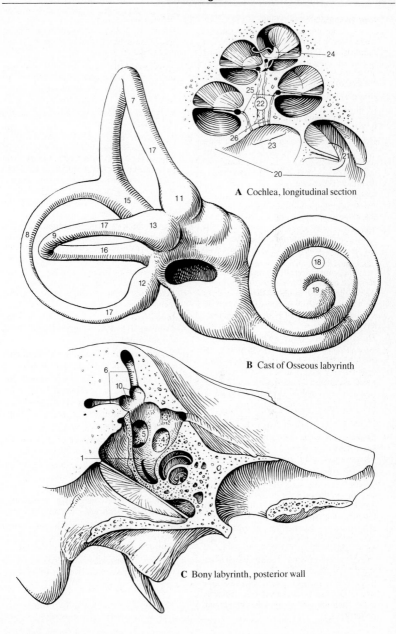

A Cochlea, longitudinal section

B Cast of Osseous labyrinth

C Bony labyrinth, posterior wall

1 **Osseous spiral lamina.** Lamina spiralis ossea. Bilayered bony plate projecting from the modiolus into the spiral canal of the cochlea in a spiral fashion. Together with the cochlear duct to which it is attached, it forms a complete partition between the scale vestibuli and scala tympani. B

2 **Hook of spiral lamina.** Hamulus laminae spiralis. Free hook-shaped upper end of the osseous spiral lamina at the apex of the cochlea. B

3 **Helicotrema.** Confluence between scala vestibuli and scala tympani at the apex of the cochlea. It exists because the osseous spiral lamina and the cochlear duct end before reaching the apex of the cochlea. B

4 **Secondary spiral lamina.** Lamina spiralis secundaria. Bony ridge situated in the lower half of the basal turn. It projects from the outer wall of the spiral canal across from the osseous spiral lamina. The inferior part of the basilar lamina is stretched out between these two spiral laminae. B

5 **Internal acoustic (auditory) meatus.** Meatus acusticus internus. Beginning at the posterior wall of the petrous temporal bone, it is about 1 cm long and transmits the vestibulocochlear and facial nerves, as well as the labyrinthine artery and vein. A

6 **Porus acusticus.** Outer opening of internal acoustic meatus into the posterior wall of the petrous temporal bone above the jugular foramen. A

7 **Fundus of internal auditory meatus.** Fundus meatus acustici interni. Floor of meatus subdivided into several fields. A

8 Transverse crest. Crista transversa. Transversely oriented ridge dividing the fundus of the internal acoustic meatus into an upper and lower field. A

9 Facial nerve area. Area nervi facialis. Field containing the beginning of the canal for the facial nerve. A

10 Cochlear area. Area cochleae. Spacious field below the transverse crest. It contains the foraminous spiral tract. A

11 *Foraminous spiral tract.* Tractus spiralis foraminosus. Field perforated by fibers of the spiral ganglion forming the cochlear part of the vestibulocochlear nerve. It corresponds to the spiral canal of the cochlea. A

12 Superior vestibular area. Area vestibularis superior. Field lying lateral to the facial canal and perforated by fibers of the utriculo-ampullar nerve. A

13 Inferior vestibular area. Area vestibularis inferior. Region located lateral to foraminous spiral tract and perforated by fibers of the saccular nerve. A

14 Small opening for the posterior ampullar nerve. Foramen singulare. It lies behind the inferior vestibular area. A

15 MIDDLE EAR. AURIS MEDIA. It comprises the tympanic (middle ear) cavity, auditory tube and mastoid air cells.

16 **Tympanic cavity.** Cavitas tympanica (cavum tympani). Laterally compressed, obliquely positioned space lying medial to the tympanic membrane (eardrum). It contains the auditory ossicles and communicates posterosuperiorly with the mastoid air cells and antero-inferiorly with the nasopharyngeal cavity via the auditory tube.

17 **Tegmental wall (tegmen tympani).** Paries tegmentalis. Thin roof of the tympanic cavity. It lies lateral to the arcuate eminence of the petrous temporal bone. C

18 Epitympanic recess (attic). Recessus epitympanicus. Dome of tympanic cavity located above the upper margin of the tympanic membrane and arching superiorly and laterally. C

19 Cupular part. Pars cupularis. Upper portion of epitympanic recess. C

20 **Jugular wall.** Paries jugularis. Floor of tympanic cavity facing the jugular fossa. C

21 Styloid prominence. Prominentia styloidea. Elevation on the floor of the tympanic cavity produced by the styloid process. C

22 **Labyrinthine wall.** Paries labyrinthicus. Medial wall of tympanic cavity. C

23 Oval window. Fenestra vestibuli [[ovalis]]. It is closed by the footplate of the stapes. C

24 Fossula fenestrae vestibuli. Small depression in medial wall of tympanic cavity between the malleus and incus. C

25 Promontory. Promontorium. Prominence caused by the basal turn of the cochlea. C

26 *Sulcus promontorii.* Groove on the promontory produced by the tympanic nerve from the tympanic plexus. C

27 *Subiculum promontorii.* Small bony ridge behind the promontory and round window. C

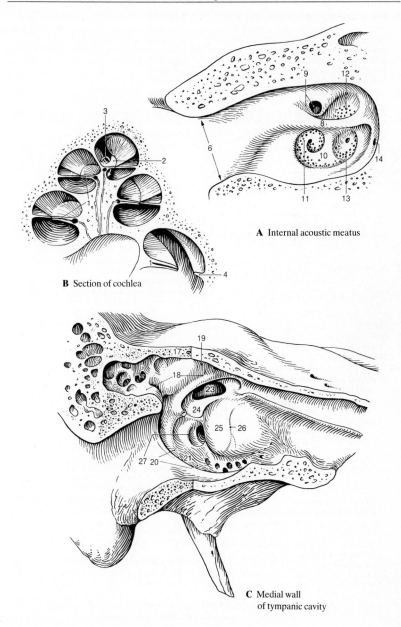

A Internal acoustic meatus

B Section of cochlea

C Medial wall
of tympanic cavity

1 Tympanic sinus. Sinus tympani. Deep fossa behind the promontory and round window. D

2 Round window (fenestra of cochlea). Fenestra cochleae [[rotunda]]. Round opening at the end of the scala tympani. It is closed by the secondary tympanic membrane. D

3 Fossula of round window. Fossula fenestrae cochleae. Small fossa leading into the round window. D

4 Crest of round window. Crista fenestrae cochleae. Bony ridge along the edge of the round window for attachment of the secondary tympanic membrane. D

5 Cochleariform process. Processus cochleariformis. Spoon-shaped bony process found above the promontory at the end of the semicanal for the tensor tympani muscle. In combination with a connective tissue loop, it serves as a pulley for the tensor tympani muscle. D

6 Secondary tympanic membrane. Membrana tympani secundaria. Stretched out across the round window, it forms a membranous partition between the scala tympani and the tympanic cavity.

7 **Mastoid wall.** Paries mastoideus [adnexa mastoidea]. Components connected with the mastoid process.

8 **Mastoid (posterior) wall.** Paries mastoideus. Posterior wall of middle ear cavity facing the mastoid process. D

9 Mastoid antrum. Antrum mastoideum. Closed space continuous with the tympanic cavity posterosuperiorly. It communicates with the mastoid air cells inferiorly. D

10 Aditus ad antrum. Entrance into the mastoid antrum from the tympanic cavity. D

11 *Prominentia canalis semicircularis lateralis.* Prominence of lateral semicircular canal. Elevation above the prominence of the facial canal. D

12 *Prominence of facial nerve canal.* Prominentia canalis facialis. Bulge lying between the oval window and prominence of the lateral semicircular canal. D

13 Pyramidal eminence (pyramid). Eminentia pyramidalis. Small pyramidal projection at the level of the oval window. Perforated at its apex, it contains the stapedius muscle the tendon of which emerges from it. D

14 Incudal fossa. Fossa incudis. Small depression in the aditus ad antrum for the posterior ligament of the incus. D

15 Sinus posterior. Small groove between the incudal fossa and pyramid. D

16 Tympanic aperture of canaliculus of chorda tympani. Apertura tympanica canaliculi chordae tympani. Opening of chorda tympani canal into tympanic cavity. It lies at the posterior margin of the tympanic membrane at the level of the pyramid. D

17 Mastoid air cells. Cellulae mastoideae. Like the tympanic cavity, they are lined by a squamous/cuboidal epithelium. D

18 Tympanic cells. Cellulae tympanicae. Small cell-like depressions in the floor of the tympanic cavity. D

19 **Carotid wall.** Paries caroticus. Anterior wall formed partly by the carotid canal, partly by the opening of the auditory tube. D

20 **Membranous wall.** Paries membranaceus. Lateral wall of tympanic cavity formed primarily by the tympanic membrane. B

21 **Tympanic membrane (eardrum).** Membrana tympanica. Obliquely oriented membrane at the end of the external acoustic meatus. Its diameter is 9–11 mm. A B

22 **Pars flaccida** [[Shrapnell's membrane]]. Smaller, more flaccid part of tympanic membrane located above the anterior and posterior mallear folds. A B

23 **Pars tensa.** Stretched out within the tympanic ring, it represents, by far, the largest part of the tympanic membrane. A B

24 **Anterior mallear fold.** Plica mallearis anterior. Located at the inner side of the tympanic membrane and concave downward, it passes anteriorly from the base of the handle of the malleus. B

25 **Posterior mallear fold.** Plica mallearis posterior. Located at the inner side of the tympanic membrane and concave downward, it passes posteriorly from the root of the handle of the malleus. B

26 **Mallear prominence.** Prominentia mallearis. Small elevation on the outside of the tympanic membrane caused by the lateral process of the malleus. A

27 **Stria mallearis.** Light band on the external surface of the tympanic membrane caused by the handle of the malleus – fused with the tympanic membrane – shining through. A

28 **Umbo of tympanic membrane.** Umbo membranae tympani. It lies at the apex of the handle of the malleus where the tympanic membrane is drawn inward, i.e., its point of greatest convexity. A

29 **Cutaneous layer.** Stratum cutaneum. External surface of tympanic membrane covered by stratified squamous epithelium. C

30 **Fibrocartilaginous ring.** Anulus fibrocartilagineus. Tissue anchoring the tympanic membrane in the tympanic sulcus. C

31 **Radiate layer.** Stratum radiatum. Group of outer, radially oriented fibers in the tympanic membrane. C

32 **Circular layer.** Stratum circulare. Inernally located fibers running circularly in the tympanic membrane. C

33 **Mucosal layer.** Stratum mucosum. Simple squamous epithelium covering the internal surface of the tympanic membrane. C

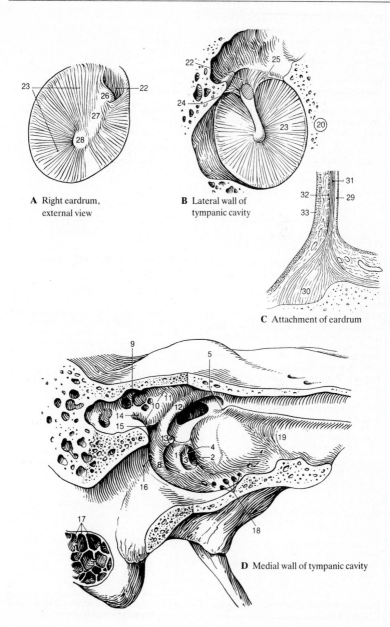

A Right eardrum, external view

B Lateral wall of tympanic cavity

C Attachment of eardrum

D Medial wall of tympanic cavity

1 **Auditory ossicles (malleus, incus and stapes).** Ossicula auditoria (auditus). They operate collectively as a bent lever system transferring sound waves from the tympanic membrane to the inner ear.

2 **Stapes** (stirrup). Its footplate (base) fits into the oval window. A B

3 Head of stapes. Caput stapedis. It lies opposite the base and articulates with the lenticular process of the incus. A B

4 Anterior crus (limb). Crus anterius. It is almost straight. A B

5 Posterior crus (limb). Crus posterius. It is somewhat curved. A B

6 Base (footplate) of stapes. Basis stapedis. It is inserted into the oval window. A B

7 **Incus** (anvil). It is found between the head of the malleus and the head of the stapes. A D

8 Body of incus. Corpus incudis. It articulates with the malleus by means of a saddle-shaped joint. A

9 Long crus (limb). Crus longum. Long process which is oriented approximately vertically downward behind the handle of the malleus and bears the lenticular process at its end. A

10 *Lenticular process.* Processus lenticularis. Very small bony projection at the end of the long crus. It articulates with the stapes. A

11 Short crus (limb). Crus breve. Small process directed posteriorly and attached to the incudal fossa by a ligament. A

12 **Malleus** [[hammer]]. It lies between the tympanic membrane and the incus. A C

13 Handle (manubrium) of malleus. Manubrium mallei. Its outer surface is fused to the tympanic membrane as far as the lateral process. A

14 Head of malleus. Caput mallei. It bears a convex articular surface for the body of the incus. A

15 Neck of malleus. Collum mallei. Connective piece between the head and handle of the malleus. A

16 Lateral process. Processus lateralis. Short process at the end of the handle. It causes the mallear prominence. A

17 Anterior process. Processus anterior. Long, very thin process. In the newborn it extends into the petrotympanic fissure; in the adult it is reduced. A

18 Articulations of auditory ossicles. Articulationes ossiculorum auditoriorum. They are not true joints but syndesmoses.

19 Incudomallear joint. Articulatio incudomallearis. Joint between the incus and malleus. It occasionally exhibits an articular cavity. A

20 Incudostapedial articulation. Articulatio incudostapedialis. Union between the lenticular process of the long crus of the incus and the stapes. A

21 Tympanostapedial syndesmosis. Syndesmosis tympanostapedialis. Connective tissue attachment of the footplate of the stapes into the oval window. It is broader anderiorly than posteriorly. B

22 **Ligaments of auditory ossicles.** Ligg. ossiculorum auditoriorum.

23 Anterior ligament of malleus. Lig. mallei anterius. Arising from the anterior process of the malleus, it lies in the anterior mallear fold and extends as far as the petrotympanic fissure. D

24 Superior ligament of malleus. Lig. mallei superius. It passes from the head of the malleus to the roof of the epitympanic recess. C D

25 Lateral ligament of malleus. Lig. mallei laterale. It unites the neck of the malleus with the upper margin of the tympanic notch. C

26 Superior ligament of incus. Lig. incudis superius. Coursing approximately parallel to the superior ligament of the malleus, it connects the body of the incus with the roof of the epitympanic recess. C D

27 Posterior ligament of incus. Lig. incudis posterius. It passes from the short limb of the incus to the lateral wall of the tympanic cavity. C D

28 Stapedial membrane. Membrana stapedialis. Thin membrane between the limbs and base of the stapes. B

29 Anular ligament of stapes. Lig. anulare stapediale. It lies between the footplate of the stapes and the margin of the oval window. It is broader anteriorly than posteriorly. B

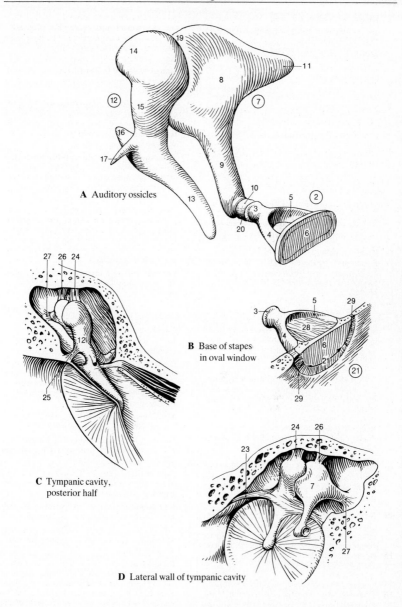

A Auditory ossicles

B Base of stapes in oval window

C Tympanic cavity, posterior half

D Lateral wall of tympanic cavity

1 **Muscles of auditory ossicles.** Musculi ossiculorum auditoriorum. The following two muscles attach to the ossicles:

2 **M. tensor tympani.** It is located in the semicanal for the tensor tympani muscle above the auditory tube. Its tendon bends laterally around the cochleariform process almost at a right angle and inserts at the base of the handle of the malleus. I: Mandibular nerve. A

3 **M. stapedius.** It originates in a bony canal on the posterior wall of the tympanic cavity and its tendon passes through an opening at the apex of the pyramid before inserting at the head of the stapes. By tilting the stapes, it exerts a dampening effect on sound vibrations reaching the inner ear. I: Nerve to stapedius from the facial nerve. B

4 **Mucous membrane of tympanic cavity.** Tunica mucosa cavitatis tympanicae. It consists of a simple squamous to cuboidal epithelium and a delicate vascular-rich lamina propria.

5 **Posterior mallear fold.** Plica mallearis posterior. Fold from the base of the handle of the malleus to the posterior, upper part of the tympanic ring. It contains the posterior portion of the chorda tympani. D

6 **Anterior mallear fold.** Plica mallearis anterior. Fold from the base of the handle of the malleus to the anterior, upper part of the tympanic ring. It contains the anterior segment of the chorda tympani, the anterior process of the malleus and the anterior ligament of the malleus. D

7 **Fold of chorda tympani.** Plica chordae tympani. Fold thrown up by the chorda tympani on the neck of the malleus between the two above mentioned folds. D

7a **Recess of tympanic membrane.** Recessus membranae tympanicae. Mucosal pouch in the tympanic cavity.

8 **Anterior recess of tympanic membrane.** Recessus [membranae tympani] anterior. Mucosal pouch between the anterior mallear fold and the tympanic membrane. D

9 **Superior recess of tympanic membrane** (Prussak's pouch). Recessus [membranae tympani] superior. It is bordered laterally by the flaccid part of the tympanic membrane, medially by the head and neck of the malleus as well as by the body of the incus. D

10 **Posterior recess of tympanic membrane.** Recessus [membranae tympani] posterior. Mucosal pouch between the posterior mallear fold and tympanic membrane. D

11 **Incudal fold.** Plica incudialis. Mucosal fold from the roof of the epitympanic recess to the head of the incus or also from the short limb of the incus to the posterior wall of the tympanic cavity. D

12 **Stapedial fold.** Plica stapedialis. Mucosal fold from the posterior wall of the tympanic cavity to the stapes. It covers the stapedius muscle and the stapes. B

13 **Auditory (pharyngotympanic, eustachian) tube.** Tuba auditoria (auditiva). Narrow 4 cm long, partly cartilaginous, partly bony tube between the middle ear and the nasopharynx for aeration of the tympanic cavity. A C

14 **Tympanic ostium of auditory tube.** Ostium tympanicum tubae auditoriae. Opening of tube at the anterior wall of the tympanic cavity. It usually lies somewhat above the floor of the tympanic cavity. A

15 **Osseous part of auditory tube.** Pars ossea tubae auditoriae. Located laterally and posterosuperiorly, it involves about $1/3$ of the tube's length, lies below the semicanal for the tensor tympani muscle and has its entrance between the carotid canal and the foramen spinosum. A

16 **Isthmus [tubae auditoriae].** Narrow portion of tube between the cartilaginous and bony segments. A

17 **Air cells.** Cellulae pneumaticae. Small fossae in the wall of the osseous part of the tube. A

18 **Cartilaginous part of tube.** Pars cartilaginea [tubae auditoriae] located anteromedially with a length of about 2.5 cm. A

19 **Cartilage of auditory tube.** Cartilago tubae auditoriae. Hook-shaped in cross section, it becomes lower lateroposteriorly and consists of elastic cartilage only in the angle between the two cartilaginous laminae. A

20 *Medial cartilaginous lamina.* Lamina (cartilaginis) medialis. Broad plate of cartilage. C

21 *Lateral cartilaginous lamina.* Lamina (cartilaginis) lateralis. Narrow plate of cartilage directed anterolaterally. C

22 **Membranous lamina.** Lamina membranacea. Membranous portion of the wall of the cartilaginous part of the auditory tube. A C

23 **Tunica mucosa.** Mucous membrane of auditory tube lined by a simple ciliated epithelium. C

24 **Glands of auditory tube.** Glandulae tubariae. Mucous glands especially in the cartilaginous extent of the tube. C

25 **Pharyngeal opening of auditory tube.** Ostium pharyngeum tubae auditoriae. Funnel-shaped to slit-like opening lying above the levator eminence at the level of the inferior nasal meatus, 1 cm lateral and anterior to the posterior wall of the pharynx. A

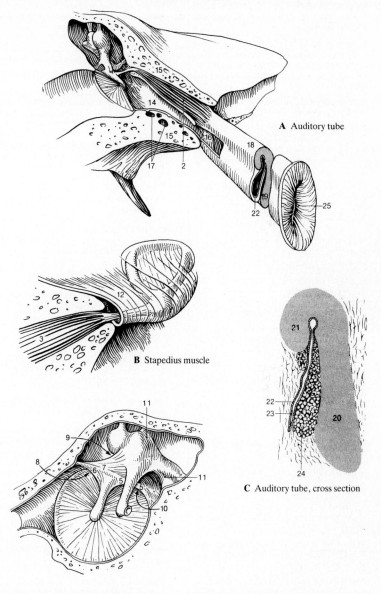

A Auditory tube

B Stapedius muscle

C Auditory tube, cross section

D Lateral wall of tympanic cavity

1 EXTERNAL EAR. AURIS EXTERNA. It consists of the auricle (pinna) and external acoustic meatus.

2 **External acoustic (auditory) meatus (canal).** Meatus acusticus externus. Flat, partly cartilaginous, partly bony, S-shaped canal about 2.4 cm long with a diameter of about 6 mm. C

3 **External opening of acoustic canal.** Porus acusticus externus. C

3 a **Tympanic notch.** Incisura tympanica. Defect between the greater and lesser tympanic spines. In the newborn, the gap superiorly between the still free ends of the tympanic ring. See 16.8

4 **Cartilaginous part of external acoustic meatus.** Meatus acusticus externus cartilagineus. Lateral, cartilaginous one-third of the external acoustic meatus. C

5 Cartilage of external acoustic meatus. Cartilago meatus acustici. United with the cartilage of the pinna, it forms a groove open superiorly and posteriorly. D

6 *Incisurae cartilaginis meatus acustici.* Two fissures in the cartilage of the external acoustic meatus. Bridged over by connective tissue, they are usually directed anteriorly. D

7 **Lamina tragi.** Lateral part of the meatal cartilage. It lies in front of the external opening of the acoustic meatus. D

8 **Auricle (pinna).** Auricula. A B

9 **Ear lobe.** Lobulus auricularis. Lower end of pinna devoid of cartilage. A B C

10 **Auricular cartilage.** Cartilago auricularis. Structural framwork of the pinna consisting of elastic cartilage. D

11 **Helix.** External, curved margin of auricle. A B C D

12 Crus of helix. Crus helicis. Beginning of helix in the cavity (concha) of the auricle. A B D

13 Spine of helix. Spina helicis. Small cartilaginous projection given off by the crus anteriorly. D

14 Tail of helix. Cauda helicis. Posterior, inferior end of the helix separated from the antitragus by an indentation. D

15 **Antihelix** [[anthelix]]. Arched projection located in front of the posterior part of the helix. A B C D

16 Triangular fossa. Fossa triangularis. Located anterosuperiorly, it is enclosed by the two crura of the antihelix. A D

17 Crura of antihelix. Crura antihelicis. Formed by the bifurcation of the antihelix superiorly, the two crura form the boundary of the triangular fossa. A D

18 **Scaphoid fossa.** Scapha. Narrow gutter situated posteriorly between the helix and antihelix. A D

19 **Concha (cavity) of auricle.** Concha auricularis. It is embraced by the antihelix, antitragus and tragus. A

20 Cymba conchalis. Upper, slit-like part of the concha between the crura of the helix and antihelix. A

21 Cavity of concha. Cavitas (Cavum) conchalis. Main part of concha located below the crus of the helix and behind the tragus. A

22 **Antitragus.** Small tubercle present on the inferior continuation of the antihelix and separated from the tragus by the intertragic incisure. A D

23 **Tragus.** Flat projection in front of the external opening of the acoustic canal. A

24 **Anterior notch.** Incisura anterior (auris). It lies between the tragus (supratragic tubercle) and the crus of the helix. A

25 **Intertragic incisure.** Incisura intertragica. Notch between tragus and antitragus. A D

26 **Auricular [[Darwin's]] tubercle.** [Tuberculum auriculare]. It is occasionally present on the anterior margin of the helix where it turns postero-inferiorly. A

27 **Apex of auricle.** [Apex auricularis]. Occasionally present, drawn out outer margin of auricular cartilage (helix) in a backward, upward and outward direction. B

28 **Posterior auricular sulcus.** Sulcus auricularis posterior. Shallow indentation between the antitragus and antihelix. A

29 **Supratragic tubercle.** [Tuberculum supratragicum]. Small tubercle occasionally present at the upper end of the tragus. A

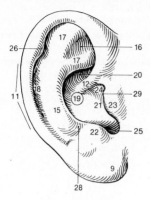

A Auricle (pinna)

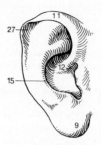

B Auricle with apex

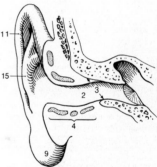

C External acoustic meatus

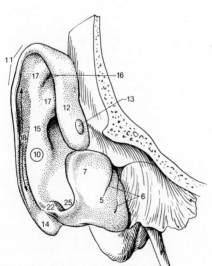

D Auricular cartilage from front

1 **Isthmus of auricular cartilage.** Isthmus cartilaginis auricularis. Narrow bridge of cartilage connecting the cartilage of the external acoustic meatus and tragic lamina with the auricular cartilage. A

2 **Terminal notch.** Incisura terminalis auricularis. Deep notch separating the lamina tragi from the auricular cartilage. A

3 **Fissura antitragohelicina.** Deep fissure separating the antitragus and helix inferiorly as well as the antihelix and helix further superiorly. A

4 **Transverse sulcus of antihelix.** [[Sulcus antihelicis transversus]]. Depression visible posteromedially between the eminence of the triangular fossa and that of the concha. A

5 **Groove of crus of helix.** Sulcus cruris helicis. Shallow furrow on the posterior surface of the auricular cartilage. It corresponds to the crus of the helix on the anterior surface. A

6 **Fossa of antihelix.** Fossa antihelicis. Furrow on posterior surface of auricular cartilage corresponding to the antihelix on the anterior surface. A

7 **Eminence of concha.** Eminentia conchae. Elevation on the posterior surface of the auricular cartilage corresponding to the cavity of the choncha. A

8 **Eminence of scaphoid fossa.** Eminentia scaphae. Curved elevation on the posterior surface of the auricular cartilage corresponding to the scaphoid fossa of the anterior surface. A

9 **Eminence of triangular fossa.** Eminentia fossae triangularis. Elevation on the posterior surface of the auricular cartilage corresponding to the triangular fossa. A

10 **Auricular ligaments.** Ligg. auricularia. Ligaments of the pinna. They attach the auricular cartilage to the temporal bone.

11 **Anterior auricular ligament.** Lig. auriculare anterius. It extends from the root of the zygomatic arch to the spine of the helix. B

12 **Superior auricular ligament.** Lig. auriculare superius. It passes from the upper margin of the osseous external auditory meatus to the spine of the helix. B

13 **Posterior auricular ligament.** Lig. auriculare posterius. It extends from the eminence of the concha to the mastoid process. C

14 **Mm. auriculares.** Muscles of the pinna.

15 **M. helicis major.** It passes upward from the spine of the helix to the helix. B

16 **M. helicis minor.** It lies on the crus of the helix. B

17 **M. tragicus.** It lies vertically on the lamina tragi. B

18 **M. pyramidalis auricularis.** Muscle fibers occasionally split off from the tragicus muscle and passing to the spine of the helix. B

19 **M. antitragicus.** Muscle fibers on the antitragus. They extend partly to the tail of the helix. B

20 **M. transversus auricularis.** Located on the posterior surface of the auricular cartilage, it spreads out between the eminence of the scaphoid fossa and that of the concha. C

21 **M. obliquus auricularis.** It lies between the eminence of the concha and that of the triangular fossa. C

22 **[M. incisurae helicis].** Muscle fibers occasionally present in the caudal continuation of transversus auricularis muscle. C

23 OLFACTORY ORGAN. ORGANUM OLFACTORIUM (OLFACTUS). Organ of smell.

24 **Nasal mucosa of the olfactory region.** Regio olfactoria tunicae mucosae nasi. Covered by olfactory epithelium, this area is about the size of a nickel and occupies the lateral and medial walls, as well as roof (below the cribriform plate) of the nasal cavity at the level of the superior nasal concha. E F

25 **Olfactory glands (of Bowman).** Glandulae olfactoriae. Serous glands found below the olfactory epithelium. Their predominantly serous secretions have the ability to enhance and wash away odorous substances. F

26 GUSTATORY ORGAN. ORGANUM GUSTATORIUM (GUSTUS). Organ of taste. It comprises all of the taste buds.

27 **Taste bud.** Caliculus gustatorius (gemma gustatoria). Occupying the full thickness of the epithelium, it consists of supporting cells and taste cells. Each of the taste cells carries microvilli on its surface as chemoreceptors. Distribution of taste buds: aggregated, in the epithelium of vallate (circumvallate) and foliate papillae; solitary, on the outside of the tongue. D

28 **Taste pore.** Porus gustatorius. Space left by the epithelium above the apex of the taste bud. Microvilli project into it. D

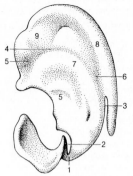

A Auricular cartilage, medial view

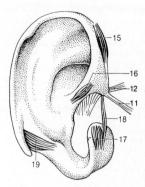

B Auricular cartilage, lateral view

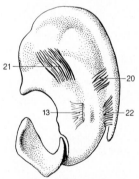

C Auricular cartilage, medial view

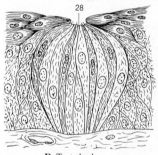

D Taste bud

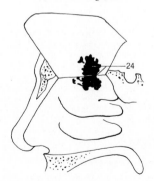

E Olfactory region

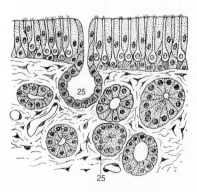

F Olfactory mucosa

1 SKIN (INTEGUMENT). INTEGUMENTUM COMMUNE. External skin consists of three layers: epidermis, dermis (corium) and subcutaneous tissue. In the adult it covers a surface of about 1.8 square meters.

2 **Cutis.** Collective designation for epidermis and dermis.

3 **Sulci of skin.** Sulci cutis. Of different dimensions on the surface of the skin, e.g., nasolabial groove, deep sulci at joints, fine furrows of skin field and furrows between ridges of thick skin. A

4 **Skin (dermal) ridges.** Cristae cutis. Produced by the underlying connective tissue papillae, they are found on the thick skin of the palmar side of hand and plantar aspect of foot. A

5 **Retinacula cutis.** Bands of connective tissue which attach the skin to the fascia or periosteum. A

6 **Tactile elevations.** Toruli tactiles. Skin fields provided with more abundant fat deposits, e.g., at the phalanges and at the thenar and hypothenar eminences. B

7 **Coccygeal foveola.** [Foveola coccygea]. Pit above the coccyx caused by the caudal retinaculum. C

8 **Caudal retinaculum.** Retinaculum caudale. Connective tissue remains of the embryonic notochord lying between the coccygeal foveola and the coccyx. C

9 **Epidermis.** Stratified squamous, keratinized epithelium covering the body. Its thickness varies between 30 μm and 4 mm or even more. A

10 **Stratum corneum.** Most superficial, cornified (keratinized) layer of the epidermis which undergoes continual desquamation. A

11 **Stratum lucidum.** Located between the stratum granulosum and stratum corneum, it is a homogeneous, strongly refractile layer rich in eleidin fibers. A

12 **Stratum granulosum.** It consists of 1–5 cell layers with degenerative nuclear changes. In it lie stongly refractory keratohyaline granules. A

13 **Stratum spinosum.** Prickle cell layer. It consists of polygonal cells with spinous processes which project from their surfaces and contact each other by means of a desmosome. They appear to bridge over relatively large intercellular spaces (shrinkage artifact). A

14 **Stratum basale [cylindricum].** Deepest, cylindrical cell layer of the epidermis. Cell proliferation occurs in this layer as well as the stratum spinosum and provides for the continual renewal of the epidermis. A

15 **Dermis (Corium).** It consists of an intimate network of collagenous and elastic fibers rich in nerves and blood vessels and devoid of fat. A

16 **Papillary layer.** Stratum papillare. Upper delicate layer of the dermis interdigitated with the epidermis by many connective tissue papillae. A

17 **Papillae.** Cones of connective tissue projecting into the epidermis. They can stand in a row (thick skin), be ramified and vary markedly in form and organization. A E

18 **Reticular layer.** Stratum reticulare. Part of dermis adjoining the papillary layer. It consists of more compact, strongly interwoven connective tissue. A

19 **Subcutaneous tissue.** Tela subcutanea. Firmly attached to the dermis, it is compartmentalized by connective tissue tracts and is displaceable with the fascia. A

20 **Panniculus adiposus.** Well-developed fat deposit in the subcutaneous tissue. A

21 **Terminal nerve corpuscles.** Corpuscula nervosa terminalia. Collective term for encapsulated nerve endings.

22 **End bulbs of Krause (bulboid corpuscles).** Corpuscula bulboidea. Oval convolutions of nerve fibers found especially in the lamina propria of the mucosa. They are considered to be cold receptors. E

23 **Lamellated [[Vater-Pacini, pacinian]] corpuscles.** Corpuscula lamellosa. Oval bodies, 2–3 mm long, with concentric layers of connective tissue surrounding an inner core (axon and Schwann cells). They are pressure receptors and lie in the subcutaneous fat tissue as well as in muscles and viscera. A

24 **Tactile [[Meissner's]] corpuscles.** Corpuscula tactus. Lying in the connective papilla of the dermis, these encapsulated sensory organs measure about 0.1 mm in length and consist of transversely placed tactile cells amid a ramified nerve network. A

25 **Genital corpuscles.** [[Corpuscula genitalia]]. Elliptical, encapsulated nerve endings similar to the end bulbs of Krause and found abundantly in the clitoris, glans and nipple. E

26 **Tactile menisci [[Merkel's discs or corpuscles]].** Menisci tractus. Flat group of light cells with intracellular neurofibrils. They occupy epithelium. D

27 **Articular corpuscles.** [[Corpuscula articularia]]. Modified pacinian corpuscles within joint capsules.

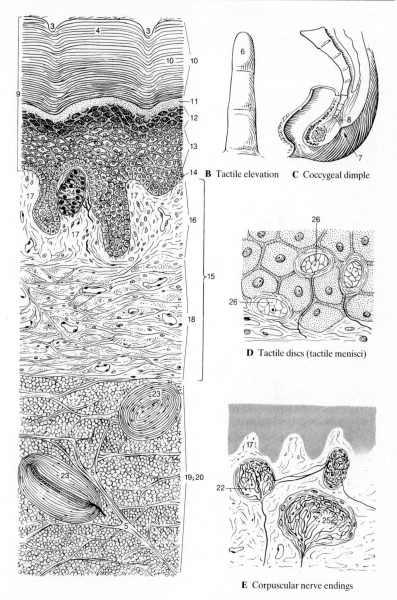

B Tactile elevation

C Coccygeal dimple

D Tactile discs (tactile menisci)

E Corpuscular nerve endings

A Skin and subcutaneous layer

1 **Pili.** Collective term for any type of filamentous appendage (hairs).

2 **Lanugo.** Fine woolly hair which is distributed over the entire body, especially in the newborn. It usually lacks a medulla.

3 **Scalp hairs.** Capilli.

4 **Hairs of eyebrow.** Supercilia.

5 **Eyelashes.** Cilia.

6 **Hairs of beard.** Barba.

7 **Hairs of external acoustic meatus.** Tragi.

8 **Hairs at the external nares.** Vibrissae.

9 **Axillary hairs.** Hirci.

10 **Pubic hairs.** Pubes.

11 **Hair follicle.** Folliculus pili. Connective tissue-epithelium covering of the hair root. A

12 **Hair papilla.** Papilla pili. Connective tissue papilla which projects into the bulb-like, distended, lowermost part of the hair root. A

13 **Hair shaft.** Scapus pili. It projects out from the skin. A

14 **Hair root.** Radix pili. A

15 **Bulb of hair.** Bulbus pili. Bulb-like enlargement at the lower end of the hair root. A

16 **Mm. arrectores pilorum.** Bundles of smooth muscle passing from the middle of the hair follicle to the papillary layer of the dermis. They are absent on hair of eyelashes, eyebrows, nose, ear and beard. Function: erect hairs (goose-pimples), probably also compression and emptying of sebaceous glands. Innervation: Sympathetic fibers from the sympathetic ganglion. A

17 **Hair streams.** Flumina pilorum. Orientational patterns of hair. B

18 **Whorled pattern of hair growth.** Vortices pilorum. B

19 **Cruciate pattern of hair growth.** Cruces pilorum. It is found at sites where the hair patterns meet one another from two directions and then go out into two new directions perpendicular to each other. B

20 **Nails.** Unguis. Fingernails and toenails. C D

21 **Nail matrix (bed).** Matrix unguis. Tissue (epidermis) upon which the nail rests (root and lunula). Nail substance is formed in the region of the lunula. D E

22 **Crests of nail matrix.** Cristae matricis unguis. Longitudinal ridges in nail bed. E

23 **Nail groove (fold).** Sulcus matricis unguis. Cutaneous slit into which the lateral nasal margins are embedded. C

24 **Nail sinus.** Sinus unguis. Deep furrow into which the root of the nail is inserted. D

25 **Wall of nail.** Vallum unguis. Cutaneous fold overlapping the sides and proximal end of the nail. C D

26 **Body of nail.** Corpus unguis. C D E

27 **Root of nail.** [[Radix unguis]]. Part of nail situated in the nail sinus. D

28 **Lunula.** Crescentic, whitish field at the posterior wall of the nail. Its anterior margin corresponds to the anterior border of the nail-forming tissue. C

29 **Margo occultus.** Proximal, posterior margin of the nail located in the depth of the nail sinus. D

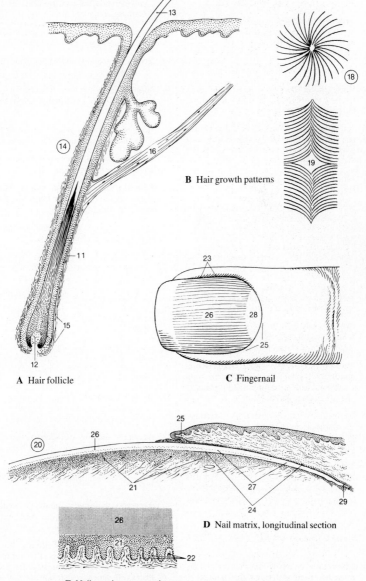

A Hair follicle

B Hair growth patterns

C Fingernail

D Nail matrix, longitudinal section

E Nail matrix, cross section

1 **Lateral margin.** Margo lateralis. Lateral margin of nail lying beneath the nail wall. B

2 **Free margin.** Margo liber. Anterior, free margin of nail. It corresponds to the abrasive or cutting edge of the nail. B

3 **Perionyx.** Projecting edge of the eponychium covering the proximal strip of the lunula. A

4 **Eponychium.** Epithelium lying on the root of the nail. It is pushed forward somewhat from the posterior nail wall. A

5 **Hyponychium.** Epithelium of nail bed located beneath the nail. Its posterior portion in the region of the lunula and nail root form the matrix. A

6 **Stratum corneum unguis.** Part of nail already cornified. A

7 **Stratum germinativum unguis.** Layer of nail bed epithelium still undergoing cell proliferation. A

8 **[[Retinacula unguis]].** Anchoring tracts of connective tissue extending from the nail bed to the periosteum of the nail segment. A

9 **Cutaneous glands.** Glandulae cutis. Glands arising from the epidermis and standing in close relationship to the skin.

10 **Sweat glands.** [[Gll. glomiformes]]. Collective term for the small eccrine sweat glands and the large apocrine sweat or odoriferous glands.

11 **Eccrine (merocrine) sweat (sudoriferous)**
~ **glands.** Gll. sudorifer merocrina (eccrina). Contrasted with apocrine sweat glands of the anal, genital and axillary regions. E

12 **Terminal secretory part.** Portio terminalis. Coiled, secretory body of the sweat gland. It lies in the subcutaneous tissue or in the deep portion of the dermis. E F

13 **Sweat gland duct.** Ductus sudorifer. Excretory duct passing to the surface. It is shaped like a corkscrew within the strongly cornified squamous epithelium of thick skin and opens on the ridges. E F

14 **Pore of sweat gland.** Porus sudorifer. Opening of excretory duct of sweat gland on the skin. E

15 **Circumanal glands.** Gll. circumanales. Large apocrine sweat glands grouped around the anus.

16 **Ceruminous glands.** Gll. ceruminosae. Apocrine, so-called ear wax glands secreting a proteinaceous material.

17 **Sebaceous glands.** Gll. sebaceae. Holocrine glands opening into the hair follicles. F

18 **Breast.** Mamma. It consists of glandular tissue, connective tissue tracts and fat. D

19 **Nipple.** Papilla mammae. It contains openings of the lactiferous ducts and is rich in smooth muscle. D

20 **Body of mammary gland.** Corpus mammae. Glandular body surrounded by adipose tissue.

21 **Mammary gland.** Glandula mammaria. Glandular tissue of female breast. D

22 **Lateral (axillary) process; axillary tail** Processus lateralis (axillaris). Glandular process extending toward the axilla.

23 Lobes of mammary gland. Lobi glandulae mammariae. 15–20 conical lobes. D

24 *Lobules of mammary gland.* Lobuli glandulae mammariae. Subdivisions of each lobe produced by connective tissue septa. D

25 Lactiferous ducts. Ductus lactiferi. Excre-
~ tory ducts, 15–20, one from each lobe. They have a diameter of 1.7–2.3 mm and open on the nipple. D

26 Lactiferous sinus. Sinus lactiferi. Spindle-shaped dilatation of the lactiferous duct with a diameter of 5–8 mm shortly before opening at the apex of the nipple. D

27 **Areola mammae.** Round, pigmented area around the nipple with a ring of small, rounded papillae produced by the areolar glands. D

28 **Areolar glands (of Montgomery).** Glandulae areolares. 10–15 apocrine glands in the region of the areola. D

29 **Male mammary gland.** Mamma masculina. Rudimentary.

30 **Accessory mammary glands.** [Mammae accessoriae]. They lie along the embryonic milk ridge. C

31 **Suspensory ligaments of breast.** Ligg. suspensoria mammaria. Tracts of connective tissue from the skin of the breast to the pectoral fascia with which they are united by a thin layer of loose displaceable tissue. D

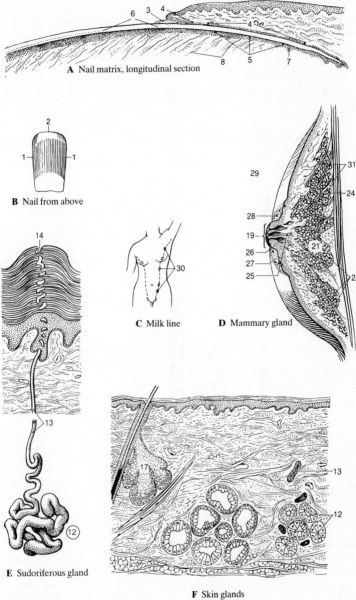

A Nail matrix, longitudinal section

B Nail from above

C Milk line

D Mammary gland

E Sudoriferous gland

F Skin glands

1   GENERAL TERMS. TERMINI GENERALES.

2   **Vertical (perpendicular).** Verticalis.

3   **Horizontal.** Horizontalis.

4   **Median.** Medianus. Lying in the midline (midsagittal plane).

5   **Coronal.** Coronalis. Lying in the plane of the coronal suture (same as frontal plane). A

6   **Sagittal.** Sagittalis. Lying in the plane of the sagittal suture. A

7   **Right.** Dexter.

8   **Left.** Sinister.

9   **Transverse.** Transversalis. Situated at right angles to the long axis of a part.

10   **Medial.** Medialis. Lying closer to the median plane.

11   **Intermediate.** Lying inbetween.

12   **Lateral.** Lateralis. Situated toward the side.

13   **Anterior.** Situated in front of.

14   **Posterior.** Situated behind.

15   **Ventral (anterior).** Ventralis. Toward the belly.

16   **Dorsal (posterior).** Dorsalis. Toward the back.

17   **Frontal.** Frontalis. 1. Pertaining to the forehead; 2. Plane separating body into front and back parts (frontal or coronal plane). A

18   **Occipital.** Occipitalis. Pertaining to the occiput.

19   **Upper.** Superior.

20   **Lower.** Inferior.

21   **Cranial.** Cranialis. Pertaining to the head; toward the head.

22   **Caudal.** Caudalis. Situated toward the tail.

23   **Rostral.** Rostralis. Located toward the rostrum of the corpus callosum.

24   **Apical.** Apicalis. Pertaining to the apex; toward the apex.

25   **Basal.** Basalis. Pertaining to the base; lying toward the base.

26   **Basilar.** Basilaris. Pertaining to the base; lying toward the base.

27   **Middle.** Medius.

28   **Transverse.** Transversus.

29   **Longitudinal.** Longitudinalis. Running longitudinally.

30   **Axialis.** Pertaining to the axis, thus the 2nd cervical vertebra; or related to an axis.

30 a   **External (outer).** Externus.

30 b   **Internal (inner).** Internus.

31   **Superficial.** Superficialis. Lying near the surface.

32   **Deep.** Profundus.

33   **Proximal.** Proximalis. Lying toward the body. B

34   **Distal.** Distalis. Lying further away from the body.

35   **Central.** Centralis. Lying in the midpoint.

36   **Peripheral.** Peripheralis. Not pertaining to the center.

36 a   **Periphery.** Periphericus.

37   **Radial.** Radialis. Pertaining to the radius and lying toward it. B

38   **Ulnar.** Ulnaris. Pertaining to the ulna and situated toward it. B

39   **Fibular.** Fibularis. Pertaining to the fibula and located on its side of the leg. B

40   **Tibial.** Tibialis. Pertaining to the tibia and its side of the leg. B

41   **Palmar.** Palmaris. Pertaining to the palmar side or lying there. B

42   **Volar.** Volaris. Same as palmar. B

43   **Plantar.** Plantaris. Pertaining to the sole of the foot and lying there. B

44   **Flexor.** A muscle that bends (flexes) a joint.

45   **Extensor.** A muscle that straightens (extends) a joint.

46   REGIONS AND PARTS OF THE BODY. REGIONES ET PARTES CORPORIS.

47   **Anterior median line.** Linea mediana anterior. Vertical plane through the middle of the trunk. C

48   **Sternal line.** Linea sternalis. It lies at the lateral margin of the sternum. C

49   **Parasternal line.** Linea parasternalis. Vertical line midway between the sternal and midclavicular lines. C

50   **Midclavicular (mammary) line.** Linea medioclavicularis. Vertical line passing through the halfway point of the clavicle. C

51   **Mammary line.** Linea mamillaris. Same as midclavicular line. C

52   **Anterior axillary line.** Linea axillaris anterior. It lies at the anterior fold of the axilla. C

53   **Axillary (midaxillary) line.** Linea axillaris media. It lies in the middle between the anterior and posterior axillary lines. C

54   **Posterior axillary line.** Linea axillaris posterior. It lies at the posterior fold of the axilla. B C

55   **Scapular line.** Linea scapularis. A vertical line through the inferior angle of the scapula. B

56   **Paravertebral line.** Linea paravertebralis. Vertical line through the ends of the transverse processes demonstrable only in radiograms. B

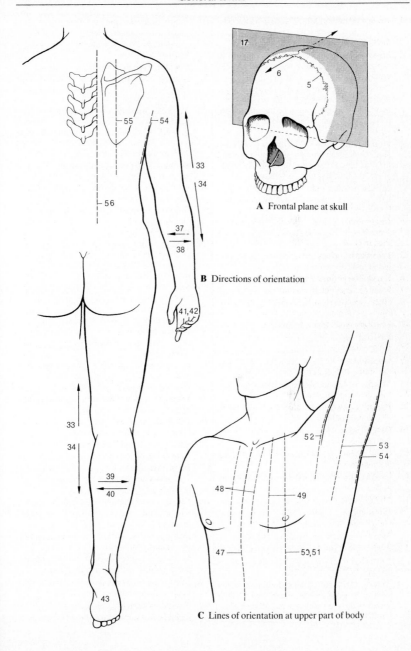

A Frontal plane at skull

B Directions of orientation

C Lines of orientation at upper part of body

1 **Posterior median line.** Linea mediana posterior. Vertical line through the median plane of the posterior trunk. B

2 **Subcostal plane.** Planum subcostale. Transverse plane through the lower edge of the 10th costal cartilage. C

3 **Transpyloric plane.** Planum transpyloricum. Horizontal plane transecting the trunk halfway between the upper margin of the pubic symphysis and the upper margin of the manubrium sterni. C

4 **Supracristal plane.** Planum supracristale. Horizontal plane through the highest point of the iliac crest. It transects the vertebral column at the level of the spinous process of L4. C

5 **Intertubercular plane.** Planum intertubercular. Transverse plane through the iliac tubercle. C

6 **Interspinal plane.** Planum interspinale. Transverse plane through the anterior superior iliac spine. C

7 **Preaxillary line.** Linea praeaxillaris. Not found in the literature at our disposal.

8 **Postaxillary line.** Linea postaxillaris. Not found in the literature at our disposal.

9 **Head regions.** Regiones capitis. Topographical fields in the head.

10 **Frontal region.** Regio frontalis. A

11 **Parietal region.** Regio parietalis. It lies over the parietal bone. A B

12 **Occipital region.** Regio occipitalis. It lies over the occipital bone. A B

13 **Temporal region.** Regio temporalis. It lies over the temporal bone. A B

14 **Facial regions.** Regiones faciales. Topogra-
~ phical areas of the face. A

15 **Orbital region.** Regio orbitalis. Area covering the orbit. A

16 **Nasal region.** Regio nasalis. Region covering the nose. A

17 **Oral region.** Regio oralis. Area around the mouth. A

18 **Mental region.** Regio mentalis. Chin area. A

19 **Infraorbital region.** Regio infraorbitalis. Field below the orbit. A

20 **Buccal region.** Regio buccalis. Cheek area. A

21 **Zygomatic region.** Regio zygomatica. A

22 **Cervical regions.** Regiones cervicales. Topographical fields of the neck.

23 **Anterior triangle of neck.** Regio cervicalis anterior (trigonum cervical anterius). Region between the midline and the sternocleidomastoid muscle.

24 **Submandibular (digastric) triangle.** Trigonum submandibulare. Field bounded by the inferior border of the mandible and the two bellies of the digastric. A

25 **Carotid triangle.** Trigonum caroticum. Triangle between the sternocleidomastoid, posterior belly of the digastric and the superior belly of the omohyoid. A

26 **Muscular (inferior carotid) triangle.** Trigonum musculare (omotracheale). Triangle between the anterior median line of neck, anterior margin of sternocleidomastoid and superior belly of the omohyoid. A

27 **Submental (suprahyoid) triangle.** Trigonum submentale. Triangle below the chin between the hyoid bone and the anterior belly of the digastric of each side. A

28 **Sternocleidomastoid region.** Regio sternocleidomastoidea. It lies on the sternocleidomastoid muscle. A

29 **Lesser supraclavicular fossa.** Fossa supraclavicularis minor. Triangular depression between the sternal and clavicular origins of the sternocleidomastoid. A

30 **Posterior triangle of neck.** Regio cervicalis lateralis (trigonum cervicale posterius). Triangle between the clavicle, anterior margin of the trapezius and posterior border of the sternocleidomastoid. A

31 **Supraclavicular (omoclavicular, subclavian) triangle.** Trigonum omoclaviculare (Fossa supraclavicular major) greater supraclavicular fossa. Triangle between the clavicle, sternocleidomastoid and omohyoid. A

32 **Posterior region of the neck (nuchal region).** Regio cervicalis posterior (Regio nuchalis). B

33 **Pectoral regions.** Regiones pectorales. Collective term for the following:

34 **Presternal region.** Regio presternalis. Area in front of the sternum. C

35 **Infraclavicular fossa.** Fossa infraclavicularis.
~ Depression produced by the clavipectoral triangle. C

36 **Clavipectoral triangle.** Trigonum clavipectorale. Triangle between the deltoid, pectoralis major and clavicle. C

37 **Pectoral region.** Regio pectoralis. Area on the pectoralis major muscle. C

38 **Mammary region.** Regio mammaria. Region corresponding to the mammary gland. C

39 **Inframammary region.** Regio inframammaria. Field below the mammary region. C

40 **Axillary region.** Regio axillaris. C

41 **Axillary fossa.** Fossa axillaris. C

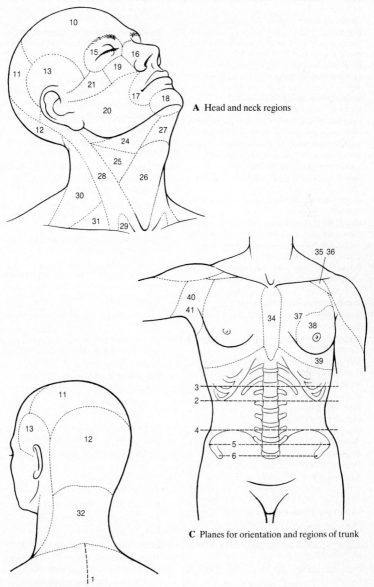

A Head and neck regions

B Head and nuchal regions

C Planes for orientation and regions of trunk

1 ABDOMINAL REGIONS. REGIONES ABDOMINALES.

2 **Hypochondriac region (hypochondrium).** Regio hypochondriaca (hypochondrium). Region lateral to midclavicular line between the pectoral region and the transpyloric plane. B

3 **Epigastric region (epigastrium).** Regio epigastrica (epigastrium). Field medial to the midclavicular line between the pectoral region and the transpyloric plane. B

4 **Lumbar (lateral) region.** Regio lateralis. Field lateral to the midclavicular line between the transpyloric and intertubercular planes. B

5 **Umbilical region.** Regio umbilicalis. Area medial to the midclavicular line between the transpyloric and intertubercular planes. B

6 **Inguinal (iliac) region.** Regio inguinalis. Region lateral to the midclavicular line between the intertubercular plane and the inguinal ligament. B

7 **Hypogastric (pubic) region.** Regio pubica (hypogastrium). Field medial to the midclavicular line between the intertubercular plane and the inguinal ligament. B

8 **Posterior (dorsal) regions.** Regiones dorsales. Topographical fields of the back.

9 **Vertebral region.** Regio vertebralis. Band over the vertebral column. A

10 **Sacral region.** Regio sacralis. It lies over the sacrum. A

11 **Scapular region.** Regio scapularis. It lies over the scapula. A

12 **Infrascapular region.** Regio infrascapularis. Area between the scapular region and the lumbar region. A

13 **Region cranial to the iliac crest.** Regio lumbaris (lumbalis). A

14 **Lumbar (Petit's) trigone.** Trigonum lumbare [[Petiti]]. Triangle above the iliac crest between the margins of the latissimus dorsi and external abdominal oblique.

15 **Perineal region.** Regio perinealis. C

16 **Anal region.** Regio analis. Area around the anus. It is bordered anteriorly by an imaginary line going through both ischial tuberosities. C

17 **Urogenital region.** Regio urogenitalis. Perineal area in front of the imaginary line between both ischial tuberosities. C

18 REGIONS OF UPPER LIMB. REGIONES MEMBRI SUPERIORIS.

19 **Deltoid region.** Regio deltoidea. It lies on the deltoid muscle. B

20 **Upper arm.** Brachium.

21 **Anterior brachial region.** Regio (facies) brachialis anterior. Anterior surface of upper arm. B

22 **Posterior brachial region.** Regio (facies) brachialis posterior. Posterior surface of upper arm. A

23 **Elbow.** Cubitus.

24 **Anterior cubital region.** Regio (facies) cubitalis anterior. Anterior surface of elbow. B

25 **Posterior cubital region.** Regio (facies) cubitalis posterior. Posterior surface of elbow. A

26 **Cubital fossa.** Fossa cutibalis. B

27 **Lateral bicipital groove.** Sulcus bicipitalis lateralis (radialis). B

28 **Medial bicipital groove.** Sulcus bicipitalis medialis (ulnaris). B

29 **Forearm.** Antebrachium.

30 **Anterior antebrachial region.** Regio (facies) antebrachialis anterior. Anterior surface of forearm. A B

31 **Posterior antebrachial region.** Regio (facies) antebrachialis posterior. Posterior surface of forearm. A B

32 **Lateral margin.** Margo lateralis (radialis).

33 **Medial margin.** Margo medialis (ulnaris).

34 **Wrist.** Carpus.

35 **Anterior carpal region.** Regio carpalis anterior. Anterior of flexor side of wrist. A

36 **Posterior carpal region.** Regio carpalis posterior. Posterior or extensor side of wrist. B

37 **Hand.** Manus.

38 **Dorsum of hand.** Dorsum manus. B

39 **Palm of hand.** Palma manus. A

40 **Thenar eminence.** Thenar (eminentia thenaris). Ball of thumb.

41 **Hypothenar eminence.** Hypothenar (eminentia hypothenaris). Ball of little finger.

42 **Metacarpus.** Part of hand between wrist and digits.

43 **Digits (fingers).** Digiti.

44 **Thumb.** Pollex (digitus primus (I)).

45 **Index finger.** Index (digitus secundus (II)).

46 **Middle finger.** Digitus medius (tertius (III)).

47 **Ring finger.** Digitus anularis (quartus IV)).

48 **Little finger.** Digitus minimus (quintus (V)).

49 **Ventral (palmar, flexor) side of fingers.** Facies digitales ventrales (palmares).

50 **Dorsal (extensor) side of fingers.** Facies digitales dorsales.

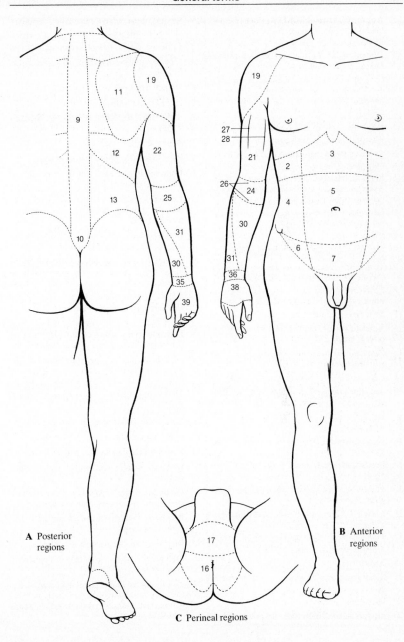

A Posterior regions

B Anterior regions

C Perineal regions

1 **Regions of lower limb.** Regiones membri inferioris. Topographical fields of the lower limb.

2 **Gluteal region.** Regio glutealis. Area over the gluteal musculature. A

3 **Gluteal fold.** Sulcus glutealis. Crease passing over the gluteus maximus and bordering the buttocks inferiorly when the hip joint is extended. A

3 a **Hip joint.** Coxa (Regio coxalis).

4 **Thigh.** Femur (Regio femoralis).

5 **Anterior thigh region.** Regio (Facies) femoralis anterior. B

6 **Femoral triangle.** Trigonum femorale. It lies in the groin and is bordered by the inguinal ligament, sartorius and adductor longus. B

7 **Posterior thigh region.** Regio (facies) femoralis posterior. A

8 **Knee.** Genus.

9 Anterior side of knee. Regio genus anterior. B

10 Posterior side of knee. Regio genus posterior. A

11 **Popliteal fossa.** Fossa poplitea. A

12 **Lower leg.** Crus.

13 **Anterior surface of lower leg.** Regio (Facies) cruralis anterior. B

14 **Posterior surface of lower leg.** Regio (Facies) cruralis posterior. A

15 **Calf.** Sura (Regio suralis). A

16 **Anterior and posterior talocrural (malleolar) regions.** Regiones talocrurales anterior et posterior.

17 **Foot.** Pes.

18 **Heel (calcaneal region).** Calx (Regio calcanea). A

19 **Dorsum of foot.** Dorsum (Regio dorsalis) pedis. B

20 **Plantar surface of foot (sole).** Planta (Regio plantaris) pedis. A

21 **Lateral (fibular, outer) margin of foot.** Margo lateralis (fibularis) pedis.

22 **Medial (tibial, inner) margin of foot.** Margo medialis (tibialis) pedis.

23 **Ankle.** Tarsus.

24 **Metatarsus.** Part of foot between ankle and toes.

25 **Toes.** Digiti.

26 **Big (great) toe.** Hallux (Digitus primus (I)).

27 **Second, third, fourth toes.** Digiti secundus, tertius, quartus (II, III, IV).

28 **Little toe.** Digitus minimus (quintus) (V).

28 a **Plantar (under) surface of toe.** Facies digitalis plantaris.

28 b **Dorsal surface of toe.** Facies digitalis dorsalis.

29 OSTEOLOGY. OSTEOLOGIA.

30 SKELETAL SYSTEM. SYSTEMA SKELETALE.

31 **Bony part.** Pars ossea.

32 **Periosteum.** External covering of bone.

33 **Endosteum.** Internal lining of bone. It also lines the marrow cavity.

34 **Cortical substance.** Substantia corticalis. Superficial layer formed by the external main lamellae of bone.

35 **Compact bone.** Substantia compacta. Dense bony substance formed by osteons.

36 **Spongy (trabecular) bone.** Substantia spongiosa (trabecularis). Loosely organized bone substance with interstices occupied by bone marrow.

37 **Cartilaginous part (of the skeleton).** Pars cartilaginosa.

38 **Perichondrium.** Connective tissue covering of cartilage. It contributes to cartilage growth.

39 AXIAL SKELETON. SKELETON AXIALE. Skeleton of the trunk.

40 APPENDICULAR SKELETON. SKELETON APPENDICULARE. Skeleton of the limbs.

41 **Long bone.** Os longum. e.g., fibula.

42 **Short bone.** Os breve. e.g., wrist bone.

43 **Flat bone.** Os planum. e.g., parietal bone.

44 **Irregular bone.** Os irregulare. e.g., spenoid bone.

45 **Pneumatic bone.** Os pneumaticum. Bone with air-containing cells, e.g., ethmoid bone.

46 **Epiphysis.** End of a long bone temporarily involved in bone growth.

47 **Diaphysis.** Middle piece (shaft) of bone.

48 **Metaphysis.** Bony region between epiphysis and diaphysis.

49 **Epiphysial cartilage.** Cartilago epiphysialis. Cartilage zone between the diaphysis and epiphysis. It is responsible for the growth in length of long bones.

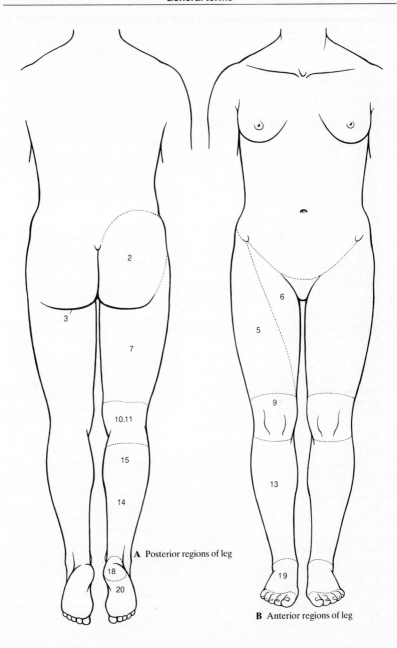

A Posterior regions of leg

B Anterior regions of leg

1 **Epiphysial line.** Linea epiphysialis. Line visible in radiograms and in sections of bone marking the former site of the epiphysial cartilage.

2 **Joint surface.** Facies articularis.

3 **Medullary cavity.** Cavitas medullaris.

4 **Yellow bone marrow.** Medulla ossium flava. It contains abundant fat.

5 **Red bone marrow.** Medulla ossium rubra. It is hemopoietic.

6 **Nutrient foramen.** Foramen nutriens. Macroscopic foramen for blood vessels nourishing mainly the bone marrow.

7 **Nutrient canal.** Canalis nutriens. Canal continuous with the nutrient foramen.

8 **Center of ossification.** Centrum ossificationis. Site of the onset of ossification in bones preformed in cartilage (endochondral ossification).

9 **Primary center of ossification.** Centrum ossificationis primarium. It forms in the diaphysis (diaphysial ossification).

10 **Secondary center of ossification.** Centrum ossificationis secondarium. It develops in the epiphysis (epiphysial ossification).

11 ARTHROLOGY. ARTHROLOGIA. Study of joints.

12 **Fibrous joints.** Articulationes fibrosae. They usually have no direct relationship to an articular cavity.

13 **Syndesmosis.** Fibrous joint with interosseous membrane or ligament.

14 **Suture.** Sutura.

15 **Dentate suture.** Sutura serrata. Serrated Suture. e.g., lambdoid suture.

16 **Squamous suture.** Sutura squamosa. e.g., at the temporal bone.

17 **Flat suture.** Sutura plana. Bony union with smooth surfaces, e.g., between zygomatic and maxilla.

18 **Schindylesis.** Union between a groove in one bone and a ridge in the other e.g. between the vomer and sphenoid.

19 CARTILAGINOUS JOINTS. ARTICULATIONES CARTILAGINEAE.

20 **Synchondrosis.** Bony union by means of hyaline cartilage.

21 **Symphysis.** Bony union, partly by means of fibrocartilage.

22 SYNOVIAL JOINTS. ARTICULATIONES SYNOVIALES. Bony union with an intervening articular cavity.

23 **Simple joint.** Articulatio simplex. It occurs between only two bones, e.g., hip joint.

24 **Composite joint.** Articulatio composita (complexa). Joint involving more than two bones, e.g., wrist joint.

25 **Plane joint.** Articulatio plana. Joint with almost smooth articular surfaces.

26 **Spheroidal joint.** Articulatio sphaeroidea (cotylica). Ball and socket joint, e.g., shoulder joint.

27 **Ellipsoidal (condylar) joint.** Articulatio ellipsoidea (condylaris). It has two axes, e.g., wrist joint.

28 **Hinge joint.** Ginglymus. It has one axis, e.g., elbow joint.

29 **Bicondylar joint.** Articulatio bicondylaris. Articulation with one main transverse axis and another axis in the longitudinal direction of a skeletal part, e.g., knee joint.

30 **Trochoidal joint.** Articulatio trochoidea. Pivot joint with one axis, e.g., radio-ulnar joint.

31 **Saddle (sellar) joint.** Articulatio sellaris. It has two axes, e.g., metacarpophalangeal joint of thumb.

32 **Ovoidal joint.** [[Articulatio ovoidalis]]. Joint with only weakly curved articular surfaces.

33 **Articular cartilage.** Cartilago articularis.

34 **Articular cavity.** Cavitas articularis. Joint cavity.

35 **Articular disc.** Discus articularis. It divides the joint cavity into two separate chambers.

36 **Meniscus.** Meniscus articularis. Ring-like articular disc, e.g., in the knee joint.

37 **Articular lip.** Labrum articulare. Rim of cartilage at the margin of a socket.

38 **Joint capsule.** Capsula articularis.

39 **Fibrous membrane.** Membrana fibrosa (Stratum fibrosum). Connective tissue layer of the capsule often reinforced by ligaments.

40 **Synovial membrane.** Membrana synovialis (Stratum synoviale). Inner layer of articular capsule lined by epithelioid connective tissue cells.

41 *Synovial fold.* Plica synovialis. Fold projecting from the capsule into the joint space.

42 *Synovial villi.* Villi synoviales.

43 **Synovia.** Synovial fluid secreted by the synovial membrane of the capsule.

44 **Articular ligaments.** Ligamenta.

45 **Extracapsular ligaments.** Ligamenta extracapsularia. They lie outside of the capsular wall, e.g. external collateral ligament of knee joint.

46 **Capsular ligaments.** Ligamenta capsularia. Reinforcing fibers residing in the capsule, e.g. collateral ligaments of the interphalangeal joints.

47 **Intracapsular ligaments.** Ligamenta intracapsularis. They are located within the joint space, e.g. cruciate ligaments of knee joint.

1 MYOLOGY. MYOLOGIA. Study of muscles.

2 **Muscle.** Musculus.

3 **Head.** Caput.

4 **Belly.** Venter.

5 **Fusiform muscle.** Musculus fusiformis. Spindle-shaped muscle.

6 **Quadrate muscle.** M. quadratus. Square-shaped muscle.

7 **Triangular muscle.** M. triangularis. Triangular-shaped muscle.

8 **Unipennate muscle.** M. unipennatus. Muscle fibers approach the tendon from one side.

9 **Bipennate muscle.** M. bipennatus. Muscle fibers approach the tendon from two sides.

10 **Multipennate muscle.** M. multipennatus. Muscle fibers approach tendon from many sides.

11 **Sphincter muscle.** M. sphincter.

11 a **Dilator muscle.** M. dilator (dilatator).

12 **Orbicular muscle.** M. orbicularis. Circular muscle.

13 **Cruciate muscle.** M. cruciatus. Its fibers cross.

14 **Articular muscle.** [[M. articularis]]. Muscle which attaches to a joint capsule.

15 **Skeletal muscle.** M. skeleti. Muscle with attachment to the skeleton in contrast to a cutaneous muscle.

16 **Cutaneous muscle.** M. cutaneus.

17 **Tendon.** Tendo.

18 **Tendon (synovial) sheath.** Vagina tendinis. Lubricated sheath for easy gliding of tendon.

19 **Fibrous layer.** Stratum fibrosum. Outer, connective tissue portion of tendon sheath.

20 **Synovial layer.** Stratum synoviale. Inner, smooth layer of tendon sheath. It secretes synovial fluid.

20 a **Synovial sheath of tendon.** Vagina synovialis tendinis.

21 **Mesotendineum.** Mesentery-like connection between tendon and tendon sheath. It carries blood vessels to the tendon.

22 **Peritendineum.** Connective tissue at the surface of a tendon.

23 **Aponeurosis.** Flat tendinous expansion.

23 a **Epimysium.** Fibrous sheath enveloping an entire muscle.

24 **Perimysium.** Fibrous sheath enclosing a bundle of muscle fibers.

25 **Endomysium.** Fibrous sheath surrounding a single muscle fiber enclosed by sarcolemma.

26 **Fascia.** External sheath of one or several muscles.

26 a **Superficial fascia.** Fascia superficialis. Annot. p. 409

26 b **Deep fascia.** Fascia profunda.

27 **Tendinous intersections.** Intersectio tendinea.

27 a **Intermediate tendon.** Tendo intermedius.

28 **Tendinous arch.** Arcus tendineus. It serves for the origin of muscle fibers.

29 **Muscular trochlea.** Trochlea muscularis. Skeletal part serving to support a muscle as it changes the direction of pull of its tendon, e. g., tendon of flexor hallucis longus at the sustentaculum tali.

30 SYNOVIAL BURSAE. BURSAE SYNOVIALES.

31 **Subcutaneous bursa.** Bursa [synovialis] subcutanea. It lies directly beneath the skin.

32 **Submuscular bursa.** Bursa [synovialis] submuscularis. It lies beneath a muscle.

33 **Subfascial bursa.** Bursa [synovialis] subfascialis. It lies beneath a fascia.

34 **Subtendinous bursa.** Bursa [synovialis] subtendinea. It lies beneath a tendon.

35 SPLANCHNOLOGY. SPLANCHNOLOGIA. Study of viscera.

36 **GENERAL TERMS.** NOMINA GENERALIA.

37 **Tunica albuginea.** Tough, whitish connective tissue sheath.

38 **Tunica fibrosa.** Fine connective tissue layer.

39 Tunica adventitia. Outermost connective tissue covering.

40 **Tunica mucosa.** Mucous membrane with its layers.

41 **Epithelium mucosae.** Epithelial cell layer of the mucosa.

42 **Lamina propria mucosae.** Lamina propria of the mucosa. Layer of reticular connective tissue extending up to the muscularis mucosae.

43 **Lamina muscularis mucosae.** Layer of smooth muscle fibers between the lamina propria and submucosa. It acts upont the mucosa.

44 **Tela submucosa.** Layer of collagenous and elastic fibers between the muscularis mucosae and the muscularis. It is the main bearer of blood vessels.

45 **Tunica muscularis.** Double layer of smooth muscle.

46 **Stratum circulare.** Circular muscle layer.

47 **Stratum longitudinale.** Longitudinal muscle layer.

48 **Tunica serosa.** Outer layer of intestinal tract wall covered by peritoneum. It glistens because of its smooth surface.

1 **Tela subserosa.** Connective tissue substrate for the serosal (peritoneal) epithelium.

2 **Parenchyma.** Specific functional elements of an organ.

3 **Stroma.** Connective tissue supporting framework of an organ.

4 **Gland.** Glandula.

5 **Lobe.** Lobus.

6 **Lobule.** Lobulus.

7 **Mucous gland.** Glandula mucosa.

8 **Serous gland.** Glandula serosa. It produces a thin, fluid secretion.

9 **Seromucous gland.** Glandula seromucosa. Mixed gland with mucous and serous secretions.

10 ANGIOLOGY. ANGIOLOGIA. Study of vessels.

11 **Arteriovenous anastomosis.** Anastomosis arteriolovenularis (arteriovenosa). Direct connection between an artery and vein.

12 **Artery.** Arteria.

13 **Nutrient artery.** Arteria nutricia (nutriens). It supplies tissues with nutrients.

14 **Arteriole.** Arteriola. Small artery directly preceding a capillary.

15 **Arterial circle.** Circulus arteriosus. Circle of anastomosing arteries.

16 **Circular connection of vessels.** Circulus vasculosus.

17 **Cistern.** Cisterna. Dilatation of a lymphatic vessel.

18 **Blood.** Haema (hema).

19 **Lymph.** Lympha.

20 **Nervi vasorum.** Nerves innervating the wall of blood vessels.

21 **Lymph node.** Nodus lymphaticus (Lymphonodus).

22 **Lymphatic nodule (follicle).** Nodulus (folliculus) lymphaticus. Circular mass of lymphocytes.

23 **Lymphatic plexus.** Plexus lymphaticus.

24 **Vascular plexus.** Plexus vasculosus.

25 **Venous plexus.** Plexus venosus.

26 **Arterial plexus.** Plexus arteriosum.

27 **Rete mirabile.** Two capillary networks lying one after another.

28 **Rete vasculosum articulare.** Network of anastomosing blood vessels around a joint.

29 **Rete venosum.** Venous network.

30 **Sinus venosus.** Venous segment devoid of a typical venous wall.

31 **Tunica externa.** Outer layer of a blood vessel wall.

32 **Tunica intima.** Inner layer of a blood vessel wall.

35 **Tunica media.** Middle layer of a blood vessel wall.

34 **Valve.** Valva. Large flap.

35 **Lymphatic valve.** Valvula lymphatica. Valve in lymphatic vessels.

36 **Valve of veins.** Valvula venosa.

37 **Anastomotic vessel.** Vas anastomoticum.

38 **Capillary.** Vas capillare.

39 **Collateral vessel.** Vas collaterale. Parallel-coursing accessory vessel.

40 **Lymphatic vessel.** Vas lymphaticum.

41 **Sinusoid.** Vas sinusoideum. Special, thin-walled vascular segment with a large lumen.

42 **Vasa vasorum.** Blood vessels supplying the walls of blood vessels.

43 **Vein.** Vena.

44 **Accompanying vein.** Vena comitans.

45 **Cutaneous vein.** Vena cutanea.

46 **Emissary vein.** Vena emissaria. Vein passing externally through foramen in the skull.

47 **Deep vein.** Vena profunda. It lies below the fascia.

48 **Superficial vein.** Vena superficialis. Cutaneous vein lying on the fascia of the limbs.

49 **Venule.** Venula. Small vein directly following capillaries.

50 CENTRAL NERVOUS SYSTEM. SYSTEMA NERVOSUM CENTRALE. It comprises the brain and spinal cord.

51 **Gray matter (nuclei and columns).** Substantia grisea [Nuclei et columnae]. It consists of an accumulation of nerve cell bodies and is gray because only a sparse amount of medullary sheath material (myelin) is present in it.

52 **White matter.** Substantia alba [Tractus et fasciculi]. It is present in the tracts and conduction bundles.

53 **Reticular formation.** Formatio (Substantia) reticularis. Scarcely definable mixture of cells and fibers, among others, with influence on movements, circulation and respiration as well as the sleeping-waking rhythm.

54 **Substantia gelatinosa.** Glia-rich, weakly stained zone at the apex of the posterior horn of the spinal cord. It serves afferent tracts.

55 **Ependyma.** Cellular lining of the cavities of the central nervous system.

1 PERIPHERAL NERVOUS SYSTEM. PARS PERIPHERICA (SYSTEM NERVOSUM PERIPHERICUM). It begins at the surface of the brain and spinal cord.

2 **Nerve.** Nervus.

3 **Endoneurium.** Delicate connective tissue sheath attaching directly to the basement membrane of an individual nerve fiber.

4 **Perineurium.** Connective tissue sheath enclosing a bundle of nerve fibers.

5 **Epineurium.** External connective tissue sheath of a nerve.

6 **Afferent nerve fibers.** Neurofibrae afferentes. Nerve fibers travelling into the central nervous system.

7 **Efferent nerve fibers.** Neurofibrae efferentes. Nerve fibers passing out of the central nervous system.

8 **Somatic nerve fibers.** Neurofibrae somaticae. They stand in contrast to autonomic, i.e. visceral nerves.

9 Autonomic (visceral) nerve fibers. Neurofibrae autonomicae (viscerales). Fibers of visceral nerves.

10 **Ganglion.** An accumulation of nerve cell bodies and thus a macroscopic thickening of a nerve.

11 **Capsule of ganglion.** Capsula ganglii (ganglionica). It is composed of connective tissue.

12 **Stroma of ganglion.** Stroma ganglii (ganglionicum). Internal connective tissue of a ganglion.

13 **Craniospinal (sensory) ganglia.** Ganglia craniospinalia (encephalospinalia sensoria). Collective term for the following two special cases.

14 **Spinal ganglia (sensory).** Ganglia spinalia (sensoria). Dorsal root ganglia.

15 **Sensory ganglia of cranial nerves.** Ganglia sensoria neuricum cranialium (gg. encephalica). Spinal ganglia equivalent of cranial nerves.

16 **Autonomic (visceral) ganglia.** Ganglia autonomica (visceralia). Ganglia of visceral nerves.

17 **Preganglionic nerve fibers.** Neurofibrae praeganglionicae. Myelinated nerve fibers passing to the ganglia of the visceral nerves.

18 **Postganglionic nerve fibers.** Neurofibrae postganglionicae. Nonmyelinated nerve fibers passing from the visceral ganglia to the viscera.

19 **Sympathetic ganglion.** Ganglion sympatheticum (sympathicum). Represented mainly by the sympathetic trunk, among others.

20 White ramus communicans. Ramus communicans alba. Connection between the spinal nerve and sympathetic trunk. It appears white on account of its myelinated preganglionic fibers.

21 Gray ramus communicans. Ramus communicans griseus. Connection between the sympathetic trunk and spinal nerve. It contains postganglionic, nonmyelinated fibers and therefore appears gray.

22 **Parasympathetic ganglion.** Gangion parasympatheticum (parasympathicum). See 348, 28–35.

23 **Spinal nerves.** Nervi spinales. They arise from the union of dorsal and ventral roots.

24 **Plexus of spinal nerves.** Plexus nervorum spinalium. It is present in the cervical, lumbar and sacral regions and gives rise to the nerves for the limbs.

1 **Cranial nerves.** Nervi craniales (encephalici). The fact that they leave the cerebrospinal covered expanse through foramina in the base of the skull defines these nerves.

2 **Cranial nerve nuclei.** Nuclei nervorum cranialium (encephalicorum).

3 Nuclei of origin. Nuclei originis. They give rise to the efferent, mostly motor, nerve fibers.

4 Nuclei of termination. Nuclei terminationis. Sensory nuclei where the afferent nerve fibers terminate and synapse with a second neuron.

5 **Mixed nerve.** Nervus mixtus (N. mixtarum neurofibrarum). Considered as a nerve containing both motor and sensory fibers, it can also refer to a nerve with somatic and visceral components.

6 **Cutaneous branches.** Rami cutanei. Cutaneous nerves or also rami going to the skin.

7 **Articular branches.** Rami articulares. Nerves or nerve rami going to joints.

8 **Muscular branches.** Rami musculares. Nerves or nerve rami passing into musculature.

9 **Motor nerve.** Nervus motorius. Nerve which only has fibers for muscles. Afferent fibers, e.g., from muscle spindles, are left out of consideration in the naming of this nerve.

10 **Sensory nerve.** Nervus sensorius. It contains afferent fibers which pass into the central nervous system from peripheral receptors.

11 **Communicating branch.** Ramus communicans.

12 **Autonomic (visceral) nerve and ramus.** Nervus et ramus autonomici (viscerales). Nerves and their rami from the region of nerve supply to the viscera.

13 **Autonomic (visceral) plexus.** Plexus autonomicus (visceralis). It is situated within the organ itself.

13a **Vascular plexus.** Plexus vascularis. Nerve plexus in the wall of vessels with sensory and autonomic components.

14 Periarterial plexus. Plexus periarteriales. Nerve plexus within the adventitia of arteries.

15 Nervi vasorum. Nerves supplying blood vessels.

16 **Vasa nervorum.** Blood vessels supplying nerves.

17 NERVOUS TISSUE. TEXTUS NERVOSUS.

18 **Neuron (nerve cell).** Neuron (Neurocytus).

19 **Nerve cell body (perikaryon).** Corpus neurale. Portion of neuron containing the nucleus but excluding the cell processes.

20 **Axon (axis cylinder).** Axon (Neuritum). Usually a long process of a neuron which, together with others, form the peripheral nerves and can be either nonmyelnated or myelinated.

21 **Dendrite.** Dendritum. One of many tree-like branched processes of a neuron. In contrast to axons, it has no special sheath.

Remarks

The new terms 188.28a; 198.25a, 216.10a–e; 298.11 and 322.20a–e have been, like others in past editions, added to the international nomenclature without any commentary from the Committee. Our attemps to obtain an explanation from the responsible parties were in vain.

The meaning of the following three terms can be safely guessed:
216.10 c   A. radicularis posterior: Artery accompanying the posterior radix of the spinal nerve.
216.10 d   A. radicularis anterior: Artery accompanying the anterior radix of the spinal nerve.
216.10 e   A. medullaris segmentalis: Segmental feeder for the longitudinal arterial system.

298.11   The thalamic nuclei are referred to in many different ways in the literature. We have retained the nomenclature used in previous editions.

405.26 a   Fascia superficialis: Superficial fascia. In English-speaking countries, this is described as consisting of the subcutaneous fat and the connective tissue—in the abdomen, fascia of Camper and Scarpa's fascia.

References

1 Ahrens, G.: Naturwissenschaftliches und medizinisches Latein, 3. Aufl. Barth, Leipzig 1963

2 Alverdes, K.: Grundlagen der Anatomie, 3. Aufl. Edition Leipzig 1963

3 Arey, L. B.: Developmental Anatomy, 5. Aufl. Saunders. Philadelphia 1949

4 Bargmann, W.: Histologie und mikroskopische Anatomie des Menschen, 6. Aufl. Thieme, Stuttgart 1967; 7. Aufl. 1977

5 Benninghoff, A., K. Goerttler: Lehrbuch der Anatomie des Menschen, 7. Aufl. Urban & Schwarzenberg, München 1964

6 Boyden, E. A.: Segmental Anatomy of the Lungs. Mc Graw-Hill, New York 1955

7 Braus, H., C. Elze: Anatomie des Menschen, 2. Aufl., Springer Berlin 1960

8 Brodal, A. Neurological Anatomy, 2nd. Ed. Oxford University Press, London 1969

9 Bucher, O.: Histologie und mikroskopische Anatomie des Menschen, 4. Aufl. Huber, Bern 1965

10 Carpenter, B. M.: Human Neuroanatomy, 7th Ed. Williams & Wilkins, Baltimore 1976

11 Clara, M.: Das Nervensystem des Menschen, 3. Aufl. Barth, Leipzig 1959

12 Corning, H. K.: Lehrbuch der Topographischen Anatomie, 20. u. 21. Aufl. Bergmann, München 1942

13 Critchley, M.: Butterworths Medical Dictionary, 2nd. Ed. Butterworths, London 1980

14 Crosby, E. C., Tr. Humphrey, E. W. Lauer: Correlative Anatomy of the Nervous System. Macmillan, New York 1962

15 Cunningham, D. J.: Textbook of Anatomy, 11th Ed. Oxford University Press, London 1972

16 Curtis, A., St. Jacobsen, E. M. Marcus. An Introduction to the Neurosciences. Saunders, Philadelphia 1972

17 Denker, A., W. Albrecht: Lehrbuch der Krankheiten des Ohres und der Luftwege, 12. u. 13. Aufl. Fischer, Jena 1932

18 Donath, T.: Erläuterndes Anatomisches Wörterbuch. Terra, Budapest 1960

19 Duus, Peter: Neurologisch-topische Diagnostik. Thieme, Stuttgart 1976; 2. Aufl. 1980

20 Duvernoy, H. M.: Human Brainstem Vessels. Springer, Berlin 1978

21 Elias, H., D. Petty: Gross anatomy of the blood vessels and ducts within the human liver. Amer. J. Anat. 90 (1952) 59–111

22 Frick, H., H. Leonhardt, D. Starck: Taschenlehrbuch der gesamten Anatomie, Bd. I: Allgemeine Anatomie. Spezielle Anatomie I, 2. Aufl. Thieme, Stuttgart 1980

23 Georges, K. E.: Ausführliches lateinisch-deutsches Handwörterbuch. Hannover u. Leipzig 1913/1918

24 Gottschick, J.: Die Leistungen des Nervensystems. Fischer, Jena 1952

25 Gray, H.: Anatomy of the Human Body, 29th Ed. Lea & Febiger, Philadelphia 1973

26 Gray's Anatomy, 36th Ed. Churchill Livingstone, Edinburgh 1980

27 Guntz, M.: Nomenclature anatomique illustrée. Masson, Paris 1975

28 Hafferl, A.: Lehrbuch der topographischen Anatomie, 2. Aufl. Springer, Berlin 1957

29 Hamilton, W. J.: Textbook of Human Anatomy, Macmillan, London 1958

30 HAMILTON, W. J., J. D. BOYD, H. W. MOSSMANN: Human Embryology, 3. Aufl. Heffer, Cambridge 1962

31 HJORTSJÖ, C.-H.: The Anatomical Foundations of Liver Surgery. Karger, Basel

32 HOFF, H., G. OSLER: Neurologie auf den Grundlagen der Physiologie. Maudirch, Wien 1957

33 HOLLINDSHEAD, W. H.: Anatomy for Surgeons. Hoeber-Harper, New York 1961

34 HORSTMANN, E.: Die Haut. In Bargmann, W.: Handbuch der mikroskopischen Anatomie des Menschen, Bd. III/3. Springer, Berlin 1957

35 KÄGI, J.: Beitrag zur Topographie der A. transversa colli. Eine Untersuchung an 134 Halshälften. Anat. Anz. 107 (1959)

36 KAHLE, W., H. LEONHARDT, W. PLATZER: Taschenatlas der Anatomie, 3 Bde. Thieme, Stuttgart 1975; 3. Aufl. 1979

37 KINCAID, O. W.: Renal Angiography. Medical Publisher, Chicago 1966

38 KNESE, K. H.: Nomina Anatomica, 5. Aufl. Thieme, Stuttgart 1957

39 KOLMER, W.: Gehörorgan. In Bargmann, W.: Handbuch der mikroskopischen Anatomie des Menschen, Bd III/1. Springer, Berlin 1927

40 KRAYENBÜHL, H., M. G. YASARGIL: Zerebrale Angiographie für Klinik und Praxis, 3. Aufl. Thieme, Stuttgart 1979

41 KRIEG, W. J. S.: Functional Neuroanatomy. Blakiston, Philadelphia 1942

42 KRÜBER, G.: Der Anatomische Wortschatz, 8. Aufl. Hirzel, Leipzig 1964

43 KUBIK, S.: Klinische Anatomie Bd. III 2. Aufl. Thieme, Stuttgart 1969

44 LAZORTHES, G.: Le systeme nerveux central, 2me Ed. Masson, Paris 1973

45 LIERSE, W.: Becken. In v. Lanz Wachsmuth: Praktische Anatomie Bd. II/8 a, Springer, Berlin 1984

46 MAC NALTY, A. S.: Butterworths Medical Dictionary. Butterworths, London 1965

47 MENGE. H., GÜTHLING: Enzyklopädisches Wörterbuch, I. Teil: Griechisch-Deutsch, 13. Aufl. Langenscheidt, Berlin 1955

48 MENGE. H. GÜTHLING: Enzyklopädisches Wörterbuch, I. Teil: Lateinisch-Deutsch, 9. Aufl. Langenscheidt, Berlin 1955

49 MEYER. W.: Die Zahn-, Mund und Kieferheilkunde. Urban & Schwarzenberg, München 1955–1960

50 MORRIS, J., J. PARSONS, SCHAEFFER: Human Anatomy, 12. Aufl, Blakiston, Philadelphia 1966

51 MÜHLREITER, E.: Anatomie des menschlichen Gebisses, 5. Aufl. Felix, Leipzig 1928

52 MUMENTHALER, M., H. SCHLIACK: Läsionen peripherer Nerven. Thieme, Stuttgart 1965; 3. Aufl. 1977

53 NETTER, F. H.: The Ciba Collection of Medical Illustrations. Ciba, New York 1954

54 NEUBERT, K.: Die Basilarmembran des Menschen und ihr Verankerungssystem. Z. Anat, Entwickl.-Gesch. 114 (1949/50) 539–588

55 Nomina anatomica, 4th Ed. Excerpta Medica, Amsterdam 1977

56 OELRICH, T. M.: The striated urogenital sphincter muscle in the female. Anat. Rec. 205 (1983)

57 OLIVEROS, L. G.: Veins of the Lungs, Salamanca 1959

58 PAPE, W.: Griechisch-Deutsches Handwörterbuch, 3. Aufl. Braunschweig 1914

59 PATURET, G.: Anatomie Humaine. Bde. I, II, III. Masson, Paris 1958

60 PEELE, T. L.: The Neuroanantomic Basis for Clinical Neurology. Mc Graw-Hill, New York 1977

61 PERNKOPF, E.: Topographische Anatomie des Menschen. Urban & Schwarzenberg, München 1960

62 PLATZER, W.: Atlas der topographischen Anatomie. Thieme, Stuttgart 1982

63 POIRIER, P., A. CHARPY: D'anatomie humaine, 3. Aufl. Masson, Paris 1920

64 RANSON, St. W., S. L. CLARK: The Anatomy of the Nervous System, 10. Aufl. Saunders, Philadelphia 1964

65 RAUBER, A., F. KOPSCH: Lehrbuch und Atlas der Anatomie des Menschen, 19. Aufl. Thieme, Stuttgart 1955

66 ROHEN, J.: Die funktionelle Gestalt des Auges und seiner Hilfsorgane. Verlag der Akademie der Wissenschaften und der Literatur, Mainz, Jg. 1953, Nr. 4

67 ROHEN, J. W.: Topographische Anatomie. Schattauer, Stuttgart 1966

68 ROHEN, J. W., F. J. RENTSCH: Zur funktionellen Morphologie des Akkommodationsapparates. In: Neure Ergebnisse zur funktionellen Morphologie. Schattauer, Stuttgart 1969

69 SEEGER, W.: Atlas of Topographical Anatomy of the Brain and Surrounding Structures. Springer, Wien 1978

70 SICHER, H.: Oral Anatomy, 4. Aufl. Mosby, Saint Louis 1965

71 SIEGLBAUER, F.: Lehrbuch der normalen Anatomie des Menschen, 8. Aufl. Urban & Schwarzenberg, München 1958

72 SOBOTTA, J. H. BECHER: Atlas der Anatomie des Menschen, 16. Aufl. Urban & Schwarzenberg, München 1962

73 SPALTENHOLZ, W., R. SPANNER: Handatlas der Anatomie des Menschen, 16. Aufl. Scheltema & Holkema, Amsterdam 1961

74 STARCK, D.: Embryologie, 2. Aufl. Thieme, Stuttgart 1965; 3. Aufl. 1975

75 STEDMAN, Th. L.: Medical Dictionary, 20. Aufl. Williams & Wilkins, Baltimore 1961

76 STEPHENS, R. B., D. L. STILLWELL: Arteries and Veins of the Human Brain. Thomas Springfield/III. 1969

77 STIEVE, H.: Nomina Anatomica, 4. Aufl. Fischer, Jena 1949

78 TABER, Cl. W.: Cyclopedic Medical Dictionary, 9. Aufl. Blackwell, Oxford 1962

79 TANDLER, J.: Lehrbuch der Systematischen Anatomie. Vogel, Leipzig 1926

80 TESTUT, L.: D'anatomie humaine, 4. Aufl. Paris 1900

81 TÖNDURY, G.: Anatomie der Lungengefäße. Ergebn. ges. Tuberk.- u. Lung.-Forsch. 14 (1958) 61–100

82 TÖNDURY, G.: Angewandte und topographische Anatomie, 3. Aufl. Thieme, Stuttgart 1965; 5. Aufl. 1981

83 TOLDT, C., F. HOCHSTETTER: Anatomischer Atlas, 23. Aufl. Urban & Schwarzenberg, Wien 1961

84 TRUEX, R. C., M. B. CARPENTER: Strong und Elwyn's Human Neuroanatomy, 5. Aufl. Williams & Wilkins, Baltimore 1964

85 VIAMONTE JR. M., RÜTTIMANN: Atlas of Lymphography. Thieme, Stuttgart 1980

86 VILLIGER, E., E. LUDWIG: Gehirn und Rückenmark, 11.–13. Aufl. Engelmann, Leipzig 1940

87 VOSS, H., R. HERRLINGER: Taschenbuch der Anatomie, 10. Aufl. Fischer, Stuttgart 1959

88 WALDEYER, A.: Anatomie des Menschen, 4. u. 5. Aufl. De Gruyter, Berlin 1967

89 WOERDEMANN, M. W.: Nomina anatomica Parisiensia (1955) et B. N. A. (1895). Oosthoek, Utrecht 1957

90 WOLF-HEIDEGGER, G.: Atlas der systematischen Anatomie des Menschen. Karger, Basel 1957

91 WOLF-HEIDEGGER, G.: Atlas der Human Anatomie, 4. Aufl. Karger, Basel 1990

92 WYBURN, G. M.: The Nervous System. Academic Press, London 1960

93 ZENKER, R., HEBERER, H.-H. LÖHR: Die Lungenresektionen. Springer, Berlin 1954

94 ZÖLLNER, F.: Anatomie, Physiologie, Pathologie und Klinik der Ohrtrompete, Springer, Berlin 1942

430   Index